Exercise, Nutrition, *and the* Older Woman
Wellness for Women Over Fifty

Exercise, Nutrition, *and the* Older Woman
Wellness for Women Over Fifty

Edited by **Maria A. Fiatarone Singh, M.D.**

Scientist I
Nutrition, Exercise Physiology and Sarcopenia Laboratory
Jean Mayer U.S. Department of Agriculture
Human Nutrition Research Center on Aging at Tufts University
Boston, Massachusetts

John Sutton Chair
Professor
School of Exercise and Sport Science
Faculty of Health Sciences
and Professor
Faculty of Medicine
University of Sydney
Sydney, Australia

CRC Press
Boca Raton London New York Washington, D.C.

Any opinions, findings, conclusions, or recommendations expressed in this publication are those of the authors, and do not necessarily reflect the view of the U.S. Department of Agriculture.

Library of Congress Cataloging-in-Publication Data

Exercise, nutrition, and the older woman : wellness for women over fifty / edited by
Maria A. Fiatarone Singh.
p. cm.
Includes bibliographical references and index.
ISBN 0-8493-0258-7 (alk. paper)
1. Middle aged women—Health and hygiene. I. Singh, Maria A. Fiatarone Singh.
RA778.A2-Z+ 2000
613.7′045—dc21

00-020810
CIP

Visit the CRC Press Web site at www.crcpress.com

Dedication

This work is dedicated to the memory of my beloved grandmother

Jeanne Marie Celine Torre Saint Gaudens
October 15, 1895–January 27, 1981

My first and greatest mentor in wellness.
For making me exercise with Jack LaLanne every afternoon,
And eat bread that was a different color than everyone else's,
But mostly for showing me the way to age with grace and wisdom;
And know the best is yet to come.

Preface

"The greatest revolution of our time is the knowledge that human beings, by changing the inner attitudes of their minds, can transform the outer aspects of their lives."

William James

Hopefully, as health care practitioners you have already embraced this concept of transformation in your work with older women in your care. Our goal in the assembly of these chapters has been to present a core of knowledge about the health of older women that will enable them to be more in control of the way they age and the speed with which they do it. But as William James suggests, it is the first step—the changing of the inner aspects of one's mind—that really matters. Once an individual has decided to exert some influence over the physical, mental, and emotional changes of aging, there is often a need for guidance from professionals with the right educational tools to effect such a transformation. The unifying goal of the authors of this book has been to facilitate the knowledge of how to change one's attitude toward aging as well as to impart specific lifestyle recommendations linked to health and well-being.

In most western countries, health promotion and disease prevention through lifestyle changes have not been the priority of individuals or the health care systems in general. Thus, it is not surprising that health care providers do not uniformly provide patients with the knowledge, access, or behavioral and financial incentives needed to effect substantial long-term changes in these areas.

There is plenty of accumulated scientific evidence that doing so would make a difference. Epidemiological studies indicate that exercise and physically active lifestyles are linked to longer life spans, less cardiovascular disease, stroke, diabetes, osteoporosis, cancer, high blood pressure, obesity, depression, and disability with age. Similarly, higher intakes of fruits, vegetables, and fiber, and lower intakes of fats and animal products are associated with lower rates of cancer, cardiovascular disease, diabetes, high blood pressure, high cholesterol, and obesity. These findings have led to numerous position papers and consensus statements over the past decade which give a central role to exercise and nutrition in health promotion at all ages.

In health promotion, as elsewhere, knowledge is power. The knowledge which has been advanced over the past century by scientific and medical research into health promotion and disease prevention is that much of what had been attributed to bad luck, bad genes, or mysterious forces of nature may instead be linked to poor lifestyle choices or environmental conditions. We clearly cannot control everything about how well people age and how long they survive; it will depend in part on their cultural and ethnic heritage, genetic endowment, environmental toxins, and socioeconomic status. Indeed, we may have limited influence over the very health care system in which we practice, and be frustrated by the lack of support for behavioral training and programs designed to optimize health rather than merely treat disease. However, it is certainly possible with the knowledge base of today to offer our older population a more optimistic and empowering alternative to years of biological degeneration and chronic disease.

As a professional working with older women, why should you concern yourself with the acquisition and dissemination of this empowering knowledge? Simple! Women now spend close to one-half of their lives in the years beyond child-bearing age. It is during these years in particular when attention to health and quality of life is critical to the maintenance of vigorous, active, and involved personal and societal roles for women. Since women currently outlive men by 6 to 8 years in most countries, women should have more and more influence over the priorities and needs driving health promotion, because they comprise an increasingly larger proportion of the population with each advancing decade. The vast majority of those over the age of 85 and those living in nursing homes are women. Thus, the specific health concerns of older women must be given greater attention in the research world, and the findings disseminated rapidly and responsibly to consumers and health care institutions by scientists and health care practitioners.

The health-related areas in which older women can often have the greatest influence over their own aging process are physical activity and nutrition. Most of the major chronic health conditions common in older women (heart disease, high blood pressure, diabetes, obesity, arthritis, osteoporosis, cancer, vascular disease, and others) can be prevented, delayed, modified, and/or treated in whole or in part by understanding the proper role of nutrition and exercise in their pathogenesis and prognosis. This is not to say that traditional medical care will not be needed in the future, but rather that the burden of disease and disability which accumulates with age may be substantially reduced by acting on this understanding. Hopefully, we are entering an era in which exercise and nutrition will be more fully integrated into the mainstream of health care practice, and the artificial distinction between traditional and non-traditional treatment can be eliminated, and replaced by complete rather than incomplete treatment options.

The benefits to the individual woman and society in general with this approach are enormous. If such diseases are prevented, or their disabling effects modified, there will be lower health care costs, regardless what system or policies are driving expenditures in the future. Individual quality of life will also benefit from achievement of optimal body weight and nutritional balance, as well as markedly improved fitness levels and physical capacities.

What might our health care system and policies look like if we really paid attention to the data available on the benefits of exercise and good nutrition? Insurance rates would be higher for those who are sedentary, just as they are for smokers. Employers would provide on-site wellness centers and wholesome food in their cafeterias, and health clubs would provide services for elderly and frail clients. Medical insurance would routinely cover long-term exercise training, nutritional counseling, exercise equipment, and transportation for those who don't drive to access these facilities. Health care providers would actually learn in detail about exercise, nutrition, and behavioral tools in medical, nursing, and other school curricula. Doctors' waiting rooms would be transformed into wellness rooms where videos, books, fitness equipment, cooking demonstrations, and stationary bikes replace the traditional line of chairs along the wall. Nursing homes would all have gymnasiums and exercise equipment in patient rooms, and staff would be trained to assist with these activities as part of their jobs.

Such scenes are currently happening in some areas, still far-fetched in others. Our purpose in this volume is to educate you, the provider of health care, to believe enough in the principles and practice of preventive health behaviors so as to start shaping the health care system of the future in your workplace today to include priorities of healthful, successful aging, enhanced by optimal fitness and good nutrition.

This book has been dedicated to the health of older women by a core of physicians and researchers who share these concerns by virtue of their own experiences as caregivers and educators. As a group, we have tried to identify in each topic area the essential tools needed by older women to change their lifestyles or expand their knowledge about the aging process in ways which will enhance their continued vitality and health throughout the years. We do not claim to have answers which our wise grandmothers did not—and in many cases you may recognize the admonitions and advice of your own matriarchs in these pages. We hope that we can simply convey the facts about how to enhance health, as well as dispel negative myths about aging or unfounded promises from the latest fountain of youth on the market.

Although knowledge is powerful, it is not sufficient. Physical activity and dietary intakes are behaviors, and behavior is shaped not only by knowledge, but also by habit, by experience, by fear, and by reward. We hope that after reading these pages you will be able to recognize and nurture in your patients and clients a readiness to change behaviors in a positive and healthful way. Even if only by one small step at a time, the habit of a physically active lifestyle and nutritious diet can be established. You may even experience subtle and not-so-subtle changes in your own attitudes, energy, mood, strength, function, optimism, and many other domains as you begin to apply this knowledge to those in your care. We hope that your fears of change, injury, or uncertainty are alleviated by the practical guidelines we have included along the way, and the reinforcing feedback you receive from women who benefit from this information.

The rewards of a newer, more robust physical, mental, and spiritual well-being may begin to be felt when one is 40 or 104. Women have much to offer the world at any age, and as health care practitioners we are in a unique position to facilitate their capacity to contribute throughout life. In the words of Goethe, "Whatever you can do, or dream you can, begin it. Boldness has genius, power and magic in it." There's never been a better time to begin than now.

Maria Antoinette Fiatarone Singh, M.D.

About the Editor

Dr. Maria A. Fiatarone Singh is a board-certified internist and geriatrician with particular interest in exercise, nutrition, and aging. She currently holds the John Sutton Chair of Exercise and Sport Science at the University of Sydney, Australia, Professorship in Medicine at the University of Sydney and an Associate Professorship, School of Nutrition Science and Policy, Tufts University, Boston.

The primary focus of Professor Maria Fiatarone Singh's research and clinical career has been to integrate the disciplines of exercise physiology and nutrition into a better understanding of both the basic biology of aging and the clinical practice of geriatric medicine. Her current active research studies include a range of issues of central importance to health and functioning in the fit and frail elderly. These topics include nutritional determinants of functional and health status in frail elders; effects of strength, power, balance, and endurance training on functional independence in older adults; utility of strength training in congestive heart failure, including changes in muscle protein turnover; comparison of changes in function after strength or aerobic training; the role of cytokines in the adaptation of muscle in heart failure; effects of long-term exercise on mitochondrial volume and density in older women; ultrastructural damage and repair in muscle after strength training; treatment of psychological depression with various intensities of strengthening exercise; anabolic adaptation to strength training to counteract the negative effects of a low protein diet for chronic renal failure; behavioral interventions to modify food group choices in the grail elderly; effects of vitamin E supplementation on immune function and resistance to influenza in nursing home residents; effect of exercise on nutritional intake in the elderly; prevention of hip fractures in the nursing home with a combined intervention of staff education, strength and balance training, and hip protectors; longitudinal analyses of the rates of change of muscle mass and function in the initially healthy elderly; and a combination of nursing rehabilitation models and exercise programming to prevent functional decline in nursing home residents.

In addition to the above specific studies of the basic mechanisms of frailty and functional decline, Professor Fiatarone Singh continues to develop and test models for the integration and implementation of exercise and nutrition in geriatric care settings, including nursing home, elderly housing, adult day care, home care, rehabilitation hospital, and outpatient clinics. This work is being done through research grant support as well as under the auspices of the Fit For Your Life Foundation, Ltd., a non-profit organization of which she is the founder and director.

Dr. Singh is the recipient of the Edward Henderson Award in Geriatric Medicine, The American Geriatrics Society New Investigator's Award, The Brookdale Foundation Fellowship, The Pfizer Award for Research in Aging, the Herbert DeVries Award for Contributions to Aging among others, and serves on the boards of numerous gerontologic organizations. She is a fellow of the Gerontological Society of America and the Royal Australian College of Physicians.

Contributors

Beth C. Bock, Ph.D.
Assistant Professor
Department of Psychiatry and Human
  Behavior
Brown University Center for Behavioral
  and Preventive Medicine
The Miriam Hospital
Providence, Rhode Island

Sharon Bortz, M.S., R.D.
Private practice
Ukiah, California

**Carmen Castaneda Sceppa, M.D.,
Ph.D.**
Assistant Professor, School of Nutrition
  Science and Policy
Scientist II
Jean Mayer USDA Human Nutrition
  Research Center on Aging
Tufts University
Boston, Massachusetts

**Peter Cistulli, MBBS, Ph.D., FRACP,
FCCP**
Director, Centre for Sleep Disorders and
  Respiratory Failure
Department of Respiratory Medicine
St. George Hospital
Sydney, Australia
and
Conjoint Senior Lecturer,
Department of Medicine
University of New South Wales
Australia

Matthew M. Clark, Ph.D.
Associate Professor
Department of Psychiatry and
  Psychology
The Mayo Clinic
Rochester, Minnesota

Barbara J. de Lateur, M.D., M.S.
Professor, Director, and Lawrence
  Cardinal Shehan Chair
Department of Physical Medicine and
  Rehabilitation
The Johns Hopkins University School
  of Medicine
Baltimore, Maryland

Karen Duvall, M.D., MPH
Assistant Clinical Professor
UCLA
Department of Family Medicine
Center for Health Promotion and
  Disease Prevention
and
Associate Director
Preventive Medicine Residency
Los Angeles, California

Christina D. Economos, Ph.D.
Assistant Professor
School of Nutrition and Policy
Scientist III
Jean Mayer USDA Human Nutrition
  Research Center on Aging
Tufts University
Boston, Massachusetts

Cynthia T. Henderson, M.D., M.P.H.
Medical Director
Oak Forest Hospital
Oak Forest, Illinois

Fran E. Kaiser, M.D.
Adjunct Professor of Medicine
St. Louis University
St. Louis, Missouri

Elizabeth Krall, Ph.D., MPH
Associate Professor
Department of Health Policy and Health
  Services Research
Boston University Goldman School of
  Dental Medicine
Boston, Massachusetts

Jennifer Layne, M.S., CCS
Nutrition, Exercise Physiology and
  Sarcopenia Laboratory
Tufts University
Boston, Massachusetts

Justus Lehmann, M.D.
Professor Emeritus
Department of Physical Medicine and
  Rehabilitation
University of Washington School of
  Medicine
Seattle, Washington

Alice H. Lichtenstein, D.Sc.
Senior Scientist
Professor of Nutrition
Jean Mayer USDA Human Nutrition
  Research Center on Aging
Tufts University
Boston, Massachusetts

Bess H. Marcus, Ph.D.
Associate Professor
Department of Psychiatry and
  Behavioral Medcine
Brown University Center for Behavioral
  and Preventive Medicine
The Miriam Hospital
Providence, Rhode Island

Timothy S. McElreavy, M.A.
Jean Mayer USDA Human Nutrition
  Research Center on Aging
Tufts University
Boston, Massachusetts

Mohsen Meydani, D.V.M., Ph.D.
Jean Mayer USDA Human Nutrition
  Research Center on Aging
Tufts University
Boston, Massachusetts

Simin Nikbin Meydani, D.V.M., Ph.D.
Chief, Nutritional Immunology
  Laboratory
Professor, Nutrition and Immunology
Jean Mayer USDA Human Nutrition
  Research Center on Aging
Tufts University
Boston, Massachusetts

Patricia A. Moore, M.A., M.Ed.
President
DesignMoore
Phoenix, Arizona

Linda Morrow, M.D.
San Jose, California

Miriam E. Nelson, Ph.D.
Associate Professor, School of Nutrition
  Science and Policy
Associate Chief, Nutrition, Exercise
  Physiology and Sarcopenia
  Laboratory
Tufts University
Boston, Massachusetts

Paddy A. Phillips
Professor and Head of Medicine
Flinders University of South Australia
Adelaide, Australia

Bernardine M. Pinto, Ph.D.
Assistant Professor
Department of Psychiatry and Human
  Behavior
Brown University Center for Behavioral
  and Preventive Medicine
The Miriam Hospital
Providence, Rhode Island

**Helen M. Rasmussen M.S., RD,
FADA**
Research Nutritionist
Metabolic Research Unit
Jean Mayer USDA Human Nutrition
  Research Center on Aging
Tufts University
Boston, Massachusetts

Susan Roberts, Ph.D.
Professor, Nutrition and Psychiatry
Chief, Energy Metabolism Laboratory
Tufts University
Boston, Massachusetts

Barbara J. Rolls, Ph.D.
Department of Nutrition
The Pennsylvania State University
University Park, Pennsylvania

K. Lea Sewell, M.D.
Assistant Professor in Medicine
Harvard Medical School
Division of Aging and Rheumatology
Beth Israel Deaconess Medical Center
Boston, Massachusetts

Maria A. Fiatarone Singh, M.D.
Professor of Medicine
John Sutton Chair of Exercise and Sport
  Science
University of Sydney
Sydney, Australia
and
Associate Professor of Medicine
School of Nutrition Science and Policy
Scientist I
Jean Mayer USDA Human Nutrition
  Research Center on Aging
Tufts University
Boston, Massachusetts

Nalin Singh, MBBS, FRACP
Staff Specialist, Geriatrics
Royal Prince Alfred Hospital
and
Balmain Hospital
Sydney, Australia

Deborah F. Tate, Postdoctoral Fellow
Department of Psychiatry and Human
  Behavior
Brown University Center for Behavioral
  and Preventive Medicine
The Miriam Hospital
Providence, Rhode Island

Jeanne Wei, M.D.
Associate Professor of Medicine
Harvard Medical School
Senior Physician, Beth Israel Deaconess
  Medical Center
Boston, Massachusetts

Contents

Section III — Exercise, Nutrition, and Chronic Disease

Section IV — Integrating the Exercise, Nutrition, and Wellness Prescription into Health Care Practice

Section I

Exercise

We begin this book by considering the role of exercise in the health and aging of older women. An appreciation of the major role played by physical activity in the structural and metabolic changes we have come to know as aging is critical for health care practitioners from all disciplines. Such an appreciation of the centrality of this role will hopefully lead to a new vision about what is inevitable, what is preventable, and what is modifiable in regard to physical aging. However, unless this view is accompanied by specific knowledge of the types of exercise possible, and the basic techniques to which we must adhere in order to produce substantive, clinically relevant adaptation, the current paradigm of inexorable physiologic cannot be successfully challenged. Finally, since health care practitioners must deal with chronic disease, nutritional imbalance, and medications in the women they counsel and treat, a discussion of the important interactions in each of these domains with the basic physical activity prescription is offered.

Since all women are not alike, a variety of options for the incorporation of these exercise recommendations into individual lifestyles and routines are suggested. The basic principles of each modality of exercise apply, whether one is 50 or 100 years of age, healthy or frail. However, it is important for health care practitioners to be able to advise women under their care as to which elements can be modified and which cannot for clinical results to accrue.

The most motivating aspect of an exercise regimen is often a perception by the participant of the physical and psychological benefits that have resulted. In the past, poorly conceptualized, non-theoretically based, or diluted exercise recommendations have frequently been proffered because of a belief that they would be safer or more palatable to the older or frailer adult. Unfortunately, this approach may be unintentionally counterproductive. Since very low intensity exercises may be stripped of most of their potential to effect real physiologic adaptation, they may result in little or no clinical improvement or perceptible benefit to the individual. This outcome is likely to reinforce the opinion, on the part of both practitioners and patients, that exercise is at best adjunctive or optional in relation to health outcomes, and therefore long-term adherence will suffer.

Therefore, our approach is to present exercise modalities and dosages that are known to be theoretically grounded and successful in combating age-related physiologic changes, preventing disease, reversing pathophysiologic changes of disuse and disease, and treating side-effects of common medical regimens. All of the exercise routines described in this section are based on many years of research and have been shown to work in younger as well as older adults, and those who are healthy as well as those with multiple chronic illnesses. Their efficacy is matched by their safety and feasibility, as demonstrated in many clinical trials involving thousands of older men and women over the past two decades.

Although exercise is much more than a medical intervention, when it *is* used as medical treatment, it should be conceptualized as a drug. What type should be taken? What is the proper indication, dosage, frequency, side-effect profile, interaction with other drugs, or nutritional considerations? What are the anticipated benefits and the expected time course of those outcomes? Hopefully, the chapters that follow will provide the kinds of information practitioners need to know to begin such a rational prescription of exercise for older women.

1 Exercise and Aging

Maria A. Fiatarone Singh

CONTENTS

EXERCISE AND THE HEALTH OF THE POPULATION

There has been a gradually growing awareness among policy makers and health care
professionals over the past several decades of the centrality of appropriate exercise
habits to major public health outcomes. For example, in the current draft of *Healthy
People 2010*, the goal suggested in the realm of physical activity is to "improve the
health, fitness, and quality of life of all Americans through the adoption and maintenance of regular, daily physical activity."[1] It has been known for decades that

3

physical activity prevents heart disease, but more recent data suggest that, on average, physically active people outlive those who are inactive[2,3] and that regular physical activity helps to maintain the functional independence of older adults and enhances the quality of life for people of all ages.

The first Surgeon General's Report on Physical Activity and Health[4] released in July 1996, concluded that regular sustained physical activity can substantially reduce the risk of developing or dying from heart disease, diabetes, colon cancer, and high blood pressure. This hallmark report was meant to provide impetus for Americans to establish an active and fit lifestyle. Unfortunately, as shown in Table 1, relatively few Americans engage in regular physical activity despite the widely reported benefits in both the scientific and popular media. Only about 10% of the U.S. adult population reports regular, vigorous physical activity three days per week, a small proportion are engaged in muscle strengthening exercise, and about 25% are completely sedentary (engaged in no physical activity).

Unfortunately, among population groups who are most at risk for diseases related to sedentariness, levels of physical activity are even lower than in the general population, thus exaggerating the negative health consequences of a sedentary lifestyle. According to the 1996 Surgeon General's Report on Physical Activity and Health,[4] demographic groups at highest risk for inactivity are the elderly, women, minorities, those with low income or less educational background, and those with disabilities or chronic health conditions. So, for example, in comparison to the figures for all adults shown in Table 1, 43% of adults aged 65 and older were sedentary in 1985, and 29% in 1991. As might be expected, these are the same demographic groups that bear a large burden of the diseases amenable to prevention and treatment with exercise, and yet often have the least access and opportunity for health promotion efforts related to physical activity. Therefore, health care practitioners should identify and understand barriers to physical activity faced by particular population groups and be prepared to develop programs and tools that address those barriers.

Previous objectives for the nation have focused primarily on physical activities designed to improve cardiorespiratory fitness and prolong life. However, it is now recognized that everyone could benefit from physical activities designed to ensure functional independence throughout life. The specific physical fitness components that provide continued physical function as individuals age also include muscle strength, muscle endurance, balance, and flexibility. The problems of mobility impairment, falls, arthritis, osteoporotic fractures, and functional status are clearly related to muscle strength and mass,[5,6] and thus strengthening activities, while important for all age groups, are particularly important for older adults. Age-related loss of strength, muscle mass, and bone density, which are most dramatic in women, may be attenuated by strengthening exercises,[7,8] and regained even long afterward with appropriate resistance training.[9] Unfortunately, national survey data indicate that women in general report lower than average adult participation levels for strength training (11 vs. 16%). Additionally, despite the evidence on safety and efficacy in even frail elders,[10–12] the prevalence rate for resistive exercise is even lower among the old (6% at ages 65–74) or the very old (4% above age 75). Individuals in this latter age group, particularly over the age of 85, are primarily women, making an understanding of the risks and benefits of exercise in this population a priority.

TABLE 1
Prevalence of Physical Activity among Adults in the U.S., Progress Toward Year 2000 Goals

Type of Activity	Percent of Adult Americans Reporting in 1985	Percent of Adult Americans Reporting in 1995	Goal for Year 2010
Light to moderate sustained physical activity for 30 minutes at least 5 days per week[a]	22%	23%	30%
Regular vigorous physical activity at least 3 days per week that promotes cardiorespiratory fitness[b]	12%	16%	25%
Sedentary lifestyle (inactive, most of time spent sitting)	24%	23%	15%
Stretching (one time/week)	No data available	27% (1991)	
Strengthening exercises (three times/week)	No data available	16% (1991)	
Access to community fitness facilities	No data available	No data available	

Data are reported in the *Draft Objectives of Healthy People 2010* (www.HealthyPeople.com) and are drawn from National Health Interview Survey, Centers for Disease Control, and National Center for Health Statistics sources.

[a] Sustained physical activity requires muscular movements and is at least equivalent to brisk walking. In addition to walking, activities may also include swimming, cycling, dancing, gardening and yardwork, and various domestic and occupational activities.

[b] Vigorous physical activities are rhythmic, repetitive physical activities that use large muscle groups at 60 percent or more of maximum heart rate for age. An exercise heart rate of 60 percent of maximum heart rate for age is about 50 percent of maximal cardiorespiratory capacity and is sufficient for cardiorespiratory conditioning. Maximum heart rate equals roughly 220 beats per minute minus age.[34] Examples of vigorous physical activities include jogging/running, lap swimming, cycling, aerobic dancing, skating, rowing, jumping rope, cross-country skiing, hiking/backpacking, racquet sports, and competitive group sports (soccer, basketball, volleyball).

Most studies suggest that physical activity counseling in a primary care setting increases physical activity behaviors, at least in the short term. However, the traditional training in most health care disciplines does not include sufficient specific knowledge in exercise physiology or behavioral science to be able to prescribe or manage such programs. In fact, clinician counseling for physical activity is even less common than it was when *Healthy People 2000* goals were established in 1991, suggesting that recent efforts to educate health care professionals in this regard have not been very successful. In addition, the needs of an older, chronically ill or disabled population in relation to physical activity are more complicated than the straightforward elements of the basic exercise prescription that may be provided to younger adults.[13] Thus, an understanding of the relationship of exercise to aging and disease, and the specificity of training adaptations which occur, is critical to the care of the older woman, and is the focus of this and subsequent chapters.

The Department of Health and Human Services is now formulating a plan to assist health care professionals in their counseling efforts toward older adults. This will include

Strategies to help caregivers advise patients about physical activity;

Increasing efforts to work within managed care organizations so that physical activity is more effectively included in reimbursed prevention activities; and

Ensuring that programs and messages are designed specifically to reach minorities and women, who are at highest risk of sedentary behavior.

It is hoped that the information in this book will contribute to this educational effort as well.

INTEGRATING DISCIPLINES

In this chapter, we will consider the interaction of habitual physical activity and chronic disease expression in the older woman, with an aim to identify the intersection of these fields as they relate to optimization of aging processes, as well as both prevention and treatment of common disease and syndromes relevant to aging. The rationale for the integration of a physical activity prescription into geriatric health care is based on four essential concepts which will be reviewed in detail in the sections that follow. First, there is a great similarity between the physiologic changes which are attributable to disuse and those that have been typically observed in aging populations, leading to the speculation that the way we age may, in fact, be greatly modulated with attention to activity levels.[14] Second, chronic diseases increase with age, and exercise has now been shown to be an independent risk factor and/or potential treatment for most of the major causes of morbidity and mortality in western societies, a potential that is vastly underutilized currently. Third, traditional medical interventions don't typically address disuse syndromes accompanying chronic disease, which may be responsible for much of their associated disability. Exercise is particularly good at targeting syndromes of disuse. Finally, many pathophysiologic aberrations that are central to a disease or its treatment are specifically addressed only by exercise, which therefore deserves a place in the mainstream of medical care, not as an optional adjunct.

It is clear that the optimum approach to successful aging or to health care in the older woman cannot ignore the overlap of these areas. In some cases, exercise can be used to avert age-related decrements in physiologic function, and thereby maximize function and quality of life in the elderly. On the other hand, the combination of exercise and sound nutrition, particularly in relation to favorable alterations in body composition, will have numerous important effects on risk factors for chronic disease as well as the disability that accompanies such conditions. Therefore, understanding the effects of aging on exercise capacity and how habitual physical activity can modify this relationship in the older woman, including its specific utility in treating medical diseases, is critical for health care practitioners of all disciplines.

RETARDING THE AGING PROCESS

BIOLOGICAL CHANGES OF AGING IMPAIR EXERCISE CAPACITY

Not all changes attributed to the aging process will impact directly on exercise capacity. For example, some of the most visible changes we recognize as aging, such as changes in hair color and volume, development of presbyopia, altered skin texture and elasticity, reductions in height, and even changes in speed of cognitive processing and retention of new information, will have little direct impact on the ability to exercise or continue to perform physical work in advanced years. However, changes in other systems will have far greater relevance to the continued performance of physical activity at high levels throughout the adult lifespan.

In most physiologic systems, the normal aging processes do not result in significant impairment or dysfunction in the absence of pathology and under resting conditions. However, in response to a stress, the age-related reduction in physiologic reserves causes a loss of homeostatic balance. This process has been termed "homeostenosis," or a lessened capacity for fine tuning of the system. So, for example, metabolic processes enable maintenance of a normal fasting glucose level in most older individuals without diabetes. However, a reduced sensitivity to insulin action (loss of reserve) causes many older adults to exhibit glucose intolerance (elevated circulating glucose levels) in response to a metabolic stress such as a meal or an oral glucose tolerance test. Tables 2 through 7 summarize the major physiologic changes which are typically observed in normal aging in various body systems and are relevant to exercise capacity in the older woman.

TABLE 2
Aging of the Cardiovascular System

Abnormalities of cardiac conduction system
Decreased capillary density in skeletal muscle
Decreased cardiac contractility
Decreased heart rate variability at rest
Decreased maximal ejection fraction
Decreased maximal heart rate
Decreased number of pacemaker cells in sinus node
Decreased sensitivity to beta-adrenergic stimulation
Decreased total blood volume
Exaggerated blood pressure response to exercise
Impaired early diastolic filling of ventricles, (myocardial stiffness and impaired relaxation)
Impaired vasodilation in peripheral vasculature
Impaired augmentation of ejection fraction during exercise
Increased arterial stiffness/afterload
Increased cardiac size, increased end systolic and end diastolic volumes

---

The effect of all of the changes noted above is twofold. On the one hand, these changes limit the maximal performance or work capacity in a given domain. This may be seen in tests of maximal muscle strength, muscle power, muscle endurance,

TABLE 3
Aging of the Pulmonary System

Decreased diffusion capacity
Decreased maximal ventilatory capacity
Decreased peak flow rates
Decreased tidal volume

TABLE 4
Age-Related Changes in Body Composition

Decrease in total body calcium
Decrease in total body nitrogen and protein content
Decrease in total body potassium
Decrease in total body water
Decreased bone mass and density
Decreased muscle mass
Increased bone fragility
Increased central and visceral adipose tissue
Increased connective tissue volume and cross-linkage
Increased total fat mass

TABLE 5
Aging of the Musculoskeletal System

Decreased oxidative and glycolytic enzyme capacity
Decreased total number of muscle fibers
Decreased water content and degenerative changes of cartilage
Degenerative structural changes of bones and joints
Increased cross-linkage of collagen and total amount of collagen
Increased intramuscular fat and connective tissue
Selective atrophy of Type 2 (fast twitch) fibers
Shortening of tendons and ligaments
Decreased tissue elasticity

aerobic capacity, static or dynamic balance, or flexibility, for example. Although such changes will be immediately noticeable and disastrous for an elite athlete,[15] they may accrue insidiously in non-athletic populations over many years without much effect on daily life. This is because most sedentary individuals rarely call upon themselves to exert maximal effort in physical domains. In fact, even the slightest evidence that maximal capacity has changed (for example, climbing a flight of stairs rapidly causes shortness of breath or aching in the thighs, or rising from a low chair

TABLE 6
Age-Related Changes in Metabolism

Decreased body protein content and protein synthesis rates
Decreased glycogen storage in muscle
Decreased sensitivity to increased serum osmolality
Decreased sweat volume
Decreased thirst sensation and delayed fluid replacement in response to dehydration or salt loading (renin/angiotension system)
Impaired temperature regulation
Insulin resistance

TABLE 7
Aging of the Nervous System

Decreased dendritic sprouting in central nervous system
Decreased number of alpha motor neurons in spinal cord
Decreased number of motor units and increased size of remaining units
Diminished proprioception
Impaired neural recruitment
Neurofibrillary plaques and tangles in cerebral cortex
Slowed nerve conduction velocity
Slowed reaction time
Type grouping of muscle fibers
Decreased accommodation in lens (presbyopia), cataract formation

feels difficult) leads most people to immediately substitute strategies to avoid such discomfort, such as taking escalators or using arms to assist with standing. Thus, subtle changes in physical activity patterns over the adult lifespan allow most people not engaged in athletic pursuits to lose a very large proportion of their physical work capacity before they even notice that something is wrong or find that they have crossed a threshold of disability.[5] Women are particularly susceptible here because their initial reserve of muscle mass is so much lower than that of men, due to gender differences in anabolic hormonal milieu.[16–18] They will therefore in most cases cross the threshold where losses of musculoskeletal capacity impact functional status at least 10 years before men do.[19]

The second consequence of age-related changes in physiologic capacity is the increased perception of effort associated with submaximal work. For example, between youth and middle age, an untrained woman may find that walking briskly results in increased blood pressure, heart rate, respiratory rate, and an earlier sense of overall and leg muscle fatigue than previously.[20] Again, this changing physical capacity has the unfortunate negative side effect of increasing the tendency to avoid activity, contributed to by changing job requirements or retirement, societal roles and expectations, and other psychosocial influences.[21] Thus a vicious cycle is set up: usual aging leading to decreasing exercise capacity, resulting in an elevated perception of effort, subsequently causing avoidance of activity, and finally feeding back to exacerbation of the age-related declines themselves that are secondary to disuse. The major decrements in exercise capacity observed in normal aging are summarized in Table 8. It is incumbent upon health care practitioners, therefore, to intervene in this pervasive process by understanding the underlying physiology, recognizing it in its early stages, separating inactivity from aging and disease, and most important, educating older women about the need for prevention and the potential for reversibility inherent in this pathway.

TABLE 8
Effects of Age-Related Changes in Physiology on Exercise Capacity

Decreased anaerobic threshold
Decreased joint range of motion (flexibility)
Decreased maximal aerobic capacity (0.5–1.0% per year)
Decreased muscle force, endurance, and power (1–2% per year)
Impaired coordination and speed of movement
Impaired static and dynamic balance
Increased cardiovascular response, perception of effort, and
   increased lactate response to submaximal aerobic work

Cardiovascular endurance capacity, or aerobic capacity, is dependent primarily upon cardiac output (stroke volume × heart rate), oxygen-carrying capacity of the blood, capillary density, extraction of oxygen by the working muscles, and oxidative capacity of the muscle fibers, including oxidative enzyme content, mitochondrial volume density, proportion of Type I (slow-twitch) fibers, and storage of glycogen for fuel. In healthy older individuals without chronic pulmonary disease, pulmonary airflow rates and oxygen-carrying capacity in the blood are not limiting factors in exercise tolerance.

There are two major reasons for reduced maximal aerobic capacity with aging. First is diminished maximal heart rate in response to exercise, which appears to be limited by an age-related decreased sensitivity of the myocardium to beta-adrenergic stimulation.[22,23] This observation has been used to roughly estimate maximal heart rate as:

$$220 - \text{age of subject,}$$

220 being the approximate maximal heart rate achievable by healthy young individuals challenged with increasing exercise loads to exhaustion. Therefore, the approximate maximal heart rate of a healthy 80-year-old woman can be estimated as only 140 beats/min. This insensitivity to sympathomimetic stimulation has not been shown to be altered by lifestyle factors such as habitual activity,[24,25] and therefore stands as a primary biological aging factor for which there is as yet no known remedy.

Musculoskeletal function (strength, power, muscle endurance) is dictated largely by the size of the muscle mass which is contracting, and to a lesser extent by changes in surrounding connective tissue in the joint (cartilage, tendons, and ligaments) and neural recruitment, conduction velocities, and fatigue patterns. Sedentary individuals lose large amounts of muscle mass over the course of adult life (20 to 50%), and this loss plays a major role in the similarly large losses in muscle strength observed in both cross-sectional and longitudinal studies.[17,26,27] However, unlike many other changes which impact exercise capacity, muscle mass cannot be maintained into old age even with habitual aerobic activities in either normals[28] or master athletes.[29] Only loading of muscle with weight-lifting exercise (resistance training) has been shown to avert losses of muscle mass (and also strength) in older individuals.[30] In his study, Klitgaard found that elderly men who swam or ran had similar measures of muscle size and strength as their sedentary peers, whereas the muscle of older men who had been weight lifting for 12 to 17 years was almost indistinguishable, and even superior in some aspects, to healthy men 40 to 50 years younger than them.

SIMILARITY OF DISUSE AND AGING

One of the major goals of gerontologic research over the past several decades has been to separate the true physiologic changes of aging from changes due to disease or environmental factors, including disuse or underuse of body systems. However, since most people in westernized societies become increasingly sedentary with age, it is difficult to pinpoint the degree to which an individual's regular level of physical activity influences the way in which he or she ages. Nevertheless, numerous studies point out the superior physical condition of those who exercise regularly compared to their more sedentary peers, even in the tenth decade of life.[31,32] On the other hand, research indicates that years of physiologic aging of diverse organ systems and metabolic functions can be mimicked by short periods of enforced inactivity such as bed rest, casting, denervation, or loss of gravitational forces. These two types of studies have led to a theory of disuse and aging suggesting that aging as we now know it in modern society is, in many ways, an exercise deficiency syndrome,[14] implying that we may have far more control over the rate and extent of the aging process than we previously thought.

ATTENUATION OF AGE-RELATED CHANGES BY HABITUAL PHYSICAL ACTIVITY

Many studies suggest that chronic adaptation to physical activity can markedly attenuate decrements in exercise capacity that would otherwise occur with aging. The major effects of training on these physiologic factors are shown in Table 9. Although the peak workload achievable is on average lower in aged individuals, the cardiovascular and musculoskeletal adaptations to chronic aerobic exercise[33-35,36-38] enable the trained older individual to sustain higher submaximal workloads with less cardiorespiratory response (heart rate, blood pressure, dyspnea), as well as less overall and musculoskeletal fatigue. Thus, apart from peak athletic performance, the adaptations to cardiovascular training can overcome most of the day-to-day functional limitations which might otherwise be imposed by the physiologic changes of aging and disuse.[25]

TABLE 9
Effect of Habitual Activity on Age-Related Changes in Exercise Capacity

Physiologic Change	Habitual Exercise Minimizes Change
Decreased glucose transport and glycogen storage capacity in skeletal muscle	Yes
Decreased capillary density in skeletal muscle	Yes
Decreased ligament and tendon strength	Yes
Decreased maximal aerobic capacity	Yes
Decreased maximal heart rate	No
Decreased maximal muscle strength	Yes
Decreased muscle endurance	Yes
Decreased muscle mass	Yes
Decreased muscle power	Yes
Decreased nerve conduction velocity	Yes
Decreased oxidative and glycolytic enzyme capacity in skeletal muscle	Yes
Decreased pulmonary flow rates	No
Decreased stroke volume augmentation during exercise	Yes[a]
Decreased tissue elasticity and joint range of motion	Yes
Decreased anaerobic threshold during submaximal exercise	Yes
Loss of motor neurons and motor units	Unknown
Increased fat mass and percent body fat	Yes

[a] Shown in men only.

Adaptations to aerobic training that have been documented in the older adult are shown in Table 10. It should be noted that there may be a slight difference in gender adaptation to cardiovascular training. Whereas older men have been shown to be able to augment stroke volume and cardiac contractility during exercise after a period of training, which would serve to enhance their peak aerobic capacity,[39] women have not yet been shown to adapt in this way. In women, the peripheral adaptations to aerobic training appear, therefore, to be the primary manner in which adaptation occurs. The reason for this gender difference in adaptation is not known at this time.

Appropriate, progressive, resistance training programs of 3 to 12 months in duration can be shown to increase muscle strength by an average of 40 to 150%, depending on the subject's characteristics and the intensity of the program, and to increase total body muscle mass by several kilograms.[11,40–44] Thus, even if some of the neural control of muscle and absolute number of motor units remaining are not affected by exercise, the adaptation to muscle loading, even in very old age, causes neural, metabolic, and structural changes in muscle which can completely compensate for the strength losses and a portion of the atrophy of aging. It is not at all unusual to see elderly individuals who after training are stronger than they have ever been, even in their youth, and stronger than their untrained sons and daughters. The physiologic adaptations documented after high-intensity, progressive resistance

---

TABLE 10
Physiologic Adaptations to Cardiovascular Exercise in the Older Adult

Decreased adipose tissue mass
Decreased arterial stiffness
Decreased exercise-induced ischemia, increased time to claudication
Decreased fibrinogen levels
Decreased heart rate and blood pressure response to submaximal exercise
Increased maximal aerobic capacity
Decreased resting pulse and blood pressure
Decreased sympathetic nervous system tone
Decreased total cholesterol, increased HDL cholesterol
Improved heart rate variability
Improved tolerance to postural blood pressure stresses
Increased arterio-venous oxygen difference
Increased blood volume
Increased bone density
Increased capacity to use fat as fuel during prolonged submaximal work
Increased capillary density in skeletal muscle
Increased gastrointestinal transit time
Increased glycogen storage, GLUT-4 receptors in muscle
Increased insulin sensitivity
Increased maximal cardiac output
Increased neural reaction time
Increased oxidative enzyme capacity
Increased stroke volume and ejection fraction with exercise

---

training are outlined in Table 11. As described in more detail in Chapter 2, the adaptations to resistance training are highly dependent on the intensity of the training, because training intensities below 50% of capacity induce little physiologic or functional adaptation. It is perhaps more correct to classify low-intensity strengthening exercises as a different form of exercise than true progressive resistance training, because the physiologic response to these kinds of activities (light weights, elastic bands, use of body weight as resistance, etc.) in fact bears little resemblance to true resistance training.

MINIMIZING RISK FACTORS FOR CHRONIC DISEASE

Apart from retarding physiologic aging itself, another way to integrate exercise into health care is to view it in light of its potential to reduce risk factors for chronic diseases. As shown in Table 12, the very large potential for exercise to act as a primary prevention tool is obvious from the kinds of risk factors and diseases included in this list. The major causes of morbidity and mortality (heart disease, stroke, diabetes, cancer, arthritis, functional dependency, hip fracture) in the older population, and in older women in particular, are all more prevalent in individuals who are sedentary as compared to their more active peers.[45] From a public health

TABLE 11
Physiologic Adaptations to Resistance Training in the Older Adult

Activation of satellite cells
Appearance of insulin-like growth factor I in muscle fibers
Decreased adipose tissue mass
Decreased aerobic exercise-induced ischemia
Improved static and dynamic balance
Improved tolerance to postural blood pressure stresses
Increased maximal aerobic capacity
Increased bone density
Increased glycogen storage, GLUT-4 receptors in muscle
Increased insulin sensitivity
Increased joint range of motion
Increased muscle fiber area, total muscle mass
Increased muscle force, endurance, and power
Increased myofibrillar protein synthesis rate, increased protein turnover
Increased nitrogen retention from diet
Increased oxidative enzyme capacity
Increased total energy expenditure (resting, activity, muscle mass, protein turnover, increased thermic effect of feeding)
Increased gastrointestinal transit time
Myofibrillar damage

TABLE 12
Benefits of Exercise in Older Women: Decreasing Risk Factors for Chronic Disease

Risk Factors	Related Diseases
Insulin Resistance	Glucose intolerance, Type II diabetes, atherosclerosis
Hyperlipidemia	Cardiovascular disease, stroke, peripheral vascular disease
Hypertension	Stroke, cardiovascular disease, congestive heart failure, chronic renal failure, peripheral vascular disease, dementia
Obesity, visceral adiposity	Hypertension, cardiovascular disease, diabetes, stroke, breast and colon cancer, arthritis, sleep apnea, functional and mobility impairment
Osteopenia	Osteoporotic fracture
Sarcopenia	Gait and balance disorders, falls, osteoporotic fracture, functional decline, immune dysfunction, malnutrition

standpoint, minimizing sedentariness or less than optimal participation in physical activities, if possible, would provide more benefit to the health of the population than any other change in behavior.[4] This is because 70 to 80% of the adult population in the U.S. is less than optimally active, and sedentariness is a potent risk factor for our major diseases, doubling risk in many cases. By contrast, smoking behavior, which also doubles the risk of cardiovascular mortality, for example, is present in only 25% of the adult population. Even obesity, at a prevalence of 30 to 40% of adults in the U.S., is only one-half as prevalent as low physical activity levels.[46] Therefore, at this stage, the problem is not in defining the risk of inactivity, but in finding ways to change behavior in sustained ways that will impact subsequent long-term morbidity and mortality.[2,47] At all ages, women are at higher risk for sedentary behavior than men, and as disability, particularly arthritis, increases after the age of 65, this disparity widens even further. Thus, any attempts at risk factor modification must be particularly sensitive to the needs of older women with disabilities. These behavioral issues are discussed further in Chapters 25 and 26.

NUTRITIONAL STATUS AND BODY COMPOSITION IN RELATION TO EXERCISE AND AGING

OVERVIEW

There are many reasons to integrate exercise into the conceptual model of healthy aging, but clearly one of the most potent pathways from physical activity to health status involves the modulation of body composition by habitual exercise patterns.

Body composition is the division of the body mass into its component parts, along the lines of physical, chemical, or other properties of the tissues. Some of the most common methods divide the body into fat and fat-free (or lean) mass, using various techniques such as hydrostatic weighing, isotopic measurements of total body water, dual energy X-ray absorptiometry (DEXA), computerized tomography, or elemental analysis of total body potassium, carbon, nitrogen, and calcium, for example.[48,49] Lean body mass includes muscle, bone, and visceral organs. Adipose tissue may be divided into its subcutaneous, truncal, appendicular, and visceral components if regional imaging techniques such as MRI or CT scanning are utilized.[50] Because aging is associated with decreased energy requirements and increased protein requirements, for the reasons shown in Table 13, there is a potential for body composition changes and adverse consequences to occur over time. For example, if energy intake is restricted due to decreased requirements, micronutrient deficiencies may arise unless nutrient density is increased to compensate for the reduced volume of food. If energy intake is not appropriately matched to needs, then obesity may result. If protein requirements are not met, then muscle wasting will occur. All of these nutritional and body composition changes will negatively impact both cardiovascular and musculoskeletal capacity for exercise, even in the absence of disease.

RELATIONSHIP OF BODY COMPOSITION TO CHRONIC DISEASE

In this conceptual model, one can categorize chronic diseases and geriatric syndromes that are potentially modifiable by exercise if an underlying derangement in body composition is addressed. For example, stabilization or increase in bone mass is achievable by either resistive or weight-bearing aerobic exercise, and will be useful for both prevention and treatment of osteoporosis and related fractures and disability.

TABLE 13
Age-Related Changes in Nutritional Requirements Related to Body Composition and Exercise Capacity

Decreased Energy Requirement	Increased Protein Requirement	Effects of Reduced Energy and Protein Intake on Exercise Capacity
Muscle mass decreases, lowering basal metabolic rate	Decreased protein synthesis rate	Decreased muscle strength and endurance
Fewer calories are used in physical activity	Decreased nitrogen retention in the face of low energy intakes	Decreased aerobic capacity
Thermic effect of meal reduced as food intake is decreased		
Potential for micronutrient deficiencies which impair performance (B vitamins, iron, zinc, vitamin D, magnesium) due to low energy intake		

Decreases in adipose tissue accumulation are achievable by both aerobic and resistive training, usually in conjunction with an energy-restricted diet. This is both preventive and therapeutic for many common chronic diseases, and preventive in the case of cancer, stroke, and vascular impotence. An increase in muscle mass, by contrast, is only achievable with progressive resistance training or generalized weight gain,[51] and with the exception of its potential role in prevention for diabetes, functional dependency, and falls and fractures, is primarily important in the treatment of chronic diseases and disabilities[16] that are accompanied by disuse and sarcopenia. It is notable that the treatment of disease-related sarcopenia with exercise is an area that is not addressed at all by the pharmacologic management of conditions such as congestive heart failure and Parkinson's disease, and therefore it is likely that such adjunctive treatment will impact significantly on related morbidity in these patients. For some diseases, like Type II diabetes mellitus, there are advantages to both minimizing fat tissue as well as maximizing muscle tissue, since these components have opposite, independent effects on insulin resistance in the elderly.[50]

DECREASING FAT MASS

Exercise does little to significantly modify body weight or total body fat as an isolated intervention in normal elders or those who are already obese,[52-55] even after one year of training. The most significant losses of weight and body fat occur in studies of men, in which relatively high doses and durations of exercise are utilized, and the response appears to be most robust in younger populations who are not morbidly obese. In a study of middle-aged obese women, Despres found that aerobic exercise resulted in preferential losses of central adiposity,[56] just as has been seen in non-obese older adults.[57,58] Other reasons to advocate such exercise in older adults include increases in aerobic fitness[59] and insulin sensitivity[60,61] which may occur with exercise independent of weight loss in the elderly.

Like aerobic training, progressive resistive exercise in the absence of dietary energy restriction appears to have only a small impact on total body weight or adipose tissue mass in young or old individuals. However, there is evidence of reduction in intra-abdominal fat stores with resistance training in two studies of normal weight elders,[62,63] which would be metabolically advantageous if achievable in those with visceral obesity.

Energy expenditure and intake, and therefore body weight, may be influenced both by aerobic and resistance training in unique ways, as shown in Table 14. Much of the benefit of exercise in terms of energy balance comes from the changes in basal energy expenditure rather than that expended in the exercise sessions themselves. Over the long term, adaptations within muscle tissue in response to resistance training may significantly affect energy balance and contribute to the maintenance of a healthful body weight while minimizing fat deposition.

TABLE 14
Changes in Energy Expenditure with Exercise

Effect	Observed with Aerobic Training in Elderly	Observed with Resistance Training in Elderly
Excess energy expenditure in exercise session	Yes	Yes
Increased spontaneous physical activity level apart from prescribed exercise	No	Yes
Increased resting metabolic rate	Variable	Yes
Increased fat oxidation	Yes	Yes
Increased thermic effect of feeding	Variable	Yes
Increased energy requirements of larger muscle mass	No	Yes
Increased protein turnover in skeletal muscle	Variable	Yes
Better adherence to hypocaloric diet	Yes	Unknown

INCREASING MUSCLE MASS

There are numerous potential etiologies for the consistently observed loss of muscle mass with aging described in the literature.[51,64,65] Likely mediators of this sarcopenia include

1. Neuronal loss or dysfunction
2. Loss of anabolic stimuli (estrogen, DHEA, testosterone, growth hormone, insulin-like growth factor I)
3. Catabolic illness (congestive heart failure, rheumatoid arthritis, chronic obstructive pulmonary disease, etc.)
4. Medications (corticosteroids)
5. Undernutrition (protein, energy, vitamin D)
6. Disuse atrophy

The approach to this problem, therefore is clearly multifactorial. The issues relevant to disuse atrophy and exercise treatment are outlined below.

There are numerous studies in normal healthy older adults which indicate that high-intensity resistance training is associated with increases in lean body mass or muscle area, usually with minimal alteration of total body weight.[40–42,66] However, the observed adaptive response of skeletal muscle to resistance training in these studies is quite variable, likely influenced by the intensity and duration of the intervention, subject characteristics, and the precision of the measurement technique itself.[40,67,68]

Unfortunately, most studies to date have included only healthy individuals,[41,43,69–71,72,73] and little clinical information other than age is given to allow insight into the wide range of muscle tissue responsiveness to weightlifting regimens. It is clear from these studies and our own,[9,11] which include frail elders, that advancing age impairs the hypertrophic response to resistance training, for reasons not yet identified. Taken together, the existing literature suggests that both exercise-related variables as well as individual characteristics contribute to the wide range of lean tissue responsiveness to resistance training. Because hypertrophy requires synthesis of new proteins and structural changes, neural adaptation is the primary cause of immediate changes in strength in response to resistance training, and longer periods of training are associated with greater gains in muscle tissue. Exercise which does not involve high loading forces on the muscle is generally ineffective with regard to gains in both strength and muscle mass. Although it is possible to see changes in whole body lean tissue with progressive resistance training even in the face of hypocaloric dieting in healthy middle-aged and older women,[74,75] in chronically diseased elderly, even eucaloric energy intake appears insufficient for muscle growth, and energy supplementation was necessary to induce significant hypertrophy with weight-lifting exercise.[76] Further research is required to separate the effects of advanced age, nutritional deficiencies, hormonal status, disease attributes, and extreme sedentariness in clinical populations which may impair their ability to augment lean tissue with this mode of exercise relative to healthy peers.

In summary, exercise is useful to combat the typical age-associated increases in fat mass and decreases in lean mass that are seen in older women. It is adjunctive to energy restriction in the treatment of generalized and central obesity, and will therefore contribute to the management of this risk factor for many chronic diseases. Resistance training, in the presence of adequate or increased energy intake, will augment muscle mass and bone density, and is therefore of central importance for the prevention of functional impairment and osteoporotic fractures in older women. Since exercise increases energy expenditure and requirements in a variety of ways, it may also counteract the risk for vitamin and mineral deficiencies which is seen in older women consuming a very small volume of food due to reduced energy requirements.

ADJUNCTIVE AND PRIMARY TREATMENT OF CHRONIC DISEASE

There are a variety of diseases in which exercise has a potential role because of its ability to directly treat the pathophysiology of the disease itself. Examples of this use of exercise are given in Table 15. In some cases, it may provide similar benefits to medications or nutritional interventions; in others, it may act through an entirely different pathway. In diabetes, for example, insulin can replace the missing endogenous hormone, whereas exercise increases sensitivity to insulin, and the ability to transport glucose into cells and store it as glycogen, without altering insulin levels. Thus the two treatments are complementary to each other, and it is possible that exercise can delay the need for insulin injections or the dosages required. In congestive heart failure, medical therapies improve fluid balance, cardiac contractility, prevent ischemia and arrhythmias, and decrease afterload, while exercise improves exercise tolerance by targeting the peripheral abnormalities (decreased capillary density, decreased mitochondrial density and oxidative enzyme capacity, and myopathy of Type I skeletal muscle fibers). Thus, again these two forms of treatment in combination may offer a far superior approach to disease management. In depression, exercise appears to have about the same potency as pharmacologic management (see Chapter 21) in that about 70% of clinically depressed older people will respond in a meaningful way to both treatments.

TABLE 15
Benefits of Exercise in Older Women:
Providing Adjunctive Treatment for
Established Diseases

Congestive heart failure
Coronary artery disease
Depression
Diabetes mellitus
Hypertension
Inflammatory arthritis
Obesity
Osteoarthritis
Parkinson's disease
Peripheral vascular disease
Stroke
Varicose veins

Thus the decision about which form of therapy to use in a given individual may depend on the constellation of other diseases present, and the risks and benefits relevant to each mode of treatment, as well as the personal preferences of the patient. In some cases, such as treatment of peripheral edema due to venous insufficiency, exercise and other mechanical interventions are preferable to pharmacologic management with diuretics, which is a suboptimal solution with many potential side effects such as dehydration, postural hypotension, and mineral deficiencies. The treatment of chronic hypertension and coronary artery disease is clearly a case for adjunctive management with standard medical treatments and exercise. Exercise may prevent secondary cardiovascular events as well as minimize the need and risk of polypharmacy or high drug dosages in these conditions. Many of the specific diseases most relevant to exercise and older women are reviewed separately in the subsequent chapters of this book.

TREATING DISUSE ACCOMPANYING CHRONIC DISEASE

For a great many diseases, gradual reduction in activity levels is a near universal accompaniment to the chronic illness. This may be due to pain, as in arthritis or osteoporosis, or exercise intolerance as in peripheral vascular disease, chronic lung disease, stroke, or congestive heart failure. In this situation, there is inevitable atrophy and disuse of many physiologic systems which will exacerbate age-related changes in these domains and thus markedly accelerate functional decline. Standard medical treatments, unfortunately, do not address these syndromes of disuse, which result in cardiovascular deconditioning, muscle atrophy and weakness, postural hypotension due to loss of baroreceptor sensitivity, venous stasis, insulin insensitivity and glucose intolerance, and immune dysfunction among other things. However, exercise retains its capacity to prevent or treat disuse in these systems, just as it does in the healthy aged individual. This may be one of the most powerful and underutilized capacities of exercise in health care practice.

The benefits are often most dramatic in individuals in whom medical treatment is already optimized and cannot be pushed further, or when the pathophysiology of the disease itself is not amenable to change. For example, in chronic obstructive pulmonary disease, once bronchospasm has been relieved and oxygen supplemented, exercise intolerance may still be very limited due to peripheral skeletal muscle atrophy and the inability from years of disuse, poor nutrition, and other factors to effectively extract oxygen and utilize it for aerobic work. However, such peripheral abnormalities can be directly and effectively targeted and treated with progressive endurance training protocols that have been shown to significantly improve exercise tolerance, functional status, and quality of life in such patients. Not using exercise as an adjunct to medical therapy, therefore, is clearly a suboptimal approach to the treatment.

Other conditions in which disuse is common and should provoke exploration of exercise treatment include peripheral vascular disease, arthritis and joint replacement, stroke, Parkinson's disease, congestive heart failure, gait and balance disorders, chronic pain syndromes, osteoporotic fracture, and anyone who has prolonged or recurrent hospitalizations or periods of bed or chair rest. Depending on the particular type of disuse that is most prominent (cardiovascular vs. musculoskeletal), exercise should be applied specifically and progressively, as outlined in Chapter 2. In most cases, if disuse has been prolonged or severe, it is prudent to begin with muscle reconditioning, as walking will not be possible in a safe fashion until sufficient strength and balance have been regained through re-training of the musculoskeletal system.

COMBATING THE SIDE EFFECTS OF DIETARY OR PHARMACOLOGICAL MANAGEMENT OF DISEASE

In addition to its usefulness in optimal aging and the prevention and treatment of disease, exercise may be considered as a specific intervention to offset adverse side effects of standard medical therapies, as summarized in Table 16. Multiple medications may be implicated in anorexia and decreased nutritional intake in the older woman, with resultant weight loss and depletion of lean tissue.

TABLE 16
Counteracting Iatrogenic Disease with Exercise

Disease Treatment	Adverse Consequences	Effective Exercise Modalities
Anorexia secondary to drug therapy (digoxin, serotonin re-uptake inhibitors, theophylline, multiple drug regimens)	Weight loss, sarcopenia	Progressive resistance exercise[a]
Corticosteroid treatment for chronic pulmonary disease, rheumatologic disease, organ transplantation	Myopathy Osteopenia, osteoporotic fracture	Progressive resistance exercise Progressive resistance exercise and endurance exercise
Hypocaloric dieting for obesity	Loss of lean body mass (muscle and bone)	Progressive resistance exercise
Low protein diet for chronic renal failure or liver failure	Weight loss, sarcopenia	Progressive resistance exercise
Postural hypotension secondary to drug therapy (diuretics, antihypertensives, Parkinsonian drugs, antidepressants)	Postural symptoms, falls, fractures	Endurance exercise[a]
Slowed gastrointestinal motility secondary to anticholinergics, narcotics, calcium channel blockers, iron therapy	Constipation, fecal impaction, reduced food intake	Progressive resistance exercise and endurance training[a]
Thyroid replacement for hypothyroidism	Osteopenia	Progressive resistance exercise and endurance exercise
Treatment with beta-blockers or alpha-methyl dopa for hypertension or heart disease	Depression	Progressive resistance training or endurance training

[a] Clinical trial evidence not yet available; based on known physiologic effects.

Progressive resistance training has been shown to allow augmentation of energy intake in frail elders with a nutritional supplement, whereas sedentary peers had no increase in total energy intake when given the same supplement.[11] Chronic corticosteroid therapy causes large losses of muscle and bone mass, as well as a proximal myopathy that is reversible with progressive resistance training, even in heart transplant recipients.[77,78] This finding has very significant implications for patients with rheumatoid arthritis, chronic lung disease, other organ transplantation, and other illnesses where long periods of immunosuppressive therapy are indicated. Restriction of energy intake in obesity[74,75] and protein intake in chronic renal failure[79] both result in losses of muscle mass and strength that can be completely offset by the concurrent prescription of progressive resistance training in the elderly.

This work has important implications for the clinical management of chronic renal failure and liver disease, in that the necessary protein restriction can be accomplished without negative consequences on health and functioning that would otherwise occur. In other older women, protein intake may be low, not due to iatrogenic prescriptions, but simply to small volumes of food consumed, avoidance of certain food groups for financial reasons or preferences, etc. In these situations as well, the tendency to waste skeletal muscle to preserve visceral protein stores for metabolism and immune function may be offset by the addition of the anabolic influence of progressive resistance training.

Improved nitrogen retention with weight lifting exercise has not been demonstrated to occur with aerobic exercise in older adults. Therefore, if this is one of the goals of the exercise prescription, it is important to advise the correct modality of exercise needed (see Chapter 2).

For some conditions (slowed gastrointestinal transit time, depression, osteopenia related to drug therapy), aerobic training may provide similar benefits to resistance training, and the choice of which modality to use may be made in the context of other clinical features and individual preferences. In general, it is advisable to think about the adjunctive use of exercise for these and other common side effects of standard treatment before beginning a second medication to treat the side effects of the first. The benefits of this approach include not only the avoidance of polypharmacy and unwanted medication interactions, but also cost savings and improved fitness levels and other health benefits attributable to exercise itself.

TREATMENT OF DISEASE CLUSTERS AND GERIATRIC SYNDROMES

Common geriatric syndromes that fall outside the boundaries of single disease entities are often ideally treated with an exercise prescription, and are at the same time often not easily treated with standard medical approaches, emphasizing the benefit of this integrated approach to care. Examples of such conditions and their suggested prescriptive elements are given in Table 17. They are some of the most common complaints and symptoms which lead older women to seek medical care, and yet they are syndromes which are often poorly treated by standard medical or even psychological approaches. This is one of the most effective ways to use exercise, but it must be done in a rational way, applied in the correct modality, dose, and time of day in some cases, in order to be effective. For example, if someone complains of weakness, it will not benefit them very much in regard to this symptom to advise taking a walk or some other low-intensity cardiovascular form of exercise. In some cases, the modality of exercise does not seem to be critical, whereas the time of day does, as in the case of insomnia (see also Chapter 20). Details on the prescription of these exercise modalities can be found in Chapter 2.

TABLE 17
Choice of Exercise for Common Geriatric Syndromes

Syndrome	Therapeutic Exercise Recommendation
Anorexia	Resistance training
Constipation	Endurance or resistance exercise
Depression, anxiety, low self-efficacy, low morale, loneliness, low self-esteem	Individual or group exercises including endurance or resistive exercises at moderate to high intensity
Fatigue	Endurance training in the morning hours, increase duration and intensity as tolerated
	Muscle endurance training
Functional dependency	Stair-climbing for endurance
	Resistance training of upper and lower extremities
	Power training
	Balance training
Incontinence (stress)	Pelvic muscle strengthening (Kegel exercises); mobility improvement with endurance, balance, and resistance training as needed
Insomnia	Endurance or resistance exercise in early to mid afternoon
Low back pain, spinal stenosis	Resistance training to strengthen the back extensor muscles, rectus abdominus, and hip and knee extensor muscle groups
Recurrent falls, gait and balance disorders	Lower extremity resistance training for hip, knee, and ankle
	Balance training, T'ai Chi, yoga, ballet
	Training in use of ambulatory device as needed
Weakness	Moderate to high intensity resistance training for all major muscle groups

Another way to consolidate treatment is to use exercise in older women who present with clusters of diseases that are all responsive in some way to appropriate levels of physical activity. For example, it would not be uncommon for an older woman with central and generalized obesity to present at age 65 with osteoarthritis, Type II diabetes, hypertension, coronary artery disease, peripheral vascular disease, varicose veins, hyperlipidemia, mobility impairment, insomnia, and depression. Even if only one drug were given for each of these conditions (often it is two or more), a list of eight to ten different medications may be quickly generated. Although exercise is unlikely to eliminate the need for all medications, it certainly has the potential to replace some and reduce dosages of others. At the same time, it will provide conditioning effects and other benefits previously unrealized with drug therapy alone. Therefore, a thorough review of all diagnoses and medications is warranted in all older patients, to see where substitutions and alterations can be made to reduce the burden of treatment and suffering and increase quality of life and functioning. More details on the nature of this screening process prior to exercise prescription and programming can be found in Chapter 25. It is critical to re-evaluate what has been prescribed every 2 to 3 months, to see whether clinical disease control and risk factors are improved with this change in management, and assess current needs.

USE OF EXERCISE IN FRAILTY AND FUNCTIONAL DECLINE

RATIONALE AND BENEFITS

In the past, exercise has been generally considered inappropriate for frail or very aged individuals, due to both low expectations of benefit as well as exaggerated fears of exercise-related injury. The past decade has seen an accumulation of scientifically generated data that for the first time dispels myths of futility, and additionally provides reassurance of the safety of exercise in the oldest old.[16]

The benefits are wide ranging, including physiologic, metabolic, psychological, and functional adaptations to physical activity that can substantially contribute to quality of life in older women with disabilities. The goals of exercise appropriate to younger adults,[80] such as prevention of cardiovascular disease cancer, or diabetes, or increases in longevity itself,[81] are replaced in the oldest old with a new set of goals which include minimizing biological changes of aging,[51] reversing disuse syndromes,[31] contributing to the control of chronic diseases,[8,82,83] maximizing psychological health,[84,85] mobility and function,[11,86] and assisting with rehabilitation from acute and chronic illnesses. For many of the geriatric syndromes common to this vulnerable population, in fact, a targeted exercise prescription offers benefits which cannot be achieved with any other therapeutic modality. It is important to understand the diverse pathophysiology of frailty in order to utilize exercise appropriately in this setting.

THE PATHWAY TO FRAILTY

A combination of biological aging, high burdens of chronic disease, malnutrition, and extreme sedentariness are the primary contributants to a final common pathway that results in the syndrome of physical frailty as summarized in Table 18. Frailty is not specific to the elderly, but is increasingly prevalent with aging, particularly after the age of 80.[19] Many of the age-related physiologic changes described in cross-sectional and longitudinal studies are in fact modifiable by exercise, even in the oldest old.[18,51] These include decreased aerobic capacity,[87,88] muscle strength,[10,11] muscle mass,[10] and bone density.[89] There is also evidence that chronic diseases and syndromes responsible for significant morbidity in the aged, such as arthritis, diabetes, coronary artery disease, congestive heart failure, chronic obstructive pulmonary disease, depression, disorders of gait and balance, falls, and insomnia respond to exercise in the elderly,[45,90] although data on those over the age of 85 are currently limited. And finally, the atrophy of muscle and bone, cardiovascular deconditioning, postural hypotension, joint stiffness, and diminished neural control of balance reflexes related to inactivity[31] may be the most responsive of all parameters studied to the re-initiation of appropriate exercise in the very sedentary older woman.

TABLE 18
The Pathway to Frailty

Biological aging
Disease
Malnutrition
Lifestyle choices
Psychosocial factors
Environmental design

Anorexia and undernutrition are commonly seen in frail sedentary elders. Exercise has been of interest as a way to boost energy requirements, and thus appetite and voluntary food intake in such individuals, thus reducing the risk of malnutrition as a contributor to frailty.[91] Aerobic exercise has been associated with higher dietary intake in free-living healthy older women.[92] However the same studies failed to demonstrate that the initiation of an endurance training program in sedentary older women resulted in higher dietary intakes at the end of several months. It is not known if a longer intervention or greater intensity of exercise would provide such benefits. The literature suggests that this is the case, since weight loss is unusual in free-living exercise studies, implying that energy intake must be increasing to maintain body weight. In institutionalized older men and women, resistance training has been shown to prevent the decrease in habitual food intake seen with administration of a liquid multi-nutrient supplement.[11] This may have important clinical implications, since the assumption is that such liquid supplements augment total caloric intake, as opposed to simply substituting one form of calories for another. It is not currently known if aerobic training would provide the same benefit in frail elders. Further studies are required to define the long-term benefit of treating undernourished individuals with a combination of weight lifting or other exercise and nutritional supplements, in comparison to supplementation alone.

SAFETY OF EXERCISE IN FRAIL ADULTS

The contraindications to exercise in this population are not different than those applicable to younger healthier adults.[13] In general, frailty or extreme age is not a contraindication to exercise, although the specific modalities may be altered to accommodate individual disabilities.[88] Acute illnesses, particularly febrile illnesses, undiagnosed or unstable chest pain, uncontrolled diabetes, hypertension, asthma, congestive heart failure, or new or undiagnosed musculoskeletal pain, weight loss, or falling episodes warrant investigation, regardless of exercise status, but certainly before a new regimen is begun. Sometimes temporary avoidance of certain kinds of exercise is required during treatment of hernias, cataracts, retinal bleeding, or joint injuries, for example. A very small number of untreatable or serious conditions are more permanent exclusions for vigorous exercise, including an inoperable enlarging aortic aneurysm, known cerebral hemorrhage or aneurysm, malignant ventricular arrhythmia, critical aortic stenosis, end-stage congestive heart failure or other rapidly terminal illness, or severe behavioral agitation in response to participation in exercise secondary to dementia, alcoholism, or neuropsychological illness. It should be noted, however, that the mere presence of cardiovascular disease, diabetes, stroke, osteoporosis, depression, dementia, chronic pulmonary disease, chronic renal failure, peripheral vascular disease, or arthritis is not by itself a contraindication to exercise. In fact, for many of these conditions, exercise will offer benefits not achievable through medication alone.

Intolerance to many medication side effects in the very old makes the search for alternative non-pharmacologic therapies such as exercise very attractive in this cohort. The literature on exercise training in the frail elderly in nursing homes, between the ages of 80 and 100, includes no reports to date of serious cardiovascular incidents, sudden death, myocardial infarction, or exacerbation of metabolic control of hypertension.[10–12,88,93–105] Exercise-related events that have been described include exacerbation of a pre-existing hernia,[10] and underlying arthritis or other joint abnormalities requiring modification of the exercises prescribed.[11] No adverse events related to resistance training with free weights in small groups have been reported in a large, randomized, controlled trial of nursing home residents who exercised over a 12-month period.[12] Sedentariness appears a far more dangerous condition than physical activity in the very old.

THE CHOICE OF EXERCISE MODALITY IN FRAIL ELDERS

The principles of specificity which apply to younger adults are of equal relevance in the frail elderly. Increases in muscle mass and strength are seen following high-intensity, progressive, resistance training (80% of the one repetition maximum),[11] whereas lower intensity regimens (body weight, elastic bands or tubing, resistance to a therapist, or light weights) result in little if any significant gains in strength.[105] Muscle weakness and atrophy are probably the most functionally relevant and reversible parameters related to exercise in this population, so attempts to reverse these deficits and minimize the clinical consequences (functional decline, immobility, poor balance, falls, low energy requirements and intake) should focus on scientifically proven strategies rather than non-specific movement programs for the aged. The rationale for the use of resistive exercise as a treatment for frailty is outlined in Table 19.

TABLE 19
Rationale for the Use of Resistance Training for Rehabilitation of the Elderly

Specificity of training principle
Targeting of age-related deficits in physiologic capacity
Relationship between muscle dysfunction and functional impairment
Treatment of syndrome of musculoskeletal disuse accompanying chronic disease

---

As summarized in Table 20, resistance training in frail elders results in a range of clinical adaptations that are relevant to the targeted disability, which is almost always a multifactorial phenomenon. Associated with gains in strength after resistance training in the frail elderly are improvements in gait velocity, balance, ability to rise from a chair, stair climbing power, aerobic capacity, performance-based tests of functional independence, self-reported disability, morale, depressive symptoms, and energy intake.[9-11,95,96,106] In healthier elderly subjects, resistance training has also been shown to increase bone density, resting metabolic rate, insulin sensitivity, gastrointestinal transit time, decrease pain and disability from arthritis, reduce body fat and central adiposity, and improve sleep quality, but it remains to be demonstrated that these adaptations, in fact, occur in the very frail as well.

TABLE 20
Clinical Improvements Associated with
Progressive Resistance Training in the Elderly

Aerobic capacity (maximal workload and submaximal tolerance)
Balance
Depression
Fall risk
Flexibility
Gait speed and stability
Mobility tasks
Morale
Muscle mass
Muscle strength and endurance
Nutritional intake
Overall physical activity level
Perceived quality of life
Self-efficacy

High-intensity aerobic training interventions have not been described in frail elderly populations. Low- to moderate-intensity aerobic activities such as walking, standing, and stationary cycling at 60% of maximal predicted heart rate have been associated with modest improvements in cardiovascular efficiency[87,88] and mobility tasks[102] (walking, standing from a chair, etc.). It should be noted, however, that the energy cost of activities for frail elders with assistive devices such as walkers and wheelchairs, joint deformities, and gait disorders may be significantly higher than standard equations would predict, and therefore until studies using indirect calorimetry to both monitor effort as well as document change are reported in this population, the exact magnitude of the physiologic benefits of aerobic training remains unclear. It is likely, however, that like younger adults, lower intensity aerobic activities may provide benefits in terms of quality of life, psychological outcomes, and relief of pain and disability, without changing cardiovascular conditioning substantively.

Exercise programs that include balance training or resistive exercises have been shown to improve clinical testing of balance in elders who were selected for mobility disorders or functional impairment. In the healthy elderly, T'ai Chi has been shown to reduce fall rates,[107] and a multicomponent intervention which included low-intensity, lower extremity resistive exercises and balance training also significantly reduced falls.[108] A meta-analysis of the various exercise studies in the FICSIT trials indicates a small protective effect of exercise, although the interventions that included only aerobic training (walking) were not protective.[109] This is in agreement with other walking studies of the elderly that, in general, do not show a balance-enhancing effect. Balance training has not been tried as an isolated intervention in the frail elderly, and there is still much debate about the exact nature of the stimulus required to best enhance balance and ultimately reduce falls.[110] These issues are discussed in more detail in Chapter 2.

Flexibility declines markedly with aging, and is associated with disability,[111–113] but no specific studies have been done to test responsiveness to standard proprioceptive neural facilitation or other techniques in this population.[114] Increases in the active range of motion involving trained muscle groups have been observed following high-intensity, progressive resistance training in the frail elderly,[11] depressed elders,[115] and cardiac rehabilitation patients,[116] but not after low-intensity resistance training[115] or aerobic interventions. It is likely that bone deformity as well as muscle weakness, tendon shortening, and tissue inelasticity from disuse contribute to the problem, thus indicating more than one approach may be needed for its resolution. In general, simple calisthenics, with holding of positions for only a few seconds, appears to offer no therapeutic benefit in regard to range of motion or function, as this is typically the control group condition in many exercise studies in the elderly.

ADAPTATIONS TO TRAINING

Very large-scale studies of training in frail elders remain to be published, but the results from the randomized clinical trials to date indicate that the gain in strength in response to high-intensity resistance training, although heterogeneous, is on average robust, and is more dependent on the intensity of the stimulus than the characteristics, age, or health status of the individual. Those with the weakest muscles but the largest reserves of lean tissue appear to have the best response,[11] which is consistent with primarily neural adaptations to training in the first three months. Advanced age appears to reduce the hypertrophic response to resistance training, however, when all of the studies including muscle biopsy analyses are evaluated.[76] Whether this is truly related to chronological age or co-existent disease is an unresolved question at this time. The data on aerobic capacity are much less clear, as very little data are available on actual physiologic changes occurring after cardiovascular interventions in the very old or frail.[87] Balance enhancement is clearly possible after training in the frail elderly, and this may be one of the most robust adaptations to exercise in this cohort.[10] As described further in Chapter 2, we are currently testing the efficacy of one year of standing resistance training exercises with reduced hand support as a means to enhance balance and prevent falls. After only 12 weeks of these exercises, frail elders in their 80s and 90s demonstrate large, clinically meaningful increases in static and dynamic balance.

SUMMARY

Many common geriatric syndromes contributing to frailty are improved after increased levels of appropriate physical activity. The major physiologic deficits which are relevant and reversible include muscle weakness, low muscle mass, low bone density, cardiovascular deconditioning, and poor balance and gait. The greatest evidence for benefit exists with programs that include resistance training and balance training, and higher intensity training is more beneficial and just as safe as lower intensity training. Therefore, all exercise programs for the frail elderly should include progressive resistance training of the major muscle groups of the upper and lower extremities and trunk. Balance training should also be incorporated, either as part of resistance training or as a separate modality if time and functional status permits. The most difficult prescription for the frail elderly is that of aerobic training. Severe gait disorders, arthritis, dementia, cardiovascular disease, podiatric and orthopedic problems, visual impairment, and incontinence are only some of the conditions which make the usual recommendation of walking for aerobic fitness often difficult or even impossible in the frail elderly. Tolerance to weight-bearing activity such as walking may be significantly improved by first improving muscle strength, joint stability, and balance, as described above.

Most frail elders live in environments and among caregivers for whom exercise is still an unfamiliar and perhaps frightening concept, and there is a great need to change the physical surroundings, recreational programming options, and staff training to allow these recommendations to be instituted in private homes, senior apartment complexes, life care communities, and nursing homes, as described further in Chapter 27. By eliminating unnecessary barriers to optimal mobility and fitness among the oldest old, substantial health benefits may be realized via both prevention of new disabilities as well as rehabilitation from chronic conditions. The short-term safety and benefits of exercise are increasingly well documented in the very aged, and the evidence for long-term improvements in function and quality of life are likely to emerge from ongoing clinical studies.

FUTURE RESEARCH AND CLINICAL PRACTICE NEEDS

Integrating exercise therapy and geriatric medicine into a holistic vision of health care for the older woman is clearly the major unmet need in this area. This will require extensive education of health care practitioners so they recognize the importance of physical activity for

- Prevention of age-related declines
- Primary risk factor prevention
- Treatment of established disease
- Treatment of accompanying disuse syndromes
- Treatment of medication/diet prescription side effects
- Benefits outside of the target disease, treatment of disease clusters and geriatric syndromes.

Optimal health and functioning of the older woman are obviously a multifactorial process, dependent upon genetic substrate, environmental design, and social/political forces, psychological factors, support networks, and lifestyle choices, among other things. Recognition of the overlapping roles played by physical activity levels and nutritional status assumes increasing importance as we seek to identify modifiable elements in this puzzle which will prevent or delay the onset of many chronic diseases and disabilities. The potential for exercise to lead to improved quality of life on many levels is evidenced by a large body of research over the past several decades. As outlined in Table 21, the challenge for gerontologists and health care providers now is to apply and integrate this knowledge into overall aspects of planning and care for the older woman, and the aged population in general.

TABLE 21
Identify Medical Goals of the Exercise Prescription

Reduce symptoms
Eliminate medications or reduce doses needed
Counteract iatrogenic side effects of medication or diet
Correct nutritional imbalance
Optimize disease control via adjunctive treatment
Treat underlying pathophysiology not addressed by standard treatment
Address previously untreated factors: disuse, other diseases, risk factors,
   age-related declines, psychological issues

REFERENCES

1. Department of Health and Human Services, *Healthy People 2010*, Draft for Public Comment, 1999. (www.healthypeople2010.com)
2. Blair, S. N., Kohl, H., Barlow, C., Paffenbarger, R. S., Gibbons, L., and Macera, C., Changes in physical fitness and all-cause mortality: A prospective study of healthy and unhealthy men, *JAMA*, 273, 1093–1098, 1995.
3. Lee, I., Hsieh, C., and Paffenbarger, R., Exercise intensity and longevity in men: the Harvard alumni health study, *JAMA*, 273, 1179–1184, 1995.
4. Department of Health and Human Services, Physical activity and health: A report of the Surgeon General, Centers for Disease Control and Prevention, National Center for Chronic Disease Prevention and Health Promotion, U.S. Department of Health and Human Services, 1996.
5. Wagnar, E. H., Lacroix, A. Z., Buchner, D. M., and Larson, E. B., Effects of physical activity on health status in older adults, *Ann. Rev. Public Health*, 13, 451–468, 1992.
6. Foldvari, M., Clark, M., Laviolette, L., Bernstein, M., Castaneda, C., Pu, C. et al., Association of muscle power with functional status in community dwelling elderly women, *J. Gerontol.*, 2000, (in press).
7. Mazzeo, R., Cavanaugh, P., Evans, W., Fiatarone, M., Hagberg, J., McAuley, E. et al., Exercise and physical activity for older adults, *Med. Sci. Sports Exerc.*, 30, 992–1008, 1998.

8. Nelson, M., Fiatarone, M., Morganti, C., Trice, I., Greenberg, R., and Evans, W., Effects of high-intensity strength training on multiple risk factors for osteoporotic fractures, *JAMA*, 272, 1909–1914, 1994.

9. Pu, C., Johnson, M., Forman, D., Piazza, L., and Fiatarone, M., High-intensity progressive resistance training in older women with chronic heart failure, *Med. Sci. Sports Exerc.*, 29, S148, 1997.

10. Fiatarone, M. A., Marks, E. C., Ryan, N. D., Meredith, C. N., Lipsitz, L. A., and Evans, W. J., High-intensity strength training in nonagenarians. Effects on skeletal muscle, *JAMA*, 263, 3029–3034, 1990.

11. Fiatarone, M. A., O'Neill, E. F., Ryan, N. D., Clements, K. M., Solares, G. R., Nelson, M. E. et al., Exercise training and nutritional supplementation for physical frailty in very elderly people, *N. Engl. J. Med.*, 330, 1769–1775, 1994.

12. Morris, J., Fiatarone, M., Kiely, D., Belleville-Taylor, P., Murphy, K., Littlehale, S. et al., Nursing rehabilitation and exercise strategies in the nursing home, *J. Gerontol.*, 54A (10), M494–500, 1999.

13. Kenner, W., Ed., American College of Sports Medicine. ACSM's Guidelines for Exercise Testing and Prescription Vol. 5th ed. Williams & Wilkins, Philadelphia, 1995.

14. Bortz, W. M., Redefining Human Aging, *J. Am. Geriatr. Soc.*, 37, 1092–1096, 1989.

15. Hagerman, F., Fielding, R., Fiatarone, M., Gault, J., Kirkendall, D., Ragg, K. et al., A 20-year longitudinal study of Olympic oarsmen, *Med. Sci. Sports Exerc.*, 28, 1150–1156, 1996.

16. Fiatarone, M. A. and Evans, W. J., Exercise in the oldest old, *Top. Geriatr. Rehab.*, 5, 63–77, 1990.

17. Frontera, W., Hughes, V., Lutz, K., and Evans, W., A cross-sectional study of muscle strength and mass in 45- to 78-yr-old men and women, *J. Appl. Physiol.*, 71, 644–650, 1991.

18. Evans, W. and Campbell, W., Sarcopenia and age-related changes in body composition and functional capacity, *J. Nutr.*, 123, 465–468, 1993.

19. Guralnik, J., LaCroix, A., Abbott, R. D., Berkman, L. F., Satterfield, S., Evans, D. A. et al., Maintaining mobility in late life, *Am. J. Epidemiol.*, 137, 845–857, 1993.

20. Zauner, C. W., Notelovitz, M., Fields, C. D., Clair, K. M., Clair, W. J., and Vogel, R. B., Cardiorespiratory efficiency at submaximal work in young and middle-aged women, *Am. J. Obstet. Gynecol.*, 150, 712–715, 1984.

21. Grembowski, D., Patrick, D., Diehr, P., Durham, M., Beresford, S., Kay, E. et al., Self-efficacy and health behavior among older adults, *J. Health Soc. Behav.*, 34, 89–104, 1993.

22. Heath, G., Hagberg, J., Ehsani, A., and Holloszy, J., A physiological comparison of young and older endurance athletes, *J. Appl. Physiol.*, 51, 634–640, 1981.

23. Lehmann, M., Schmid, P., and Keul, J., Age- and exercise-related sympathetic activity in untrained volunteers, trained athletes and patients with impaired left-ventricular contractility, *Europ. Heart J.*, 5, 1–7, 1984.

24. Stratton, J. R., Cerqueira, M. D., Schwartz, R. S., Levy, W. C., Veith, R. C., Kahn, S. E. et al., Differences in cardiovascular responses to isopreterenol in relation to age and exercise training in healthy men, *Circulation*, 86, 504–512, 1992.

25. Panton, L. B., Guillen, G. J., Williams, L., Graves, J. E., Vivas, C., Cediel, M. et al., The lack of effect of aerobic exercise training on propranolol pharmacokinetics in young and elderly adults, *J. Clin. Pharmacol.*, 35, 885–894, 1995.

26. Asmussen, E. and Heeboll-Nielsen, S., Isometric muscle strength of adult men and women, in *Community Testing Observation Inst.*, Asmussen, E., Fredsted, A., and Ryge, E., Eds., Danish Nat. Assoc. Infantile Paralysis. Vol. 11, 1–43, 1961.

27. Larsson, L. G., Grimby, G., and Karlsson, J., Muscle strength and speed of movement in relation to age and muscle morphology, *J. Appl. Physiol.*, 46, 451–456, 1979.

28. Pollock, M., Miller, H., Janeway, R., Linnerud, A., Robertson, B., and Valentino, R., Effects of walking on body composition and cardiovascular function of middle-aged men, *J. Appl. Physiol.*, 30, 126–130, 1971.

29. Pollock, M. L., Foster, C., Knapp, D., Rod, J. L., and Schmidt, D. H., Effect of age and training on aerobic capacity and body composition of master athletes, *J. Appl. Physiol.*, 62, 725–731, 1987.

30. Klitgaard, H., Mantoni, M., Schiaffino, S., Ausoni, S., Gorza, L., Laurent-Winter, C. et al., Function, morphology and protein expression of ageing skeletal muscle: a cross-sectional study of elderly men with different training backgrounds, *Acta Physiol. Scand.*, 140, 41–54, 1990.

31. Bortz, W. M., Disuse and aging, *JAMA*, 248, 1203–1208, 1982.

32. Rickli, R. and Jones, J., Development and validation of a functional fitness test for community-residing older adults, *J. Aging Phys. Activity*, 7, 129–161, 1999.

33. Mazzeo, R. S., Brooks, G. A., and Horvath, S. M., Effects of age on metabolic responses to endurance training in rats, *J. Appl. Physiol.: Respir., Environ. Exerc. Physiol.*, 57, 1369–1374, 1984.

34. Meredith, C. N., Zackin, M. J., Frontera, W. R., and Evans, W. J., Body composition and aerobic capacity in young and middle-aged endurance-trained men, *Med. Sci. Sports Exerc.*, 19, 557–563, 1987.

35. Meredith, C., Frontera, W., Fisher, E., and Hughes, V., Peripheral effects of endurance training in young and old subjects, *J. Appl. Physiol.*, 66, 2844–2849, 1989.

36. Rogers, M. A., Hagberg, J. M., III, Martin, W. H., Ehsani, A. A., and Holloszy, J. O., Decline in VO_2 max with aging master athletes and sedentary men, *J. Appl. Physiol.*, 68, 2195–2199, 1990.

37. Seals, D. R., Hagberg, J. M., Hurley, B. F., Ehsani, A. A., and Holloszy, J. O., Endurance training in older men and women. I. Cardiovascular responses to training, *J. Appl. Physiol.*, 57, 1024–1029, 1984.

38. Poulin, M. J., Paterson, D. H., Govindasamy, D., and Cunningham, D. A., Endurance training of older men: responses to submaximal exercise, *J. Appl. Physiol.*, 73, 452–457, 1992.

39. Ehsani, A. A., Ogawa, T., Miller, T. R., Spina, R. J., and Jilka, S. M., Exercise training improved left ventricular systolic function in older men, *Circulation*, 83, 96–103, 1991.

40. Cartee, G. D., Aging skeletal muscle, response to exercise, *Exerc. Sport Sci. Revs.*, 22, 91–120, 1994.

41. Charette, S., McEvoy, L., Pyka, G., Snow-Harter, C., Guido, D., Wiswell, R. et al., Muscle hypertrophy response to resistance training in older women, *J. Appl. Physiol.*, 70, 1912–1916, 1991.

42. McCartney, N., Hicks, A., Martin, J., and Webber, C., Long-term resistance training in the elderly: effects on dynamic strength, exercise capacity, muscle, and bone, *J. Gerontol.*, 50A, B97–B104, 1995.

43. Pyka, G., Taaffe, D. R., and Marcus, R., Effect of a sustained program of resistance training on the acute growth hormone response to resistance exercise in older adults, *Horm. Metab. Res.*, 26, 330–333, 1994.

44. Skelton, D. A., Young, A., Greig, C. A., and Malbut, K. E., Effects of resistance training on strength, power, and selected functional abilities of women aged 75 and older. *J. Am. Geriatr. Soc.*, 43, 1081–1087, 1995.

45. Pate, R. R., Pratt, M., Blair, S. N., Haskell, W. L. et al., Physical activity and public health: a recommendation from the Centers for Disease Control and Prevention and the American College of Sports Medicine, *JAMA*, 273, 402–407, 1995.

46. Blair, S., Kohl, H., and Barlow, C., Physical activity, physical fitness, and all-cause mortality in women: do women need to be active? *J. Am. Coll. Nutr.*, 12, 368–371, 1993.

47. Dunn, A., Marcus, B., Kampert, J., Garcia, M., Kohl, H., and Blair, S., Comparison of lifestyle and structured interventions to increase physical activity and cardiorespiratory fitness: A randomized trial, *JAMA*, 281, 327–340, 1999.

48. Lohman, T., *Advances in Body Composition Assessment*, Vol. 3, Human Kinetics Publishers, Champaign, IL, 1992, 150.

49. Going, S., Williams, D., and Lohman, T., Aging and body composition: Biological changes and methodological issues, *Ex. Sports Sci. Rev.*, 22, 411–458, 1994.

50. Despres, J.-P., Body fat distribution, exercise and nutrition: Implications for prevention of atherogenic dyslipidemia, coronary heart disease, and non-insulin dependent diabetes mellitus, in *Perspectives in Exercise Science and Sports Medicine, Exercise, Nutrition and Weight Control*, Vol. 11, Lamb, D. and Murray, R., Eds., Cooper Publishing Group, Carmel, IN, 1998, 107–150.

51. Fiatarone, M. and Evans, W., The etiology and reversibility of muscle dysfunction in the elderly, *J. Gerontol.*, 48, 77–83, 1993.

52. Epstein, L. and Wing, R., Aerobic exercise and weight, *Addict. Behav.*, 5, 371–388, 1980.

53. Thompson, J., Jarvic, G., and Lahey, R., Exercise and obesity, etiology, physiology and intervention, *Psych. Bull.*, 91, 55–79, 1982.

54. Ballor, D. and Keesey, R., A meta-analysis of the factors affecting exercise-induced changes in body mass, fat mass, and fat-free mass in males and females, *Int. J. Obesity*, 15, 717–726, 1991.

55. King, A., Haskell, W., Taylor, C., Kraemer, H., and DeBusk, R., Group- vs. home-based exercise training in healthy older men and women: A community-based clinical trial, *JAMA*, 266, 1535–1542, 1991.

56. Despres, J.-P., Pouliot, M., and Moorjani, S., Loss of abdominal fat and metabolic response to exercise training in obese women, *Am. J. Physiol.*, 24, E159–167, 1991.

57. Kohrt, W. M., Obert, K. A., and Holloszy, J. O., Exercise training improves fat distribution patterns in 60- to 70-year-old men and women, *J. Gerontol.*, 47, M99–105, 1992.

58. Schwartz, R. S., Shuman, W. P., Larson, V., Cain, K. C., Fellingham, G. W., Beard, J. C. et al., The effect of intensive endurance exercise training on body fat distribution in young and older men, *Metabol.: Clin. Exper.*, 40, 545–551, 1991.

59. Ruoti, R. G., Troup, J. T., and Berger, R. A., The effects of nonswimming water exercises on older adults, *J. Orthopaed. Sports Phys. Therap.*, 19, 140–145, 1994.

60. Hersey, W. Cr., Graves, J. E., Pollock, M. L., Gingerich, R., Shireman, R. B., Heath, G. W. et al., Endurance exercise training improves body composition and plasma insulin responses in 70- to 79-year-old men and women, *Metabol.: Clin. Exper.*, 43, 847–854, 1994.

61. Katzel, L. I., Bleecker, E. R., Colman, E. G., Rogus, E. M., Sorkin, J. D., and Goldberg, A. P., Effects of weight loss vs. aerobic exercise training on risk factors for coronary disease in healthy, obese, middle-aged and older men. A randomized controlled trial [see comments], *JAMA*, 274, 1915–1921, 1995.

62. Treuth, M., Hunter, G., Szabo, T., Weinsier, R., Goran, M., and Berland, L., Reduction in intra-abdominal adipose tissue after strength training in older women, *J. Appl. Physiol.*, 78, 1425–1431, 1995.
63. Treuth, M., Ryan, A., Pratley, R., Rubin, M., Miller, J., Nicklas, B. et al., Effects of strength training on total and regional body composition in older men, *J. Appl. Physiol.*, 77, 614–620, 1994.
64. Baumgartner, R., Koehler, K., Gallager, D., Romero, L., Heymsfield, S., Ross, R. et al., Epidemiology of sarcopenia among the elderly in New Mexico, *Am. J. Epidemiol.*, 147, 755–763, 1998.
65. Chumlea, W., Guo, S., Glaser, R., and Vellas, B., Sarcopenia, function and health, *Nutr. Health Aging*, 1, 7–12, 1997.
66. Lillegard, W. A. and Terrio, J. D., Appropriate strength training, *Med. Clinics N. Am.*, 78, 457–477, 1994.
67. Nelson, M., Fiatarone, M., Layne, J., Trice, I., Economos, C., Fielding, R. et al., Analysis of body-composition techniques and models for detecting change in soft tissue with strength training, *Am. J. Clin. Nutr.*, 63, 678–686, 1996.
68. Evans, W. J., Reversing sarcopenia: how weight training can build strength and vitality, *Geriatrics*, 51, 46–47, 51–54, 1996.
69. Frontera, W. R., Meredith, C. N., O'Reilly, K. P., Knuttgen, H. G., and Evans, W. J., Strength conditioning in older men: skeletal muscle hypertrophy and improved function, *J. Appl. Physiol.*, 64, 1038–1044, 1988.
70. Larsson, L., Physical training effects on muscle morphology in sedentary males at different ages, *Med. Sci. Sports Exerc.*, 14, 203–206, 1982.
71. Lexell, J., Downham, D., Larsson, Y., Bruhn, E., and Morsing, B., Heavy-resistance training in older Scandinavian men and women: short- and long-term effects on arm and leg muscles, *Scand. J. Med. Sci. Sports*, 5, 329–341, 1995.
72. Campbell, W. W., Crim, M. C., Young, V. R., and Evans, W. J., Increased energy requirements and changes in body composition with resistance training in older adults, *Am. J. Clin. Nutr.*, 60, 167–175, 1994.
73. Brown, A., McCartney, N., and Sale, D., Positive adaptations to weight-lifting training in the elderly, *J. Appl. Physiol.*, 69, 1725–1733, 1990.
74. Ballor, D. L., Katch, V. L., Becque, M. D., and Marks, C. R., Resistance weight training during caloric restriction enhances lean body weight maintenance, *Am. J. Clin. Nutr.*, 47, 19–25, 1988.
75. Ballor, D. L., Harvey-Berino, J. R., Ades, P. A., Cryan, J., and Calles-Escandon, J., Contrasting effects of resistance and aerobic training on body composition and metabolism after diet-induced weight loss, *Metab.: Clin. Exper.*, 45, 179–183, 1996.
76. Fiatarone Singh, M., Ding, W., Manfredi, T., Solares, G., O'Neill, E. et al., Insulin-like growth factor I in skeletal muscle after weight-lifting exercise in frail elders, *Am. J. Physiol.*, 277, E136–143, 1999.
77. Braith, R., Welsch, M., Mills, R., Keller, J., and Pollock, M., Resistance exercise prevents glucocorticoid-induced myopathy in heart transplant recipients, *Med. Sci. Sports Exerc.*, 30, 1998.
78. Braith, R., Mills, R., Welsch, M., Keller, J., and Pollock, M., Resistance exercise training restores bone mineral density in heart transplant recipients, *J. Am. Coll. Coariol.*, 28, 1471–1477, 1996.
79. Castaneda, C., Gordon, P., Uhlin, K., Kehayias, J., Levey, A., Dwyer, J. et al., Resistance training prevents muscle wasting in renal disease, *FASEB*, 13 (5), A877, 1999.
80. Goldberg, T. and Chavin, S., Preventive medicine and screening for older adults, *J. Am. Geriatr. Soc.*, 45, 344–354, 1997.

81. LaCroix, A., Leveille, S., and Hecht, J., Does walking decrease the risk of cardio-vascular disease, hospitalizations and death in older adults? *J. Am. Geriatr. Soc.*, 44, 1113–1220, 1996.

82. Oddis, C., New perspectives on osteoarthritis, *Am. J. Med.*, 100, 2A10S–15S, 1996.

83. Evans, W., Hughes, V., Ferrara, C., Fielding, R., Fiatarone, M., Fisher, E. et al., Effects of training intensity on glucose homeostasis in glucose intolerant adults, *Med. Sci. Sports Exerc.*, 23, 51–52, 1991.

84. Singh, N. A., Clements, K. M., and Fiatarone, M. A., A randomised controlled trial of the effect of exercise on sleep, *Sleep*, 20, 95–101, 1997.

85. Singh, N. A., Clements, K. M., and Fiatarone, M. A., A randomized controlled trial of progressive resistance training in depressed elders, *J. Gerontol.*, 52A, M27–35, 1997.

86. Ory, M. G., Schecthman, K. B., Miller, P., Hadley, E., Fiatarone, M. A. et al., Frailty and injuries in later life: the FICSIT trials, *J. Am. Geriatr. Soc.*, 41, 283–296, 1993.

87. Stamford, B., Effects of chronic institutionalization on the physical working capacity and trainability of geriatric men, *J. Gerontol.*, 28, 441–446, 1973.

88. Naso, F., Carner, E., and Blankfort-Doyle, K. C., Endurance training in the elderly nursing home patient, *Arch. Phys. Med. Rehabil.*, 71, 241–243, 1990.

89. Smith, E. L., Jr. and Reddan, W., Physical activity and calcium modalities for bone mineral increase in aged women, *Med. Sci. Sports Exerc.*, 13, 60–64, 1981.

90. Bouchard, C., *Physical Activity, Fitness, and Health, International Proceedings and Consensus Statement*, Human Kinetics Publisher, Champaign, IL, 1994, 1055.

91. Morley, J., Anorexia in older persons: Epidemiology and optimal treatment, *Drugs & Aging*, 8, 134–155, 1996.

92. Butterworth, D., Nieman, D., and Warren, B., Exercise training and nutrient intake in elderly women, *J. Am. Diet Assoc.*, 93, 653–657, 1993.

93. Stamford, B. A., Hambacker, W., and Fallica, A., Effects of daily physical exercise on the psychiatric state of institutionalized geriatric mental patients, *Res. Quart.*, 45, 1974.

94. Blankfort-Doyle, W., Waxman, H., and Coughey, K., An exercise program for nursing home residents, in *Aging and Motor Behavior*, Ostrow, A. C., Ed., Benchmark Press, Indianapolis, 201–206, 1989.

95. Fisher, N., Pendergast, D., and Calkins, E., Muscle rehabilitation in impaired elderly nursing home residents, *Arch. Phys. Med. Rehabil.*, 72, 181–185, 1991.

96. Sauvage, L. R., Jr., Myklebust, B. M., Crow-Pan, J., Novak, S., Millington, P., Hoffman, M. D. et al., A clinical trial of strengthening and aerobic exercise to improve gait and balance in elderly male nursing home residents, *Am. J. Phys. Med. Rehab.*, 71, 333–342, 1992.

97. Carl, C. A., The effects of an exercise program on self-care activities for the institutionalized elderly, *J. Gerontol.*, 8, 282–285, 1982.

98. McMurdo, M. E. and Renne, L. M., Improvements in quadriceps strength with regular seated exercise in the institutionalized elderly, *Arch. Phys. Med. Rehabil.*, 75, 600–603, 1994.

99. Molloy, D., Delaquerriere-Richardson, L., and Crilly, R., The effects of a three-month exercise programme on neuropsychological function in elderly institutionalized women: a randomized controlled trial, *Age Ageing*, 17, 303–310, 1988.

100. Friedman, R. and Tappen, R., Effect of planned walking on communication in Alzheimer's disease, *J. Am. Geriatr. Soc.*, 39, 650–654, 1991.

101. Jirovec, M., The impact of daily exercise on the mobility, balance, and urine control of cognitively impaired nursing home residents, *Int. J. Nurs. Stud.*, 28, 145–151, 1991.

102. Schnelle, J., MacRae, P., Ouslander, J., Simmons, S., and Nitta, M., Functional incidental training, mobility performance, and incontinence care with nursing home residents, *J. Am. Geriatr. Soc.*, 43, 1356–1362, 1995.
103. Perkins, K., Rapp, S., Carlson, C., and Wallace, C., Behavioral interventions to increase exercise, *Gerontologist*, 26, 479–481, 1986.
104. Lindemuth, G. and Moose, B., Improving cognitive abilities of elderly Alzheimer's disease patients with intense exercise therapy, *Am. J. Alzheimer's Care Rel. Disord. Res.*, 5, 31–33, 1990.
105. Mulrow, C., Gerety, M., Kanten, C., DeNino, L., and Cornell, J., A randomized trial of physical rehabilitation for very frail nursing home residents, *JAMA*, 271, 519–524, 1994.
106. Nelson, M., Layne, J., Nuernberger, A., Allen, M., Judge, J., Kaliton, D. et al., Home-based exercise training in the frail elderly: Effects on physical performance, *Med. Sci. Sports Exerc.*, S110, 1997.
107. Wolf, S., Jutner, N., Green, R., and McNeely, E., The Atlanta FICSIT study: two exercise interventions to reduce frailty in elders, *J. Am. Geriatr. Soc.*, 41, 329–332, 1993.
108. Tinetti, M., Baker, D., and McAvay, G., A multifactorial intervention to reduce the risk of falling among elderly people living in the community, *N. Eng. J. Med.*, 331, 821–827, 1994.
109. Province, M., Hadley, E., Hornbrook, M., Lipsitz, L., Miller, J., Mulrow, C. et al., The effects of exercise on falls in elderly patients, *JAMA*, 273, 1341–1347, 1995.
110. Shumway-Cook, A., Gruber, W., Baldwin, M., and Liao, S., The effect of multidimensional exercises on balance, mobility, and fall risk in community-dwelling older adults, *Phys. Ther.*, 77, 46–57, 1997.
111. Bassey, E. J., Morgan, K., Dallosso, H. M. et al., Flexibility of the shoulder joint measured as a range of abduction in a large representative sample of men and women over 65 years of age, *Eur. J. Appl. Physiol.*, 58, 353–360, 1989.
112. Gehlsen, G. M. and Whaley, M. H., Falls in the elderly: Part II. Balance, strength, and flexibility, *Arch. Phys. Med. Rehabil.*, 71, 739–741, 1990.
113. Jette, A. M. and Branch, L. G., Impairment and disability in the aged, *J. Chron. Dis.*, 38, 59–65, 1985.
114. Bandy, W. and Irion, J., The effects of time on static stretch on the flexibility of the hamstring muscles, *Phys. Ther.*, 74, 845–852, 1994.
115. Stavrinos, T., Scarbek, Y., Galambos, G., Fiatarone Singh, M., and Singh, N., The effects of low intensity versus high intensity progressive resistance weight training on shoulder function in the elderly, *Aust. Soc. Geriat. Med. Ann. Mtg.*, 1999.
116. Beniamini, Y., Rubenstein, J., Faigenbaum, A., Lichtenstein, A., and Crim, M., High-intensity strength training of patients enrolled in an outpatient cardiac rehabilitation program, *J. Cardiopulmonary Rehabil.*, 19, 8–17, 1999.

2 The Exercise Prescription

Maria A. Fiatarone Singh

CONTENTS

INTRODUCTION TO THE EXERCISE PRESCRIPTION

There has been considerable debate recently over the appropriateness of a standard exercise prescription as opposed to counseling individuals about the assumption of a generally more active lifestyle. The genesis of this controversy is twofold. On one hand, the exercise prescription based on laboratory data emphasizing the robust physiologic adaptation to various modalities of exercise is quite precise in its formulation of recommendations. On the other hand, the epidemiological data linking physically active lifestyles to chronic disease prevalence or longevity are often based on histories of physically active occupations, or walking most days, but not necessarily participation in specific exercises or sports.[1] Second, despite widespread public health campaigns to encourage exercise in adults of all ages, the physical activity level of the population is not rising in any age category. This is thought to be related to a cultural and behavioral aversion to vigorous exercise. Therefore, recommendations to simply become more active in daily life have been formulated, in the hope that this will be more appealing and successful in long-term behavior change.[2]

There is now evidence from clinical trials that the lifestyle approach for increasing physical activity is approximately as effective in changing exercise behavior in middle-aged adults as a traditional, structured exercise prescription, but it is not *more* effective as had been postulated.[3] Additionally, the physiologic adaptation to this type of behavioral program in terms of maximal aerobic capacity is less robust than anticipated, and less than that achieved with structured exercise. There are no data yet that this lifestyle approach is efficacious in older adults or those with chronic diseases.

In the older adult with established disease, therefore, caution must be used in applying this new recommendation for an active lifestyle to the treatment of disease or prevention of functional decline in old age. There are several important reasons for this.

1. A more active lifestyle is generally translated into more walking and related activities. There is no evidence that such activities will reverse deficits in muscle mass, muscle strength, tissue elasticity, or balance. If

these physiologic maladaptations underlie the target disease or disability in an older adult, then a more specific structured exercise prescription must be made to effect the desired outcome (e.g., prevention of falls, treatment of sarcopenia).

2. The treatment of established disease usually requires a more intensive intervention than the prevention of the same disease, whether that intervention is exercise, dietary manipulation, or medications. Therefore, it is unlikely that very low intensity or modest changes in physical activity patterns will have a significant impact on established risk factors or diseases. For example, in a trial of aerobic or resistive exercise for osteoarthritis, marginal clinical improvements in function (about 10% after 18 months) were seen after the adoption of low intensity exercise which did not produce physiologic adaptation, and achieved relatively low long-term compliance.[4]

3. The opportunities for changing lifestyle may, in fact, be quite limited for older adults in settings where instrumental activities of daily living are done for them, with no occupational pursuits, fewer opportunities for social interaction, and environmental barriers to such a recommendation. It may be easier, in fact, to give such individuals a structured prescription that can be carried out simply and routinely in their place of residence.

Therefore, in light of these considerations, this chapter will outline the elements of a prescription designed to stimulate robust adaptation within the major physiologic domains that can be modified by exercise: strength, cardiovascular endurance, flexibility, and balance, as recommended by the American College of Sports Medicine and endorsed by most major medical consensus groups.[5,6] These elements are discussed separately, because in most cases exercise training is quite specific in its effects, and little cross-over will be seen. For example, balance training will not increase one's aerobic capacity or strength. Resistance training is unique in this regard, as it has been shown to benefit all of these domains to some extent, with its most powerful effect in the realms of muscle strength and muscle endurance (Table 1).

Next, the clinical diseases and syndromes that are appropriately targeted by each of these elements of the exercise prescription are summarized, and risks of each mode of exercise outlined. Suggestions for prioritizing the elements of the exercise prescription depending on the characteristics and desires of the older woman are offered. Finally, an approach to lifestyle counseling that should supplement the basic prescription by addressing ways to introduce physiologic adaptations into activities of daily living is provided.

PROGRESSIVE RESISTANCE TRAINING

DEFINITION

Progressive resistance training (PRT) is the process of challenging the skeletal muscle with an unaccustomed stimulus, or load, such that neural and muscle tissue adaptations take place, leading ultimately to increased muscle force producing capacity (strength) and muscle mass.[7] In this kind of exercise, the muscle is contracted slowly

TABLE 1
General Exercise Recommendations for Older Women

Modality	Resistance Training	Cardiovascular Endurance Training	Flexibility Training	Balance Training
Dose				
Frequency	2–3 days/wk	3–7 days/wk	2–7 days/wk	1–7 days/wk
Volume	1–3 sets of 8–12 repetitions, 8–10 major muscle groups	20–60 min	4 repetitions, 30 sec/stretch, 6–10 major muscle groups	1–2 sets of 4–10 different exercises including static and dynamic postures[a] Progressive difficulty as tolerated[b]
Intensity	15–17 on Borg Scale (80% 1RM), 10 sec/repetition	11–14 on Borg Scale (45–80% maximal heart rate reserve)	Stretch to maximal pain-free distance and hold, relax, and stretch slightly further	
Requirements for safety and maximal efficacy	Slow speed Good form No breath holding Increase weight progressively	Low impact activity Weight-bearing if possible	Non-ballistic movements	Safe environment or monitoring Gradual increase in difficulty

[a] Examples of balance-enhancing activities include T'ai Chi movements, standing yoga or ballet postures, tandem standing and walking, standing on one leg, stepping over objects, climbing up and down steps slowly, turning, standing on heels and toes.

[b] Intensity is increased by decreasing the base of support (e.g., progressing from standing on two feet while holding onto the back of a chair to standing on one foot with no hand support); by decreasing other sensory input (e.g., closing eyes or standing on a foam pillow); or by perturbing the center of mass (e.g., holding a heavy object out to one side while maintaining balance, standing on one leg while lifting the other leg behind body, or leaning forward as far as possible without falling or moving feet).

just a few times in each session against a relatively heavy load. Any muscle may be trained in this way, although 6 to 12 major muscle groups with clinical relevance are usually trained, for a balanced and functional outcome.

EQUIPMENT

There are many ways to carry out progressive resistance training. Equipment may range from only body weight to technologically sophisticated pneumatic or hydraulic resistance training machines. A listing of the general types of equipment available and considerations for their use is presented in Table 2. In general, in the older adult, machine-based training allows the most robust adaptations to be achieved, offers maximum safety, and requires less technique be learned. Free weights, on the other hand, offer significant advantages in terms of cost and flexibility in programming, and may provide a better stimulus for motor coordination and balance, and are the only option in most home and limited space settings. An example of a system of

TABLE 2
Types of Resistance Training Equipment

Category	Advantages	Disadvantages
Body weight	Free Always available	Difficult to monitor intensity or progression Isometric rather than dynamic in most cases
Free weights	Inexpensive More exercises possible Stimulate postural control muscles and coordination more than machines	Difficult to progress to high loads with the lower extremities Safety may be a problem in unsupervised settings Need to learn more technique than with machines
Elastic bands	Inexpensive Light, portable	Difficult to increase intensity appropriately Elasticity lost over time Difficult to reinforce eccentric phase of contraction
Weight stack machines	Allow precise prescription of load and progression Form guided by machine Many muscle groups available	Expensive Requires training in use Some machines do not provide adequate back support or adjustments for elderly users May require supervision for safety Not portable Increments in load limited by the size of the weight plates Momentum can be used to complete lifts inappropriately Not all machines easily accessible for frail individuals
Pneumatic resistance machines	Allow exact prescription of load and progression; increments in load not limited by the size of weight plates Form guided by machine Many muscle groups available Smooth, low impact loading Inability to overcome resistance with poor technique (momentum)	Expensive Requires training in use May require supervision for safety Not portable Not all machines easily accessible for frail adults

free weights we have used in many of our home-based and nursing home trials is shown in Figures 1 and 2.

GENERAL TECHNIQUE

Muscle strengthening exercise is accomplished by contracting muscles against an external form of resistance (as noted above) so as to move the object or resistance

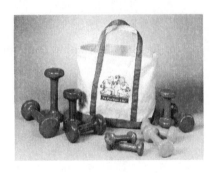

FIGURE 1   Sample system of dumbbells for upper body and arm exercises. Available in 1 lb increments from 1 to 15 lb, vinyl coated and color coded

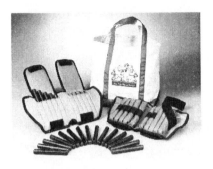

FIGURE 2   Sample system of leg weights for lower body exercises. Pouch fastens with Velcro around ankle. Lead weights available in 0.5 and 1.0 lb increments up to 20 lbs per leg.

through space. This is referred to as *dynamic* muscle contraction. Although muscles can be exercised by contracting them without movement (*isometric*, or *static* contraction), this is advised only when the joint is too painful or inflamed to move, or no appropriate equipment is available. Dynamic movements are in general more functional, simulate real-life activities, and lead to improvements in strength throughout the range of motion. In addition, they can increase range of motion across the joint, which is often an important goal in older persons as well. Therefore, the general technique is to move the muscle group slowly through its entire pain-free range of motion. Initially, the movement should be performed with no added resistance, until the technique is mastered. At that point, the resistance should be gradually increased so a constant stimulus to adaptation is maintained.

The speed of movement during this form of exercise is quite slow, as the adaptations in the muscle are related to the total time that the muscle is under tension. It should take 6 to 10 seconds for each repetition (lift), with one-half to two-thirds of the time spent in the lowering phase of the repetition. This slow speed is difficult to reinforce, particularly during the lowering of the weight, but it is critical for optimal adaptation and hypertrophy of the muscle.

Each movement should come to a complete stop before the next repetition begins. If it doesn't, then the person will be using the stored energy in the system as momentum rather than generating the full force during the next lift. This tendency to swing the weight will be particularly evident in very weak individuals or those attempting to lift a weight that exceeds their current capacity. Clinically, this technique of using momentum to compensate for limited strength is used to enable very frail or arthritic adults to rise from a chair by rocking the resistance (their body weight) back and forth until the rise is accomplished. It is evident from this discussion, however, that such compensatory tricks, although they work, do not address the underlying problem of the muscle weakness itself, and will ultimately encourage rather than treat muscle atrophy. They should not be substituted for therapeutic interventions, but rather used in the transition phase as mobility skills are regained through appropriate resistive and balance training, or in those in whom irreversible deficits in muscle function are present (motor neuron disease, muscular dystrophy, hemiparesis, etc.).

During each lift, it is important to breathe in before lifting the weight, breathe out during the "concentric" or lifting phase, and then breathe in again during the "eccentric" or lowering phase. Most people will have an impulse to hold their breath or perform a Valsalva maneuver during the lifting phase, particularly if the weight is heavy. This should be watched for and discouraged, as it may be associated with ischemia, elevated blood pressure, and cardiac conduction disturbances in those with underlying heart disease (particularly heart block). The easiest way to reinforce this technique in supervised sessions is to ask individuals to count out during the lift. In this way the appropriate speed is reinforced, and breath holding is impossible.

It is important not to substitute other muscle groups for the one that is meant to be targeted (isolated) by each exercise. Such isolation will encourage maximum recruitment of the trained muscle, as well as minimize the potential for injury in other muscle groups due to poor body mechanics. Again, the weaker the individual, the more likely he/she will be to substitute stronger muscles for weaker ones when attempting to complete a lift. For example, the shoulder will be elevated when attempting a biceps curl, or the hip flexors will be used to assist the quadriceps muscle in extending the knee or the hip abductors in abducting the leg. This is why form should be perfected with no resistance, and only then should weights be added. Machine-based training tends to minimize substitution of muscle groups by virtue of the positioning and mechanics of the equipment itself. This is why free weight training is more difficult in terms of technique, and more likely to cause injuries if technique is disregarded.

These general principles of resistance training are summarized in Table 3.

TABLE 3
General Techniques of Progressive Resistance Training

Factor	Recommendation
Muscle groups	Clinically or functionally relevant, 6–10 total per session
	Balance right and left, front and back, trunk and extremities
Contraction	Dynamic concentric (lifting, shortening) and eccentric (lowering, lengthening) contractions; use isometric when joint symptoms preclude dynamic training
Speed	Slow, 6–10 seconds per repetition; don't use momentum
Breathing	Breathe out when lifting, in when lowering the resistance
	Don't perform Valsalva maneuver or hold breath
Isolation	Master technique before adding resistance; don't move other body parts

INTENSITY

The most important element of the resistance training prescription is the intensity of the load used. This point cannot be overemphasized, as it is the most common reason that strength training programs fail to increase strength in clinically meaningful ways. Intensity refers to the relative force that must be generated by the muscle to overcome or move the resistance through space. In isometric exercise, there is no external movement, but relative degrees of intensity can be attainted by contracting the muscle group against a fixed resistance with various amounts of force. It is evident from many decades of research and clinical practice that muscle strength and size are only increased significantly when the muscle is loaded at a moderate or high intensity. Loads which are equivalent to at least 60% of the maximal capacity (the one repetition maximum, or 1RM) of the muscle are needed for adaptation. In general, the higher the intensity, the more robust the adaptation, with a range from 60 to 90% of the 1RM usually appropriate. Thus, if you test someone's strength and they can lift ten pounds, then the appropriate stimulus for training (as soon as the technique is mastered) is six to nine pounds for that muscle group.

If strength itself cannot be measured, there is an option that is commonly used to rate effort during a lift, using a scale of perceived exertion, such as the Borg scale.[8] On this scale from 6 to 20, a rating of 15 to 17 (Hard to Very Hard) is equivalent to 80% of maximum lifting capacity in studies we have conducted in young and older adults, and is therefore an appropriate training goal. The technique is as follows. As soon as the person performs the lift with the first weight selected, he/she should be asked to rate how difficult it was to lift. If it's given a score less than 15, then the next higher weight available can be used, until the appropriate range is reached. If a weight that is too heavy is selected, as long as proper form and breathing and speed of lifting are adhered to, the only thing that can happen is that the person will be unable to cover the full range of motion or complete a full set of repetitions. Older adults, particularly older women, rarely if ever voluntarily choose weights that are too heavy. On the other hand, there is a great tendency to choose weights that are far too light to be optimally therapeutic. This reluctance is at least as great on the part of therapists as it is on the part of exercisers. The negative effects of exercising at a sub-therapeutic intensity are many: discouragement at lack of progress, delayed recovery from atrophy and illness, limited improvements in arthritis, mobility, balance, and other outcomes, and in the end, this approach is quite counterproductive. There is, in fact, no evidence that the often presumed positive benefits of using lighter than recommended weights (prevention of injury, minimizing dropout, addressing fears of lifting heavy objects, avoiding cardiovascular events, etc.) actually occur.

Several authors have recommended that elderly or frail adults use a lower intensity (approximately 60% of the 1RM, or a weight that can be lifted 12 to 15 times before fatiguing).[9] Although these suggestions are made as though they resulted from experimental trials or clinical experience, in fact, all of the randomized controlled trials of resistance training in the elderly that have resulted in large gains in strength have used an intensity of approximately 80% of the 1RM. There is no evidence that this intensity is unsafe or poorly tolerated in men or women, healthy or frail, up to 100 years of age,[10] or even those in early outpatient cardiac rehabilitation.[11] By contrast, low intensity training results in negligible or modest gains in strength[12] and associated clinical benefits, and cannot therefore be recommended if the primary intent of training is to increase muscle size and strength.

Intrinsic to the concept of appropriate intensity is the principle of progression, giving rise to the name *progressive resistance training*, as the most effective muscle strengthening technique. This system requires that the absolute load lifted must be progressively and continuously increased to maintain a constant relative intensity as strength increases. Since about half of the strength gains at one year are achieved within the first 12 weeks, it is important not to undermine this potential for substantial early adaptation by waiting too long to increase the weight. The best method is to instruct the person to rate the difficulty of the lift at each session, using the Borg scale as described above. As soon as his/her rating falls below 15 (Hard), the weight should be increased, assuming pain or medical issues don't dictate otherwise. Some authors advocate changing the resistance when more than 12 or 15 repetitions of an exercise can be performed without fatigue. However, elderly individuals are quite heterogeneous with respect to the number of repetitions that they can perform with a weight of a given relative intensity. Therefore, this method is quite unreliable and difficult to standardize. A simpler and quicker technique is to increase the weight whenever the lift is no longer perceived to be hard.

VOLUME

The volume of resistance training refers to the frequency of sessions, and the number of sets and repetitions (lifts) performed during each session for each muscle group. This subject has generated a great deal of debate among scientists, trainers, and athletes. However, a review of the existing scientific data does allow some useful conclusions to be drawn.

Frequency

Training for one to four days per week will result in increased strength in a dose-dependent fashion, assuming that the required intensity is achieved (see above). This has led most consensus panels to recommend 2 days per week training schedules for weight lifting exercise as a compromise between efficacy and likelihood of compliance with more time-consuming regimens. It is of note that in the case of cervical and lumbar muscle resistance training, much of the literature has been published on once-a-week training regimens, and these truncal muscles appear to respond more robustly to such reduced volume training than is the case for appendicular muscle groups.[13] Training frequencies greater than 4 days per week are not recommended, as the skeletal muscle needs time to recover from the damage induced by loading during the previous session.[14] This damage is thought to be linked to a repair process that results ultimately in fiber hypertrophy.

Depending on the access to training, motivation of the individual, and other circumstances, training frequency should therefore be tailored to maximize adherence, without compromising physiologic and clinical benefits. We have found that it is most effective to recommend training frequencies of 3 days per week in the older adult. Since compliance generally does not exceed 60 to 70% of recommended sessions long term unless entirely supervised, this level of compliance will still result in 2 sessions per week on average.[5] Thus a reasonable physiologic response is achievable. If there is only one session a week planned, and it is missed due to intercurrent illness, vacation, or other activities, then 2 full weeks will elapse between training, which may result in lost strength, disruption of progress, soreness, or loss of commitment to the new behavior in the interval. In addition, with only one session a week (with the exception of truncal muscle training perhaps) it will take longer for a level of competence and clinical benefit to be reached that will lead to sustained adherence.

We have found that some individuals like to train every day, particularly if they notice psychological benefits from participation. This can be accomplished by exercising different muscle groups on different days. For example, arm exercises on Monday, Wednesday, Friday, and leg exercises on Tuesday, Thursday, Saturday. This still allows individual muscle groups to recover between training sessions, but provides an activity for the person six days per week. Such shorter sessions (15 minutes or so) may fit better into some schedules than a few long sessions each week and may thus enhance overall compliance. A similar approach has been advocated with cardiovascular training (see below), as intermittent short bouts of exercise appear to be as beneficial in most ways as longer sessions. In all cases, a balance must be achieved between preferences, convenience, barriers such as time or transportation, access to trainers or equipment, and known physiologic requirements before a rational prescription can be formulated which maximizes compliance and adaptation.

Sets and Repetitions

The other component related to the volume of training is the number of sets and repetitions of a particular exercise that are performed at each session. At the recommended intensity (see above), only 8 lifts or so can be completed before fatigue occurs or form is compromised. This number has therefore traditionally been referred to as a *set* during high intensity progressive resistance training (loads of 70 to 90% of the 1RM). It is evident from controlled trials that increasing the number of sets from one to three does not meaningfully increase the adaptation in terms of strength, although it may result in slightly more hypertrophy. Thus, for most general purposes related to health and aging rather than bodybuilding, one set of 8 repetitions for 8 to 10 different muscle groups will produce marked musculoskeletal benefit with a minimum time commitment. There is no harm in prescribing more sets if time, equipment, and desire allow, but they should not be considered essential.

Unfortunately it is often the approach of trainers to minimize intensity in favor of volume when advising older clients, thinking that this will be safer and equally efficacious. This is not the case. Volume cannot substitute for intensity in the outcome of strength or hypertrophy, and there is no evidence that low-intensity, high-volume resistance training is safer than low-volume, high-intensity training. Thus, the most time-efficient approach is clearly one set (8 repetitions) at high intensity, and this should require only about 30 minutes to complete (2 minutes per set, 10 exercises, 1 minute rest between exercises). This is ideal in clinical settings where staff time and space are at a premium, when several modes of exercise are to be carried out at the same session, or when individuals are working or otherwise quite busy.

SETTING AND SUPERVISION

Resistance training is a novel activity for most older women, and supervision is recommended in some form initially to ensure proper technique, provide confidence, and, most important, ensure progression to appropriate levels of intensity. This supervision may take the form of hands-on training, or a combination of visits, videos, telephone calls, mail, or feedback on activity logs. Most unsupervised weight lifting programs in the elderly suffer more from low intensity than from low compliance, and this will markedly limit the adaptation that accrues, and therefore needs to be addressed in any program implementation or exercise prescription. Success in getting older adults to progress to higher weights requires continuous supervision, although this may gradually shift from direct supervision to more remote means of providing feedback.

Given adherence to the principles of intensity, form, and volume outlined above, the setting is quite flexible, and will primarily depend on issues such as cost, transportation, availability of trainers, spouse or other dependent needs at home, living situation, health status, cognition, and functional or mobility impairments. Cognitive impairment does not preclude training, but it does mandate long-term supervision. It has been demonstrated that compliance is highest when older adults are allowed to choose the setting in which they wish to exercise, and that not all older adults want to exercise in a group, as has sometimes been wrongly assumed.[15] Even in the nursing home, we have seen that one of the major factors that predicts lack of involvement in a nursing home ward exercise program is the patient characteristic of not participating in groups of any kind as assessed by the nursing staff.[16] Therefore, determination of such barriers to adoption and preferences for setting is crucial to successful behavior change in relation to all modes of exercise (see also Chapter 26).

BENEFITS

The physiologic adaptation to strength training is summarized in Table 4. The increases in muscle size and strength are not seen with other forms of exercise, and are also not obtainable with low-intensity progressive resistance training. Therefore, if a primary goal of exercise is to prevent or treat sarcopenia, then there is no effective substitute for this modality of exercise.

The hypertrophic response to training does appear to be affected by health status, anabolic hormonal milieu, nutritional substrate availability, changes in protein synthesis with age, and other factors yet to be identified. Previous suggestions that women do not undergo hypertrophy as effectively as men appear to be related to differences in training intensity and age of the subjects in these trials rather than reflecting a true gender difference in training adaptation.[17] It is clear that exogenous anabolic steroids can augment the hypertrophic response to resistive exercise in young men. However, the role of exogenous anabolic steroids in the resistance training prescription for older adults remains to be clarified. Trials with growth hormone or its secretagogues, however, have thus far largely failed to show benefit in terms of muscle mass or strength in older adults when given alone or in combination with resistance training.[18] The major factors predictive of hypertrophy after training are summarized in Table 5.

TABLE 4
Primary Physiologic Adaptations to Resistance Training

Types I and II fiber hypertrophy

Increased protein synthesis, amino acid uptake into muscle cells

Increased blood flow to muscle

Increased oxidative enzyme capacity in muscle

Increased GLUT-4 receptors on skeletal muscle

Increased glycogen storage capacity

IGF-1 appearance in skeletal muscle

Activation of satellite cells

Myofibrillar damage

Appearance of developmental myosin isoforms

Variable effect on capillary density (no change, increase, decrease reported)

Increased glucose disposal rate

Increased recruitment of muscle fibers

Increased strength of ligaments

TABLE 5
Factors Associated with Greater Muscle Hypertrophy during Resistance Training

Training Variables	Subject Characteristics
Higher intensity (load)	Healthy
Eccentric (lengthening) contractions	Young
Longer duration of training	Previously untrained
	Positive energy balance during training

The other physiologic adaptations listed in Table 4 and the clinical benefits listed in Table 6 have not been sufficiently studied in relation to resistance training intensity or volume to be able to define a clear dose-response curve. Therefore, at this time it is advised that all physiologic adaptations to resistance training are best achieved by adhering to standard training techniques that are optimally effective for strength gain. However, there is a great need for good methodological studies in this area to refine the prescription for specific clinical purposes relevant to older women. For example, it is not known whether intensity is the only factor important for changes in bone density, or whether training volume, speed, or other factors need to be emphasized as well.

TABLE 6
Major Clinical Outcomes Associated
with Resistance Training

Decreased depressive symptoms
Decreased protein requirements
Decreased symptoms of coronary artery disease
Decreased visceral and total body fat
Improved arthritis signs and symptoms
Improved static and dynamic balance
Improved gait velocity
Improved morale
Improved sleep
Increased bone density
Increased capacity for aerobic work
Increased energy intake from food
Increased functional independence
Increased insulin sensitivity
Increased muscle mass, strength, endurance
Increased overall physical activity level
Increased range of motion and joint function
Increased self-efficacy
Increased total energy expenditure

RISKS

Progressive resistance training has been thought of as a relatively risky form of exercise in the past, and has therefore sometimes been avoided by health care professionals in their counseling of older adults. However, a wealth of literature over the past ten years indicates that this modality of exercise is, in fact, quite safe, and is more feasible in many groups of patients and frail elders than is cardiovascular exercise, as illustrated in Table 7. There are relatively few medical contraindications to progressive resistance training, as outlined in Table 8. Apart from these specific circumstances, resistance training is a realistic option even in very frail elderly individuals. Frailty is not a contraindication to strength training, but conversely one of the most important reasons to prescribe it.

The potential risks of resistance training are primarily musculoskeletal injury and cardiovascular events. Musculoskeletal injury is almost entirely preventable with attention to the following points:

- Adherence to proper form
- Isolation of the targeted muscle group
- Slow velocity of lifting
- Limitation of range of motion to the pain-free arc of movement
- Avoidance of use of momentum and ballistic movements to complete a lift
- Use of machines or chairs with good back support, and
- Observation of rest periods between sets and rest days between sessions

TABLE 7
Choosing Resistance Training over Aerobic Training

Severe arthritis preventing weight-bearing activity
Lower extremity fracture with casting
Inability to support body weight
Foot ulceration or ankle injury
Severe balance disorder or recurrent falls precluding safe standing or walking
Amputation of lower extremities without prostheses
Chronic lung disease and hypoxia with aerobic exercise
Angina precluding aerobic exercise
Claudication precluding aerobic exercise

TABLE 8
Medical Contraindications to Resistance Training

Unstable angina, untreated severe left main coronary artery disease
Angina, hypotension, or arrhythmias provoked by resistance training
Significant exacerbation of musculoskeletal pain with resistance training
End-stage congestive heart failure
Failure to thrive, terminal illness
Severe valvular heart disease
Malignant or unstable arrhythmias[a]
Large or expanding aortic aneurysm, known cerebral aneurysm
Recent intracerebral or subdural hemorrhage
Uncontrolled systemic diseases[b]
Symptomatic or large abdominal or inguinal hernias, hemorrhoids
Unstable or acutely injured joints, ligaments, tendons
Severe dementia/behavioral disturbance
Acute alcohol or drug intoxication
Acute retinal bleeding/detachment
Recent ophthalmologic surgery[c]

[a] Ventricular tachycardia, complete heart block without pacemaker, atrial flutter, junctional rhythms.
[b] For example, diabetes, hypertension, thyroid disease, congestive heart failure, inflammatory arthritis, multiple sclerosis, sepsis, acute illnesses, and fevers.
[c] Laser, cataract extraction, retinal surgery, glaucoma surgery, etc.

A distinction should be made between delayed onset muscle soreness (DOMS), a normal response to the initiation or increase in intensity of PRT, and an acute musculoskeletal injury due to training, such as a ligament tear, sprain, or hernia, or muscle rupture. DOMS presents as a dull, diffuse aching sensation over the trained muscle group that starts the day following exercise and peaks about 48 hours after the session, but may take several days to completely resolve. This symptom complex gradually diminishes and disappears in the first few weeks of continuous training, but will resurface after interruptions to the training schedule. It is related to the damage caused to the muscle by mechanical stretch and loading, which in turn stimulates a reactive inflammatory response, characterized by damage to muscle cell membranes, cytokine elevations, intracellular edema, and leukocyte infiltrates.[19,20] Ultimately, this process is not harmful, and does not need to be suppressed or treated, as the attempt to repair this damage results in a desirable adaptation of increased protein synthesis and fiber hypertrophy. It is thought that the eccentric (lowering, lengthening) contraction is what produces most of the damage. However, since the damage ultimately leads to hypertrophy, eccentric contractions should not be avoided, but emphasized in training programs for older adults with low muscle mass.

An acute injury, by contrast, will be felt during or just after the exercise session itself, and is more likely to be perceived as sudden in onset, sharp, easily localizable, often allowing identification of the exact site of injury. Such events should always provoke a response known as "RICE":

- Rest
- Ice
- Compression
- Elevation

Ice can be applied via use of a cold pack for 15 to 20 minutes every hour in the acute phase. Compression with an elastic bandage to limit fluid accumulation will minimize pain, as does elevating the arm or leg if possible. Such a protocol serves to immobilize the affected joint and lessen the edema and inflammatory infiltrate which will otherwise occur. Additionally, if there is a dislocation, fracture, or other serious injury, stabilization of the bones and ligaments is crucial prior to definitive diagnosis and treatment. Weight-bearing and all other activity should be minimized until appropriate medical care is available.

In patients with pre-existing arthritis, there may be intermittent exacerbations of joint symptoms or inflammation with the initiation of PRT. However, the overall effect of training is to decrease chronic arthritis pain over time.[4,21] During periods of disease flare, it may be necessary to switch to isometric contractions, lower the weight lifted, limit the range of motion through which the load is lifted, or insert additional days of rest between training. It is advisable to continue isometric contractions if nothing else, as this will prevent loss of strength, and will not further increase pain. Once the symptoms have lessened, normal exercise sessions may resume.

The circulatory response to PRT has been a matter of fear and controversy, and there is much misperception about the actual changes that occur. The blood pressure changes are difficult to measure during PRT because of the transient nature of the rises, and the fact that blood pressure falls to normal almost immediately after a repetition is completed. This makes monitoring of intra-arterial pressure the only accurate way to gather such information.

The best study of these factors has been completed in older men by Benn[22] and additional reviews of the literature provided by McCartney.[23] The heart rate response to PRT is in general lower than that due to aerobic exercise such as walking up an incline or stair climbing, whereas the increase in systolic blood pressure tends to be greater than walking, but less than stair climbing. Diastolic pressure elevations are greater with PRT than aerobic exercise, thus increasing mean arterial pressure to a greater degree. The double product (the product of systolic blood pressure and heart rate), which is felt to be representative of myocardial oxygen demand, is greatest for stair climbing, followed by weight lifting and walking. The authors concluded from these studies that older adults engaged in high-intensity weight lifting exercise are exposed to no greater peak circulatory stress than that created by a few minutes of inclined walking, and much less than that which is elicited by climbing 3 to 4 flights of stairs. In addition, it has been pointed out that although the double product during weight lifting and some forms of aerobic work is similar, the contribution of heart rate is much higher in aerobic work, whereas the mean pressure is higher in weight lifting. The slower heart rate and increased diastolic pressure during PRT compared to aerobic work would facilitate diastolic filling and coronary artery perfusion, both desirable outcomes in an older individual, particularly someone with diastolic dysfunction (impaired relaxation and filling) or coronary artery disease. Consistent with these observations are the reports of patients who exhibit ischemia or angina during treadmill work, but not during weight-lifting exercises at a similar elevation of the double product.[23] In the largest series of maximum strength tests yet reported, in 26,000 individuals undergoing testing, not a single cardiovascular event occurred.[24] Additionally, the literature consistently documents a reduction in ischemic signs and symptoms after PRT in cardiac patients, attesting to the safety of this form of exercise even in high risk individuals.

In contrast to typical weight-lifting regimens, the response to a sustained isometric contraction of a small muscle mass is a more substantial increase in arterial pressure, and therefore, this mode of training is not recommended unless joint pain temporarily precludes dynamic training. Circulatory responses increase with the intensity of the relative load and the number of repetitions in a set. The augmentation in blood pressure is also contributed to by increased intrathoracic pressure during a Valsalva maneuver that is transmitted directly to the arterial vasculature, causing a rise in pressure. The Valsalva maneuver is difficult to avoid when lifting loads greater than 85% of the 1RM, and is invoked with lower loads when muscles are fatigued. Thus, keeping lifting intensity at about 80% of the 1RM and limiting sets to 8 repetitions (rather than "to fatigue" as has sometimes been suggested) should minimize the contribution of the Valsalva to circulatory stress. The circulatory response is least during the eccentric (lowering) phase of the repetition, and highest during the static and early part of the concentric phase. Thus, emphasizing the duration of the eccentric contraction will both moderate cardiovascular stress and maximize adaptations that lead to hypertrophy (see above) and is thus highly recommended for older adults in particular. A summary of the major factors related to circulatory responses in weight-lifting exercise is presented in Table 9.

A review of the use of resistive exercise in patients with coronary artery disease, congestive heart failure, and hypertension may be found in Chapter 14. Patients with unstable cardiovascular signs and symptoms, as noted in Table 8, should not begin any exercise regimen, including weight lifting, without medical evaluation.

TABLE 9
Factors Related to Increased Circulatory
Stress During Resistance Training

Higher relative intensity of load lifted
Static contractions
Early phase of concentric contraction
Greater muscle mass used
Performance of a Valsalva maneuver
Increasing number of repetitions
Fatigue of muscles

Note: Circulatory Stress = increase of heart rate and
blood pressure in response to resistive exercise

SPECIAL CONSIDERATIONS IN OLDER WOMEN

There is no need to change the specifics of the exercise prescription given above to be more suitable for older women. They will lift lower absolute loads than men due to their generally smaller muscle mass, but the relative load recommended is exactly the same. Their adaptations should be similar if this principle is observed.

Special consideration should be given to erector spinae and upper back muscles, which contribute to back extension. Stimulation of these muscle groups will increase bone density of the thoracic and lumbar spine and counteract the forces promoting osteopenic vertebral compression fractures in postmenopausal women.

Disorders of gait and balance and falls are more prevalent in older women and therefore training programs should always include the ankle dorsiflexors and plantar flexors, hip abductors, hip extensors, and knee extensors and flexors if possible. Those who are already wheelchair bound or nearly so will benefit from triceps and shoulder exercises to increase independence in transfers and wheelchair mobility.

Abdominal muscle strengthening is of interest to many older women for aesthetic reasons (even in 90-year-old nursing home residents in our experience), and to therapists for its contribution to good posture, balance, and control of low back pain symptoms due to degenerative changes in the spine and surrounding tissues.

MONITORING PROGRESS

It is imperative to monitor progress in PRT, as adaptation is dependent upon maintenance of the training stimulus, which means continuous increases in absolute load. Many techniques suitable for enhancing compliance are discussed in Chapter 26, but in regard to this modality of training in particular, the need for documentation of the training load (by the individual or the trainer) is paramount. Providing this feedback in graphical form is particularly useful for reinforcing the presence or absence of appropriate progression, as training loads should be increasing steadily and continuously if appropriate technique is being followed. For some individuals it may also be important to monitor target symptoms or functions that may change during the course of training, such as angina, shortness of breath, falls, insomnia, depressive symptoms, ability to climb stairs, use of assistive devices, fear of falling, blood glucose levels, waist, arm, or calf circumference, etc.

Deciding what goals are important and realistic in the beginning, and monitoring progress in domains that are meaningful to the older woman will provide the most effective motivation. Since strength increases themselves are usually the most dramatic outcome, periodically testing maximum strength is a good idea if equipment is available. If it isn't, a simple test such as recording the amount of time it takes the woman to stand up and sit down 10 times in a row will provide a proxy index of lower extremity muscle strength and endurance. In addition, the perceived exertion in response to lifting the weights that were used in the first week of training can be re-measured over time to demonstrate how much easier tasks which once seemed difficult are after training. Any adverse events attributable to the exercise should also be tracked on activity logs so that appropriate investigation and/or adjustments in training regimens can be made.

Specific Exercises

As noted earlier, there are many types of equipment available for PRT, and specific exercises will be determined by the availability of such equipment. In this section, we will outline a program utilizing free weights for the arms and legs which covers all of the major muscle groups relevant to health and functioning in older adults. These exercises are illustrated in Figures 3 to 52. The body positions of these exercises have been specifically chosen to provide maximum feasibility for all women, including those who may have physical limitations that preclude them from lying on the floor or in a prone position. In addition, they are designed for maximum stabilization and protection of the lower back, a vulnerable zone in poorly designed or supervised weight lifting programs for any age group. A standard routine would be comprised of 8 to 10 different exercises, including some for the upper and lower extremities, as well as the trunk. It is wise to train the back and the front of a body part and muscles on both sides of a joint for overall clinical utility and maintenance of appropriate body alignment and mechanics. A sample routine might include, for example,

- Biceps
- Triceps
- Side shoulder raise
- Upper back
- Abdomen
- Hip extensors
- Hip abductors
- Knee extensors
- Knee flexors
- Plantar flexors

For some exercises there is more than one way to exercise the muscle group suggested (e.g., triceps) depending on the initial range of motion in the shoulder and strength of the individual. It is appropriate in some cases to start with just 1 to 3 exercises and add others as tolerance and confidence increase in tentative individuals. For variety, different exercises that include similar muscle groups (around the shoulder, for example) can be substituted over time to maximize neural and musculoskeletal adaptation and provide novelty to the routine. Specific tips for each exercise illustrated are provided in the legends accompanying each figure.

ENHANCING BALANCE WITH RESISTANCE TRAINING

As has been noted, standard high intensity PRT has been shown to improve mobility and balance. We have recently tested the feasibility and efficacy of a specific balance-enhancing technique incorporated directly into the PRT routine in a group of older adults of average age 84 with a history of falling or gait and balance problems. As outlined in Table 10, and illustrated in Figures 53 to 57, they were instructed to gradually reduce hand support during their standing weight lifting exercises, but otherwise follow the general principles outlined above. They exercised 3 days per week over a 12-week period. The exercises in which these balance-enhancing postures were included were the hip extensors, hip flexors, hip abductors, knee flexors, and plantar flexors. This training regimen resulted in large improvements in static and dynamic balance, as follows:

Usual gait speed:	6% increase
Maximal gait speed:	10% increase
Tandem stand time:	162% increase
One-legged stand time:	126% increase
Tandem walk time:	6% increase
Errors made during tandem walk:	55% decrease.

The ability to incorporate such balance-enhancing postures into PRT is a distinct advantage of free-weight modes of training, as it is not possible using seated machine-based training for these same muscle groups. Even if a woman does not have balance impairments at the time of initial prescription, it is prudent to instruct her in this adaptation of standard technique for standing exercises, as it does not take any extra time to complete the session, and may prevent decrements in balance from occurring in the future. Studies are continuing on the long-term adaptations to this enhanced form of resistance training.

INTEGRATION OF STRENGTH TRAINING INTO DAILY ACTIVITIES

Although PRT is usually conceptualized as a discreet exercise activity, there are, in fact, ways to incorporate elements of PRT into daily life in the same way as aerobic activities. The guiding principles underlying such incorporation are

To use the smallest possible muscle mass to accomplish a given task.
To resist gravity rather than relying on it to make tasks easier.
To avoid use of momentum and strive for slow development of force instead to move an object or body weight through space.
To perform static muscle contractions for 10 seconds periodically during resting periods.

Examples of the practical application of each of these principles are given in Table 11.

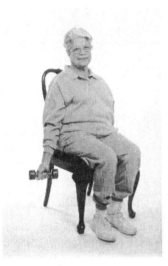

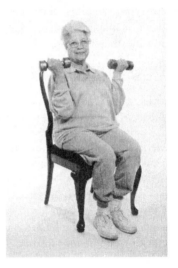

FIGURE 3   Biceps curl. Strengthens the muscles which flex the elbow. Sit erect with arms at your sides holding the dumbbells.

FIGURE 4   Bend arms at the elbow to lift the dumbbell toward your shoulder. Don't move the upper arm or shoulder during the lift. Lower slowly and return to the starting position. May be done by alternating arms as well.

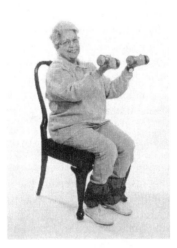

FIGURE 5   Incorrect   biceps   form. Upper arm is being brought forward during the lift instead of tucking elbow into the waist.

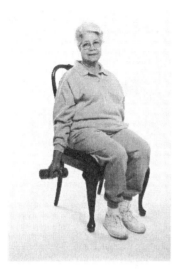

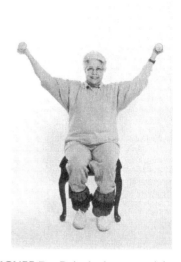

FIGURE 6 Shoulders. Strengthens the upper arm, back, and shoulder muscles. Sit erect in chair with your arms hanging at your sides holding dumbbells, with palms facing away from your body.

FIGURE 7 Raise both arms straight out to your side and try to touch your hands over your head.

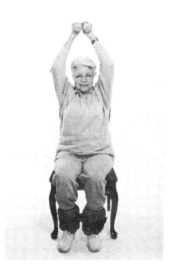

FIGURE 8 If you cannot bring your hands all the way up, lift the weights as high as you can without pain and then return to the starting position.

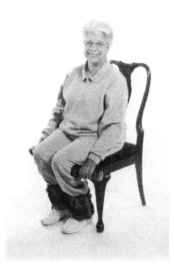

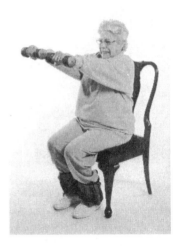

FIGURE 9   Anterior deltoid. Strengthens the muscles at the front of the shoulder that bring the arm forward. Start with your hands hanging down by your sides holding dumbbells with palms facing in.

FIGURE 10 Lift arms until they are parallel to the ground, then slowly lower to the starting position. May be done by alternating arms as well.

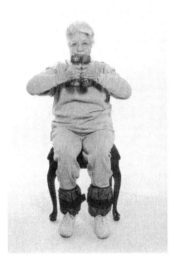

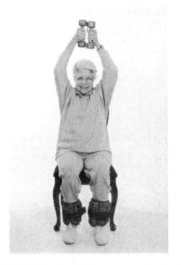

FIGURE 11 Triceps. Strengthens the muscles that straighten the elbow, for those who do not have enough range of motion in the shoulder to reach behind the neck. Sit erect in a chair holding your dumbbells in front of your chest with your elbows pointing directly out to the sides.

FIGURE 12 Straighten arms with hands touching so that the dumbbells are lifted just in front of your face and end up directly over your head. Weights may be rested on lap between repetitions if necessary.

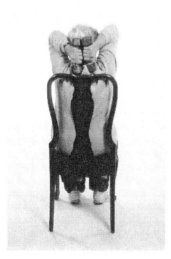 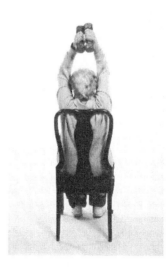

FIGURE 13 Triceps, for those with more shoulder flexibility (preferable position). Sit erect in a chair with dumbbells in hands resting on back of neck and elbows as close to head as possible.

FIGURE 14 Raise arms until dumbbells are straight overhead, keeping elbows close to head at all times. Slowly lower weights to the starting position.

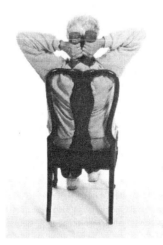

FIGURE 15 Incorrect triceps position. Elbows are pointing out to the side instead of touching the head.

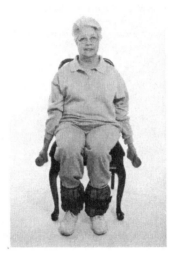

FIGURE 16   Side   shoulder   raise.
Strengthens the deltoid muscles that lift
the arm out to the side. Sit erect with your
arms hanging by your sides holding dumbbells, palms facing inwards.

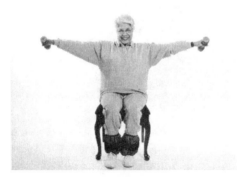

FIGURE 17   Raise both arms without bending
elbows, until your arms are parallel to the ground,
then slowly return to the starting position. If you
cannot lift arms all the way up, go as far as you can
without pain.

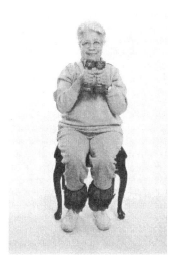

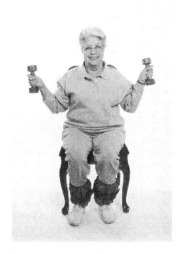

FIGURE 18 Shoulders and upper back. Strengthens muscles of the upper torso for good posture and balance. Move forward in the chair while sitting erect to leave about 6 inches clear behind your back. Hold the dumbbells perpendicular to the ground with your elbows bent so that the weights are touching a few inches in front of your chest.

FIGURE 19 Slowly bring your arms out to the side in an arc while trying to squeeze your shoulder blades together in the back.

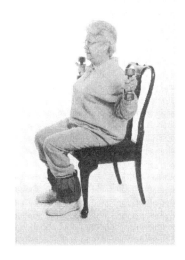

FIGURE 20 Bring weights back to the starting position, trying to return along the same path. Dumbbells can be rested on the lap between repetitions if necessary.

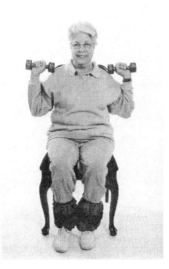

FIGURE 21 Overhead press. Strengthens the triceps and shoulder muscles that allow you to reach overhead. Sit erect in the chair holding the dumbbells at shoulder level, with palms facing forward.

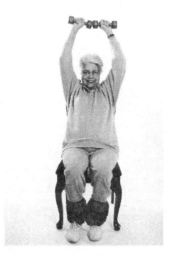

FIGURE 22 Slowly lift both arms straight overhead until elbows are fully extended and dumbbells are touching over your head. Lower to starting position. Dumbbells may be rested in lap between repetitions if necessary.

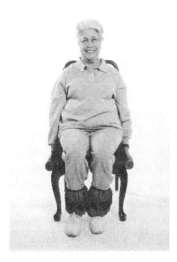

FIGURE 23 Knee extension. Strengthens the quadriceps muscles at the front of the thigh. Sit erect with the weights strapped around your ankles and the back of your knees resting against the chair seat.

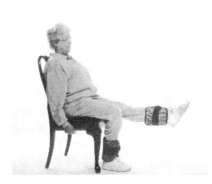

FIGURE 24 Raise one leg at a time until the knee is as straight as possible with the toe pointing forward.

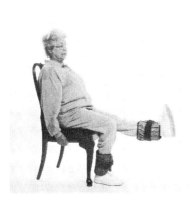

FIGURE 25 While holding the leg in the fully extended position, flex the foot toward your body as far as possible, then slowly lower leg to the starting position. Alternate legs.

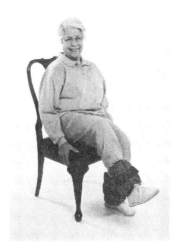

FIGURE 26 Incorrect knee extensor position. Hip is flexed instead of keeping thigh fixed on the chair seat.

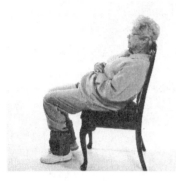

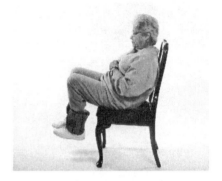

FIGURE 27 Seated abdominal crunch. Strengthens the muscles of the upper and lower abdomen. Wearing leg weights. Slide forward in the chair so that your buttocks are near the front edge of the chair seat and arms are crossed in front of your chest.

FIGURE 28 At the same time, lift feet several inches off the ground while lifting shoulders and back away from the support of the chair. If this is too difficult, just lift legs initially, or do the exercise without leg weights.

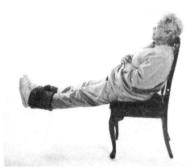

FIGURE 29 Straighten out your legs, holding them together out in front of you for several seconds, then slowly lower legs back to the starting position.

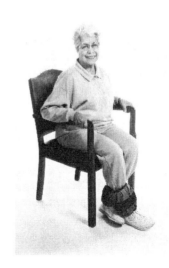

FIGURE 30 Triceps dip. Strengthens the muscle at the back of the upper arm to assist in transfers and reaching. Sit slightly forward but erect in a chair with solid armrests. Put your hands at the ends of the armrests, so that your hands are in line with your torso. Bend knees so that your feet are slightly underneath the chair seat and your weight is resting lightly on your toes.

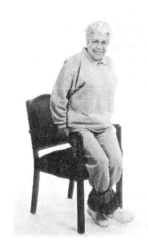

FIGURE 31 Slowly lift your body weight out of the chair using arms rather than legs to do this, until your elbows are nearly straight or you have risen as high as you can. Slowly lower yourself with your arms to the starting position. When this becomes too easy, advance by keeping just one foot on the ground or cross feet at the ankles and do the exercise with both feet off the ground.

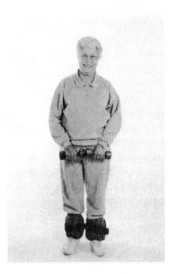

FIGURE 32 Upright row. Strengthens the muscles of the shoulders and upper back. Start by standing with dumbbells in hands hanging straight down in front of you.

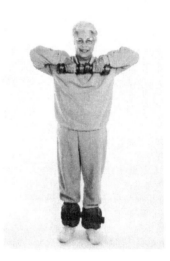

FIGURE 33 Lift dumbbells together with elbows pointing out to the side until they are at the level of your collarbone, keeping the weights touching and your back straight at all times. Slowly lower weights to the starting position.

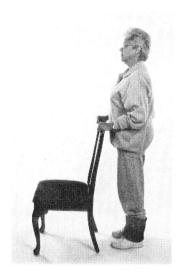

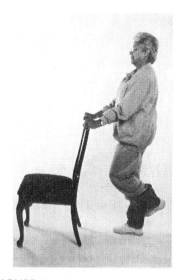

FIGURE 34 Plantar flexors. Strengthens the muscles at the back of the calf. With ankle weights in place, stand erect holding onto the back of a chair.

FIGURE 35 Raise your body up as high as possible on your toes and then slowly lower to the starting position.

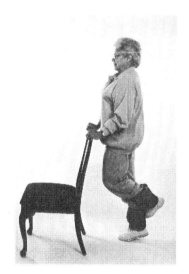

FIGURE 36 When it is too easy with two feet, lift one foot slightly off the floor or hook it around your other ankle during the exercise. Alternate legs between sets.

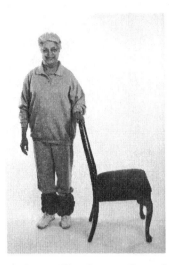

FIGURE 37 Hip flexors. Strengthens the muscles that bring the knee toward the chest. With ankle weights in place, stand sideways next to a chair.

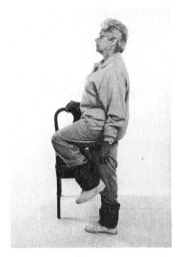

FIGURE 38 Without bending at the waist, bring one knee at a time as close to the chest as possible, and then lower to the starting position. Alternate legs between repetitions or sets. This exercise may be done in the seated position if balance or strength is not sufficient for a standing posture.

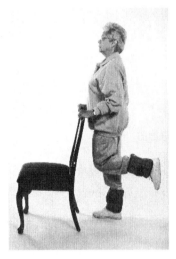

FIGURE 39 Knee flexors. Strengthens the hamstring muscles at the back of the upper thigh. With ankle weights in place, stand close behind a chair. Without moving your thigh at all, bend one knee back until your foot is as close to the back of the thigh as possible. Lower leg slowly and alternate between repetitions.

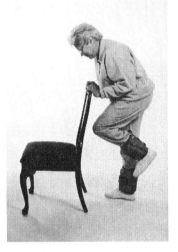

FIGURE 40 Incorrect knee flexion. Don't allow your thigh to come forward during the movement. The knees should be touching at all times during the lifting and lowering phases.

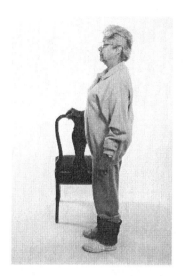

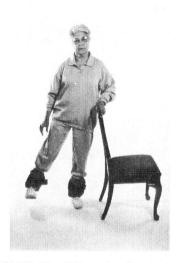

FIGURE 41 Hip abduction. Strengthens the muscles at the side of the thigh that move the leg to the side. With ankle weights in place, stand erect holding onto the back of a chair.

FIGURE 42 Without bending the knee or waist, bring one leg out to the side about 8 to 12 inches with toes always pointing forward. Slowly lower back to the starting position and alternate legs between sets.

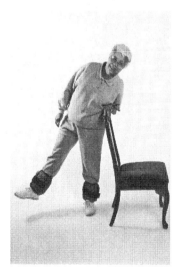

FIGURE 43 Incorrect hip abduction. Toes are allowed to point outward rather than straight ahead during the lift. Waist is bent toward chair.

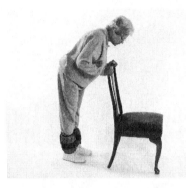

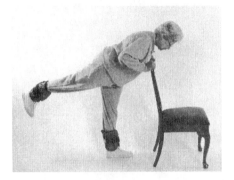

FIGURE 44 Hip extension. Strengthens the muscles of the buttocks and hamstrings. With ankle weights in place, stand holding onto the back of a chair and bend forward about 45 degrees at the waist.

FIGURE 45 Lift one leg straight out behind you as high as possible without bending your knees or moving your upper body closer to the chair. Slowly lower to the starting position and alternate legs between repetitions.

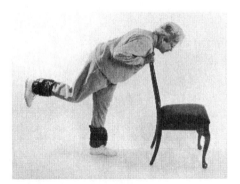

FIGURE 46 Incorrect hip extension. Knee is bent and upper body has moved closer to the chair.

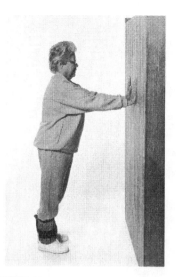

FIGURE 47 Wall push-ups. Strengthens the muscles of the chest and upper arm. Stand facing a wall so that arms are extended in front of you at shoulder height with palms against the wall and elbows straight.

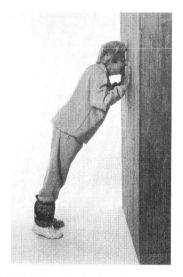

FIGURE 48 Slowly bend elbows until your nose touches the wall, then return to the starting position. As you improve, move feet slightly farther away from the wall.

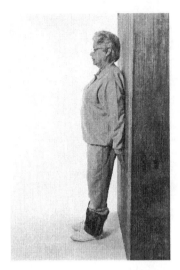

FIGURE 49 Wall squats. Strengthens the quadriceps muscle at the front of the thigh. Stand with your back to a wall, palms against the wall by your sides, feet about 6 to 8 inches away from the wall.

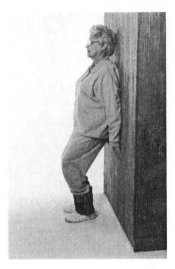

FIGURE 50 Slowly slide down the wall until your knees are bent about 45 degrees and hold this position for several seconds before returning to the starting position.

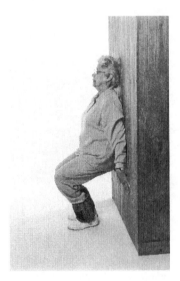

FIGURE 51 Advance by holding one foot off the ground and performing the exercise with one leg. Alternate between sets. You may also advance by deepening the squat to 90° of knee flexion, as shown.

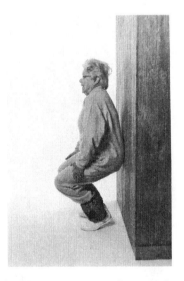

FIGURE 52 Incorrect wall squats. Squat is done too deeply, too much strain is put on the knee joint, and balance may be lost.

TABLE 10
Adding Balance Training to Resistive Exercises

Step 1:   Hold onto chair or table with two hands during standing resistive exercises (hip flexion, hip abduction, hip extension, knee flexion, plantar flexion)
Step 2:   Hold on with one hand only
Step 3:   Hold on with one fingertip only
Step 4:   Keep both hands two inches above chair or table
Step 5:   Close eyes, keep both hands two inches above chair or table

Note: These postures are illustrated in Figures 53 to 57.

CARDIOVASCULAR ENDURANCE TRAINING

DEFINITION

Cardiovascular endurance training refers to exercise in which large muscle groups contract many times (thousands of times at a single session) against little or no resistance other than that imposed by gravity. The purpose of this type of training is to increase the maximal amount of aerobic work that can be carried out, as well as to decrease the physiologic response and perceived difficulty of submaximal aerobic workloads. Extensive adaptations in the cardiopulmonary system, peripheral skeletal muscle, circulation, and metabolism are responsible for these changes in exercise capacity and tolerance.

Many different kinds of exercise fall into this category, including walking and its derivatives (hiking, running, dancing, stair climbing, biking, swimming, ball sports, etc.). The key distinguishing features between activities which are primarily aerobic vs. resistive in nature are listed in Table 12. Obviously, there may be some overlap if aerobic activities are altered to increase the loading to muscle, as in resisted stationary cycling or stair-climbing machines. However, such activities are still primarily aerobic in nature, as they do not cause fatigue within a very few contractions as PRT does, and they therefore do not cause the kinds of adaptations in the nervous system and muscle which lead to marked strength gain and hypertrophy.

MODES OF EXERCISE

There are many more kinds of cardiovascular exercise available than is the case for strengthening exercise. The decision about how to train aerobically depends on factors such as preference, access, likelihood of injury, and health-related restrictions or desired benefits. In general, although there are differences in oxygen consumption among various kinds of aerobic exercise, unless one is training for a particular sport, personal preference can provide much of the direction in this regard, as long-term compliance will require that an enjoyable pursuit has been selected. Given attention to the intensity and volume requirements below, most activities can

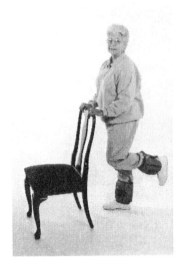

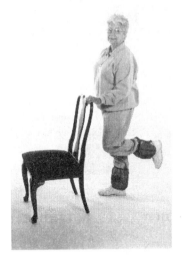

FIGURE 53 Balance sequence. When doing hip flexion, knee flexion, hip abduction, hip extension, and plantar flexion exercises, begin by holding onto the back of a chair with two hands (STEP 1).

FIGURE 54 Decrease hand support to one hand as soon as step one is mastered (STEP 2).

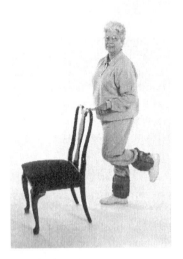

FIGURE 55 Decrease hand support to one fingertip (STEP 3).

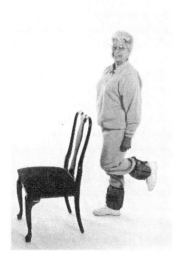

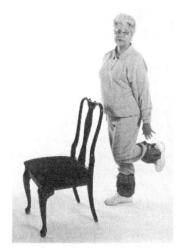

FIGURE 56 Remove all hand support but keep hands close to the back of the chair for safety (STEP 4).

FIGURE 57 Perform exercise as in STEP 4 but with eyes closed (STEP 5)

TABLE 11
Incorporating Strengthening Into Daily Activities

Principle	Examples
Use smallest possible muscle mass to accomplish task	Rise from a chair without using arms to assist
	Lift heavy objects with one arm instead of two
	Stand on one leg
	Climb stairs, only lightly using hands on rails for balance
Resist gravity	Sit down slowly
	Lower body weight slowly up and down stairs
	Lower packages slowly
Do not use momentum to assist with tasks	Lift slowly rather than swing objects into position
	Don't rock body to rise from a low chair or sofa
Perform isometric contractions when resting	Push down on floor with toes when sitting
	Hook toes under sofa and pull up while sitting
	Stand on one leg in line
	Push against chair arms with forearms and upper arm while sitting
	Extend spine against back of chair while sitting
	Press legs together when sitting or lying
	Do abdominal crunches while riding in cars or buses
	Place hands, palms up, under desk and pull up while sitting
	Push head back against high-backed seat
	Perform Kegel (pelvic floor) exercises any time

TABLE 12
Characteristics of Aerobic vs. Resistive Exercise

Feature	Aerobic Exercise	Resistive Exercise
Muscle groups	Most large, appendicular +/– truncal	Any, large or small
Contractions	Many	Few
Mechanical loading of muscle	Low, gravity or light resistance only	High, moderate to heavy resistance (60–90% of maximal tolerable load)
Speed of contractions	Fast	Slow[a]
Pulse response	Large increase (to 60–85% of maximum)	Small increase, non-sustained between contractions
Blood pressure response	Primarily systolic, diastolic may decrease; dependent on intensity of workload	Systolic, diastolic, and mean pressure increase, dependent on intensity of load, mass of muscle involved, duration of contractions; non-sustained between contractions
Primary physiologic responses	Increased maximal aerobic capacity Decreased cardiovascular response, fatigue, and perceived exertion during fixed submaximal workloads	Increased muscle strength, size, and endurance; smaller effect on increased tolerance to aerobic work

[a] Exception is muscle power training, which requires high-force, high-velocity contractions.

contribute to improvements in cardiovascular efficiency, reduction of metabolic risk factors, and reduced risk of many chronic diseases.

Two other factors assume importance in older adults, and older women in particular. The first is the beneficial effects of weight-bearing aerobic activities on bone density. The loading of bone is critical to this outcome;[25,26] non-weight-bearing aerobic activities (such as swimming and biking) have not been shown to maintain or increase bone density, whereas walking, jogging, and stepping have positive effects in cross-sectional and longitudinal studies.[27–32] Second, high-impact activities such as jogging, jumping, and running have been associated with very high rates of knee and ankle injuries, even in healthy older adults.[33] In older women with pre-existing arthritis, such high-impact activities are neither feasible nor recommended, as they are even more likely to result in injuries and exacerbations of arthritis in this cohort.

Balancing the skeletal need for weight-bearing or loading and the safety requirements of the joints and connective tissues for low impact, one would favor exercises such as walking, dancing, hiking, or stair climbing over running, step aerobics, or jumping rope in older women. Younger women may safely perform high impact activities as long as muscle and ligament strength and joint structure are normal. It has been suggested anecdotally that concurrent PRT may prevent much of the joint problems and injuries incurred during typical high-impact aerobic pursuits, but this remains to be shown experimentally.

Overall, walking and its derivations surface as the most widely studied, feasible, safe, accessible, and economical mode of aerobic training for women of most ages and states of health. It does not require special equipment or locations, and does not need to be taught or supervised (except in the cognitively impaired, very frail, or medically unstable individual). Walking bears a natural relationship to ordinary activities of daily living, making it easier than any other mode of exercise to integrate into lifestyle and functional tasks. Therefore, it is theoretically more likely to translate into improved functional independence and mobility than other modes of exercise.

INTENSITY

The intensity of aerobic exercise refers to the amount of oxygen consumed (VO_2), or energy expended, per minute while performing the activity, which will vary from about 5 kcal/min for light activities, to 7.5 kcal/minute for moderate activities, to 10–12 kcal/min for very heavy activities. Energy expenditure increases with increasing body weight for weight-bearing aerobic activities, as well as with inclusion of larger muscle mass, and increased work (force × distance) and power output (work/time) demands of the activity. Therefore, the most intensive activities are those which involve the muscles of the arms, legs, and trunk simultaneously, necessitate moving the full body weight through space, and are done at a rapid pace (e.g., cross-country skiing). Adding extra loading to the body weight (backpack, weight belt, wrist weights) increases the force needed to move the body part through space, and therefore increases the aerobic intensity of the work performed.

The intensity of aerobic work can be calculated by measuring the actual consumption of oxygen using indirect calorimetry of inspired and expired gases, which are analyzed for the oxygen and carbon dioxide content. Since this method is normally only available in research facilities, estimations are usually made by assessing cardiovascular responses or subjective rating of effort by the participant. Rise in heart rate is directly proportional in normal individuals in sinus rhythm to increasing oxygen consumption or aerobic workload. Thus, monitoring heart rate has traditionally been a primary means of both prescribing appropriate intensity levels as well as following training adaptations when direct measurements of oxygen consumption are not available. The relative heart rate reserve (HRR) is the most useful estimate of intensity based on heart rate, and training intensity is normally recommended at approximately 60 to 80% of the HRR. This is calculated as follows:

HRR = (Maximal heart rate – resting heart rate) + resting heart rate

60 to 80% HRR = .6–.8(Max HR – resting HR) + resting HR

If someone has had a true maximal aerobic capacity test, the peak heart rate achieved during that test may be used in the above formula. If this is not available, or the test was terminated prematurely, then maximal HR can be estimated from the following equation:

$$\text{Maximal HR} = 220 - \text{age}$$

However, it should be recognized that this estimation is rather crude, becomes more imprecise with advancing age, and may err by 10 to 20 beats on either side in a given individual. Other difficulties with an intensity prescription based on heart rate in the older adult include the presence of arrhythmias, pacemakers, or beta-blockers (systemic or ophthalmologic) which will alter the heart rate response to exercise.[34]

Therefore, a more easily obtainable and reliable estimate of aerobic intensity is to prescribe a level of "somewhat hard," or 12 to 14 on the Borg scale which runs from 6 to 20.[8] At this level, the exerciser should note increased pulse and respiratory rate, but still be able to talk. This scale has been validated for use in men and women, young and old, those with coronary disease and normals, and in many other clinical situations, and is therefore of widespread applicability. It is easy to teach, and is a means to supervise training intensity from afar, by means of written diaries or telephone calls, making it cost-effective in community programs and health care settings. Usually, a visual representation of the Borg Scale is used to increase accuracy, but assessment can even be done without this prop in patients who are blind or cannot read.

All of the major benefits of aerobic exercise (i.e., increased cardiovascular fitness, decreased mortality, decreased incidence of chronic diseases, improved insulin sensitivity, blood pressure, and cholesterol) are attainable with this moderately intense level of aerobic training.[35] Therefore, the only reason to prescribe higher intensity training (16 to 18 on the Borg scale, >85% HRR) would be for greater improvements in aerobic capacity or elite athletic performance requirements. For most individuals, the increased risk of cardiovascular events or musculoskeletal injuries is not worth these performance outcomes. There is evidence that even training levels as low as 40 to 60% of the HRR have some physiologic and clinical benefit, so individuals who may have health problems precluding higher levels of effort can still reap health benefits from participation.[36]

As is the case with all other forms of exercise, in order to maintain the same relative training intensity over time, the absolute training load must be increased as fitness improves. In younger individuals, walking may be changed to jogging and then running to increase intensity as needed. More appropriate in older women are progressive alterations in workload which increase energy expenditure without converting to a high-impact form of activity. Examples of how to prescribe such progression for various modes of aerobic exercise are given in Table 13. The workloads should progress based on ratings of effort at each training session. Once the perceived exertion slips below 12, the intensity of the regimen should be increased to maintain the physiologic stimulus for optimal rates of adaptation. As with PRT, the most common error in aerobic training is failure to progress, which results in an early submaximal plateau in cardiovascular and metabolic improvement.

TABLE 13
Increasing the Intensity of Aerobic Exercise

Mode of Exercise	Ways to Increase Intensity
Walking	Add small weights around wrists
	Swing arms
	Use race walking style
	Add inclines, hills, stairs
	Carry weighted backpack or waist belt[a]
	Push a wheelchair or stroller (with someone in it)
Cycling	Increase pedaling speed
	Increase resistance to pedals
	Add hills
	Add backpack[a]
	Add child carrier to back of bike
Water activities	Use arms and legs in strokes
	Add resistive equipment for water
	Increase pace
Tennis	Convert from doubles to singles game
Golf	Carry clubs[a]
	Eliminate golf cart
Dance	Increase pace of movements
	Add more arm and leg movements

[a] Avoid flexing the spine when doing this to prevent excessive compressive forces on the thoracic spine

VOLUME

Frequency and duration combine to describe the volume of aerobic exercise performed. There has been a great deal of controversy over this part of the prescription, and the range recommended has varied from as little as 20 minutes, 3 days per week to 30 minutes, most days per week.[2] As with intensity, the exact dosage required depends on the outcomes one wishes to achieve. Cardiovascular protection and risk factor reduction appear to require 20 to 30 minutes, 3 days per week, as does improvement in aerobic capacity.[5,37-39] Peak athletic performance will usually require higher volumes of training than this, as will expenditures of large amounts of energy to aid in weight and adipose tissue losses from diet.[40] Improvements in glucose homeostasis (glucose disposal rate, insulin sensitivity, etc.) appear to require an exercise session every 72 hours, as the metabolic effects begin to diminish after this,[41,42] even in those who are chronically trained. Epidemiological studies of mortality suggest that walking about 1 mile per day (presumably about 20 minutes at average pace) or expending about 2000 kcal/week in physical activities[43,44] is protective, again pointing to the moderate levels that are needed for major health outcomes. It has been shown that exercise does not need to be carried out at a single session to provide training effects, and may be broken up into sessions of 10 minutes at a time.[2] Shorter duration sessions than this have not been evaluated for efficacy, although public health recommendations for integrating short sessions of even 5 minutes into the daily routine have been made recently.

Overall, a session or sessions of exercise at least once every three days adding up to about 90 minutes a week appears to be the minimal prescription justifiable based on the available literature. Higher volumes than this (30 minutes per day, most days per week) are frequently recommended, and should fit into most life-styles. Exercise in very long sessions once or twice a week is not recommended as an alternative, as this is likely to result in muscle soreness and injuries. The risk of sudden death during physical activity appears to be limited to those who do not exercise on a regular basis (at least one hour per week), which is another reason for advocating regular, moderate doses of exercise rather than periodic high-volume training.

SUPERVISION AND SETTING

Most people will be familiar with the basic principles of common forms of aerobic exercise (walking, biking, swimming, etc.), so this modality of exercise is fre-quently carried out in unsupervised settings. Exceptions to this general rule may be made in special circumstances, such as in cardiac rehabilitation settings or for frail adults where safety may be a concern. In addition, when new techniques are introduced (aerobic dance, aqua aerobics, etc.) or when compliance needs to be more intensively monitored for efficacy (as in the treatment of obesity or diabetes), supervision may be required. It is often possible to graduate to a partially monitored program after a new routine has been established, to increase flexibility and yet maintain reinforcing contact and supervision. It should be remembered that a group setting or supervised program does not automatically ensure higher exercise compliance in older adults.[15] King has stated that *choice* is the most important determinant of compliance, and if barriers to supervised participation away from home (such as dislike of group exercise, need to care for a family member, lack of transportation, financial costs, inclement weather, inconvenient scheduling or work commitments) outweigh the benefits (perceived safety, access to trainers, support of group members, socialization), then there is no advantage to prescribing center-based, supervised exercise. Assessing an older woman's preferences in this regard is most important early in the prescriptive process to avoid failure and behavioral relapse.

MONITORING PROGRESS

The best way to monitor progress in an aerobic training program is to review an activity log kept by the participant, including frequency, duration, and ratings of perceived exertion (RPE) of exercise sessions. This can be simply recorded on an ordinary calendar posted on the refrigerator in the spaces for each day of the month, as follows:

Walking, 20 minutes, RPE 14

If such monthly calendars are reviewed periodically by an appropriate member of the health care team, advice can be given on a timely basis about patterns, volume, and intensity of exercise to enhance compliance and optimize efficacy. For example, if a diabetic is noted to be exercising in long bouts at intervals 5 days apart on average, advice may be given to change to shorter bouts every 3 days. Events which typically trigger long bouts of non-compliance (illness, injury, depression, work commitments, vacation, baby-sitting responsibilities, etc.) can be identified and relapse prevention strategies put into place to avert such patterns (see also Chapter 26).

Most health outcomes appear to be related to the accumulated volume of exercise, and so monitoring compliance as above will theoretically provide evidence that the benefits are occurring. However, there may also be benefit in monitoring the improvements in cardiovascular fitness from training, as aerobic capacity itself has an even stronger relationship to mortality than the level of physical activity. Documenting improvements in fitness may have a reinforcing effect on long-term behavioral adaptations as well. Improved fitness may be shown by

- Improved measurements of maximal aerobic capacity.
- Decreased heart rate and blood pressure response to a fixed submaximal workload.
- Decreased rate of perceived exertion for a fixed submaximal workload.

Since treadmill testing and indirect calorimetry are not typically available to the health care practitioner, field estimates of aerobic capacity and cardiovascular responses are usually substituted. A simple way to do this in clinical practice that requires minimal equipment is the 6-minute walk test. This test has been used as an index of rehabilitation in cardiac and pulmonary patients, and is known to improve with effective interventions. The test is performed on a flat indoor course without obstacles as follows:

Step 1: Take pulse and BP after a 5-minute rest period.
Step 2: Instruct the woman to cover as much ground as possible in 6 minutes without breaking into a run. During this time the examiner will be following along behind with a stopwatch and measuring wheel, and encouraging maximal performance every 30 seconds.
Step 3: At the end of 6 minutes, the woman is asked to stop and a rating of perceived exertion (RPE), pulse, and BP are taken immediately.
Step 4: The total distance covered is recorded in meters from the measuring wheel, or by noting the number of laps of known distance completed, etc.

With training, RPE, pulse, and blood pressure at six minutes should decrease, and distance covered should increase. In young or very fit individuals, a running test is usually needed, as they do not have room for much improvement on a walking test. Alternatives to the 6-minute walk are climbing multiple flights of stairs as rapidly as possible or stepping up and down a single step for several minutes, followed by the measurements above. Availability of stairs and the potential for musculoskeletal injury due to balance, hip and knee arthritis, or vision problems make rapid stepping tests less desirable in the older adult.

In evaluating the responses above, it should be noted that in general the reduced fatigue during submaximal exercise will be of greater magnitude than the increase in maximal aerobic capacity, if this is measured. Since most activities of daily living take place at submaximal workloads, this benefit should be readily appreciated by the older woman as well. Large improvements in maximal aerobic capacity are not seen in lifestyle approaches to aerobic exercise and are likely to occur only after structured, moderate- to high-intensity progressive aerobic training.[3] Therefore, to avoid discouraging a compliant woman who is doing an appropriate volume of exercise to achieve health benefits, but perhaps not at an intensity required for improvements in maximal aerobic capacity, it is best to concentrate on the improved tolerance for submaximal workloads that is likely to have accrued instead. In addition to clinical testing for such improved tolerance, it is a good idea to ask a woman to provide her current RPE for a series of tasks performed at home at regular intervals, as shown in Table 14. Providing this as written or visual proof of progress over the course of several months will reinforce the positive change in behavior that has occurred and emphasize the relevance of the exercise prescription to daily life.

BENEFITS

The benefits of aerobic exercise have been studied extensively over the past 40 years, and the most important of these for older adults are listed in Table 15. They include

---

TABLE 14
Measuring the Benefit of Aerobic Training

Activity	RPE Month 1	RPE Month 2	RPE Month 3	RPE Month 4	RPE Month 5	RPE Month 6
Walking up 1 flight of stairs						
Walking up 3 flights of stairs						
Washing windows						
Vacuuming						
Carrying load of laundry up stairs						
Making a bed						
Other activities: (list)						
_____						
_____						

Instructions: Rate your perceived exertion during each activity currently, or note "Unable" if you are physically unable to perform this activity. Use the Borg Scale, from 6 to 20, where 7 is very, very light and 19 is very, very hard.

a broad range of physiologic adaptations that are, in general, opposite to the effects of aging on most body systems, as well as major health-related clinical outcomes. Many of these effects are reviewed in Chapter 1 as well. The health conditions that are responsive to aerobic exercise include most of those of concern to older women: osteoporosis, heart disease, stroke, breast cancer, diabetes, obesity, hypertension, arthritis, depression, and insomnia. These physiologic and clinical benefits form the basis for the inclusion of aerobic exercise as an essential component of the overall physical activity prescription for healthy aging.

RISKS

The major potential risks of aerobic exercise are listed in Table 16. Most of these adverse events are preventable with attention to the underlying medical conditions present, appropriate choices in regard to the modality of exercise used, avoiding exercise during extreme environmental conditions, wearing proper footwear and

TABLE 15
Benefits of Aerobic Exercise

Physiologic Adaptation	Prevention or Treatment of Disease
Increased bone density	Arthritis
Decreased total body and visceral adipose tissue	Breast cancer
Decreased fibrinogen levels	Chronic insomnia
Decreased sympathetic and hormonal response to exercise	Colon cancer
Decreased LDL, increased HDL levels	Coronary artery disease
Decreased postural blood pressure response to stressors	Depression
Increased heart rate variability	Hyperlipidemia
Increased neural reaction time	Hypertension
Increased blood volume and hematocrit	Impotence
Increased energy expenditure	Obesity
Increased glycogen storage in skeletal muscle	Osteoporosis
Increased oxidative enzyme capacity in skeletal muscle	Overall and cardiovascular mortality
Increased glucose disposal rate	Peripheral vascular disease
Increased mitochondrial volume density in skeletal muscle	Prostate cancer
Decreased resting heart rate and blood pressure	Stroke
Increased GLUT-4 receptors in skeletal muscle	Type II diabetes mellitus
Decreased arterial stiffness	
Increased maximal aerobic capacity	
Increased stroke volume during exercise[a]	
Increased capillary density in skeletal muscle	
Increased insulin sensitivity	
Improved glucose tolerance	
Increased cardiac contractility during exercise[a]	
Decreased heart rate/BP response to submaximal exercise	
Increased oxygen extraction by skeletal muscle	

[a] Observed only in older endurance-trained men thus far.

TABLE 16
The Risks of Aerobic Exercise in the Older Woman

Musculoskeletal	Cardiovascular	Metabolic
Falls	Arrhythmia	Dehydration
Foot ulceration or laceration	Cardiac failure	Electrolyte imbalance
Fracture, osteoporotic or traumatic	Hypertension	Energy imbalance
Hemorrhoids[a]	Hypotension	Heat stroke
Hernia[a]	Ischemia	Hyperglycemia
Joint or bursa inflammation, exacerbation of arthritis	Pulmonary embolism	Hypoglycemia
Ligament or tendon strain or rupture	Retinal hemorrhage or detachment, lens detachment	Hypothermia
Muscle soreness or tear	Ruptured cerebral or other aneurysm	Seizures
Stress incontinence	Syncope or postural symptoms	

[a] Primarily associated with increased intra-abdominal pressure during resistive exercise, but may occur if Valsalva maneuver occurs during aerobic activities.

clothing, and minimizing or avoiding exercise during acute illness or in the presence of new, undefined symptoms. All older adults should have yearly ophthalmologic exams for glaucoma and retinal changes, and to avoid complications exercise programming should be delayed until this routine health screen has been completed. If someone has had recent ophthalmologic surgery, exercise is contraindicated for several weeks to avoid raising intraocular pressure, and in these cases the exact recommendations should be gotten from the ophthalmologist. Metabolic complications are rare unless diabetes is out of control at the time exercise is initiated, or dehydration or acute illness are present. Most fluid balance problems can be handled by only exercising in reasonable temperature and humidity and drinking extra fluid on exercise days.

Cardiovascular complications are most likely if ischemic heart disease is not well-controlled medically or surgically prior to exercise initiation, if warning signs are ignored, or if sudden, vigorous exercise is tried in a previously completely sedentary individual. When done properly, both aerobic and resistance training have been shown to reduce the incidence of angina and medication use in cardiac rehabilitation settings, and are indicated as part of standard medical management of coronary artery disease.[46,47] Although claudication is mentioned as a possible adverse side effect of exercise in those with peripheral vascular disease, there is an important treatment caveat here. It has been shown that aerobic exercise significantly increases exercise tolerance in patients with peripheral vascular disease (i.e., time to claudication). However, it works optimally if walking is continued for about 30 to 90 seconds if possible after the onset of claudication, and then a rest period taken. This is different from angina or any of the other symptoms listed in Table 16, for which exercise should be stopped immediately if they occur.

Musculoskeletal problems are more common than any other risk of aerobic exercise, particularly in the novice or very frail woman. If significant weakness or balance impairment is present, it is often best to avoid aerobic exercise altogether until strength and balance have been improved sufficiently with specific training, to allow safe weight-bearing exercise such as walking. If this is not done, falls, arthritis pain, fear of falling, and muscle fatigue will be so limiting that effective aerobic training is precluded. Warming up muscles gently with slow movements prior to aerobic routines is important to avoid soft tissue injury. The most important point is to avoid high-impact activities (such as jumping, step aerobics, jogging) in those with pre-existing arthritis or weak muscles and ligaments, as this is the cause of most sports-related injury.

SPECIAL CONSIDERATIONS IN THE OLDER WOMAN

Women respond as well as men to aerobic training, given the same level of training. Less robust responses in terms of aerobic capacity or weight loss appear to be due to reduced volume and/or intensity of training in many studies involving women. There does appear to be a difference in the way in which men and women adapt to cardiovascular training, however. Endurance-trained older men have been shown to increase exercise-related cardiac contractility and stroke volume during aerobic work, whereas this central adaptation has not yet been observed in older women. Older women adapt to aerobic training with peripheral changes, such as increased oxidative enzyme capacity, mitochondrial volume density, and capillary density in skeletal muscle, and these peripheral changes are responsible for the overall increase in maximal oxygen consumption achieved.

Another consideration in older women that may escape detection is exercise-induced or exacerbated urinary incontinence. This symptom may be so limiting that it precludes exercise participation entirely in some women, and should be considered when compliance is low despite delivery of appropriate training and behavioral methods. Incontinence in this case is usually stress incontinence related to weakened pelvic floor muscles and collagen due to the low estrogenic state of postmenopausal women not on hormone replacement therapy, aging, and birth trauma primarily.

Although a complete discussion of urinary incontinence is beyond the scope of this chapter, a few points are worth emphasizing. Loss of urine when standing, coughing, sneezing, or initiating exercise is often due to stress incontinence secondary to the rise in intra-abdominal pressure caused by these activities. The presence of such symptoms should be part of the pre-exercise assessment of the older woman. If there are any other urinary symptoms, such as dysuria, frequency, urge incontinence, hematuria, etc., then referral for medical evaluation is necessary. If not, then the simple measures outlined in Table 17 can be instituted to minimize the occurrence of incontinent episodes. Pelvic floor muscle exercises are essentially isometric resistance training for the levator ani muscles which prevent the urethra

---

TABLE 17
Steps to Minimize Urinary Incontinence Related to Exercise

Void prior to activity
Drink extra fluid after exercise, rather than before or during sessions
Avoid all caffeine- and alcohol-containing foods and beverages for at least 3 hours before exercise
Minimize breath holding and use of Valsalva maneuver during exercise
Practice pelvic muscle strengthening exercises
Minimize high impact activities
Use intra-vaginal support or external pad during exercise
Review medications and dosing schedule with physician

---

from descending in response to increases in intra-abdominal pressure as noted above. A proven effective regimen is as follows:

- Hold a maximal contraction of levator ani muscles (without Valsalva) for 5 seconds; these muscles can be identified during pelvic exam or as the muscles which are used voluntarily to stop the stream of urine.
- Rest for 10 seconds.
- Repeat above steps for a total of 10 minutes.
- Complete this 10-minute session 4 times per day every day.

Success rates for pelvic muscle exercises vary widely (30 to 60%), most likely because compliance with such a 40-minute regimen every day is quite low, and contractions are submaximal. Biofeedback has been used as a way to show women when they are effectively producing contractile force with these muscles. An approach to compliance that may be behaviorally attractive is to tell women with stress incontinence to perform the pelvic muscle contractions whenever they are sitting at rest or driving, or during rest periods between sets of a weight lifting regimen. In this way, the pelvic training does not actually take any extra time during the day, and will become automatic once the habit is established. If the problem is not resolved with these simple measures, referral to a specialist is indicated for more specific treatment or medication management.

Finally, the generally lower muscle mass and tendency for gait disorders and falls seen in older women compared to men mean that aerobic training is rarely indicated as an isolated exercise prescription in this population. The older and more frail the individual, the more this is true. It is reasonable, therefore, to start with strength and balance training, and add aerobic training only when there has been some improvement in these other areas. It should be remembered that there is no scientific evidence that aerobic training improves strength, muscle mass, or balance, although such statements are often made in general exercise guidelines for the older adult or health care provider. The most important guideline is to assess each woman prior to the exercise prescription in terms of her preferences, health status, risk factors for disease or injury, and current fitness level. This will allow prioritization among the various choices and modalities of exercise available.

INTEGRATION OF CARDIOVASCULAR EXERCISE INTO DAILY ACTIVITIES

Among all the modalities of exercise, cardiovascular exercise is perhaps the easiest to integrate into daily activities. It simple requires a few behavioral decisions be made that can be adhered to with reasonable success. For example, decisions could be made to

> Never use an escalator or elevator when stairs are available.
> Never take the car for errands that can be accomplished via a 10-minute walk or less.
> Do not use remote control devices.
> Substitute manual devices (lawn mowers, electric mixers, brooms) for mechanical devices whenever possible.
> Park in the most remote corner of the parking lot whenever shopping.

If some of these things appear too difficult initially (such as climbing 5 flights of stairs while carrying the groceries), they can be gradually added. For example, a woman might start by taking the elevator 4 flights, and walking the final flight, and advance to walking the entire way. This approach is very effective because it adheres to both the behavioral principle of *shaping*—taking small steps at a time—as well as the physiologic principle of incremental progression of volume and intensity of training. Immediate feedback on fitness is available to the woman as well, as she notes her ability to climb all 5 flights of stairs with minimal effort after a few short weeks. Although it may seem that all of these alterations in routine are time-consuming, the advantage is that no additional time is required for a discreet endurance training session of 20 to 30 minutes during the course of the day. Often, waiting for a busy elevator actually takes longer than climbing the flight of stairs, and the time taken circling the parking lot looking for a close space could have been better and less stressfully spent walking the extra distance.

The key to successful integration is to assess the woman's current routine, access to endurance training opportunities such as stairs and household tasks, and preferences for discreet or integrated activities. Some people do not feel as though they are really exercising unless they don a leotard and tights and go to a gym-like setting, and it may be best to recommend structured exercise sessions for such individuals. For others, being able to complete their training with minimal disruption to an already busy schedule is more appealing and likely to succeed.

Institutionalized elders present a special problem in this regard. In a nursing home patient, it is difficult to find stairs to climb or lawns to mow, so walking groups initiated around regularly scheduled activities when staff are available already (such as going to the dining room for meals or other activities) may have the best chance of success. As residents improve in fitness, instead of walking directly to the dining room, extra laps around the ward can be added to extend the walk to at least 10 minutes for those who are able. Three such walks a day will complete a 30-minute aerobic regimen 7 days a week with minimal time commitment or extra resources needed. The most fit residents should be encouraged to push wheelchair-bound residents on these walks, as this will free staff to help less-able residents ambulate, and will also increase the aerobic intensity of the walk for the fitter residents. Additionally, the psychological benefits of increased self-esteem and morale may be substantial when residents are encouraged to do this, as they are given back an essential caregiving role which may have been lost on entry to the long-term care facility. Some basic suggestions for carrying out walking groups in a nursing home setting are outlined in Table 18.

TABLE 18
Conducting Walking Groups in Frail Elders

Check feet and footwear
Use corrective lenses and hearing aids
Toilet before walk
Use assistive devices for ambulation
Organize walkers by skill level
Time medications to prevent arthritis pain or exercise-induced angina or dyspnea if necessary, avoid side effects such as postural hypotension or incontinence
Increase duration by one-minute intervals as tolerated
Increase intensity by adding inclines, stairs, objects to push or carry rather than speed
Have more able-bodied residents push wheelchair-bound residents on walks
Increase intensity for residents using walkers by adding weights to the bag or basket on the front of the walker

---

FLEXIBILITY TRAINING

DEFINITION

Flexibility training includes movements or positions designed to increase range of motion across joints. Such range of motion is determined by both soft tissue factors (muscle strength, muscle and ligament length, scarring from surgery or trauma, joint and bursa fluid, synovial tissue thickness and inflammation, ligament laxity, tissue elasticity, degenerative changes of cartilage, temperature of tissues) and bony structure (deformities, arthritic and degenerative changes in bone, surgical devices). Obviously, only some of these abnormalities are amenable to exercise intervention, and these will be discussed below. In general, the effect of stretching the soft tissues around a joint slowly and consistently over time is to increase the pain-free range of motion that is possible for that joint.

Although ranging can be done by a therapist or other person (passive stretching), this is not as desirable as actively ranging the joint by the individual. Passive ranging should be used when neurologic disease (stroke, Parkinson's disease, dementia, brain injury, muscular dystrophy, multiple sclerosis, etc.) or arthritic deformity (rheumatoid arthritis) or other conditions make active ranging difficult or impossible to do effectively.

EQUIPMENT

Flexibility may be enhanced without the use of any specialized equipment. There are devices made which allow placement of arms and legs on bars or tubing while stretches are completed. Although these devices may increase the motivation to stretch or remind people to do it and thus serve a motivational purpose, they are not essential for the actual performance of flexibility exercise. It is often helpful, however, to have a thin mat available for those postures that are best done while stretched out on the floor. For adults who are not comfortable getting down on the floor, or who find it too difficult to get up, it is perfectly satisfactory to use a chair, sofa, or bed for leg and back stretches. Other props which may be helpful include a ballet bar or handrail along a wall, or parallel bars in a physical therapy department. A towel or cane can be held overhead to assist with shoulder and upper back stretches, and a towel around the dorsum of the foot will also assist with plantar flexor (calf) stretches.

GENERAL TECHNIQUE

The most effective technique for increasing flexibility is to extend a body part as fully as possible without pain, and hold this fully extended position for 20 to 30 seconds. The key requirement is to complete the movement slowly (without any bouncing or ballistic movements). Contrary to popular opinion, such bouncing does not increase efficacy and range of motion, but instead may cause muscle contraction that limits the range achievable. A technique known as proprioceptive neural facilitation (PNF) will maximize stretching effectiveness.

Once the body part has been stretched as far as possible, the muscle groups around the joint should then be completely relaxed, while still maintaining the stretch. Next, an attempt is made to stretch a little further, which is usually possible. This final position is then held for about 20 to 30 seconds before returning to the initial position. PNF serves to counteract the involuntary resistance to overextension of a joint caused by a feedback loop of receptors within the muscle tissue that are activated by mechanical stretch.

Flexibility exercise is part of many other forms of exercise such as ballet and modern dance, yoga, T'ai Chi, and resistance training, because in all of these pursuits the muscle groups are slowly extended to their full range and held before relaxing, just as in PNF technique. In comparison to regular stretching exercises, it has been shown that resistance training can also result in significant and similar improvements in range of motion.[11] It is likely that the mechanism of benefit is slightly different, but the magnitude of effect was similar in this randomized trial comparing the two methodologies in an older group undergoing cardiac rehabilitation. Earlier anecdotal reports that resistance training impairs flexibility appear to be unfounded. Using a high-intensity form of PRT appears to be more effective than lifting very light loads in terms of resultant increases in shoulder range of motion and function in older adults.[48] Aerobic training has no specific effect on tissue elasticity or flexibility by itself, but stretching is often combined with aerobic exercise as an appropriate cool-down modality.

Thus there are a variety of ways to improve flexibility by itself or in conjunction with other components of the exercise prescription. The exact way in which it is recommended will depend to some extent on the other medical concerns relevant to the individual, the most pressing physiologic deficits requiring intervention, the likelihood of compliance with a multimodal exercise prescription, and the amount of time individuals are willing to commit to this outcome. There is great benefit in an approach to prescribing exercise in the elderly that is similar to pharmacological management. In other words, consolidating treatment goals into the fewest possible agents (or exercise modalities) is the most efficient, safe, and feasible approach. It is unlikely that one would encounter older women who do not need improvement in strength, balance, and endurance capacity, and are only in need of improved flexibility. However, in clinical and recreational settings where exercise is conducted with the elderly, particularly frail elderly, flexibility is often the only form of exercise practiced. This appears to stem from an unfounded belief that other forms of exercise are too vigorous, unsafe, or unnecessary in the old. A review of the scientific data would, in fact, lead to quite different findings.

There is a good deal of evidence that resistance training, aerobic training, and balance training are both necessary and feasible in the aged; and

Stretching and light calisthenics usually have no significant impact on psychological, physical, or functional outcomes in the elderly (which is why they often appear as the attention control or placebo arm of an experimental trial).

Thus it is hard to rationalize the isolated use of stretching as an exercise modality in the older adult, except in the case of the demented or bed-bound patient in whom passive stretching is the only appropriate approach. What is even more unfortunate is that the stretching technique utilized in senior exercise classes is often so poor (holding stretches for less than five seconds, not stretching through the full range of motion, no use of PNF technique, relying on ballistic movements, etc.) that improvements in flexibility do not even occur. There is a need for better data on the clinical benefits resulting from true flexibility exercise and the relationship between functional impairment and deficits in range of motion at various joints. In this way the exercise prescription can be based on scientific rationale, as it is with the other exercise modalities.

INTENSITY

Intensity in the domain of flexibility training refers to the degree or distance to which the body part or joint is stretched. Here the appropriate range is just to the point before any pain occurs. It is not recommended to force a stretch beyond the point of pain, as this may result in injury to soft tissue structures and ultimately worsen function. As with all forms of exercise, as the range of motion increases over time, it is appropriate and necessary to continuously increase the distance the joint is moved so that progress is maintained.

VOLUME AND FREQUENCY

The exact volume of stretching needed for optimal efficacy has not been systematically studied. Recommended regimens have ranged from daily to once a week. Since stretching is most effective when the tissues are first warmed in temperature by other forms of exercise, it is often suggested that stretching follow other exercise routines, 3 or more days per week. Vigorously stretching a cold muscle may cause muscle or tendon tears or ruptures and should be avoided. Unfortunately, common practice is often to recommend stretching prior to weight lifting or aerobic exercise. This is both ineffective and potentially harmful. Instead, the following sequence is suggested:

- Warm-up the musculoskeletal and cardiovascular system for strength and aerobic training with gentle movements of the trunk and extremities through their range of motion for several minutes. This is not meant to increase tissue elasticity, but rather to gradually increase heart rate and blood pressure and increase the temperature of the muscles.
- Next, proceed with the prescribed strength or aerobic training.
- Finally, cool-down by carrying out the PNF stretching technique outlined above for all major muscle groups. This is meant to gradually lower pulse and blood pressure, and induce physiologic adaptations in muscle and connective tissue that will gradually and safely increase flexibility.

Three days-per-week regimens do result in significant improvements in range of motion due to either stretching or resistance training exercises, so this appears to be a reasonable frequency to recommend. No harm is done by more frequent stretching, however, and it is likely that a dose-response effect exists here. If range of motion is particularly impaired, or is likely to deteriorate due to disease such as stroke, arthritis, or Parkinson's disease, for example, then higher frequencies of training may be beneficial. Again, no good data exist on the minimum effective frequency for flexibility training.

Each major muscle group should be stretched using a single stretch to the maximally extended position and held for 30 seconds. It has been demonstrated that holding a stretch for 10 seconds or less does not significantly increase range of motion,[49] so multiple, short, ballistic (bouncing) stretches, which are what is usually done, are to be discouraged because they are generally ineffective. Thus minimal time requirements of 5 to 6 minutes per session (30 seconds per muscle group for 10 to 12 muscle groups) will provide substantial flexibility benefit.

SPECIAL CONSIDERATIONS IN THE OLDER WOMAN

Maintenance of flexibility at the ankle joint is thought to be very important for balance and falls prevention, and therefore of special interest to older women.[50] The ankle should be moved in all positions (flexion, extension, eversion, inversion, rotation) as the response to perturbations of balance requires maximal mobility in all directions.

In general, joints affected by arthritis, including the cervical and lumbar spine, hips, knees, ankles, wrists, and fingers, will benefit from preservation of maximal soft tissue elasticity, tendon length, and muscle strength, all of which will serve to optimize joint range of motion, function, and minimize pain and stiffness. Even joints that appear to be predominately limited by bony structural changes and hypertrophic osteoarthropy rather than soft tissue problems will benefit from flexibility training.

If nocturnal leg muscle cramps are a problem, advise stretching the plantar flexors just before bedtime, which may relieve this symptom complex far more effectively than medications such as quinine. This may be done standing leaning into a wall with the front leg flexed at the knee and hip and the back leg straight, with both feet flat on the floor. This exercise targets both the gastrocnemius and the soleus muscles, and is the most effective way to stretch the calf muscles. If this standing stretch is not possible, a towel can be secured around the dorsum of the foot while the woman is lying supine in bed and the foot pulled toward the head for the stretch.

BENEFITS

The physiologic benefit of flexibility exercise is increased range of motion across joints. There is some evidence that range of motion is related to functional independence in activities of daily living, posture, balance, and gait characteristics in the older adults as well as pain and disability and quality of life in arthritis. Flexibility training itself does not result in improved strength or endurance, or marked improvements in balance. Therefore, it is best conceived as an accessory to other forms of exercise that contribute to overall exercise and functional capacity. To the extent that pain, fear of falling, mobility, and function are improved, quality of life may improve as well. There is a need for much better quantitative research on effective doses and long-term benefits of this mode of exercise in the elderly.

RISKS

When performed properly, there is almost no risk to flexibility training. However, it can possibly cause soft tissue injuries such as rotator cuff tears, tendon rupture, muscle tears, ligament strains, cartilage tears, herniated discs, or exacerbation of joint inflammation is susceptible individuals. This is most likely in the case of pre-existing degenerative, inflammatory, or surgical abnormalities of the joint or surrounding soft tissues. The lower back, shoulders, neck, and knee joints are the likely sites of injury. Most such injuries can be successfully avoided by adherence to the following principles:

- Always do stretching after muscles have been warmed up in temperature by gentle movements or other forms of exercise, end each weight lifting and aerobic training session with a stretch for each of the involved muscle groups as noted above;
- Limit stretching to the pain-free range of motion;
- Avoid vigorous stretching during recovery from acute injuries such as muscle and ligament tears, fractures, and dislocations. Stretching will be part of the rehabilitation process, but it must be supervised by an experienced therapist and gradually introduced in these situations.

There is no evidence that flexibility training is associated with any adverse cardiovascular or metabolic events. It is important to remind people not to hold their breath, contract muscles isometrically, or perform a Valsalva maneuver during a static stretch of 20 to 30 seconds, however, as such deviations from recommended technique could result in increases in blood pressure and undesirable alterations in cardiac hemodynamics.

MONITORING PROGRESS

Progress in flexibility training can be easily tracked by measuring joint range of motion with a goniometer or timing observed functional tasks such as fastening a brassiere or buttons in the back of a garment, bending over to pick up an object, placing something on a high shelf, etc. It is important to choose a functional outcome that is both impaired at baseline and has some intrinsic value for the individual. Such functional outcomes are not solely related to flexibility, as they may also depend on fine motor coordination, strength, and balance to some extent, but they may be more relevant and motivating to the individual than changes in degrees measured on a goniometer. Repeating measurements at frequent intervals will stimulate compliance or perhaps uncover aberrations in technique that are limiting progress in this domain.

INTEGRATION OF FLEXIBILITY TRAINING INTO DAILY ACTIVITIES

Since stretching can be done anywhere without equipment in a very limited amount of time, it is ideal for incorporation into other activities or resting periods during the day. Examples include time spent watching television or movies, reading, knitting, before rising from bed, while sitting in a car, bus, or plane, etc. Opportunities to stretch may also be added to everyday activities if one thinks about it. For example, place objects on shelves that are just slightly out of reach so that a stretch of the arms and ankles is required to get them down. Move the clothesline up a notch so that you have to stretch to reach the clothespins or take down clothes. Stretch while you are in the bath or shower where the heat will increase tissue mobility and minimize arthritis pain, allowing more effective stretching. For similar reasons, a heated pool or whirlpool (as opposed to a cold ocean) can provide a good opportunity to stretch joints without pain. providing the PNF principles are followed.

BALANCE TRAINING

DEFINITION

Balance training is probably the least defined of the various exercise modalities. Despite the use for decades of balance-enhancing modalities by physical therapists and others working with adults and children with developmental or degenerative neurological diseases affecting balance, only recently have there been well-controlled formalized studies of techniques and outcomes. The recognition that balance impairment is a risk factor for falls and hip fracture even in adults without identifiable neurologic disease has expanded the potential target population for balance training to the general aging cohort. The pressing need for definitive outcome data on feasibility and efficacy of various intervention techniques has stimulated quantitative research that will assist in the development of clinical protocols. In the meantime, the balance prescription must be formulated from a variety of evidence collected in epidemiological studies, experimental trials, and clinical practice. It should be noted that in many cases, it is difficult to compare the results across trials, as investigators have used unique training interventions and different outcome measures.

Any activity that increases one's ability to maintain balance in the face of stressors may be considered a balance-enhancing activity. Stressors include decreased base of support, perturbation of the ground support, decrease in proprioception, vision, or vestibular system input, increased compliance of the support surface, or movement of the center of mass of the body. In real life, stressors may also include things such as environmental hazards to traverse, postural hypotension, and drugs that affect central nervous system function. The plethora of conditions that contribute to gait and balance abnormalities in older women requires a multi-factorial approach to falls prevention, as outlined in Chapter 13 in more detail. What is presented below is a summary of exercise techniques that have favorable effects on this syndrome, and therefore form an important part of the exercise prescription for older women.

Balance-enhancing activities impact the central nervous system control of balance and coordination of movement, or augment the peripheral neuromuscular system response to signals that balance is threatened. Resistance training likely improves balance by specifically enhancing the strength of postural control muscles of the trunk and lower extremities, particularly ankles, hips, and knees, so the person is able to mount a more robust response to a given stressor. It is not known whether or not resistance training also changes the neural recruitment of these muscles in response to perturbations in balance so they are activated more quickly or in better sequence, but this may be an additional mode of action. Even when only seated resistance training is performed, improvements in static and dynamic balance can be demonstrated in the elderly.[10,51,52] Inclusion of standing postures, particularly if hand support is gradually withdrawn as shown in Figures 53 to 57, has an even more potent effect on balance.[53]

GENERAL TECHNIQUE

The general approach to the enhancement of balance should rely on theoretical principles which are designed to elicit adaptations in the central neurological control of posture and equilibrium. The basic idea is to progressively challenge the system with stressors of increasing difficulty in three different domains.

1. Narrowing the base of support for the center of mass of the body;
2. Displacing the center of mass to the limits of tolerance;
3. Removing or minimizing contributions of visual, vestibular, and proprioceptive pathways to balance.

Each of these will be considered in turn.

Narrowing the Base of Support

This is one of the most commonly used techniques and is quite effective. The person is instructed to stand in postures of increasing difficulty, as follows:

- Feet apart with assistive device
- Feet apart without assistive device
- Feet together (touching along entire length)
- Semitandem stand (feet touching but the toe of one foot is at the instep of the other foot)
- Tandem stand (toe of one foot is touching the heel of the foot in front)
- One-legged stand (one foot only is on the ground)
- Toe stand (standing on tip-toe with both or only one foot)
- Heel stand (standing on both heels)

These postures have been presented in order of increasing difficulty, with the possible exception of the final two postures (toe stand and heel stand) which may present variable challenges to an individual depending not only on balance capacity, but also on muscle strength, presence of arthritis, peripheral edema, range of motion in the ankle, and other podiatric problems. In order to prescribe such exercise, each of the above postures should be tried under direct supervision, to see where clients begin to have difficulties maintaining balance in this hierarchy. A useful technique is to ask them to hold the desired posture for 15 seconds. If they can do this successfully (without moving feet, grabbing for support, falling, etc.), then the next more difficult posture is tried. Obviously, it is essential that the examiner be close to the person at all times to prevent a fall. Wherever difficulty is first noted (defined as inability to hold the stance for the full 15 seconds), this is the level that is prescribed as the initial training posture. Training involves practicing this posture (see below for volume) until it is mastered, and then progressing to the next higher level of difficulty. We have seen, for example, that community-dwelling men and women of average age 85 begin to have difficulty at the level of the tandem stand. By contrast, frailer individuals in a nursing home may find the feet together position initially difficult or impossible.

In addition to the static postures noted above, the principle of narrowing the base of support can be applied to dynamic movements as well, such as during tandem (heel-to-toe) walking. This can be taken to a higher level of difficulty by tandem walking backwards or with the eyes closed, or on a flat board 3 to 4 inches wide which can serve as a balance beam.

As long as the basic principle is followed, it does not matter whether the stances are done by themselves as a discreet training session, are incorporated into strength training sessions, are practiced while carrying out daily activities such as standing in line, cooking, doing housework, talking on the phone, etc., or form part of a more extensive routine of yoga, T'ai Chi, or dance. The essential feature is progress driven by challenging persons with tasks that are slightly beyond their reach to induce favorable adaptations.

Displacing the Center of Mass

The goal of this mode of training is to move the body weight through space toward the limits of sway, just short of where balance is lost. All movement involves some displacement of the center of mass, even simple walking, but as a person's resources improve, more difficult and challenging displacement tasks can be mastered. In its simplest form, a person can be asked to stand still with his or her feet slightly apart, and keeping the body rigid, lean forward, backward, and to each side as far as possible without moving his or her feet to maintain balance. Other ways of displacing the center of mass include

- Turning in a circle
- Shifting weight from side to side
- Stepping over obstacles such as a step or book
- Turning or leaning while holding a heavy object such as a book or dumbbell in front of the chest
- Cross-over walking, sideways walking, heel walking
- Moving weighted arms or legs to the front or side (as in standing resistive exercises with free weights)
- Balancing on a large ball or rocker platform (available in many physical therapy settings)

Practicing T'ai Chi and yoga involves many postures which perturb the center of mass as well as diminish the base of support in simple or more complex movements, and thus these exercises fall into the above theoretical constructs as well. If complicated forms of these exercises cannot be mastered, there are simpler versions which have been distilled and tested and found to be feasible and effective in older adults, resulting in reduced fall rates, as well as decreased fear of falling.[54] By contrast, training using sophisticated balance platfoms has not yet been shown to improve these clinical outcomes, although improvements in balance capacity tested on the same machine may be seen.[55] Exercise classes including T'ai Chi are now available in many senior centers and local gyms and are thus economical and highly accessible to many older adults. Compared to the high cost and lack of access to computerized balance-training systems, as well as perhaps greater efficacy in falls prevention, T'ai Chi or other kinds of functional balance-stressing movements are, therefore, recommended in preference to balance-platform training at this point to meet the balance needs of most older adults. However, it is recognized that there are many groups of clinical patients, such as those with Parkinson's disease, stroke, brain injury, or other neurologic conditions who may benefit from balance platform training in an acute rehabilitation setting. There is a need for research into appropriate transition protocols for such clinical populations, which may involve use of the low-tech methods outlined above for more chronic rehabilitation or home settings.

Minimizing Contributions of Visual and Proprioceptive Pathways

The ability to tolerate a narrowed base of support or shift in the center of mass will be markedly impaired if sensory inputs to balance control are reduced. This is most simply accomplished by closing the eyes during any of the movements mentioned in the preceding two sections. This should be done only after the posture in question has already been completely mastered with eyes open. It is also best to try this under direct supervision of a trainer or another exerciser, particularly in high risk adults. In lieu of this, positioning between a wall and a chair, for example, is recommended.

Decreased proprioceptive input can be accomplished by practicing standing postures on a highly compliant surface such as a pillow, piece of foam, mattress, or quilt. Using a mattress has the added advantage of providing a safety net should balance be lost during the attempt. This should allow safer progression to higher levels of difficulty without fear of injury. It is a good idea to teach adults strategies on how to get up from a fall prior to undertaking any balance training so the fear of this outcome is reduced. Again, no progression to reduced proprioceptive input should be made until the standard movements can be completed competently (without loss of balance). Obviously, the combination of decreased vision and proprioception will be even more difficult than either adaptation alone. Proprioceptive input can be lessened in stages by inserting foam or mattresses of increasing thickness under the feet during training. A simple log sheet can be made to track the postures and these additional modifications on a weekly basis to monitor progress.

All balance movements should be done slowly and with deliberation, as this stresses the control systems more and produces better physiologic adaptation. As with resistance training, increased speed serves to substitute momentum for the appropriate physiologic domain (strength, balance), and therefore undercuts desired stress on the system. One of the outcomes of the T'ai Chi intervention reported above was that the older participants walked and moved more slowly after training, and their deliberation in movement was felt to be related to their reduced fear of falling and subsequent fall rates.[54]

INTENSITY

Intensity in balance training refers to the degree of difficulty of the postures, movements, or routines practiced. The appropriate level of difficulty or intensity for any balance-enhancing exercise is the highest level which can be tolerated without inducing a fall or near-fall. In a supervised session, the individual can be pushed to the limits of such tolerance, as safety is assured by the physical presence of the trainer. In an unsupervised setting, the person should be told to try movements only up to the level that they fail to master. For example, if the goal is to hold the tandem stand for 15 seconds, then if someone can only hold the posture for 10 seconds before grabbing the wall for support, this is the appropriate initial training intensity. Progression in intensity is the key to improvement, as in other exercise domains, but this concept of mastery of the previous level before progression must be adhered to for safety. This is particularly important in older women, who are at highest risk for falls and osteoporotic fractures.

Volume and Frequency

No definite statement can be made at this time about the minimum effective dose of balance-training techniques described above. Regimens have ranged from 1 to 7 days per week, and from once a day to several times per day. A reasonable recommendation would appear to be 2 to 3 days per week, but it is noted that this is more a matter of convention rather than an evidence-based recommendation. It is likely that as with other forms of training, a dose-response relationship exists, although thresholds have not been defined. There is no evidence that any negative effects are seen with high-volume training. Therefore, for women with significant balance impairments that require intervention, training 3 to 7 days per week may be advantageous. On the other hand, healthy, normal women may require only preventive practice 1 day a week for maintenance of function. Many more studies are needed in this area to define the recommendation further.

Choose several different exercises within the basic types of exercises (narrowed base of support, displacement of center of mass) and repeat each exercise 2 to 3 times at the most difficult level which does not result in a loss of balance. It is unlikely that increasing the number of repetitions of a task which can be easily accomplished (for example, the semitandem stand) will lead to improvements in balance, whereas just a few repetitions of a difficult task (such as standing on one leg for 15 seconds) will lead to favorable adaptations. As with PRT, the emphasis should be on progression to higher degrees of difficulty rather than high volumes of training. T'ai Chi and similar forms of exercise have been successfully prescribed for 45 minutes to one hour, 2 to 3 days per week, but, again, minimum effective doses are unknown.

SUPERVISION AND SETTING

Balance training can generally be accomplished without the need for specialized equipment, which means that it can be done anywhere. The only supervision requirement relates to safety considerations and the individual's level of risk for a fall during training. In the case of T'ai Chi or yoga, an instructor may be needed for a length of time to teach the discipline and assure correct form. Practicing balance on a carpeted or other soft surface (such as a lawn) is desirable if available. If balance is impaired to begin with, supervision is highly recommended until capacity improves. Progression to each higher level of intensity should be attempted only after verification by a trainer or other individual that mastery has been achieved.

A group setting is convenient, as exercisers can learn from each other's form and provide supervision and encouragement, and thereby challenge each other to progress with more confidence. Many trainers have used such group settings not only to teach balance exercises, but to deliver psychological interventions designed to reduce fear of falling and increase self-efficacy, talk about the safety enhancements of the home environment, practice techniques for getting up from a fall, discuss ways to get help in an emergency, and uncover other fall and fracture risks (postural hypotension, impaired vision, nutritional habits, etc.) which may benefit from treatment. Thus, the multifactorial nature of falls makes the use of a group setting for balance exercise delivery perhaps more important than it is in other modalities of exercise.

BENEFITS

Balance training has been shown to result in improved balance performance, decreased fear of falling, decreased incidence of falls, and increased ability to participate in other activities that may have been limited by gait and balance difficulties. It is expected, although not proven, that such changes would ultimately lead to improvements in functional independence, reduced hip fractures and other serious injuries, and improved overall quality of life. Such long-term outcomes will require larger studies of longer duration than those that have been reported to date. In particular, there is a need for data on the feasibility and efficacy of balance training in the very old and frail, in whom deficits are larger, fall risk is usually multifactorial, and cognitive impairments or degenerative neurological diseases exist. All of these factors may alter the robustness of the physiologic adaptation achieved with training. Although T'ai Chi and yoga have been said to be associated with many other kinds of physiologic and clinical benefits apart from their contribution to balance, a review of all of these potential benefits is beyond the scope of this chapter.

Balance training does not generally result in increased strength or aerobic capacity by itself; however, there may be some maintenance of muscle strength from the isometric contractions that occur during many of the balance-enhancing and one-legged postures and the bent-knee stance during T'ai Chi. In addition, to the extent that balance training results in increased overall physical activity and mobility, these other activities may lead to improvements in strength and endurance.

RISKS

The only real risk of balance training is loss of balance, resulting in a fall or injury or increased fear of falling. This is preventable with attention to the factors governing progression, intensity, setting, and supervision discussed above. There is little or no elevation in pulse or blood pressure during these kinds of exercises, so cardiovascular events are not an expected or reported consequence. Musculoskeletal injury, other than that resulting from a fall, would also be unlikely.

It should be noted that there may be exacerbation of pre-existing arthritic pain or inflammation of the knee during prolonged one-legged standing or T'ai Chi postures requiring a semi-crouched stance. These positions may have to be adapted or avoided in women with significant weight-bearing pain in the joint. However, once quadriceps muscle strength improves with appropriate resistive exercises (see above), these kinds of movements may be tolerable. Impaired flexibility may also limit some T'ai Chi or yoga postures initially, and may lead to injury if range of motion is forced in the beginning. Gradual progression over time in the complexity of postures should prevent most injuries to soft tissues.

INTEGRATING THE BALANCE PRESCRIPTION INTO DAILY LIFE

Many activities in daily life can be turned into a balance-enhancing movement or position with a little creativity, making balance training one of the easiest modalities of exercise to integrate. Some examples of how this can be accomplished are listed below.

- Every time you are standing in line, cooking, combing your hair, doing dishes, etc., move your feet closer together, or stand on one leg if possible during the task; alternate legs every 15 to 30 seconds.
- When crossing a room or other short distance, tandem, heel, toe, cross-over, or sideways walk for 10 to 20 feet instead of normal walking.
- Carry small items (books, cartons of milk) by holding them out at arm's length while you walk (without bending the spine).
- Close your eyes or stand on one leg while riding a moving bus or train (lightly hold onto a bar for support).

As with balance training sessions, none of these integrated exercises should be tried if they are beyond the current capacity of the individual.

With time, these habits will become reinforced, and more and more opportunities to improve balance will appear throughout the normal daily routines of older women. Challenge groups who are training together to think of creative ways to modify tasks and activities that are relevant to them. Such group participation in exercise recommendations will serve as a motivational tool to increase overall training volume and optimally enhance the functional benefits of this modality of exercise.

SUMMARY

Physiologic aging, retirement, societal expectations, accumulated diseases, and medication and nutritional effects conspire to produce deficits in strength, balance, aerobic capacity, and flexibility in older women. Fortunately, there is increasing evidence of the reversibility of many of these deficits with a targeted exercise prescription. There is still work to be done in refining the prescription, particularly in terms of the doses of flexibility and balance training needed for optimal efficacy. In addition, there is a need for well-controlled, long-term studies on clinically important outcomes such as treatment of cardiovascular disease and stroke, prevention and treatment of hip fracture, prevention of diabetic complications, reduction in nursing home admission rates, and moderation of disability from arthritis. An active lifestyle may be the most desirable public health approach to the maintenance of function and the prevention of disease in healthy persons. However, it is likely that the use of exercise for treatment of pre-existing diseases and geriatric syndromes will always need to incorporate elements of a traditional exercise prescription as outlined in this chapter, as well as behavioral approaches to more fully integrate appropriate physical activity habits into daily life.

REFERENCES

1. Blair, S. N., Kohl, H., Barlow, C., Paffenbarger, R. S., Gibbons, L., and Macera, C., Changes in physical fitness and all-cause mortality: A prospective study of healthy and unhealthy men, *JAMA*, 273, 1093–1098, 1995.
2. Pate, R. R., Pratt, M., Blair, S. N., Haskell, W. L. et al., Physical Activity and Public Health: A Recommendation From the Centers for Disease Control and Prevention and the American College of Sports Medicine, *JAMA*, 273, 402–407, 1995.
3. Dunn, A., Marcus, B., Kampert, J., Garcia, M., Kohl, H., and Blair, S., Comparison of lifestyle and structured interventions to increase physical activity and cardiorespiratory fitness: A randomized trial, *JAMA*, 281, 327–340, 1999.
4. Ettinger, W., Burns, R., Messler, S., Applegate, W., Rajeski, J., Morgan, T., Shumaker, S., Berry, M., O'Toole, M., Monu, J. et al. A randomized trial comparing aerobic exercise and resistance exercise with a health education program in older adults with knee osteoarthritis: The Fitness Arthritis and Seniors Trial (FAST), *JAMA*, 277, 25–31, 1997.
5. Pollock, M., Gaesser, G., Butcher, J., Despres, J.-P., Dishman, R., Franklin, B., and Garber, C., The recommended quantity and quality of exercise for developing and maintaining cardiorespiratory and muscular fitness, and flexibility in healthy adults, *Med. Sci. Sports Exerc.*, 30, 975–991, 1998.
6. Mazzeo, R., Cavanaugh, P., Evans, W., Fiatarone, M., Hagberg, J., McAuley, E., and Startzell, J., Exercise and physical activity for older adults, *Med. Sci. Sports Exerc.*, 30, 992–1008, 1998.
7. Delorme, T. L., Restoration of muscle power by heavy resistance exercises, *J. Bone Joint Surg.*, 27, 645–667, 1945.
8. Borg, G. and Linderholme, H., Exercise performance and perceived exertion in patients with coronary insufficiency, arterial hypertension and vasoregulatory asthenia, *Acta Med. Scand.*, 187, 17–26, 1970.
9. Verrill, D. E., Resistive exercise training in cardiac patients, *Sports Med.*, 13, 172–193, 1992.
10. Fiatarone, M. A., O'Neill, E. F., Ryan, N. D., Clements, K. M., Solares, G. R., Nelson, M. E., Roberts, S. R., Kehayias, J. K., Lipsitz, L. A., and Evans, W. J., Exercise training and nutritional supplementation for physical frailty in very elderly people, *N. Engl. J. Med.*, 330, 1769–1775, 1994.
11. Beniamini, Y., Rubenstein, J., Faigenbaum, A., Lichtenstein, A., and Crim, M., High-intensity strength training of patients enrolled in an outpatient cardiac rehabilitation program, *J. Cardiopulmonary Rehabil.*, 19, 8–17, 1999.
12. Evans, W. J., Reversing sarcopenia: how weight training can build strength and vitality, *Geriatrics*, 51, 46–7, 51–3, 1996.
13. Nelson, B., Carpenter, D., Dreisinger, T., Mitchell, M., Kelly, C., and Wegner, J., Can spinal surgery be prevented by aggressive strengthening exercises? A prospective study of cervical and lumbar patients, *Arch. Phys. Med. Rehabil.*, 80, 20–25, 1999.
14. Evans, W. J., Muscle damage: nutritional considerations, *Int. J. Sports Nutr.*, 1, 214–224, 1991.
15. King, A., Haskell, W., Taylor, C., Kraemer, H., and DeBusk, R., Group- vs. home-based exercise training in healthy older men and women: A community-based clinical trial, *JAMA*, 266, 1535–1542, 1991.

16. Morris, J., Fiatarone, M., Kiely, D., Belleville-Taylor, P., Murphy, K., Littlehale, S., Ooi, W., O'Neill, E., and Doyle, N., Nursing rehabilitation and exercise strategies in the nursing home, *J. Gerontol.*, 54A (10), M494–500, 1999.

17. Fiatarone Singh, M., Ding, W., Manfredi, T., Solares, G., O'Neill, E., Clements, K., Ryan, N., Kehayias, J., Fielding, R. et al., Insulin-like growth factor I in skeletal muscle after weight-lifting exercise in frail elders, *Am. J. Physiol.*, 277, E136–143, 1999.

18. Wolfe, J., Growth hormone: A physiological fountain of youth? *J. Anti-Aging Med.*, 1, 9–25, 1998.

19. Cannon, J. G., Meydani, S. N., Fielding, R. A., Fiatarone, M. A., Meydani, M., Farhangmehr, M., Orencole, S. F., Blumberg, J. B., and Evans, W. J., Acute phase response in exercise. II. Associations between vitamin E, cytokines, and muscle proteolysis, *Am. J. Physiol.*, 260, R1235–R1240, 1991.

20. Fielding, R. A., Manfredi, T. J., Ding, W., Fiatarone, M. A., Evans, W. J., and Cannon, J. G., Acute phase Response in exercise. III. Intramuscular mediators of inflammatory injury, *Am. J. Physiol.*, 265, R166–R172, 1993.

21. Oddis, C. V., New perspectives on osteoarthritis, *Am. J. Med.*, 100, 10S–15S, 1996.

22. Benn, S., McCartney, N., and McKelvie, R., Circulatory responses to weight lifting, walking and stair climbing in older males, *J. Am. Geriatr. Soc.*, 44, 121–125, 1996.

23. McCartney, N., Acute responses to resistance training and safety, *Med. Sci. Sports Exerc.*, 31, 31–37, 1999.

24. Gordon, N., Kohl, H., Pollock, M., Vaandrager, H., Gibbons, S., and Blair, S., Cardiovascular safety of maximal strength testing in healthy adults, *Am. J. Cardiol.*, 76, 851–853, 1995.

25. Beverly, M. C., Rider, T. A., Evans, M. J., and Smith, R., Local bone mineral response to brief exercise that stresses the skeleton, *Br. Med. J.*, 299, 233–5, 1989.

26. Barengolts, E. I., Curry, D. J., Bapna, M. S., and Kukreja, S. C., Effects of two non-endurance exercise protocols on established bone loss in ovariectomized adult rats, *Calcified Tissue Int.*, 52, 239–43, 1993.

27. Aloia, J., Cohn, S., Ostuni, J., Cane, R., and Ellis, K., Prevention of involutional bone loss by exercise, *Ann. Intern. Med.*, 89, 356–358, 1978.

28. Ayalon, J., Simkin, A., Leichter, I., and Raifman, S., Dynamic bone loading exercises for postmenopausal women: effect on the density of the distal radius, *Arch. Phys. Med. Rehabil.*, 68, 280–282, 1987.

29. Dalsky, G., Stocke, K., Ehsani, A., Slatopolsky, E., Lee, W., and Birge, S., Weight-bearing exercise training and lumbar bone mineral content in postmenopausal women, *Ann. Intern. Med.*, 108, 824–828, 1988.

30. Kohrt, W. M., Snead, D. B., Slatopolsky, E., and Birge, S. J., Jr., Additive effects of weight-bearing exercise and estrogen on bone mineral density in older women, *J. Bone Mineral Res.*, 10, 1303–11, 1995.

31. Krall, E. A. and Dawson-Hughes, B., Walking is related to bone density and rates of bone loss, *Am. J. Med.*, 96, 20–26, 1994.

32. Nelson, M., Fisher, E., Dilmanian, F., Dallal, G., and Evans, W., A 1-y walking program and increased dietary calcium in postmenopausal women: effects on bone, *Am. J. Clin. Nutr.*, 53, 1394–11, 1991.

33. Pollock, M., Miller, H., Janeway, R., Linnerud, A., Robertson, B., and Valentino, R., Effects of walking on body composition and cardiovascular function of middle-aged men, *J. Appl. Physiol.*, 30, 126–30, 1971.

34. Arkins, J., Rugh, B., and Timewell, R., Cardiovascular effects of topical beta-blockers during exercise, *Am. J. Ophthalmol.*, 99, 173–75, 1985.

35. Helmrich, S. P., Ragland, D. R., Leung, R. W., and Paffenbarger, R. S., Physical activity and reduced occurrence of non-insulin-dependent diabetes mellitus, *N. Engl. J. Med.*, 325, 147–52, 1991.

36. MacRae, P., Asplund, L., Schnelle, J., Ouslander, J., Abrahamse, A., and Morris, C., A walking program for nursing home residents: Effects on walk endurance, physical activity, mobility, and quality of life, *J. Am. Geriatr. Soc.*, 44, 175–180, 1996.

37. Poulin, M. J., Paterson, D. H., Govindasamy, D., and Cunningham D. A., Endurance training of older men: responses to submaximal exercise, *J. Appl. Physiol.*, 73, 452–7, 1992.

38. Pollock, M. L., Foster, C., Knapp, D., Rod, J. L., and Schmidt, D. H., Effect of age and training on aerobic capacity and body composition of master athletes, *J. Appl. Physiol.*, 62, 725-31, 1987.

39. Hagberg, J. M., Graves, J. E., and Limacher, M., Cardiovascular responses of 70–79 year old men and women to exercise training, *J. Appl. Physiol.*, 66, 2589–2594, 1989.

40. Green, J. S. and Crouse, S. F., Endurance training, cardiovascular function and the aged, *Sports Med.*, 16, 331–341, 1993.

41. Holloszy, J. O., Schultz, J., Kusnierkiewicz, J., Hagberg, J. M., and Ehsani, A. A., Effects of exercise on glucose tolerance and insulin resistance, *Acta Med. Scand.* (Suppl.), 711, 55–65, 1986.

42. Hersey, W. Cr., Graves, J. E., Pollock, M. L., Gingerich, R., Shireman, R. B., Heath, G. W., Spierto, F., McCole, S. D., and Hagberg, J. M., Endurance exercise training improves body composition and plasma insulin responses in 70- to 79-year-old men and women, *Metabol.: Clin. Exper.*, 43, 847–54, 1994.

43. Paffenbarger, R. S., Jr., Hyde, R. T., Wing, A. L., Lee, I. M., Jung, D. L., and Kampert, J. B., The association of changes in physical-activity level and other lifestyle characteristics with mortality among men [see comments], *N. Engl. J. Med.*, 328, 538–45, 1993.

44. Lee, I., Hsieh, C., and Paffenbarger, R., Exercise intensity and longevity in men: the Harvard alumni health study, *JAMA*, 273, 1179–1184, 1995.

45. Blair, S., Kohl, H., and Barlow, C., Physical activity, physical fitness, and all-cause mortality in women: do women need to be active? *J. Am. Coll. Nutr.*, 12, 368–371, 1993.

46. Oldridge, N., Guyatt, G. H., Fisher, M., and Rimm, A. A., Cardiac rehabilitation after myocardial infarction. Combined experience of randomized clinical trials, *JAMA*, 260, 945–950, 1988.

47. Wenger, N. K., Froelicher, E. S., Smith, L. K., Ades, P. A., Berra, K., Blumenthal, J. A., Certo, C. M., Dattilo, A. M., Davis, D., DeBusk, R. F. et al., Cardiac rehabilitation as secondary prevention. Agency for Health Care Policy and Research and National Heart, Lung, and Blood Institute, Clinical Practice Guideline – Quick Reference Guide for Clinicians, 1995, 1–23.

48. Stavrinos, T., Scarbek, Y., Galambos, G., Fiatarone Singh, M., and Singh, N., The effects of low intensity versus high intensity progressive resistance weight training on shoulder function in the elderly, *Aust. N. Zeal., J. Med.*, 1999.

49. Bandy, W. and Irion, J., The effects of time on static stretch on the flexibility of the hamstring muscles, *Phys. Ther.*, 74, 845–852, 1994.

50. Gehlsen, G. M. and Whaley, M. H., Falls in the elderly: Part II. Balance, strength, and flexibility, *Arch. Phys. Med. Rehabil.*, 71, 739–41, 1990.

51. Nelson, M., Fiatarone, M., Morganti, C., Trice, I., Greenberg, R., and Evans, W., Effects of high-intensity strength training on multiple risk factors for osteoporotic fractures, *JAMA*, 272, 1909–1914, 1994.

52. Pu, C., Johnson, M., Forman, D., Piazza, L., and Fiatarone, M., Performance-based functional changes after strength training in elderly women with heart failure, *J. Am. Geriatr. Soc.*, 45, S3, 1997.
53. Fiatarone Singh, M. and O'Neill, E., Enhancing balance with modified resistance training technique in frail elders at risk for falls (unpublished observations of authors).
54. Wolf, S., Jutner, N., Green, R., and McNeely, E., The Atlanta FICSIT study: two exercise interventions to reduce frailty in elders, *J. Am. Geriatr. Soc.*, 41, 329–332, 1993.
55. Judge, J. O., Whipple, R. H., and Wolfson, L. I., Effects of resistive and balance exercises on isokinetic strength in older persons, *J. Am. Geriatr. Soc.*, 42, 937–946, 1994.

3 Exercise, Nutrition, and Medications

Maria A. Fiatarone Singh

CONTENTS

EXERCISE AND MEDICATIONS

A variety of medications, both prescription and over-the-counter, may have effects upon a woman's exercise capacity, physical responses during exercise testing or training, or the safety and efficacy of the exercise prescription itself.[1] Since the older population consumes the vast majority of medications, it is important for both consumers and health care providers to be aware of these medication-exercise interactions.

First of all, it is important to remember that there are no medications that preclude physical activity. Rather, there are intended *direct* effects of drugs as well as potential *side* effects that may either alter the normal physiologic response to exertion, or increase the likelihood of adverse events during exercise testing or training. Knowledge of these potential interactions will be helpful in planning the timing of exercise sessions relative to medication ingestion. In some cases the status of a chronic medical condition needs to be monitored as exercise habits are adopted, as they may require adjustment of prescribed medications. For example, if hypertension is normally controlled with two different drugs, regular aerobic or resistive exercise, especially if it is accompanied by significant weight loss, may mean that only one drug will be required in the future. Such medication reduction through exercise represents a major potential benefit in terms of health, quality of life, compliance, and personal and societal health care costs and burdens. In this chapter, major categories of drugs and their potential interactions with exercise will be described. Listings of the most common agents in each class are given in the Appendix by both the generic and major brand names.

DRUGS USED FOR DIABETES MELLITUS

Diabetes mellitus in adults may be treated with either insulin by injection or oral hypoglycemic medications. There are several important interactions to consider with this class of agents. As an immediate consideration, it has been reported that exercise initiated after the subcutaneous injection of insulin may increase the rate of insulin absorption into the circulation, thus potentially leading to a more rapid fall in blood glucose than normal.[2] In insulin-dependent diabetics who are in poor metabolic control, prolonged exercise sessions may lead to either hyperglycemia or hypoglycemia. If insulin or oral hypoglycemics are taken immediately before exercise without eating first, dangerously low blood glucose levels could result.

In addition to these rapid changes in the control of blood sugar around the time of exercise, long-term increases in the expenditure of calories through physical activity and elevations in metabolic rate at rest, particularly when this results in loss of weight and visceral fat mass, may decrease requirements for insulin and/or oral hypoglycemics.

There are several ways in which the occurrence of these interactions can be minimized. The best overall recommendation is to attempt to keep to a regular schedule of medication, meals, and exercise as much as possible, particularly in the insulin-dependent or brittle diabetic. It is recommended that insulin be injected at sites away from exercising limbs (e.g., over the abdomen) on days when exercise is to be performed close to the time of insulin administration. For all diabetics, timing exercise sessions one and one-half to two hours after a meal will coincide with peak rises in blood sugar, but will not be so close to the meal as to interfere with digestion. Because the exercise will be fueled from the carbohydrate and fat in the meal, the exaggerated rise in blood glucose after meals seen in diabetics will be minimized, allowing for smoother metabolic control. This should lessen the highs and lows which may be responsible for fatigue, mood swings, or decreased ability to concentrate.

Strenuous exercise should be avoided in diabetics during periods of acute illness or fever from any cause (such as respiratory illness, influenza, urinary tract infection, etc.) when glucose regulation is likely to be abnormal or unpredictable, and dietary intake deviates from normal patterns. If in doubt, it is always better to avoid exercise than risk metabolic derangement or abnormal cardiac stress in diabetics at high risk for ischemic disease.

In terms of long-term control of diabetes after the initiation of a new exercise regimen, it is recommended that monitoring frequency be increased until a new pattern is established. During the first few weeks of any new exercise routine, you may advise checking fasting and 2-hour post-prandial blood glucose levels at home every 2 to 3 days, to see if any major changes are occurring. Very abnormal values should be confirmed by laboratory testing as well, and exercise stopped until the situation stabilizes.

If any marked changes in weight occur, either planned or unplanned, additional measurements should be taken at that point. Weight losses of only 10% of body weight have been associated with significant improvement in glucose homeostasis, so it is very possible that slow, steady weight loss accompanying exercise regimens will reduce medication dosages over time. However, if a woman unintentionally loses a large amount of weight, it is unlikely to be due to any form of exercise, and probably represents an underlying illness (cancer, hyperthyroidism, depression, etc.). In this situation, diabetic control is again unpredictable, and close monitoring and further medical follow-up are indicated. Again, this is not a time to initiate new or vigorous exercise routines.

BETA-BLOCKERS

Beta-blockers are a large class of medications used in the treatment of hypertension, atherosclerotic heart disease, cardiac arrhythmias, valvular heart disease, migraines, tremor, and glaucoma. They are important because they are widely prescribed in older men and women, and have many potential interactions with exercise capacity, testing, and prescription. Even ophthalmologic (eye drop) preparations of beta-blockers used for glaucoma may have significant cardiovascular side effects since they are absorbed into the systemic circulation after application.[3] Many patients may be on both oral and ophthalmologic preparations of beta-blockers, which will compound the side effects outlined below.

The most important property in relation to exercise is the ability of beta-bloclers to attenuate the normal postural, exercise- or stress-induced increase in heart rate.[1] Patients who are on sufficient doses of these agents to be "beta-blocked" will usually have a resting pulse of 50 to 60 beats per minute, which is atypical unless someone is a very well-trained endurance athlete, or has some other intrinsic or drug-induced conduction disturbance. In addition, these patients will have a smaller than normal rise in pulse in response to exercise. In order to maintain tissue perfusion during exercise when the tachycardic response is thus blocked, there may be an exaggerated rise in systolic blood pressure. Therefore, one cannot reliably measure exercise intensity or cardiac stress by monitoring the pulse in patients on therapeutic doses of beta-blockers. Other symptoms of exertion, such as breathlessness, sweating, fatigue, and overall level of perceived exertion will need to be used. Perceived exertion remains an accurate index of relative exercise intensity, regardless of the pulse response, underlying cardiac rhythm, age, or medical condition of the individual, and is therefore recommended as the primary method of prescribing and monitoring aerobic exercise intensity in older adults (see Chapter 2).

Another effect of beta-blockers is to reduce cardiac contractility, which is beneficial for the prevention and treatment of coronary artery disease, and reduction in cardiovascular mortality because it lessens cardiac oxygen consumption. However, in some cases, this may reduce cardiac output at rest or during exercise to a degree that impairs function and exercise tolerance.[4] Such beta-blocker-related exercise intolerance would be manifested by fatigue or dyspnea during activities of daily living or exercise that were formerly completed without significant effort.

In some patients who are already prone to postural hypotension for intrinsic or extrinsic reasons, the addition of a beta-blocker, which limits the tachycardic response to standing, will result in postural symptoms (dizziness, lightheadedness, weakness) or falls. Patients at risk for postural symptoms during beta-blockade include those with an autonomic neuropathy associated with diabetes or Parkinson's disease, dehydration, chronic diuretic therapy, or other medications that can cause postural hypotension, such as nitrates, calcium channel blockers, alpha-blockers, tricyclic antidepressants, levo-dopa, bromocriptine, and others. Thus, sudden changes in position at the initiation of exercise may be hazardous, particularly in individuals who are also frail or have poor balance. It is a good idea to measure blood pressure in the supine and standing positions if postural hypotension is suspected in individuals on beta-blockers. If a 20 mmHg or greater drop in systolic pressure is noted when changing from quiet supine rest to a standing posture at 2 minutes, then precautions should be taken when giving the exercise prescription. These include

1. Drink 1 to 2 glasses of fluid within the half-hour before exercise, more on hot days.
2. Rise slowly and allow one minute or longer for equilibration in the standing position prior to beginning exercise.
3. Cool down slowly from aerobic exercise for 5 to 10 minutes while slowly moving the arms and legs. If you stop exercising suddenly, blood pools in the lower extremities rather than returning to the systemic circulation, thus exacerbating postural symptoms and potentially causing cardiac ischemia as well. Since patients with underlying cardiac disease are often the ones prescribed beta-blockers, this side effect is of particular importance in this population.

Some older individuals will have post-prandial hypotension that occurs on standing shortly after a meal. The same precautions noted for postural hypotension apply here. It makes sense to avoid exercise immediately after eating for this reason, as well as others related to the metabolic and vascular demands of food absorption and metabolism, which should not have to compete with musculoskeletal needs for oxygen, fuel, and blood flow during exercise.

Beta-blockers may also cause bronchospasm in susceptible individuals, which may only become noticeable as wheezing or shortness of breath during aerobic exercise or heavy housework, with no symptoms at rest. This is most commonly seen in patients with chronic obstructive pulmonary disease or asthma by history, in whom beta-blockers are often contraindicated. In a patient with both systolic heart failure and chronic lung disease, it may be difficult to tell on the basis of symptoms which disease process is responsible, and physician examination and follow-up are essential. Exercise should be halted if exercise tolerance appears to be worsening rather than improving over time in such patients, as medication-exercise interaction may be responsible. Full evaluation is necessary before adequate training can be instituted, and this may sometimes require a monitored setting such as a cardiac rehabilitation program until clarified.

Because beta-blockers can mask signs of adrenalin such as tremor and sweating, the classic symptoms of hypoglycemia may not be obvious in diabetics taking these agents. This decreased ability to control body temperature through sweating is seen in all older adults to some degree, but is exaggerated by beta-blockade. Therefore, these patients in particular should not exercise in extremely hot or humid environments, and avoid hot baths, saunas, or showers immediately after exercise. Use of hot saunas or whirlpools after exercise in adults with underlying cardiac disease has been associated with sudden death and myocardial infarction and is best avoided in the elderly in general.

It is sometimes possible to adjust the type or dosage of beta-blocking medication, or even switch to a different class of drugs if the above side effects become very limiting. For example, if beta-blockers exacerbate claudication (a symptom of peripheral vascular disease), switching to a cardio-selective beta-blocker may allow exercise tolerance to improve by minimizing claudication. However, beta-blockers must always be tapered slowly rather than withdrawn all at once due to the up-regulation of beta-receptors that they have induced during chronic exposure. The individual will then be much more sensitive to sympathetic stimulation, and may develop angina, arrhythmias, or tachycardia during the withdrawal phase.

The major difference in the exercise prescription for women taking beta-blockers is the target heart rate at which they should work during endurance-building activities. Rather than using a percentage of the estimated maximal heart rate, instructions for using the Borg scale of relative perceived exertion, as outlined in Chapter 3, should be given.[5] This scale remains an accurate indicator of cardiac stress even when the heart rate cannot be followed due to beta-blockade. For most older women, a level of 11 to 14 on this visual scale from 6 to 20 will provide the appropriate endurance stimulus during training sessions. It is important to recognize that beta-blockade does *not* preclude endurance or strength training in most cases, and in fact such exercise may be beneficial for many of the underlying conditions (e.g., hypertension, atherosclerosis) for which beta-blockers are prescribed. Resistance training is unlikely to produce the level of tachycardia that endurance training does, and therefore, beta-blockers will have a less noticeable effect during this kind of exercise.

DIURETICS

Diuretics are a diverse group of drugs that are used for the regulation of fluid balance, primarily in the treatment of hypertension, congestive heart failure, and edema. With any of the agents, chronic usage of moderate or high dosages may pre-dispose someone to dehydration, as the intravascular fluid volume is already reduced. This effect is most likely to occur after prolonged exercise in high temperatures when adequate oral fluid replacement is not taken.[6] Because older adults have a decreased ability to sense alterations in blood volume and osmolar content, they may not perceive increased fluid needs as thirst until after clinical dehydration occurs.[7] Intravascular salt and water depletion may also increase the risk of heat stroke during prolonged exercise in a hot environment. These problems can usually be avoided by advising extra fluid intake (water or electrolyte replacement drinks) on exercise days, even if there is no sense of thirst at the time. Symptoms of lightheadedness or dizziness, dysequilibrium, giddiness, or a change in mental status may be indicative of present or impending dehydration or heat stroke. Exercise should be stopped and a supine posture assumed while fluid is given and vital signs are monitored.

Some diuretics also increase the renal excretion of potassium, magnesium, calcium, and/or zinc. Although losses of calcium and zinc (from loop diuretics) have important nutritional considerations, it is the losses of magnesium and potassium from thiazide and loop diuretics which are more directly related to the exercise prescription. Prolonged exposure to these medications can lead to clinically important intracellular depletion of potassium and magnesium.[8–10] Such abnormalities have been associated with muscle weakness, cramps, fatigue, exercise intolerance, and cardiac arrhythmias, particularly in patients on digoxin. Therefore, if any of these symptoms occur in someone who is chronically prescribed non-potassium sparing diuretics, physician evaluation and laboratory testing will be needed to detect and correct the imbalance. Although it is common to replace potassium in patients on thiazide-type diuretics, magnesium losses are often ignored in this setting. However, serum magnesium levels do not fall until intracellular magnesium is already quite low. Without magnesium, potassium cannot effectively replete its intracellular stores, and so the potassium supplements will be only partially effective. Patients who have hypokalemia or hypomagnesemia, or who are suspected of such on the basis of history, should be evaluated prior to initiating or continuing vigorous exercise.

Finally, some women take diuretics for many years for simple peripheral edema that is the result of varicose veins or too much sitting in a chair, rather than a true volume overload because of cardiac or renal problems. This practice is not recommended unless medical complications of the swelling are present, such as cellulitis, dermatitis, pain, immobility, or ulceration. Such mechanical pooling of fluid is best treated by exercise itself and elevation of the legs, thus avoiding the potential side effects of unneeded diuretics. Any exercise which causes the calf muscles to contract (walking, biking, toe stands, stepping, dancing, weight-lifting, etc.) will help to prevent and treat peripheral edema from venous stasis or insufficiency.

SYMPATHOMIMETICS

Drugs which primarily stimulate the alpha receptors of the sympathetic nervous system are used in many over-the-counter and prescription cough and cold preparations, allergy sinus-congestion treatments, stimulants, appetite suppressants, and for other miscellaneous conditions. These medications may occasionally aggravate high blood pressure, increase pulse rates, or cause palpitations.[1] They have the potential to cause angina or arrhythmias because they stimulate increased oxygen demand by the heart.

However, these agents are sometimes used to enhance exercise performance by athletes in sports where they are not regulated, since they have been shown to reduce fatigue and increase endurance capacity. They do this by allowing the body to rely more on plentiful stores of fat for fuel rather than the limited stores of carbohydrates available in muscles and circulation. It is not recommended that older women use these medications prior to exercise, either intentionally to enhance performance or unintentionally when prescribed for another purpose, because of the potential for cardiac complications in those with underlying cardiovascular disease. These drugs can alter the heart rate response to exercise, thus leading to an erroneous target heart rate prescription. They may also accentuate the blood pressure rise during exercise to abnormally high levels, thus compromising safety. They may increase the risk of musculoskeletal or cardiovascular strain or injuries during exercise, because persons taking these medications may become slightly euphoric, tolerant to pain and fatigue which would otherwise limit exertion, and thus have an impaired ability to recognize safe limits.

Since these medications are almost always self-prescribed for self-limited conditions, they can almost always be discontinued without the fear of adverse effects. It is recommended that these medications be withheld for 12 hours prior to regular exercise workouts if they cannot be stopped. If the medications cannot be discontinued, for example, in cases of severe allergic rhinitis, then blood pressure and pulse monitoring during initial exercise training sessions may be required to ensure that safe cardiovascular parameters are not exceeded.

BRONCHODILATORS

A variety of medications are used in the treatment of asthma or chronic obstructive pulmonary disease to prevent or treat bronchospasm. These medications may be prescribed several times per day or used only as needed for symptomatic wheezing. Some women use inhaled forms of these agents prophylactically just prior to an activity such as exercise, which they know by experience may exacerbate their pulmonary symptoms. Because these drugs stimulate the beta receptors of the sympathetic nervous system, their side effects may include tachycardia, arrhythmias, increased blood pressure, cardiac ischemia, tremor, sweating, or anxiety. Since it is often not possible (nor desirable) to exercise remote from dosing schedules for these drugs (as in the case of exercise-induced asthma), the above side effects should be monitored closely in the initial stages of the exercise activity. The stimulating effect of exercise itself will combine with the sympathetic stimulation secondary to the drugs, and may produce unsafe cardiovascular stresses. Women who are also at risk for low potassium or magnesium from diuretics (see above) should watch for signs of cardiac arrhythmias (irregular pulse, palpitations, dizziness, or hypotension during or after exercise), since mineral deficiencies will increase the arrthymogenic potential associated with bronchodilators.[9] These medications, when taken properly, can be very effective in allowing someone with even moderate or severe lung disease to exercise safely and increase their strength and endurance. Therefore, it is recommended that the timing and dosage of these medications be carefully scripted *into* the exercise prescription, rather than posing a barrier to increased physical activity participation.

GLUCOCORTICOIDS

These medications are used for diseases associated with chronic inflammation, such as rheumatoid arthritis or systemic lupus erythematosis, as well as for chronic lung disease and psoriasis. Prednisone and other glucocorticoids (steroids) taken chronically may lead to a proximal myopathy of skeletal muscle and excess bone resorption, thus increasing the risk of muscle weakness, atrophy, and osteoporotic fractures. The bone loss may not be obvious for many years, as it is quite insidious, but muscle weakness, particularly of the upper arms and thighs may become debilitating after even a short time. If a woman has the onset of difficulty reaching over her head, putting on a jacket, lifting a grandchild or a bag of groceries, getting out of a sofa, the bathtub, or the car, this may be the first sign of a clinically significant steroid myopathy.

Recognition of these side effects of chronic corticosteroid therapy is also important for the prescription of an appropriate exercise regimen that will help to preserve muscle and bone mass, if steroid therapy cannot be discontinued or reduced. Resistance training has been shown to prevent the very rapid loss of bone and muscle seen after corticosteroid therapy is begun.[11,12] Aerobic training does not have this ability. Thus, resistance training, as described in Chapter 2, should be emphasized as a priority area in any woman who needs long-term glucocorticoid therapy in addition to calcium and vitamin D supplementation.[13] The potential for fracture of osteopenic bones should also be minimized by avoiding spinal flexion exercises and movements (e.g., bowling, bending over to lift a load, sitting slumped in a chair), and improving balance if abnormalities in gait are present[14] (see Chapter 2). Although these steroids are also available in topical and inhalational forms, only oral administration has been shown to produce systemic levels sufficient to induce significant atrophy of muscle and bone. However, precautions may be warranted in chronic users of high doses of inhalational steroids (oral or nasal) for asthma or allergic rhinitis, who may be at risk as well.

As is the case with beta-blockers, corticosteroids can never be stopped suddenly due to the suppression of the endogenous glucocorticoid axis which they induce over time. Exercising in the setting of glucocorticoid insufficiency could result in serious or fatal consequences, hypotension, dehydration, and/or collapse. Exercise, acute illness, or fever may provoke clinical signs of deficiency in someone who is apparently normal at rest, due to the physiologic stress of such events. Persons at risk for such an occurence would be those who had recently stopped a prolonged course of systemic corticosteroids after a relatively short weaning period, or did not have their dosages increased during an acute serious illness.

CARDIOVASCULAR MEDICATIONS

In addition to the beta-blockers and diuretics mentioned above, other medications used for hypertension, angina, congestive heart failure, or arrhythmias may need to be re-evaluated if the adoption of an exercise regimen causes significant cardiovascular adaptations such as reduced resting blood pressures or decreased frequency of angina. The most prudent course in such individuals is to monitor blood pressure and pulse frequently during the initial stages of training, and periodically as endurance capacity improves. Since many of these medications may be associated with a drop in blood pressure upon standing (orthostatic hypotension), watching for symptoms such as dizziness associated with rapid changes in position is important. It may also become important to note the time of administration of these medications so that acute changes in blood pressure secondary to vasodilating medications, for example, will not be falsely interpreted as a sign of intolerance to exercise or significant coronary disease.

For all cardiovascular medications, no doses should be withheld on exercise testing or training days, and, if possible, sessions should not be started less than one hour after a standard dose. An exception may be made in the case of sublingual nitroglycerin which is sometimes prescribed just prior to exertion to prevent known, predictable angina in susceptible women. However, if starting a new exercise program of any kind causes a change in the usual pattern of angina, or new onset chest pain, exercise should be stopped immediately, and referral made to a physician for further evaluation. In patients with chronic stable angina, exercise has been associated with both reductions in the chronic level of anginal symptoms (frequency and intensity of pain) as well as the need for anti-anginal medications. Therefore, a worsening of angina in response to exercise is neither expected nor acceptable. Patients who cannot exercise at reasonable levels of effort (11 to 14 on the Borg scale) may require additional medications, angiography, echocardiography, and/or surgical correction of significant valvular or coronary artery lesions before they can safely exercise.

DRUGS WITH CENTRAL NERVOUS SYSTEM ACTIVITY

Many drugs have effects on the central nervous system (CNS), either as their desired therapeutic action, or as an unwanted side effect. Because there are so many of these individual agents, they are not listed separately in the Appendix.

There are several types of interactions to consider in the exercising woman. Any drug which causes sedation (e.g., sleeping pills, anti-anxiety agents, some anti-depressants, anti-histamines, narcotics) may increase the potential for falls or injuries or limit tolerance for physical exertion of any sort. Exercising at alert times of day and minimizing or avoiding use of these agents on exercising days is recommended.

The other neurologic symptom to be aware of is an impairment of neuromuscular coordination, gait, and balance which is sometimes associated with the acute or chronic use of benzodiazepines, a group of drugs used primarily in the treatment of anxiety and insomnia (e.g., Valium, Halcion, Serax). Even if taken the night before exercise, these medications may have residual effects on the central nervous system the following day. It is important in women taking these drugs to watch closely for signs of poor balance, incoordination, or sedation, particularly when they are exercising alone, using resistance training or other machine-based equipment, treadmills or other activities requiring maintenance of balance or fine motor movement.

Finally, it should also be remembered that drugs which affect the CNS may also reduce compliance or motivation to participate in exercise activities. Asking about prescribed or non-prescribed drug usage is an important part of the medical history and assessment of the kinds of behavioral supports which must be built into the exercise prescription (see Chapter 25).

THE INTERACTION OF EXERCISE AND NUTRITIONAL STATUS

Exercise may be related to nutritional status in older women in a number of ways that influence the capacity to exercise, the treatment of disease, and the specifics of the exercise prescription and the nutritional requirements in this population. For this reason, it is important to assess the medical conditions and medications present that may place the individual at risk for nutritional disorders before formulating the exercise prescription. This assessment process may lead to the specific use of exercise to treat nutrition-related diseases or medication or diet-related side effects. On the other hand, it may indicate the need to delay or modify exercise until nutritional concerns are addressed. The impact of exercise itself on the nutritional requirements of the older woman can be defined relatively simply in most cases with attention to basic principles.

NUTRITIONAL DISORDERS AND THEIR IMPACT ON EXERCISE CAPACITY

Physiologic aging and chronic disease are not the only factors that limit functional capacity in the elderly. If nutritional deficiencies exist as well, the potential for clinically overt consequences for functional independence and exercise capacity is even greater. Protein-calorie malnutrition alone, or in combination with catabolic diseases, will lead to loss of lean body mass. Loss of muscle mass may result in weakness, gait and balance disorders, falls and fractures, functional decline, immune system impairment, and insulin insensitivity, and is thus one of the most important sequelae of malnutrition in the elderly.[15]

Many diseases and medications are associated with anorexia and weight loss. It is often difficult to treat such patients with nutritional interventions alone, as their energy requirements are markedly blunted by both low muscle mass and basal metabolic rate, as well as restricted energy expenditure in physical activity. Attempts at nutritional supplementation with additional energy are often not successful in these situations, whereas individuals who begin an exercise regimen along with supplementation have been shown to be able to augment their total energy intake significantly.[16] Further studies and long-term trials need to be completed in this realm to establish the clinical utility of exercise as a co-treatment for anorexia and weight loss, utilizing its potentially positive effects on appetite and energy requirements. It should be noted, however, that some individuals who are quite ill or who have no access to additional food sources may not be able to appropriately increase their energy intake in response to exercise. In these individuals, weight loss may increase even further due to the uncompensated increased energy expenditure of the exercise itself.

Protein deficiency is usually seen in the setting of low energy intakes; although it can occur by itself, if severe catabolic stress occurs (trauma, surgery, burns, systemic inflammation, etc.), if dietary habits are unusual, or if medically prescribed diets have been imposed. This is most typically seen in relation to chronic renal failure or chronic liver disease, in which the low protein diet is used to minimize the clinical progression or expression of the underlying disease. Insufficient protein intake or negative balance due to excessive losses (surgery, proteinuria, catabolic illness, burns, malabsorption) of protein will result in muscle wasting in an attempt to preserve visceral protein stores and metabolic functions. This loss of muscle mass will impair all exercise capacities, including strength, power, balance, and aerobic.

It was previously thought that resistance training increased protein requirements, and thus a large industry has been created around protein formulas thought to enhance muscle hypertrophy and/or performance. In actuality, resistance training is an anabolic stimulus for the body, meaning that it increases, *not decreases*, the body's capacity to retain nitrogen from protein sources in the diet.[17] Thus, for the same amount of dietary protein intake, individuals who are practicing weight-lifting exercise are in a more positive protein balance. We have used this phenomenon clinically to treat the muscle wasting that accompanies a low protein diet prescribed for chronic renal failure in older persons.[18]

Carbohydrates are necessary to supply fuel for exercise, and insufficient storage of carbohydrate as glycogen in skeletal muscle in older persons may lead to early fatigue and poor cardiovascular and musculoskeletal endurance. People with impaired glucose tolerance and Type II diabetes have lower than normal glycogen stores, which can be improved over time by aerobic exercise training.[19] Very high intakes of carbohydrates as a proportion of total calories are sometimes consumed prior to endurance events in athletes to maximize glycogen storage and thus improve performance. There is no need for excessive carbohydrate intake (greater than 55% of calories) in older adults who are engaged in typical exercise training programs.

Micronutrient status is also important for physical function and exercise capacity. Skeletal muscle expresses receptors for 1,25-dihydroxyvitamin D, which appears to be necessary for the rapid intracellular re-uptake of calcium into the sarcoplasmic reticulum in the relaxation phase of myofilament contraction.[20] Muscle that cannot fully relax in this way cannot subsequently produce maximal force during the contractile phase, and this cycle results in clinical muscle weakness, particularly of the proximal muscles of the lower extremities. The proximal myopathy of osteomalacia is also associated with pain and atrophy in the affected muscle groups, but is reversible with vitamin D repletion. Individuals at high risk for this condition include homebound or institutionalized elders; those chronically receiving corticosteroids, dilantin, or phenytoin; those living in countries where dairy products or other food items are not fortified with vitamin D; or individuals abstaining from dairy products due to lactose intolerance or other reasons.

Other nutritional deficiencies that impair muscle contractile activity and result in clinical weakness include the minerals calcium, magnesium, and potassium, as noted in the section on exercise–medication interactions above. Patients with no other definable cause for muscle weakness and fatigue, who have risk factors for these mineral losses, should be considered candidates for replacement or alternative drug therapy if possible.

Sometimes, in the elderly, fatigue may be a more prominent complaint than actual muscle weakness in these conditions, so a thorough history and a high index of suspicion are essential to early diagnosis and treatment. Magnesium and potassium deficiencies may also result in potentially serious cardiac arrhythmias during exercise, particularly in the setting of concurrent digoxin treatment. Clinical deficiencies of calcium that are severe and acute may lead to impairments of muscle contraction or arrhythmias. Chronical, small losses of calcium in excess of intake will result in negative calcium balance and adversely affect bone mineral mass and density.

Vitamin B_{12} may be low in the elderly due to problems in absorption of this nutrient secondary to achlorhydria (atrophic gastritis) or pernicious anemia. This deficiency may result in a peripheral neuropathy leading to impairment in gait and balance, or to an anemia, which may limit aerobic capacity or overall exercise tolerance.

Thiamin deficiency is usually seen in conjunction with very low energy intake or excessive alcohol intake and poor diets. Thiamin deficiency can cause a proximal myopathy and cardiac failure when severe.

Iron deficiency in the elderly is almost always related to blood loss, particularly from the gastrointestinal tract. Iron deficiency results in an anemia that may be manifested as exercise intolerance, fatigue, dizziness, shortness of breath, increased angina, or worsening of chronic lung disease. A sudden onset or change in these symptoms should raise the suspicion of anemia of this or other etiologies. Exercise should not be initiated or continued at vigorous levels until this deficiency has been evaluated and treated. Occult malignancy is always a consideration in this setting.

NUTRITIONAL RECOMMENDATIONS FOR THE PHYSICALLY ACTIVE OLDER ADULT

In general, physically active older adults should follow the general nutritional guidelines that apply to the majority of older adults (see Chapter 4). However, there are a few caveats outlined below that will maximize exercise safety and effectiveness.

FLUID REPLACEMENT

Water is an essential nutrient that is often consumed in sub-optimal quantities in the elderly. Therefore, it is important to encourage extra water intake (500 to 1000 ml) on exercise days, especially in individuals prescribed diuretics or very low sodium diets, during high ambient temperatures or humid conditions, or after recovery from dehydrating illnesses or fevers. Specific "sport drink" formulations are unnecessary for fluid replacement under normal conditions and in non-competitive athletes. They are absorbed more quickly and have concentrations of electrolytes meant to replace losses in sweat more precisely than other fluids. These factors may offer some performance benefits and may reduce the incidence of gastrointestinal side effects (bloating, diarrhea) that may occur with consumption of other fluids during prolonged endurance events. However, for the non-competitive older woman engaging in typical walking, sport weight-lifting, or other recreational activities, water or juice offer adequate fluid replacement. The high cost of specialized sports drinks relative to water or other drinks is difficult to justify in normal circumstances; they may offer a behavioral incentive for some individuals that helps to maintain fluid status or promotes exercise at higher levels due to their palatability, association with youth, health and fitness, or advertising claims. If so, the behavioral benefits attained may be worth the extra cost.

Often the most difficult part of the fluid prescription in older adults is the fear of incontinence which may result. This is particularly important in those taking diuretics, nursing home residents, or in women with stress incontinence. Often the exercise itself may precipitate stress incontinence in a woman with weak pelvic floor muscles, simply due to the assumption of an upright posture, or to increased abdominal pressure during resistive exercise. It is not uncommon for older adults participating in an exercise activity, which they know by experience may lead to incontinence, to withold their diuretics, refrain from fluids, or restrict activity duration or intensity substantially. Sensitivity to this issue is critical for exercise leaders, as the true reasons for withdrawal or refusal to participate will usually require private discussion with the individual rather than group encouragement. Some suggestions that may be offered in this situation are given in Table 1.

TABLE 1
Fluid Replacement in Adults with Exercise-Related Incontinence

Time usage of diuretics for after exercise sessions if possible

Avoid all caffeine-containing foods and beverages on the day of exercise

Empty bladder just prior to exercise and during exercise if longer than one hour

Avoid breath holding and Valsalva maneuver during resistance training exercises

Add pelvic floor exercises in women to exercise routine (Kegel exercises); these can be done during rest periods between other exercises

Replace fluid after rather than before or during exercise sessions

Consult with physician if incontinence is not resolved with the above measures

---

MAINTAINING OR ALTERING WEIGHT AND BODY COMPOSITION

If the goal during the adoption of a new program of physical activity is weight maintenance, there is usually little that needs to be done in healthy adults. This is because there is a spontaneous increase in *ad libitium* dietary intake that occurs in healthy adults in response to the change in energy expenditure in order to maintain energy balance. Cross-sectional studies indicate that physically active adults consume more calories than sedentary age-matched peers. Older adults who begin an exercise program that is not part of a weight loss plan usually maintain their body weight in this way. It has been suggested, although not proven, that encouraging physical activity is a good way to improve the quality of the diet in older individuals, because they will then consume more food, and perhaps food of a greater variety. Dietary diversity, or variety, is positively related to better nutritional status in relation to recommended daily allowances and body composition. However, more research remains to be done to determine how this change in food intake after exercise is controlled, whether dietary composition or diversity is altered by physical activity itself, and whether or not this is indeed a good strategy to promote healthy nutrition. Individuals who wish to maintain body weight should be counseled if needed to increase energy intake with normal ratios of fat/carbohydrate/protein) as *food* rather than as "sports" supplements. Consuming a variety of food sources is the best way to meet micronutrient and trace element needs.

ALTERATIONS IN BODY COMPOSITION WITH EXERCISE

One of the important nutritional considerations with exercise is the ability to modulate body composition, or the ratio of lean to fat tissue with new or increased levels of training. Such alterations may be desirable for aesthetic, fitness, or health-related considerations in older women. Such goals may form the primary reason for the exercise prescription (e.g., in the obese diabetic) or they may be a non-targeted but desirable side effect (e.g., improved strength and balance in a frail elderly woman being treated with resistance training for depression). Many chronic diseases and geriatric syndromes are, in fact, related to body composition, so that altering the amounts of fat and muscle tissue with exercise may have very important medical implications. Important relationships in this regard are shown in Table 2.

LOSING BODY WEIGHT AND FAT MASS

Exercise by itself is unlikely to cause substantial weight loss in an obese individual (see Chapter 17). Therefore, if a goal of the exercise prescription is fat or weight loss, then you will need to combine exercise with a balanced hypocaloric diet. Energy expenditure must exceed energy intake by about 500 calories per day in order to achieve slow, sustained changes in weight and body composition of about one-half pound to one pound per week. It is usually recommended to supplement a hypocaloric diet with a standard multivitamin at RDA levels. Large doses of micronutrients that are often given in conjunction with commercial weight loss plans and formulas are unnecessary. They neither accelerate the rate of fat loss nor do they provide extra energy as is sometimes claimed. Loss of energy when dieting is usually related to an overly restrictive caloric intake, which is not recommended in the setting of a newly adopted physical activity program in the elderly, particularly those with chronic diseases. Excessive fatigue, discouragement, and/or injuries are likely to result from such a combination, and these patterns are not sustainable long term, thus leading to high rates of relapse.

GAINING WEIGHT AND MUSCLE MASS

For some older individuals, one of the goals of an exercise program may be weight gain, along with hypertrophy of skeletal muscle. This may be appropriate in very thin or sarcopenic (wasted) elders, frail individuals with mobility impairment and falls, and those who have lost weight due to disease or anorexia from other causes. Older women in institutionalized or isolated settings may often end up in this category. Exercise is used in this case to increase appetite and thereby improve body

TABLE 2
Clinical Syndromes Related to Modulation of Body Composition

Low Body Fat/Protective	Reduced Body Fat/Therapeutic	High Muscle Mass/Protective	Increased Muscle Mass/Therapeutic
Atherosclerosis	Atherosclerosis		Chronic obstructive pulmonary disease
Breast cancer			Chronic renal failure
Colon Cancer			Congestive heart failure
Degenerative arthritis	Degenerative arthritis		Type II Diabetes mellitus
Type II Diabetes mellitus	Type II Diabetes mellitus	Frailty, functional decline	Frailty, functional decline
Gout	Gout	Gait and balance disorders, falls	Gait and balance disorders, falls
Hyperlipidemia	Hyperlipidemia		HIV infection
Hypertension	Hypertension	Low back pain	Low back pain
Low back pain	Low back pain		Neuromuscular disease
Low self-esteem	Low self-esteem	Osteoporosis	Osteoporosis
Mobility impairment, disability	Mobility impairment, disability		Parkinson's disease
Peripheral vascular disease	Peripheral vascular disease		Protein-calorie malnutrition, marasmus
Sleep apnea	Sleep apnea		Rheumatoid arthritis
Stroke			Stroke
Vascular impotence			
Venous disease	Venous disease		

mass and add muscle bulk. This interaction depends upon the availability of increased food supplies, and the metabolic, cognitive, affective, and behavioral competence of the undernourished individual to sense and respond to the cues to increase dietary intake. Approaches that may be taken are to add nutrient and calorically dense food snacks between meals and after exercise sessions and provide increased support for shopping, cooking, and/or feeding as appropriate. Concluding exercise sessions with an ice cream social, pizza party, or other treat is an excellent way to encourage increased food intake and physical activity patterns in institutional settings or senior citizen centers.

Generalized gain in weight usually results in some lean and some fat tissue increases. However, if the primary aim is to increase muscle mass through exercise, then it is necessary to use resistance training (see Chapter 2) as the mode of exercise, as aerobic training has little affect in this regard. It has been shown that the amount of muscle hypertrophy that occurs in response to weight lifting exercise is quite variable in the elderly. It is more likely to occur robustly when the intensity of the training is high, the duration is greater than 3 months, and the participants are younger, well-nourished at the start of training, and given extra calories during the training program.[21-23]

Although there has been much debate over the issue of protein supplementation during weight-lifting exercise as a means to promote muscle hypertrophy, there is no evidence from controlled clinical trials that this is necessary. The gain in muscle tissue is not affected by either high (twice the RDA)[24] or moderate (an extra 20%) protein supplementation[16,23] during resistance training in either the healthy or frail elderly. Resistance training actually decreases the protein requirements of the elderly, as noted above. Therefore, there is no need to supplement protein beyond 1.0 to 1.2 g/kg/day, a level which can be achieved with diverse dietary sources rather than expensive isolated amino acid or protein supplements.

EXERCISE FOR DIABETICS

Diabetics can participate in all modalities of exercise. Both resistive and aerobic exercises offer benefit in terms of insulin sensitivity. When combined with weight loss in obese diabetics, exercise may be associated with substantial improvements in metabolic control. Loss of weight is a far more important consideration than alteration of the fiber or simple sugar content of the diet in obese Type II diabetics, particularly those who are not insulin-dependent. Therefore, restriction of fat intake in conjunction with exercise is the most efficacious combination of interventions in this setting.

In diabetic patients, time exercise sessions for the post-prandial peaks in blood glucose (1.5 to 2 hours after a meal) in order to minimize excursions of blood glucose. As noted above, exercise should be avoided right after an insulin injection, and injections kept away from the exercising limbs if possible. High carbohydrate and concentrated sugar snacks should be available during exercise sessions for brittle or insulin-dependent diabetics in particular, but it is a good idea in all diabetics to be prepared for unexpected hypoglycemic events as well. No diabetic patients should exercise after prolonged fasting or skipping meals, or during an acute systemic illness or febrile episode of any kind, as erratic glucose regulation may occur in these situations.

EXERCISE AND MINERAL LOSSES

As noted above, some patients on diuretics may be at risk for mineral deficiencies that could increase their risk for acute exercise-related cardiovascular events or chronic muscle contractile problems. It is prudent to advise an increase in dietary sources of potassium and magnesium if levels are marginal or low, particularly in high-risk coronary artery disease or arrhythmia-prone patients on diuretics or digoxin. However, this is contraindicated in patients with renal failure or diabetes-related Type IV renal tubular acidosis who cannot excrete excessive loads of these minerals and may become hyperkalemic. Never advise alterations of diet in this direction unless it is done in consultation with a physician and after appropriate laboratory evaluation of renal function and electrolyte and mineral status.

REFERENCES

1. Rosenbloom, D. and Sutton, J., Drugs and exercise, *Med. Clin. N. Am.*, 69, 177–87, 1985.
2. Koivista, V., Felig, P., and Ainman, B., Effects of leg exercise on insulin absorption in diabetic patients, *NEJM*, 298, 79–83, 1979.
3. Arkins, J., Rugh, B., and Timewell, R., Cardiovascular effects of topical beta-blockers during exercise, *Am. J. Ophthalmol.*, 99, 173–75, 1985.
4. Sable, D., Brammel, D., and Sheehan, W. E. A., Attenuation of exercise conditioning by beta-adrenergic blockage, *Circulation*, 65, 79–83, 1982.
5. Borg, G. and Linderholm, H., Perceived exertion and pulse rate during graded exercise in various age group, *Acta Med. Scand.*, 472(Suppl), 194–206, 1970.
6. Sarnquist, F. and Larson, P., Drug-induced heat stroke, *Anesthesiology*, 39, 330–48, 1973.
7. Philips, P. et al., Reduced thirst after water deprivation in healthy elderly men, *N. Engl. J. Med.*, 311, 753–759, 1984.
8. Dorup, I. et al., Reduced concentrations of potassium, magnesium, and sodium-potassium pumps in human skeletal muscle during treatment with diuretics, *Brit. Med. J.*, 296, 455–458, 1988.
9. Whelton, P. and Watson, A., Diuretic-induced hypokalemia and cardiac arrhythmias, *Am. J. Cardiol.*, 58, 5A–10A, 1986.
10. Stendig-Lindberg, G., Bergstrom, J., and Hultman, E., Hypomagnesemia and muscle electrolytes and metabolites, *Acta Med. Scand.*, 201, 273–80, 1977.
11. Braith, R. et al., Resistance exercise prevents glucocorticoid-induced myopathy in heart transplant recipients, *Med. Sci. Sports Exerc.*, 30, 483–489, 1998.
12. Braith, R. et al., Resistance exercise training restores bone mineral density in heart transplant recipients, *J. Am. Coll. Coariol.*, 28(6), 1471–1477, 1996.
13. Czerwinski, S., Kurowski, T., and O'Neill, T. E. A., Initiating regular exercise protects against muscle atrophy from glucocorticoids, *J. Appl. Physiol.*, 63, 1504–10, 1987.
14. Sinaki, M. and Mikkelsen, B., Postmenopausal spinal osteoporosis: flexion versus extension exercises, *Arch. Phys. Med. Rehabil.*, 65, 593–596, 1984.
15. Fiatarone, M. and Evans, W., The etiology and reversibility of muscle dysfunction in the elderly, *J. Gerontol.*, 48, 77–83, 1993.
16. Fiatarone, M. A. et al., Exercise training and nutritional supplementation for physical frailty in very elderly people, *N. Engl. J. Med.*, 330, 1769–1775, 1994.
17. Campbell, W. et al., Increased protein requirements in the elderly: new data and retrospective reassessments, *Am. J. Clin. Nutr.*, 60, 501–509, 1994.
18. Castaneda, C. et al., Resistance training prevents muscle wasting in renal disease, *FASEB*, 1998.
19. Hughes, V. A. et al., Exercise increases muscle GLUT-4 levels and insulin action in subjects with impaired glucose tolerance, *Am. J. Physiol.*, 264(6 Pt 1), E855–62, 1993.
20. Jeejeebhoy, K. N., Muscle function and nutrition, *Gut*, 27(Suppl. 1), 25–39, 1986.
21. Meredith, C. N., Frontera, W. R., and Evans, W. J., Body composition in elderly men: Effect of dietary modification during strength training, *J. Am. Geriatr. Soc.*, 40, 155–162, 1992.
22. Frontera, W. R. et al., Strength conditioning in older men: skeletal muscle hypertrophy and improved function, *J. Appl. Physiol.*, 64, 1038–1044, 1988.
23. Fiatarone Singh, M. et al., Insulin-like growth factor I in skeletal muscle after weight-lifting exercise in frail elders, *Am. J. Physiol.*, 277, E136–143, 1999.
24. Campbell, W. W. et al., Increased energy requirements and changes in body composition with resistance training in older adults, *Am. J. Clin. Nutr.*, 60(2), 167–75, 1994.

MEDICATION–EXERCISE INTERACTIONS APPENDIX

Generic and brand names of drugs available in the U.S. in the relevant categories were compiled from *Facts and Comparisons*, Olin, B. R., Ed., Facts and Comparisons, Inc., St. Louis, MO, 1992. Each list is presented in alphabetical order, with a single pharmaceutical agent represented by one generic and one or more brand names in most cases. Brand names are capitalized. For certain drugs, such as decongestants in cold preparations, not every brand name was listed because of the very large number of such products on the market; only the generic component is listed. After the individual listing by therapeutic class (e.g., anti-diabetic agents), the drug names are alphabetized in a single list with a reference number indicating to which category they belong (e.g., insulin [1]).

THERAPEUTIC CLASSIFICATIONS

Antidiabetic Agents
  acetohexamide
  chlorpropamide
  Diabenase
  Diabeta
  Dymelor
  glipizide
  Glucotrol
  glyburide
  insulin (many brands)
  Micronase
  Orinase
  tolazemide
  tolbutamide
  Tolinase

Beta-blockers
  acebutolol
  atenolol
  Betagan
  betaxolol
  Betoptic
  Blocadren
  carteolol
  Cartrol
  celiprolol
  Corgard
  Inderal
  Inderide
  Kerlone
  labetalol

Levatol
levobunolol
Lopressor
metipranolol
metoprolol
nadolol
Normodyne
Normozide
Optipranolol
penbutolol
pindolol
propranolol
Sectral
Selecor
Tenormin
Timolide
timolol
Timoptic
Trandate
Visken

Diuretics
  acetazolamide
  Aldactazide
  Aldactone
  Aldoclor
  Aldoril
  amiloride
  amiloride/hydrochlorothi-
    azide
  Anhydron

Apresazide
bendroflumethiazide
benzthiazide
bumetanide
Bumex
Capozide
chlorothiazide
chlorthalidone
Combipres
cyclothiazide
Diamox
Diulo
Diupres
Diuril
Diutensen
Dyazide
Dyrenium
Edecrin
Enduron
Esidrix
Esimil
ethacrynic acid
Exna
flumethiazide
furosemide
hydrochlorothiazide
Hydrodiuril
hydroflumethiazide
Hydromox
Hydropres
Hygroton
indapamide
Inderide
Lasix
Lozol
Maxide
Metahydrin
methychlothiazide
metolazone
Midamor
minizide
Moduretic
Naqua
Naquival
Naturetin
Normozide

Oreticyl
polythiazide
quinethazone
Rauzide
Regroton
Renese
Saluron
Salutensin
Ser-Ap-Es
spironolactone
spironolactone/hydrochlo-
    rothiazide
Tenoretic
Timolide
Trandate/HCT
triamterene
triamterene/hydrochlorothi-
    azide
trichlormethiazide
Vaseretic
Zarololyn

Sympathomimetics
    Acutrim
    Afrinol
    amphetamine
    Biphetamine
    caffeine
    decongestants (many cough
        and cold preparations)
    Desoxyn
    Dexatrim
    Dexedrine
    dextroamphetamine
    Didrex
    diethylpropion
    ephedrine
    Fastine
    fenfluramine
    Ionamin
    mazindol
    methamphetamine
    Obetrol
    phendimetrazine
    phenmetrazine
    phentermine

phenylephrine
phenylpropanolamine
Plegine
Pondimin
Preludin
pseudoephedrine
Sanorex
Sudafed
Tenuate
Tepanil

Bronchodilators
  albuterol
  Alupent
  aminophylline
  bitolterol
  Brethine
  Bricanyl
  Bronkaid
  Choledyl
  dyphylline
  epinephrine
  isoetharine
  Isuprel
  Maxair
  Metaprel
  metaproterenol
  oxtriphylline
  pirbuterol
  Primatene
  Proventil
  Slo-phyllin
  terbutaline
  Theo-dur
  theophylline
  Tornalate
  Ventolin

Glucocorticoids
  betamethasone
  Celestone
  cortisone
  Decadron
  dexamethasone
  hydrocortisone
  Medrol

methylprednisolone
prednisolone
prednisone
triamcinolone

Cardiovascular Drugs
  Accupril
  Adalat
  Aldoclor
  Aldomet
  Aldoril
  Altale
  amlodipine
  Apresazide
  Apresoline
  benazepril
  bepridil
  Cadene
  Calan
  Capoten
  Capozide
  captopril
  Cardilate
  Cardizem
  Cardura
  Catapres
  cilazapril
  clonidine
  Combipres
  Dibenzyline
  diltiazem
  Diupres
  Diutensen
  doxazosin
  Dynacirc
  enalapril
  erthrityl tetranitrate
  Esimil
  Eutonyl
  felodipine
  fosinopril
  guanabenz
  guanadrel
  guanethidine
  guanfacine
  hydralazine

Hydropres
Hylurel
Hytrin
Inhibale
Inversine
Ismelin
Isoptin
Isordil
isosorbide dinitrate
isradipine
lisinopril
Loniten
Lotensin
mecamylamine
methyldopa
Minipress
minizide
minoxidil
Monopril
Naquival
nicardipine
nifedipine
nimodipine
Nimotop
Nitro-Bid
nitroglycerin
Norvasc
Oreticyl
pargyline

pentaerythritol tetranitrate
Peritrate
phenoxybenzamine
Plendil
prazosin
Prinivil
Procardia
quinapril
ramipril
Raudixin
rauwolfia
Rauzide
Regroton
reserpine
Salutensin
Ser-Ap-Es
Serpasil
Sorbitrate
Tenex
Tenoretic
terazosin
Transderm-Nitro
Vascor
Vaseretic
Vasotec
verapamil
Wytensin
Zestril

ALPHABETIZED GENERIC AND BRAND NAME LISTING

Reference numbers refer to the drug category discussed in the text chapter. Drugs may be referenced to more than one class of agents if appropriate.

Anti-diabetic agents = 1
Beta-blockers = 2
Diuretics = 3
Sympathomimetics = 4
Bronchodilators = 5
Glucocorticoids = 6
Cardiovascular drugs = 7
    Accupril[7]
    acebutolol[2]
    acetazolamide[3]

acetohexamide[1]
Acutrim [4]
Adalat[7]
Afrinol[4]
albuterol[5]
Aldactazide[3]
Aldactone[3]
Aldoclor[3]
Aldoclor[7]
Aldomet[7]

Aldoril[3,7]
Altale[7]
Alupent[5]
amiloride[3]
amiloride/hydrochlorothiaz-
　　ide[3]
aminophylline[5]
amlodipine[7]
amphetamine[4]
Anhydron[3]
Apresazide[3,7]
Apresoline[7]
atenolol[2]
benazepril[7]
bendroflumethiazide[3]
benzthiazide[3]
bepridil[7]
Betagan[2]
betamethasone[6]
betaxolol[2]
Betoptic[2]
Biphetamine[4]
bitolterol[5]
Blocadren[2]
Brethine[5]
Bricanyl[5]
Bronkaid[5]
bumetanide[3]
Bumex[3]
Cadene[7]
caffeine[4]
Calan[7]
Capoten[7]
Capozide[3,7]
captopril[7]
Cardilate[7]
Cardizem[7]
Cardura[7]
carteolol[2]
Cartrol[2]
Catapres[7]
Celestone[6]
celiprolol[2]
chlorothiazide[3]
chlorpropamide[1]
chlorthalidone[3]

Choledyl[5]
cilazapril[7]
clonidine[7]
Combipres[3,7]
Corgard[2]
cortisone[6]
cyclothiazide[3]
Decadron[6]
decongestants[4]
Desoxyn[4]
dexamethasone[6]
Dexatrim[4]
Dexedrine[4]
dextroamphetamine[4]
Diabenase[1]
Diabeta[1]
Diamox[3]
Dibenzyline[7]
Didrex[4]
diethylpropion[4]
diltiazem[7]
Diulo[3]
Diupres[3]
Diupres[7]
Diuril[3]
Diutensen[3,7]
doxazosin[7]
Dyazide[3]
Dymelor[1]
Dynacirc[7]
dyphylline[5]
Dyrenium[3]
Edecrin[3]
enalapril[7]
Enduron[3]
ephedrine[4]
epinephrine[5]
erthrityl tetranitrate[7]
Esidrix[3]
Esimil[3,7]
ethacrynic acid[3]
Eutonyl[7]
Exna[3]
Fastine[4]
felodipine[7]
fenfluramine[4]

flumethiazide[3]

fosinopril[7]

furosemide[3]

glipizide[1]

Glucotrol[1]

glyburide[1]

guanabenz[7]

guanadrel[7]

guanethidine[7]

guanfacine[7]

hydralazine[7]

hydrochlorothiazide[3]

hydrocortisone[6]

Hydrodiuril[3]

hydroflumethiazide[3]

Hydromox[3]

Hydropres[3,7]

Hygroton[3]

Hylurel[7]

Hytrin[7]

indapamide[3]

Inderal[2]

Inderide[2,3]

Inhibale[7]

insulin (many brands)[1]

Inversine[7]

Ionamin[4]

Ismelin[7]

isoetharine[5]

Isoptin [7]

Isordil[7]

isosorbide dinitrate[7]

isradipine[7]

Isuprel [5]

Kerlone[2]

labetalol[2]

Lasix[3]

Levatol[2]

levobunolol[2]

lisinopril[7]

Loniten[7]

Lopressor[2]

Lotensin[7]

Lozol[3]

Maxair[5]

Maxide[3]

mazindol[4]

mecamylamine[7]

Medrol[6]

Metahydrin[3]

Metaprel[5]

metaproterenol[5]

methamphetamine[4]

methychlothiazide[3]

methyldopa[7]

methylprednisolone[6]

metipranolol[2]

metolazone[3]

metoprolol[2]

Micronase[1]

Midamor[3]

Minipress[7]

minizide[3,7]

minoxidil[7]

Moduretic[3]

Monopril[7]

nadolol[2]

Naqua[3]

Naquival[3,7]

Naturetin[3]

nicardipine[7]

nifedipine[7]

nimodipine[7]

Nimotop[7]

Nitro-Bid[7]

nitroglycerin[7]

Normodyne[2]

Normozide[2,3]

Norvasc[7]

Obetrol[4]

Optipranolol[2]

Oreticyl[3,7]

Orinase[1]

oxtriphylline[5]

pargyline[7]

penbutolol[2]

pentaerythritol tetranitrate[7]

Peritrate [7]

phendimetrazine[4]

phenmetrazine[4]

phenoxybenzamine[7]

phentermine[4]

phenylephrine[4]
phenylpropanolamine[4]
pindolol[2]
pirbuterol[5]
Plegine[4]
Plendil[7]
polythiazide[3]
Pondimin[4]
prazosin[7]
prednisolone[6]
prednisone[6]
Preludin[4]
Primatene [5]
Prinivil[7]
Procardia[7]
propranolol[2]
Proventil[5]
pseudoephedrine[4]
quinapril[7]
quinethazone[3]
ramipril[7]
Raudixin [7]
rauwolfia[7]
Rauzide[3,7]
Regroton[3,7]
Renese[3]
reserpine[7]
Saluron[3]
Salutensin[3,7]
Sanorex[4]
Sectral[2]
Selecor[2]
Ser-Ap-Es[3,7]
Serpasil [7]
Slo-phyllin [5]
Sorbitrate [7]
spironolactone[3]

spironolactone/hydrochlo-
    rothiazide[3]
Sudafed[4]
Tenex[7]
Tenoretic[3,7]
Tenormin[2]
Tenuate[4]
Tepanil[4]
terazosin[7]
terbutaline[5]
Theo-dur[5]
theophylline[5]
Timolide[2,3]
timolol[2]
Timoptic[2]
tolazemide[1]
tolbutamide[1]
Tolinase[1]
Tornalate[5]
Trandate/HCT[3]
Trandate[2]
Transderm-Nitro[7]
triamcinolone[6]
triamterene[3]
triamterene/hydrochlorothi-
    azide[3]
trichlormethiazide[3]
Vascor[7]
Vaseretic[3,7]
Vasotec[7]
Ventolin[5]
verapamil[7]
Visken[2]
Wytensin[7]
Zarololyn[3]
Zestril[7]

Section II

Nutrition

In this section, we begin with an overview of the general nutritional guidelines that have been developed by the major government and scientific organizations for the promotion of health and prevention of disease in the adult population. Next, some of the most important areas of nutritional health relevant to older women in particular are presented. Rather than extensively review every possible nutrient individually, we have chosen to focus on particular nutrients that deserve emphasis by virtue of their relationship to age-related physiologic changes (energy, protein) and diseases (atherosclerosis, osteoporosis) which significantly affect older women. In addition, nutrients that are typically problematic with regard to attainment of appropriate intake (e.g., fat, calcium, vitamin D) are highlighted. Finally, a look at nutrient intake as a pathway to optimization of health rather than simply prevention of disease or deficiency states is explored in depth in the chapter on vitamin E and other antioxidants. Such nutrients span the gulf between pharmacology and nutrition in many ways, as their utility is explored for the prevention and treatment of such diverse pathological conditions as dementia, Parkinson's disease, cataracts, infectious disease and immune response, cancer, arthritis, and heart disease.

Such a broad approach to nutritional intake is consistent with the newly developed Dietary Reference Intakes (DRIs) that are now being released by the Standing Committee on the Scientific Evaluation of Dietary Reference Intakes of the Food and Nutrition Board, Institute of Medicine, National Academy of Sciences and Health Canada. This new approach, which was requested by the National Institute of Health, the U.S. Food and Drug Administration, and the Agricultural Research Service of the U.S. Department of Agriculture, replaces the 1989 Recommended Daily Allowances (RDAs) that have been published in several revised formats since 1941.

The DRIs are new in that they encompass several levels of recommended intake for the population at different ages. They include the Estimated Average Requirement

(EAR), the Recommended Daily Allowance (RDA), the Adequate Intake (AI), and the Tolerable Upper Limit Intake Level (UL) to provide ranges for both adequacy and toxicity when data are available. The RDA and AI nutrient intake levels are those that have been estimated to decrease the risk of developing a condition related to a nutrient or associated with a negative functional outcome in a healthy general population. Intake at these levels would not, however, necessarily be sufficient to replete currently malnourished individuals nor to treat active disease. In these cases, specific adaptations of the general provisions are recommended in collaboration with relevant health care professionals. More detail on the specifics of these new guidelines is given in Chapter 23. It should be noted that some nutritional requirements are changing as new experimental and epidemiological data are analyzed, and differences among age groups are better defined. The nutrients presented in this section are those for which a reasonable amount of solid scientific evidence exists, and for which clear linkages can be made between health status and nutrient intake in older women.

4 General Nutrition

Christina D. Economos

CONTENTS

GENERAL INFORMATION

Today's mature woman is part of the unique Baby Boomer cohort that shares a life expectancy of close to 80 years, greater than any generation in history. She is concerned about her health, but unlike previous generations, she is individualistic, solution-oriented, and ready to take charge. Although she will experience the predictable physiologic changes in taste, smell, chewing, and digestion that occur with aging, she has the advantage of new research which demonstrates that improving eating habits and nutritional intake is effective at any age. In addition, a better understanding of an older woman's nutritional needs has made remaining healthy with age entirely possible. Since food choice affects multiple aspects of health including physical and mental performance and the ability to battle illness, deal with stress, and prevent disease, the importance of an adequate or perhaps optimal nutritional intake should not be underestimated.

A healthy diet begins with a sound foundation, and to build it, the right tools, or in this case, the nutritional know-how is required. There is no perfect or exact time to establish the foundation. Taking the right steps is advisable at any point in life. Important to understand, however, is the fact that we choose foods based on our eating habits, which have developed over time and throughout life. The longer eating habits have been followed, the harder they are to change. Understanding the complex personal and societal influences on eating habits such as flavor, cost, familiarity, availability, knowledge, occupation, income, religious beliefs, health status, cultural background, advertising, and lifestyle, will help change them to a healthier form.

Nutrition is more than just the food we choose to eat. The science of nutrition encompasses all the interactions that occur between living organisms and the nutrients in food. These include the body's ingestion, digestion, absorption, transport, metabolism, storage, and excretion of nutrients. Nutrients are chemical substances that provide energy, structure, and regulation of body processes. To date, approximately 45 nutrients must be supplied by the diet and are known as essential for human life. The six classes of nutrients are carbohydrate, fat, protein, vitamins, minerals, and water. When food is metabolized in the body, carbohydrate, fat, and protein are broken down to yield energy, measured in calories, which supports all of the activities we perform. The carbohydrate and protein in food supply 4 calories per gram, and fat supplies 9 calories per gram. The vitamins, minerals, and water do not provide energy, but help in metabolic, structural, and regulatory processes in the body.

NUTRITIONAL RECOMMENDATIONS AND GUIDELINES

Practicing good nutrition requires an understanding of which types of foods and how much of these foods you need. To aid in this process, the federal government and various non-profit agencies convene national committees of nutrition experts to assume responsibility for defining the types and amounts of dietary factors that best support health. Currently, the nutritional recommendations for the public focus on health promotion and chronic disease prevention. Recommendations provide outlines of optimal dietary intakes, which, if followed consistently, will reduce the chance of developing a diet-related disease. This is quite different from the turn of the century, when nutrition scientists were concerned with nutritional deficiencies due to inadequate nutrient consumption and the safety of the food supply. These shifts reflect the many advances that have occurred in the field of nutrition over the years.

The dietary standards in the United States are the Recommended Dietary Allowances (RDAs), originally developed in 1940.[1] The RDAs are revised at regular intervals based on the latest information in the scientific literature. RDAs for protein, vitamins, and minerals are determined by estimating the average requirement of a nutrient in a population and then adding a margin of safety to allow for variability among individuals. They are not minimum or optimal requirements, but are designed to meet the needs of practically all healthy persons. RDAs are standards used to define food and nutrition regulations, plan and develop nutrition education programs, and evaluate adequacy of the U.S. food supply. Although these standards are still used today, a variety of new recommendations are more appropriate for individuals to plan and construct healthy diets.

The *Dietary Guidelines for Americans* were established in 1980 by the U.S. Department of Agriculture (USDA) and the Department of Health and Human Services (DHHS) and have been updated every five years to reflect current research.[2] The *Guidelines* are designed to help direct food choices over the course of a day or week. The current dietary guidelines are

- Eat a variety of foods.
- Balance the food you eat with physical activity to maintain or improve your weight.
- Choose a diet with plenty of grain products, vegetables, and fruits.

- Choose a diet low in fat, saturated fat, and cholesterol.
- Choose a diet moderate in sugars.
- Choose a diet moderate in salt and sodium.
- If you drink alcoholic beverages, do so in moderation.

In an effort to provide practical information, *The Food Guide Pyramid: A Guide to Daily Food Choices* was developed in 1992, also by the USDA and the DHHS.[3] The pyramid (Figure 1) provides an outline of what to eat each day based on the *Guidelines*, and allows people to individualize their dietary intakes.

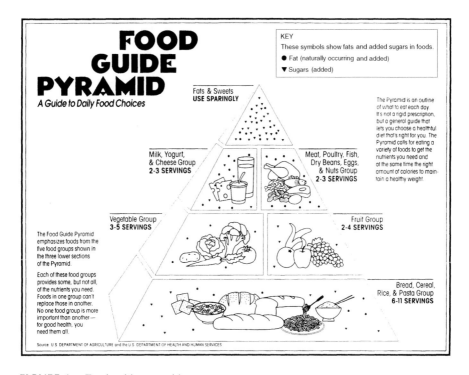

FIGURE 1   Food guide pyramid.

A GUIDE TO DAILY FOOD CHOICES

The pyramid is not a rigid prescription, but a general guide that encourages individuals to choose a healthful diet that is right for you. The pyramid calls for eating a variety of foods to get the nutrients you need, balancing the right amount of calories to maintain a healthy weight, and practicing moderation. It shows that it is best to eat more foods from the bottom and fewer from the top and illustrates the number of servings needed from the five sections. The pyramid promotes a plant-based diet with the target intake being 55% of daily calories from carbohydrate, 15% of calories from protein and, at the most, 30% of calories from fat with saturated fat making up no more than one third of total fat (or less than 10% of daily calories). Plants contain significant amounts of fiber, vitamins, and minerals. They contain no cholesterol, and, in general, supply protein and a healthy, unsaturated form of fat.

Eating a variety of foods is the key to good nutrition and to providing different textures, flavors, colors, and odors, which are all important components of food. Choosing different foods from each group (grain products, fruits, vegetables, milk and milk products, and meats and meat alternatives) provides the body with the different nutrients it needs for good health and guarantees variety. Older women require the same variety of foods as younger individuals, but some nutrients are needed in higher amounts. For example, the withdrawal of estrogen at menopause increases an older woman's need for calcium and vitamin D, which makes her requirement for calcium-rich foods such as dairy products high. The pyramid also promotes choosing nutrient-dense foods meaning that there is a relatively rich supply of nutrients in comparison with energy content.

HOW MANY CALORIES DOES THE OLDER WOMAN NEED?

To simplify things, the pyramid deals with the number of servings rather than the percentages of calories from each energy-yielding nutrient. The number of servings consumed depends on how many calories you need, but almost everyone should have the lowest number of servings in the ranges. A woman's activity level plays a large role in determining her energy (calorie) requirements: 1200 to 1600 calories are about right for most inactive to moderately active older women, 1800 to 2200 calories are about right for active to very active older women, 2400 to 2800 calories are about right for extremely active older women. It is important to realize that at the same time an older woman's energy requirements decrease, due to lower levels of activity, her nutrient requirements increase, leading to a need for a more nutrient-dense diet. In other words, the food that she does eat should be wholesome and highly nutritious. Table 1 shows sample daily diets for different calorie levels.

TABLE 1
Sample Daily Diets

Number of Servings from	Low 1200–1600	Moderate 1800–2200	High 2400–2800
Bread group	6	9	11
Vegetable group	3	4	5
Fruit group	2	3	4
Milk group	2–3*	2–3*	2–3*
Meat and meat alternative group (ounces)	5	6	7
Total fat (grams)	53	73	93
Total added sugars (tsp.)	6	12	18

*Teenagers and young adults, women who are pregnant or breast-feeding and women past menopause are advised to have 3 servings.

THE TIP OF THE PYRAMID

Certain foods need to be kept under control or consumed in moderation. The tip of the pyramid shows that fats, oils, and sweets fall under this classification. Foods like salad dressings, cream, butter, margarine, sugars, soft drinks, and colas, candies, and sweet deserts, along with alcoholic beverages, may tantalize the taste buds but when consumed in excess, can wreak havoc on a balanced diet. In general, these foods are low in nutritional value, but if they currently have a place in the older woman's diet, deprivation may not be the answer. It makes more sense to advise moderation; shaping behavior by reducing rather than totally eliminating these foods. Never say never to favorite foods; neither health nor weight is largely affected by minor eating indiscretions. It is the habitual indulgences that lead to inability to maintain a health body weight or increase the risk for chronic diseases. Balancing poor food choices with nutrient-wise choices at the next meal is a good approach. There are no good foods and bad foods; in fact, there is room for most foods in the diet. To maintain a healthy diet, how much and how often particular foods are consumed is the main issue.

A few other guidelines for general health and disease prevention have been issued within the last decade and continue to drive current recommendations and policy. These include *Healthy People 2000: National Health Promotion and Disease Prevention Objectives* (1990),[4,5] the *Five a Day for Better Health Program* (1991),[6] *Diet and Health: Implications for Reducing Chronic Disease Risk* (1989),[7] and the *Surgeon General's Report on Nutrition and Health* (1988).[8] These reports overlap considerably and share a number of themes, as they are based on the same research findings. In general, the common guidelines include consuming more complex carbohydrate and plant food with adequate fiber, less high fat animal food, sodium, sugar, and alcohol, and maintaining a healthy body weight through appropriate food consumption and adequate exercise. Their main objectives are to promote healthful lifestyles and reduce preventable death and disability for all Americans.

REFERENCES

1. National Research Council, *Recommended Dietary Allowances*, 10th ed., National Academy Press, Washington, D.C., 1990.
2. USDA, *Dietary Guidelines for Americans*, Government Printing Office, Washington, D.C., 1996.
3. USDA, *Food Pyramid: A Guide to Daily Food Choices*, U.S. Department of Agriculture, Human Information Service, Washington, D.C., 1992.
4. Public Health Service, *Healthy People 2000: National Health Promotion and Disease Prevention Objectives*. Full report with commentary, U.S. Department of Health and Human Services, Washington, D.C., 1991.
5. National Center for Health Statistics, *Healthy People 2000 Review, 1995–96*, Public Health Service, Hyattsville, MD, 1996.
6. Institute, NC, *5 A Day for Better Health*, National Cancer Institute Office of Communications, Washington, D.C., 1991.
7. National Research Council/Food and Nutrition Board, *Diet and Health: Implications for Reducing Chronic Disease Risk*, National Academy Press, Washington, D.C., 1989.
8. Public Health Service, *Surgeon General's Report on Nutrition and Health*, Washington, D.C., 1988.

5 Energy

Susan B. Roberts

CONTENTS

ENERGY BASICS

How many calories does an older woman really need? A calorie is a unit of energy, and to a scientist the terms "caloric needs" and "energy requirements" mean the same thing. In the past, the seemingly simple question of "How much energy does a person require" has been answered by scientists asking healthy weight-stable people what they usually eat. However, this approach tends to *underestimate* normal caloric requirements because some people are embarrassed to admit to all the bad foods they consume and, in addition, the very act of recording food consumption makes many people subconsciously consume less than they normally do.

A better way to provide guidelines on caloric requirements is to estimate *energy expenditure*—the calories one actually burns for different essential needs. If an individual is not gaining or losing weight, this implies a balanced energy equation, in which total energy expenditure will be the same as caloric intake. Total energy expenditure is often divided into three major categories. *Basal energy expenditure* is the energy one expends when lying down completely at rest and represents energy needs for someone who never moves, eats, or gets out of bed. In most young adults this component of total energy expenditure represents about half of the total energy expenditure. The second largest component of total energy expenditure, about 40% of total energy expenditure, is the *energy expenditure for physical activity*—this is the energy expended for all movement, whether strenuous or not. Finally, there is a third component of total energy expenditure, called the *thermic effect of feeding*. This component, which contributes about 10% to the total energy expenditure, is the energy used to do the work of digesting, processing, and storing consumed food.

As people get older, there is a strong tendency for the total energy expenditure to decrease. This decrease happens in both women and men because of decreases in energy expenditure for all the three major components of energy expenditure. Basal energy expenditure decreases because muscle mass is lost, as does energy expenditure for physical activity and also for the thermic effect of feeding, since the total amount of food eaten and processed is generally less. In addition, however, there is a disproportionate decrease in energy expenditure for physical activity. As shown in Figure 1 below, in a typical woman aged 60 years, basal metabolism represents nearly two thirds of the total energy expenditure, the thermic effect of feeding about 10%, and the remainder, only 23%, is energy expenditure for physical activity. If a woman decreases energy expenditure in physical activity in this way without a concomitant decrease in energy intake, the result can only be an energy imbalance, in which more is consumed than needed. Excess calories consumed are stored as fat, and the prevalence of such imbalances are attested to by the many studies reporting an increase in adipose tissue mass and obesity with age.

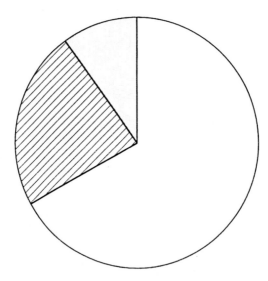

FIGURE 1   Pie chart showing how total energy expenditure is divided in typical sedentary women. An estimated 67% of total energy expenditure is used for basal energy expenditure, 23% is used for energy expenditure for physical activity, and 10% is used for the thermic effect of feeding.

INDIVIDUAL VARIABILITY

The values given in Section 1 are for the average person. However, very few people are average, and there is a lot of individual variability in energy needs. Many factors contribute to the determination of whether someone's energy needs are high or low relative to this average. In particular, several factors are important.

- *Gender.* Women have lower energy needs than men, secondary to lower basal metabolic rates, lower muscle mass, and lower energy expenditure in physical activity on average.
- *Body weight.* If an individual weighs less than average (because they are short or thin), their energy needs will be less than someone who is heavy.

- *Physical activity.* The more active one is, the more energy expended. Activities that are not too strenuous and are part of everyday activities of daily living (for example, walking) can often contribute more to total energy expenditure than very vigorous activities, because they are done more often and for longer periods of time. All physical activity is not alike with respect to its effect on the components of energy expenditure. Exercise which is anabolic in nature (such as weight-lifting exercise) can cause hypertrophy of the skeletal muscle to offset the decline in basal metabolic rate seen with age. In addition, this type of exercise has been known to increase basal metabolism apart from any changes in measurable muscle mass thought to be related to changes in muscle protein turnover. It also has a caloric expenditure of its own (approximately 100 to 150 calories per hour) increasing the thermic effect of feeding slightly, and has been shown to produce ease in spontaneous physical activities and walking apart from the exercise session itself. This combination of effects makes resistance training an attractive option for favorably influencing energy balance in the older woman. Aerobic activities by contrast do not increase muscle mass, have a variable effect on basal metabolic rate, and have not been shown to increase other forms of physical activity through-out the week.
- *Genetics.* There are significant genetic influences on both basal energy expenditure and energy expenditure for physical activity. Some families simply expend less energy than others or metabolize fat less efficiently, for reasons that are not yet clear. It should be remembered, however, that these genetic differences in metabolism are usually small compared to the large energy imbalances caused by excess intake relative to needs and reduced energy expenditure in physical activity.
- *Body composition.* People with a high percentage of fat in their body expend less energy than leaner individuals. This happens for two reasons. First, fat is not very metabolically active—in other words, it does not need as much energy to keep working as other body components such as muscle. Second, people who have a lot of fat tend to be less physically active, because physical activity is more difficult for them, and so also expend less energy for this component of energy needs.
- *Age.* With advancing age, basal energy expenditure decreases even if body weight stays the same, primarily due to the decline in lean body mass and muscle mass with age. Energy expenditure for physical activity also typically decreases although this change is not inevitable at all, but rather related to societal expectations, lack of role models, retirement, reduced opportunities for exposure to appropriate activities, and in some cases, an increasing burden of chronic diseases and disabilities. Some, but not all, research studies also suggest that menopause causes a decrease in basal energy expenditure and energy expenditure for phys-ical activity.

- *Disease.* Chronic diseases may also affect energy requirements beyond those attributable to the above factors. Some diseases increase energy requirements either due to effects on basal metabolism (e.g., hyperthyroidism) or neuromuscular activity (Parkinson's disease or causes of tremor). Wasting may result if caloric intake cannot match these requirements, and this is often the case clinically. Other diseases characterized by a high level of cytokines such as rheumatoid arthritis and congestive heart failure may also result in elevated metabolic rates and wasting of skeletal muscle. Many diseases are accompanied by reduced energy needs secondary to the disability, muscle atrophy, and disuse which accompany them, leading to low levels of physical activity, and ultimately, lower than normal caloric requirements for weight maintenance. However, because these same disease processes and the medications used to treat them are often associated with anorexia or reduced appetite, weight loss rather than weight gain is often the clinical sequel of prolonged chronic illness.

PHYSICAL ACTIVITY REVISITED

As explained above, physical activity is not usually the biggest component of total energy expenditure. However, it is the component that we can do most to change. If you expend more energy through increasing physical activity, your energy needs will be higher and you will be more easily able to maintain a stable weight while eating a generous diet. Moreover, as explained in other chapters, physical activity builds muscles, strengthens bones, and has a variety of other beneficial effects on body metabolism. For this reason, it is important to know what is expended for different activities. Table 1 lists common activities and their energy costs. The costs are expressed as multiples of basal energy expenditure, actual caloric equivalents, as well as food equivalents. Thus, cooking typically uses only 80% more than lying in bed, while walking slowly uses three times as much. It can be seen, however, that it is quite difficult to offset large volumes of food consumption with exercise alone, which is why weight reduction programs must focus on a combination of caloric restriction plus physical activity.

Physical activity also has effects on energy expenditure in addition to the immediate costs of the activities. In particular, physical activity helps to build muscle, if it involves resistive activities, and this muscle needs energy to function. Thus, there is an increase in basal energy expenditure when regular physical activity increases muscle mass. In addition, recent studies have shown that regular physical activity actually "revs up" basal metabolism quite independent of any change in body size or composition. This is as true in older individuals as in younger ones. Finally, physical activity helps the body to oxidize dietary fat. Many scientists believe that an inability to oxidize dietary fat is an important cause of obesity in both the young and the old.

TABLE 1
Energy Costs of Different Activities Conducted for One Hour[a]

Activity	Energy Cost (Calories Above Basal Metabolism)	Food Equivalent	Energy Cost (Multiple of Basal Metabolism)
Sedentary Activities			
Sleeping	0	$1/4$ small cookie	1.0
Lying down awake	10	$1/4$ small cookie	1.2
Sitting quietly	10	$1/2$ small cookie	1.2
Sitting plus activity, e.g., sewing	20	$1/2$ small cookie	1.4
Standing	25	$1/2$ small cookie	1.5
Walking			
Walking slowly	100	2 $1/4$ small cookies	3.0
Walking at normal pace	120	2 $1/2$ small cookies	3.4
Walking normally and carrying heavy load	155	3 $1/2$ small cookies	4.0
Walking uphill at normal pace	185	4 small cookies	4.6
Walking downhill at normal pace	100	2 $1/4$ small cookies	3.0
Household			
Light cleaning	85	2 small cookies	2.7
Sweeping	100	2 $1/4$ small cookies	3.0
Ironing	25	$1/2$ small cookie	1.5
Cooking	40	1 small cookie	1.8
Recreational Sports			
Light activities (golf, bowling, sailing)	60–175	1 $3/4$–4 small cookies	2.2–4.4
Moderate activities (dancing, swimming, tennis)	175–285	4–6 $1/3$ small cookies	4.4–6.6
Heavy activities	285+	6 $1/3$ small cookies+	6.6+

[a] Data recalculated from WHO, Energy and Protein Requirements. Technical Report Series 724, 1985.

HOW TO ESTIMATE TOTAL ENERGY NEEDS

Total energy needs can be predicted based on one's age, gender, weight, and estimated activity level. Although this does not take into account genetic history, it can give the best assessment of individual energy needs. As shown in Tables 2 and 3 (which are for healthy 55- and 70-year-old women), depending on weight and activity level, energy requirements can differ by nearly 100%. Note that these values are quite a lot less than the energy requirements of men, primarily because men have larger bodies with more muscle mass and this larger size increases caloric requirements. Many women will have activity patterns that make them suitable for the light activity category; they do not do regular vigorous exercise and do not regularly walk for exercise or climb stairs. If an older woman currently fits this category, she can move up to the moderate activity category and at the same time improve her health by including exercise of a moderate intensity (walking, dancing, gardening, swimming, biking) several times per week. With a regular vigorous program of exercise (jogging, singles tennis, high-intensity weight lifting, stairclimbing, powerwalking, etc.), she may even move up to the heavy activity category.

TABLE 2
Expected Total Energy Requirements for Women at Age 55

Weight (lb)	Basal Metabolism	Light Activity	Moderate Activity	Heavy Activity
100	1224	1714	1958	2203
110	1264	1770	2022	2275
120	1304	1826	2086	2347
130	1343	1880	2149	2417
140	1383	1936	2213	2489
150	1422	1991	2275	2560
160	1462	2047	2339	2632
170	1501	2104	2402	2702
180	1541	2157	2466	2774
190	1580	2212	2528	2844
200	1620	2268	2592	2916
210	1659	2323	2654	2986
220	1699	2379	2718	3058
230	1739	2435	2782	3130
240	1778	2489	2845	3200
250	1818	2545	2909	3272

Finally, an important point for older women to remember is that age is sometimes associated with loss of the ability to accurately regulate body weight. Young women and men have internal sensors for how many calories they should be eating. Scientists don't know how these sensors work but they are clearly very valuable. Recent research has indicated that the sensors can be lost in some older persons. Sometimes this is due to factors such as depression or a loss of taste sensitivity. In addition, some scientists believe that the bodily mechanisms that govern food intake actually get lost with advancing age. These factors can, in turn, make it easier to gain weight or even lose weight (also potentially dangerous), depending on life circumstances, and necessitate an increased vigilance over what food is consumed. While advising someone to watch caloric intake, also remember that fat calories are not the same as carbohydrate calories. There is a very slight tendency for the body to store fat calories more readily than carbohydrate calories, therefore limiting the proportion of the diet that is consumed as fat calories, as well as the total energy intake, may

TABLE 3
Expected Total Energy Requirements for Women at Age 70

Weight (lb)	Basal Metabolism	Light Activity	Moderate Activity	Heavy Activity
100	1073	1502	1663	1824
110	1121	1569	1738	1906
120	1169	1637	1812	1987
130	1216	1702	1885	2067
140	1264	1770	1959	2149
150	1312	1836	2034	2230
160	1360	1904	2108	2312
170	1407	1970	2181	2392
180	1455	2037	2255	2474
190	1503	2104	2330	2555
200	1551	2171	2404	2637
210	1598	2237	2477	2717
220	1646	2304	2551	2798
230	1694	2372	2626	2880
240	1741	2437	2699	2960
250	1789	2505	2773	3041

be important for weight control. In addition, many scientists believe that eating a high fat diet will encourage overeating by increasing hunger. Behaviorally, as well as metabolically, the caloric density of high fat foods makes it much easier to consume calories in this compact form, compared to the low caloric density of a high carbohydrate diet.

In conclusion, an understanding of the components of energy expenditure and their changes with age will help develop guidelines for older women to achieve and maintain a stable body weight and composition. Despite genetic influences on energy balance beyond our control, there are clearly modifiable components in this equation related to optimal body composition, modalities and quantities of physical activity recommended, and dietary composition that can be addressed with lifestyle changes.

REFERENCES

1. FAO, WHO, UNU, Energy and protein requirements, Report of a joint FAO/WHO/UNU expert consultation, Technical Report Series 724, in Geneva: World Health Organization, 1985.
2. Poehlman, E. T., Melby, C. L., Badylak, S. F., and Calles, J., Aerobic fitness and resting energy expenditure in young adult males, *Metab.*, 38, 85–90, 1989.
3. Poehlman, E. T., McAuliffe, T. L., Van Houten, D. R., and Danforth, E. J., Influence of age and endurance training on metabolic rate and hormones in healthy men, *Am. J. Physiol.*, 259, E66–E72, 1990.

4. Roberts, S. B., Young, V. R., Fuss, P., Heyman, M. B., Fiatarone, M. A., Dallal, G. E., and Evans, W. J., What are the dietary energy needs of elderly adults? *Int. J. Obesity,* 16, 969–976, 1992.

5. Roberts, S. B., Fuss, P., Heyman, M. B., Evans, W. J., Tsay, R., Rasmussen, H., Fiatarone, M., Cortiella, J., Dallal, G. E., and Young, V. R., Control of food intake in older men, *JAMA,* 272, 1601–1606, 1994.

6. Sawaya, A. L., Saltzman, E., Fuss, P., Young, V. R., and Roberts, S. B., Dietary energy requirements of young and older women, determined by using the doubly labeled water method, *Am. J. Clin. Nutr.,* 62, 338–344, 1995.

6 Protein

Carmen Castaneda Sceppa

CONTENTS

PROTEIN AND AGING

Aging affects muscle mass, physiologic function, metabolism, and nutrient requirements.[1a] As people age there is a decline in basal metabolic rate and physical activity, with a corresponding reduction in energy needs. Aging is also associated with a greater susceptibility to nutritional deficiencies. Body protein content is particularly affected during the aging process due to decreased food intake, impaired absorption and retention of dietary protein, and decreased body protein synthesis. These factors lead to a significant decrease in total body protein, with skeletal muscle reserves being primarily affected.[1b] During the course of adult life, body protein in the form of muscle mass diminishes progressively while body fat increases (Figure 1),[1b] so body weight may not necessarily change. The muscle of older women represents about 27% of total body weight compared to 45% observed in women at a younger age.[2,3]

    The age-related physiologic changes the body experiences, in particular the loss of muscle mass as age progresses, may in fact be associated with decreases in health, vitality, vigor, and independence. This is true because the threshold at which muscle strength determines function gets closer to the known age-related decrease in muscle mass. At advanced age muscle mass, translated into muscle size and muscle strength, becomes a prime determinant of function.[4] However, physiologic as well as disease-related changes that occur with aging are variable and potentially modifiable or reversible, by controlling environmental and lifestyle factors, such as diet and physical activity.[5] This approach will have an effect on health promotion and disease prevention with the ultimate aim of improving quality of life at older age.

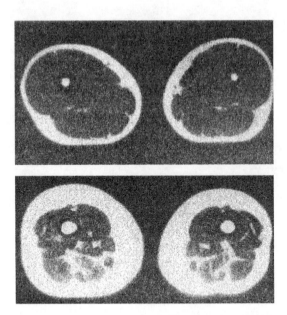

FIGURE 1   These two magnetic resonance images show the proportion of muscle versus fat in young and older women. Top. A 20-year-old athlete. Bottom. A sedentary 64-year-old woman. (From Katz, H., Ed., *Biomarkers. The 10 Determinants of Aging You Can Control*, Simon & Schuster, New York, 1991, 39–84. With permission.)

PROTEIN NEEDS

Different nutrients are needed for the body to maintain health and vitality. Protein is one of those nutrients. Twenty percent of the body is formed by or utilizes protein in one or another form, from holding bones and organs together, maintaining daily metabolic functions (e.g., digestion of foods, menstrual cycle, blood clotting, visual processes, immune function, etc.) to repairing and/or replacing tissues.[6] The proteins the body uses for all these functions are located in skeletal muscle and in visceral organs such as liver, kidneys, heart, and brain. The body does not store excess protein like it does fat as adipose tissue or carbohydrates as glycogen in muscle. If protein is plentiful in the diet, the body will use what it requires for daily functions, and the excess will be eliminated through urine, fecal matter, expired air, sweat, etc.[7] On the other hand, if someone does not eat enough protein to meet his/her bodily needs, the body will "steal" the protein contained in skeletal muscle and viscera to make up for this need. This will result in detrimental effects in the body's daily functions.[8] Thus, for body growth and maintenance, amino acids must be constantly supplied from foods.

The role of protein in food is to supply amino acids, the building blocks of proteins, from which the body can make its own proteins. For this to happen, dietary protein has to be of good quality.[9] There are about twenty different types of amino acids, most of which the body can make from scratch, and thus are referred to as non-essential. There are, however, nine of these amino acids that the body is unable to make; they can be obtained only through the diet. This group of amino acids is called essential because the body cannot make them, but they are very important constituents of the proteins needed for the body to function adequately.[9]

Good quality protein refers to protein in food that contains all nine essential amino acids. Animal protein by definition is considered good quality protein, with eggs being the reference protein to which any other protein is compared.[10] Dietary protein coming from a single plant source such as grains, cereals, legumes, and nuts may not necessarily be considered good quality protein. Individual plant protein sources, unlike animal protein sources, lack one or more essential amino acids. Thus eating just one plant protein source may not be good enough to provide all essential amino acids to the human body. Vegetarians who eat eggs, milk, and dairy products do not have a problem getting dietary protein of good quality. However, strict vegetarians referred to as "vegans," who do not eat milk or eggs, have to plan their food menus very carefully to make sure they eat different plant sources to get good quality protein in a day's worth of meals. This practice will assure that there is an adequate sustained supply of essential amino acids to be used in the long term. Mixed diets generally provide good quality protein because a complementary protein pattern results from it.[11]

If an individual does not get enough protein in the diet, the question arises as to whether or not amino acid supplementation is advisable, since the digestive system overall will handle whole body protein better than predigested protein from supplements. The body breaks down protein in foods and absorbs amino acids at rates that are optimal, thus facilitating the body's later use of amino acids to make proteins as needed. Protein and amino acid supplements may create an imbalance of the amino acids received from the diet. Amino acid supplements may, in fact, compete with food amino acids for absorption in the gastrointestinal tract, and subsequent usage in different tissues and organs. Amino acid supplements can also be toxic to the body if ingested in large quantities. A rare blood disorder called eosinophilia-myalgia has been linked to the use of supplements of the amino acid tryptophan. This condition leads to severe muscle and joint pain, swelling in the limbs, skin rash, and fever.[11] Thus, it may be safer to obtain the essential amino acids through rich-protein food sources that also contain other important nutrients which facilitate the use of amino acids by the body.

PROTEIN REQUIREMENTS

The next logical question, after having determined the importance of providing good quality amino acids in the diet, is how much dietary protein is considered adequate to maintain health and vitality. The Recommended Dietary Allowance or RDA for protein has been defined by the National Research Council as the lowest level of dietary protein intake needed to maintain adequate body protein in 97.5% of healthy individuals.[10] The RDA for protein based on a mixed American diet is estimated to be 0.8 grams per kilogram body weight per day. The reference women over 50 years of age with an approximate body weight of 60 kilograms (equivalent to 132 pounds) should eat about 48 grams of protein per day. In setting the RDA, a scientific advisory committee has assumed that people are healthy; that the protein eaten is of good quality; that the protein represents between 12 to 15% of the total energy intake, with sufficient energy coming from carbohydrates and fat; and that people's physical activity is light-to-moderate, that is, sitting, standing, and walking around to household tasks and playing.[9] A survey done in the Boston area showed that older women eating a typical American diet consume between 1.0 and 1.2 grams of protein per kilogram body weight per day or well above the RDA.[12]

There are too many assumptions regarding the RDA for protein. The fact of the matter is that older women who tend to be smaller than men and are more likely to be on weight loss diets, eating less calories and proteins, are at higher risk for muscle loss as well as functional consquences of muscle loss. It is important to remember that as a result of getting older there is already a loss of protein, mostly in the form of skeletal muscle mass associated with the aging process. Thus, any additional loss will jeopardize older women's health and vitality. Modifying environmental and lifestyle practices such as diet and physical activity will help prevent or counteract these losses regardless of age.[13]

As for diet, good quality protein sources are found in animal and plant foodstuffs. Animal protein sources such as meat, milk, and eggs have always been thought of as the best source of protein. However, these protein sources are very high in saturated fat and cholesterol content. Alternative food exchanges are skim milk, low-fat dairy products, skinned meat, etc., which provide good quality protein and at the same time are low in saturated fat content. Other good sources of protein come from plants, such as legumes (garden peas; green, lime, pinto, and garbanzo beans; lentils and soybean), grains, seeds, and nuts. These not only contribute to an adequate protein intake but also vitamins, minerals, and dietary fiber, all of which are very important and needed nutrients for the body. Legumes and cereals are also low-fat food sources. Table 1 shows an example of non-meat food mixtures that provide good quality protein based on the Recommended Dietary Allowance.

Too Little Protein

If dietary protein (mainly an exogenous source of essential amino acids) is not enough or adequate, the body will "steal" protein from muscle mass and vital organs (endogenous) to maintain important metabolic functions. In other words, the body will adapt to a less than adequate dietary protein intake by using up some of the amino acids present in active metabolic tissues such as skeletal muscle and viscera. If the lack of enough dietary protein is very large or sustained for weeks or months, there is no way the body can continue functioning without using almost all its endogenous protein. This process is called *accommodation*. Accommodation is defined as the body's effort to maintain a steady state at the expense of its own protein constituents (e.g., muscle and viscera) ultimately resulting in inadequate physical and immune function.[9,14] This phenomena has also been observed under experimental conditions in healthy elderly women fed marginal protein diets of approximately half the RDA for a period of 10 weeks.[15,16]

Sustained protein deficiency, usually accompanied by energy deficiency, leads to protein-energy malnutrition (PEM), the most widespread form of malnutrition worldwide. PEM is mostly prevalent in developing countries. In the U.S. it is not commonly seen, except in some subpopulations such as minorities, poor inner cities, and rural

TABLE 1
Non-Meat Dietary Protein Sources[a]

Food and Serving Sizes[b]	Lacto-Ovo Vegetarian[c]	Vegan[d]
Grains, Legumes, Nuts, and Seeds	7+ servings	11+ servings plus
1 slice bread or ½-¾ cup rice or pasta		2–3 servings legumes
1 ounce ready-to-eat cereal or ½-¾ cup cooked cereal		plus 2 servings nuts/seeds
1-1 ½ cups cooked dry beans or 1 ½-1 cup nuts or 2 tablespoons peanut butter		
Vegetables	3+ servings	5+ servings
1 cup raw leafy vegetables (include one dark green or leafy)		
½ cup raw or cooked vegetables or 3-4 small crackers		
Fruits	2+ servings	3+ servings
¼ cup dried fruit or ½ cup cooked fruit or ¾ cup juice		
1 whole piece fruit or 1 melon wedge		
Milk, Yogurt, Cheese	2+ servings	None
1 cup milk or yogurt or 1 ½ cups ice cream or 1 cup custard or pudding		
1 ½ ounces cheese or 2 ounces processed cheese or 2 cups cottage cheese		

[a] These menus contain approximately 1.5 times the RDA for protein.
[b] Serving sizes are based on the Food Guide Pyramid.
[c] Contains about 75 grams of protein in 1650 calories.
[d] Contains about 79 grams of protein in 1800 calories.

From Wardlaw, G. M. et al., *Contemporary Nutrition, Issues and Insights*, Mosby, Baltimore, 1994. With permission.

areas. There is evidence though that a large number of older women consume diets low in protein. The NHANES II indicates that the diets of 10 to 25% of American women over 55 years of age contain less than 30 grams of protein per day.[17] Adult PEM is also present in hospitalized patients suffering from cancer, tuberculosis, AIDS, kidney and liver disease, or in self-starvation disorders such as anorexia nervosa.

Although too little protein is a concern among very selected subpopulations in the United States, it may be a potentially dangerous problem which has a simple solution. PEM can be reversible as long as the underlying medical cause of the deficiency is treated or an adequate dietary protein supply is provided. Therefore, an amount equivalent to the RDA for protein is important in order to maintain metabolic processes, thereby decreasing the risk of infections, disease, and eventually death.[18] An adequate amount of dietary protein will help maintain good health, as well as youth, vitality, vigor, and independence of older women. All these are very important factors of healthy aging.

Too Much Protein

The majority of the American population, consuming a typical American diet, eat one to two times the RDA for protein. This is equivalent to 0.8 to 1.6 grams of protein per kilogram body weight per day. No detrimental effects have been identified with intakes of protein as high as twice the RDA; however, diets too high in protein offer no benefits. Protein-rich foods are often fat-rich foods with high content of cholesterol and saturated fats, as mentioned before. The higher a person's intake of animal protein-rich foods, the lower the amount of plant protein sources, which also provide other important nutrients such as vitamins, minerals, and fiber.[11]

There is some evidence that excess dietary protein intake stresses kidney function, and may increase the age-related changes in kidney function.[19] Protecting the kidney is important for healthy people in general, but it is especially important in people suffering from hypertension, recurrent bladder infections, diabetes, liver, and kidney diseases. In fact, many doctors may prescribe a low protein diet to patients with renal failure for therapeutic reasons.[20] In addition to kidney function, epidemiological studies have shown an association between colon cancer and high intake of meat. However, it is not clear whether this association is due to the protein content alone, or due to the saturated fat sources in meat.[21] Finally, very high intakes of dietary protein may ultimately affect other nutrients such as vitamin B_6 and calcium. Researchers have suggested that excess protein intake increases the need for vitamin B_6, a vitamin extensively involved in amino acid metabolism. It also may promote urinary calcium losses which, in turn, may affect bone mineral mass and predispose to osteoporosis.[1,8]

Current levels of dietary protein intake in United States, based on the typical American diet, that provide the RDA or twice the RDA do not seem to represent a risk.[22]

PROTEIN AND EXERCISE

In addition to adequate, good quality, dietary protein intake, exercise and higher levels of physical activity have been found to be beneficial. High physical activity levels have been shown to improve food intake and protein utilization allowing for maintenance of body protein and muscle mass.[23] They are associated with improvements in physical functioning with positive effects on aerobic capacity, flexibility, and muscle strength.[24] Exercise may also improve physical functioning and other health indicators through enhancing confidence in one's ability to be more active and/or improving mood and motivation. Resistance or strength exercise training, in particular, has beneficial effects in reversing some of the age-related physiologic changes in body composition such as the loss of muscle mass and physiologic function.[25] An example of the association between muscle strength and muscle function and mobility is shown in Figure 2.[25b]

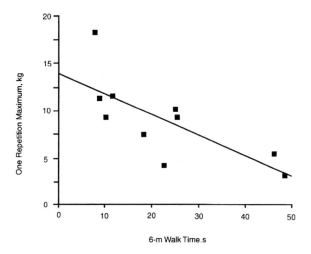

FIGURE 2   Relationship between muscle strength as assessed by one repetition maximum and mobility as assessed by length of time, in seconds, needed to walk 6 meters. This figure shows that the stronger you are, the faster you walk at very advanced ages where strength and muscle size become prime determinants of function and mobility. (From Fiatarone, M. S., Marks, E. C. et al., *JAMA*, 263, 3029–3034. Copyright 1990, American Medical Association. With permission.)

There is controversial information regarding whether or not individuals with very high physical activity levels should eat more protein than the RDA.[26] Physically active people consuming a typical American diet, who are not purposely losing weight, are eating enough protein. There is evidence that this protein will be better utilized because of the activity level itself.[23] Thus, there is no reason to consume excessive dietary protein (more than twice the RDA), or amino acid supplements, provided there is not an increased protein demand due to illness or a catabolic state. Enough good quality protein is available in animal and/or plant food sources for all healthy women, regardless of age.

The evidence derived from research demonstrates that, on one hand, physical activity is influenced by dietary protein intake; that is, eating enough protein results in stronger and bigger muscles, thus increasing strength. On the other hand, physical activity influences protein nutrition by increasing energy intake and protein utilization (i.e., protein digestion and absorption in the gut) and by increasing muscle mass and thus increasing the body's protein content.[13] The bottom line is that at any age, and in particular at an older age, there is a need to incorporate some element of physical activity in our daily lives to both improve the usage of all nutrients, including protein, and to maintain adequate reserves of protein and amino acids as major constituents of skeletal muscle and viscera. This is particularly important during the aging process when disease onset may be a high risk.

SUMMARY

In summary, protein is one of the many important nutrients the body needs to maintain health and vitality. Eating enough good quality protein is not very difficult if consuming a typical American diet, and if the sources of protein-rich foods of animal and vegetable origin are known and used. Special attention has to be paid in particular cases where dietary practices, acute or chronic diseases, physical activity patterns, and economic factors could interfere with protein nurtiture. There are nutrition education programs available through health professionals, senior citizens centers, congregate meal sites, and churches; and nutrition education programs for older adults are usually offered by dietitians, nutritionists, or geriatric health care practitioners. The goal of nutrition counseling is to influence individuals to consume an adquate diet based on the U.S. Dietary Guidelines. It is also important to be aware that in the case of disease specialized nutritional counseling is required regarding which foods to consume, how to prepare them, the need to modify dietary habits, the importance of interactions between food and medications, etc. Nutrition counseling for healthy older women is also important in making lifestyle changes oriented towards better eating habits, increasing physical activity levels, and reducing stress.

REFERENCES

1a. Munro, H. N., Aging, in *Nutrition and Metabolism in Patient Care*, Kinney, J. M., Ed., W.B. Saunders, Philadelphia, 145–166, 1988.

1b. Evan, W. J., Rosenberg, I. H. et al., The Ten Biomarkers of Vitality, in *Biomarkers. The 10 Determinants of Aging You Can Control*, Katz, H., Ed., Simon & Schuster, New York, 39–84, 1991.

2. Forbes, G. B. and Reina, J. C., Adult lean body mass declines with age: some longitudinal observations, *Metabolism*, 19(9), 653–663, 1970.

3. Kehayias, J. J. et al., Total body potassium and body fat: relevance to aging, *Am. J. Clin. Nutr.*, 66, 904–910, 1997.

4. Lexell, J. and Downham, D. Y., What is the effect of aging in type II muscle fibers? *J. Neurol. Sci.*, 107, 250–251, 1992.

5. Pate, R. R. et al., Physical Activity and Public Health. A Recommendation from the Center for Disease Control and Prevention and the American College of Sports Medicine, *JAMA*, 273(5), 402–407, 1995.

6. Crim, M. C. and Munro, H., Proteins and amino acids, in *Modern Nutrition in Health and Disease*, Shils, M.E., Olson, J. A., and Shike, M., Eds., Lea and Febiger, Philadelphia, 1–30, 1994.

7. Young, V. R., Amino acids and protein in relation to the nutrition of elderly people, *Age and Aging*, 19, 510–524, 1990.

8. Munro, H., Protein nurtiture and requirements of the elderly, in *Human Nutrition a Comprehensive Treatise. Nutrition, Aging, and the Elderly*, Munro, H. and Danford, D., Eds., Plenum Press, New York, 153–181, 1989.

9. WHO/FAO/UNU, *Energy and Protein Metabolism*. Technical report series no. 724, Geneva, World Health Organization, 1985.

10. National Research Council, *Recommended Dietary Allowances*, 10th ed., National Academy Press, Washington, D.C., 1989.

11. Wardlaw, G. M., Insel, P. M., and Seyler, M. F., Proteins, in *Contemporary Nutrition. Issues and Insights*, Mosby, Baltimore, 192–220, 1994.

12. Munro, H. et al., Protein nutriture of a group of free-living elderly, *Am. J. Clin. Nutr.*, 46, 585–592, 1987.

13. Evans, W. J. and Cy-Campbell, D., Nutrition, exercise, and healthy aging, *J. Am. Diet. Assoc.*, 97, 632–638, 1997.

14. Young, V. R. and Marchini, S., Mechanisms and nutritional significance of metabolic responses to altered intakes of protein and amino acids, with reference to nutritional adaptation in humans, *Am. J. Clin. Nutr.*, 51, 270–289, 1990.

15. Castaneda, C. et al., Elderly women accommodate to a low protein diet with losses of body composition, muscle function, and immune response, *Am. J. Clin. Nutr.*, 62, 30–39, 1995.

16. Castaneda, C. et al., Protein turnover and energy metabolism of elderly women chronically fed a low protein diet, *Am. J. Clin. Nutr.*, 62, 40–48, 1995.

17. National Center for Health Statistics, NCHS dietary intake source data: United States 1976–1980, Vital and Health Statistics, Vol. 231, U.S. Department of Health, Washington, D.C., 149–151, 1980.

18. Libow, L., Interaction of medical, biologic, and behavioral factors on aging, adaptation, and survival, *Geriatrics*, 29, 75–88, 1974.

19. Kopple, J. D., Nutrition, Diet, and the Kidney, *in Modern Nutrition in Health and Disease*, Shils, M. E., Olson, J. A., and Shike, M., Eds., Lea and Febiger, Philadelphia, 1102–1134, 1994.

20. Pedrini, M. T. et al., The effect of dietary protein restriction on the progression of diabetic and nondiabetic renal disease: a meta-analysis, *Ann. Intern. Med.*, 124, 627–632, 1996.

21. Blair, S. N. et al., Physical activity, nutrition, and chronic disease, *Med. Sci. Sports Exerc.*, 28(3), 335–349, 1996.

22. Wright, H. S., The 1987–1988 nationwide food consumption survey: an update on the nutrient intake of respondents, *Nutr. Today*, 21–27, 1991.

23. Butterfield, G., Whole-body protein utilization in humans, *Med. Sci. Sports Exerc.*, 19(5), 5157–5165, 1987.

24. Buchner, D. M. et al., Effects of physical activity on health status in older adults II: intervention studies, *Ann. Rev. Public Health*, 13, 469–488, 1992.

25a. Fielding, R. A., The role of progressive resistance training and nutrition in the preservation of lean body mass in the elderly, *J. Am. Coll. Nutr.*, 14(6), 587–594, 1995.

25b. Fiatarone, M. S., Marks, E. C. et al., High-intensity strength training in nonagenarians: Effects on skeletal muscle, *JAMA*, 263, 3029–3034, 1990.

26. Tarnopolsky, M. A., MacDougall, J. D., and Atkinson, S. A., Influence of protein intake and training status on nitrogen balance and lean body mass, *J. Appl. Physiol.*, 64(1), 187–193, 1988.

7 Fat and Cholesterol

Alice H. Lichtenstein

CONTENTS

INTRODUCTION

Fat is classically defined as a group of compounds that are insoluble in water. The most common type of fat in the body and in the foods we eat is triglyceride or triacylglycerol. However, there are many other types of substances in the body and food that are also classified as fat, as listed in Table 1. Some of these include essential nutrients such as the fat soluble vitamins (vitamins A, D, E, K) and essential fatty acids (linoleic and linolenic acids). Fat serves important physiologic, structural, and metabolic functions in the body. Like carbohydrate and protein, fat

155

is made up of carbon, oxygen, and hydrogen atoms. Unlike protein, fat does not contain nitrogen. Due to the way the carbon, oxygen, and hydrogen atoms are bonded together and the relative proportion of each to the other, fat has certain properties that sets it apart from carbohydrate and protein. One property immediately apparent is that it is hydrophobic or "water hating." This property dictates that fat be handled differently from carbohydrate and protein in the aqueous milieu of the body. Another property is that fat serves as a compact source of energy, providing 9 calories per gram. Therefore, weight for weight, fat has a little more than two times the amount of energy as either carbohydrate or protein (each supplying 4 calories per gram). Although not a particularly appealing attribute if one is trying to teleologically limit energy intake, the high energy density of fat has been advantageous with regard to survival. This chapter specifically addresses issues related to dietary fatty acids, triglycerides, and cholesterol, and the impact of these compounds on health and disease.

TABLE 1
Compounds
Classified as Fat

Fatty acids
Triglyceride
Phospholipid
Cholesterol
Cholesteryl ester
Vitamin A
Vitamin D
Vitamin E
Vitamin K
Carotinoids

FATTY ACIDS

Fatty acids are small units of fat that are used as building blocks, at least in part, of larger molecules such as triglycerides, phospholipids, cholesteryl esters, and in the case of arachidonic acid, the synthesis of biologically active compounds. Individual fatty acids are composed of chains of carbon atoms combined with hydrogen atoms, a methyl group at one end and carboxyl (acid) group at the other. These carbon atoms are linked together by either a single or double bond. The presence of a double bond limits the number of hydrogen atoms that can bind to the carbon atom. If all the carbon atoms are linked together by a single bond, the fatty acid is referred to as a saturated fatty acid (saturated with respect to the amount of hydrogen that can potentially combine with the carbon). If there are one or more double bonds in the chain of carbon atoms, the fatty acid is referred to as unsaturated. Unsaturated fatty acids are frequently divided into two groups: monounsaturated, having one double bond, and polyunsaturated, having two or more double bonds. There are multiple ways to classify fatty acids, many of which are in common usage. The following are descriptions of the systems most frequently used.

COMMON, CODE, AND FORMULA NAMES

Fatty acids may be identified by their code, common, or formula names, as listed in Table 2. Both the code and common names are shorthand notations. The code name is composed as follows: the first number denotes the number of carbon atoms in the chain, the second number denotes the number of double bonds in the chain, the n-3 or n-6 designation (see below) indicates the position of the first double bond counting from the methyl end of the acyl chain and the subsequent numbers the position of additional double bonds, if present. An alternate number system starts from the carboxyl end of the acyl chain. In that system, the position of the first double bond is preceded by a delta and subsequent numbers denote the position of additional double bonds, if present.

ESSENTIAL FATTY ACIDS

Fatty acids can be classified as to whether or not they are essential for humans. Essential fatty acids are those that cannot be synthesized in the human body and, therefore, must be derived from the diet. Linoleic (18:2n-6) and linolenic (α-linolenic acid; 18:3n-3) acids are essential fatty acids. Essential fatty acids are important because they are used to synthesize regulatory compounds, for example, prostaglandins, thromboxanes, prostacyclins, and leukotrienes. Different forms of these compounds regulate a wide range of functions such as inflammation, platelet aggregation, blood vessel contractility, uterine contractions, and dermal and renal integrity. A clinical manifestation of essential fatty acid deficiency is dermatitis which responds to essential fatty acids. This clinical manifestation has been directly attributable to the need for linoleic acid to form part of the lipid bilayers (lamellae) that fill the intercellular space in the upper part of the epidermis (stratum corium). Other fatty acids, arachidonic (20:4n-6), eicosapentaenoic (20:5n-3), and docosahexaenoic (22:6n-3) acids, are metabolic products of linoleic and linolenic acids, and can partially substitute for these fatty acids in the diet.

OMEGA-3 (N-3) AND OMEGA-6 (N-6) FATTY ACIDS

Unsaturated fatty acids can be classified with regard to the position of the first double bond, counting from the methyl end of the acyl chain. The two major series are n-3 and n-6. Although some fatty acids may have an identical number of carbons and degree of unsaturation, if they differ in the location of the double bonds (n-3 or n-6) they are handled differently. The enzymes active in the conversion of fatty acids to metabolically active products (i.e., cycloxygenase and lipoxygenases) are specific, and different isomers of the same fatty acid will have different metabolic products, and hence biological effects. N-3 fatty acids have a role in the regulation of immune response and platelet aggregation. The optimal ratio of n-3 to n-6 fatty acids in the human diet has yet to be defined.

TABLE 2
Common Fatty Acids

Code	Common Name	Formula
		Saturated
12:0	Lauric acid	$CH_3(CH_2)_{10}COOH$
14:0	Myristic acid	$CH_3(CH_2)_{12}COOH$
16:0	Palmitic acid	$CH_3(CH_2)_{14}COOH$
18:0	Stearic acid	$CH_3(CH_2)_{16}COOH$
		Monounsaturated
16:1n-7 *cis*	Palmitoleic acid	$CH_3(CH_2)_5CH=(c)CH(CH_2)_7COOH$
18:1n-9 *cis*	Oleic acid	$CH_3(CH_2)_7CH=(c)CH(CH_2)_7COOH$
18:1n-9 *trans*	Elaidic acid	$CH_3(CH_2)_7CH=(t)CH(CH_2)_7COOH$
		Polyunsaturated
18:2n-6,9 all *cis*	Linoleic acid	$CH_3(CH_2)_4CH=(c)CHCH_2CH=(c)CH(CH_2)_7COOH$
18:3n-3,6,9 all *cis*	α-linolenic acid	$CH_3CH_2CH=(c)CHCH_2CH=(c)CHCH_2C= (c)CH(CH_2)_7COOH$
18:3n-6,9,12 all *cis*	α-linolenic acid	$CH_3(CH_2)_4CH=(c)CHCH_2CH=(c)CHCH_2CH=(c)CH(CH_2)_4COOH$
20:4n-6,9,12,15 all *cis*	Arachidonic acid	$CH_3(CH_2)_4CH=(c)CHCH_2CH=(c)CHCH_2CH=(c)CHCH_2CH=(c)CH(CH_2)_3COOH$
20:5n-3,6,9,12,15 all *cis*	Eicosapentaenoic acid	$CH_3CH_2CH=(c)CH_5(CH_2)_3COOH$
22:6n-3,6,9,12,15,18 all *cis*	Docosahexaenoic acid	$CH_3(CH_2CH=(c)CH)_6(CH_2)_2COOH$

CIS AND TRANS FATTY ACIDS

Double bonds occur naturally in two conformations or physical forms, commonly referred to as *cis* or *trans*. For the more common *cis* form, the hydrogen atoms bound to the carbon atoms that form the double bond are located on opposite sides of the acyl chain. For the *trans* form, the hydrogen atoms bound to the carbon atoms that form the double bond are located on the same side of the acyl chain. The presence of a *trans* double bond results in a more linear conformation than that of a *cis* double bond. With regard to plasma lipid levels, despite being classified as unsaturated fatty acids, these *trans* fatty acids behave more like saturated fatty acids.

SATURATED, MONOUNSATURATED, AND POLYUNSATURATED FAT

Dietary fat is sometimes referred to as saturated, monounsaturated, or polyunsaturated. In contrast to individual fatty acids where the classification is made on the basis of the acyl chain length, and position and number of double bonds, dietary fat is frequently classified on the basis of the predominant fatty acids that make up the triglyceride molecules. Examples of common sources of saturated fats are dairy and animal fat, monounsaturated fats are olive and canola oils, and polyunsaturated fats are corn and soybean oils. A simple way to tell saturated from unsaturated fats by appearance is their physical form at room temperature. Saturated fat tends to be solid (e.g., butter or lard) whereas unsaturated fat tends to be liquid (vegetable oils). Notable exceptions to this rule are what are commonly referred to as the tropical oils (coconut, palm, and palm kernel oils), as they are composed of saturated fatty acids but are liquid at room temperature due to the predominance of short-chain saturated fatty acids making up the triglyceride.

CHOLESTEROL

Cholesterol is a fat soluble compound that is either derived from foods of animal origin or produced endogenously. It belongs to a class of compounds called sterols. Cholesterol is critical for the formation of cell membranes and particles that transport fat within the circulation, and is used for the synthesis of vitamin D, bile acids, and steroid hormones. Cholesterol is essential for optimal body functioning; however, it is not an essential nutrient because our bodies can make it in adequate amounts. Unfortunately, when blood cholesterol levels are elevated cholesterol can accumulate in blood vessel walls, resulting in plaque formation, narrowing of arteries, and ultimately, arteriosclerosis. The extreme outcomes are strokes, myocardial infarctions, and peripheral vascular disease. Although it would seem logical to assume that dietary cholesterol is the primary determinant of plasma cholesterol levels, the primary determinant is actually saturated fat with dietary cholesterol having a somewhat lesser effect.

DIETARY FAT AND HEALTH

The popular press continually emphasizes the need to limit fat intake, food advertisements tend to stress the fat-free or low-fat nature of their products, and fitness centers claim to be able to reduce the content of fat in your body. This would lead one to speculate that fat is intrinsically bad. Although excess body fat is detrimental from both a health and in some cultures an aesthetic point of view, fat serves many critical functions in the human body.

Fat physically insulates the body to minimize heat loss, thus preserving energy for other uses (i.e., movement). This function is very relevant clinically in the elderly, who are less able to regulate core body temperature than younger individuals. It is known that an additional risk factor for hypothermia in low ambient temperature is the presence of marasmus or protein calorie malnutrition, and its associated low levels of body fat. Fat (visceral and subcutaneous) also serves a mechanical purpose, as it protects or cushions internal organs from damage due to day-to-day activity. Externally, it attenuates the kinetic energy transmitted to bone after a fall, and may thus prevent injury. The amount of fat over the greater trochanter has been shown to be protective against hip fracture in the elderly, apparently working as an endogenous hip pad. On a cellular level, certain types of fat (phospholipids and cholesterol) form the structure of cellular membranes.

Metabolically, fat provides a compact source of energy (calories). Although this may not appear to be an advantage in wealthier societies where food security is not an issue for most people, this ability was critical for survival during earlier times and in developing nations when "feast and famine" cycles were common. It enabled individuals to survive in times of scarcity. This survival benefit (at least until midlife and during the reproductive years) may explain its evolutionary preservation in the face of its association with undesirable metabolic consequences later in life.

Fat ingestion is necessary for the absorption and transport of fat soluble vitamins, and serves as a storage depot for these vitamins as well. Thus, day-to-day fluctuations in fat intake are not as critical as they are with water soluble vitamins, which do not have such large tissue stores (with the exception of vitamin B_{12} in the liver). Adipose tissue can also serve as a reservoir for essential fatty acids. Finally, adipose tissue in women is a site for the peripheral conversion of androgenic precursors to estrogen, and this capacity is thought to be one of the reasons that obese women have higher bone density. Unfortunately, this places them at higher risk of developing breast cancer than their leaner counterparts.

DIETARY FAT RECOMMENDATIONS

TOTAL FAT

For all of the reasons outlined above, fat is a necessary dietary constituent. Additionally, it is virtually impossible to formulate a diet of natural foods that is totally devoid of fat yet adequate in all of the other essential nutrients. The World Health Organization has recommended that between 15 and 30% of calories come from fat. Similar recommendations regarding upper limits of total fat intake are made by the American Heart Association, the Dietary Guidelines for Americans (choose a diet low in fat, saturated fat, and cholesterol), and the National Cholesterol Education Program (NCEP) Expert Panel on Detection, Evaluation, and Treatment of High Blood Cholesterol in Adults. There appears to be little advantage for most individuals to consume an extremely low fat diet (less than 15% of calories), such as have been popularized in various forms recently for the prevention and/or treatment of heart disease and other chronic diseases. These diets can be extremely difficult to adhere to for extended periods of time, and often delay the institution of more moderate dietary modifications that can be incorporated into habitual dietary patterns. In addition, in certain individuals, very low fat diets may result in an increase in blood triglyceride and a decrease in high density lipoprotein levels.

Consumption of a diet at or below 30% of calories may be beneficial with respect to blood lipid levels and cardiovascular risk profile, but also with respect to dietary diversity, micronutrient intake, and possibly weight control. These potential improvements in the diet are most likely achieved when the fat content of the diet is reduced commensurate with an increase in the consumption of nutrient dense foods such as fruits, vegetables, and complex carbohydrates. When such changes occur, there is often an increase in the fiber content of the diet, which may have benefits in terms of gastrointestinal function and cancer risk. Conversely, if the fat content of the diet is reduced and replaced with high simple carbohydrate, low nutrient-dense foods, it is unlikely that these benefits will be realized.

The terms *Step 1* and *Step 2* diets are frequently incorporated into health messages. These diets were originally formulated by NCEP for the treatment of individuals with elevated levels of blood cholesterol. Step 1 diets have now been recommended for the general population over the age of two. Step 2 diets are generally recommended to individuals with hyperlipidemia who have not obtained adequate lower blood cholesterol after following a Step 1 diet. The criteria for Step 1 and Step 2 diets are presented in Table 3.

TABLE 3
Recommended Diets to Reduce Blood Cholesterol Levels

Dietary Factor	Step 1	Step 2
Total Fat	≤ 30% energy	≤ 30% energy
Saturated Fat	8–10% energy	< 7% energy
Cholesterol	< 300 mg/day	< 200 mg/day
Carbohydrate	≥ 55% energy	≥ 55% energy
Protein	15% energy	15% energy

Type of Fat

Saturated Fat

The general recommendation is that saturated fat should make up less than 10% of calories (Table 3). This is because of the relationship of saturated fat with elevated blood cholesterol levels. There are situations, such as inadequate response to dietary modification in hyperlipidemic individuals, where the recommendation is that saturated fat should make up less than 7% of calories. However, this recommendation is not a general population-wide goal.

Saturated fat intake can be reduced by decreasing the consumption of products containing dairy and animal fats. Given the wide range of non-fat and reduced-fat dairy, and the leaner cuts and types of meat products available in the market, these goals should not be difficult to achieve. Since it appears that *trans* fatty acids have a similar effect on blood cholesterol levels as saturated fatty acids, it would now appear prudent to limit the intake of both *trans* as well as saturated fatty acids. A reduction in *trans* fatty acid intake can be achieved by replacing stick margarine and hydrogenated cooking shortenings with the softer margarines and oil in the liquid state and commercially prepared fried and baked products made thereof. Common sources of saturated fat are shown in Table 4.

TABLE 4
Examples of Foods High in Specific Dietary Fats

Saturated Fat	Monounsaturated Fat	Polyunsaturated Fat	Cholesterol
Meat fats	Canola oil	Soybean oil	Eggs
Dairy fats	Olive oil	Corn oil	Meat
Tropical oils	Peanut oil	Sunflower oil	Full fat dairy products
		Safflower oil	Organ meat

Unsaturated Fat

Currently, the recommendation is that polyunsaturated fatty acids should not make up more than 10% of total calories and monounsaturated fatty acids should make up between 10 to 15% of calories (Table 3). Good sources of monounsaturated and polyunsaturated fats are shown in Table 4. The issue of whether one or the other is better has been a controversial topic for a number of years. At this point there is no clear advantage to consuming one over the other. The debate continues and will be resolved only when adequate data are available. At this point the most responsible advance is to include sources of both in the diet. Good sources of monounsaturated and polyunsaturated fat are presented in Table 4.

Cholesterol Intake

Strictly speaking, cholesterol does not need to be consumed for optimal body functioning because the human body has the capacity to make adequate amounts of cholesterol for all essential functions. Additionally, too high, rather than too low, blood cholesterol levels give reason for concern. The evidence generally indicates that for normal individuals consuming moderate levels of dietary cholesterol, 300 mg or less per day, does not adversely effect plasma cholesterol levels (Table 3). This is the level recommended for all Americans over the age of 2 years by NCEP, the Dietary Guidelines, and the American Heart Association. The recommendation to limit cholesterol intake to less than 200 mg per day is made for individuals who have elevated total cholesterol levels that do not respond to the general guidelines, in conjunction with the other components of the Step 2 diet presented in Table 3. Sources of cholesterol are shown in Table 4.

Dietary Fats of Special Consideration

Trans Fatty Acids/Hydrogenated Fat

As noted above, the presence of a *cis* or *trans* double bond impacts the conformation of the fatty acid acyl chains. *Trans* fatty acids occur naturally in dairy fat and meat. They result from the fermentation in ruminant animals such as cows. Additionally, *trans* fatty acids are also formed during the hydrogenation of fat, a process used to transform oil from a liquid to semi-solid state. The conversion of *cis* to *trans* double bonds results in a fatty acid with a straighter conformation, more similar to a saturated fatty acid. Hydrogenated fat is used to make margarines and vegetable shortenings (for home use and in the preparation of commercially baked and fried foods). Similar to saturated fatty acids, trans fatty acids have been associated with elevated plasma cholesterol levels.

Omega-3 (n-3) Fatty Acids

Long chain n-3 fatty acids (20:5n-3 and 22:6n-3) occur at relatively high levels in fish and marine products. α-linolenic acid (18:3n-3) occurs at relatively high levels in soybean and canola oils. N-3 fatty acids have been demonstrated to lower triglyceride levels in hypertriglyceridemic individuals and in some cases have been associated with reduced risk of cardiovascular disease. At this point it is unclear whether or not the biological effects attributable to the longer chain n-3 fatty acids (20:5n-3 and 22:6n-3) can also be attributed to linolenic acid when consumed at levels normally present in the diet. N-3 fatty acids have little if any effect on blood cholesterol levels.

DIETARY FAT AND CHRONIC DISEASE

Cardiovascular Disease

There are a number of established risk factors for cardiovascular disease, as shown in Table 5. These include elevated blood cholesterol levels (200 mg/dl); age (> 55 years in females, > 45 years in males); family history of premature heart disease (> 65 years in female and > 55 years in male first degree relative); current cigarette smoking; hypertension; low high-density lipoprotein (HDL) cholesterol levels (< 35 mg/dl); and insulin resistance or diabetes mellitus. Other risk factors that have been identified but are not formally used to determine risk include low levels of physical activity and central obesity (apple shape vs. pear shape). Offsetting these risk factors is a high HDL cholesterol level (> 60 mg/dl). Some of these risk factors are modifiable (i.e., blood cholesterol levels, smoking, physical activity, body weight) and others are not (i.e., age, family history). The major risk factors that can be potentially modified by diet are blood cholesterol levels, blood pressure, and body weight, and by life style, physical activity and smoking. For most individuals, the determining dietary factor with respect to blood cholesterol levels is saturated fat intake. The lower the dietary saturated fat, the lower the plasma cholesterol level. The second factor is dietary cholesterol intake. Above a minimum level of intake, the lower the dietary cholesterol, the lower the plasma cholesterol level.

TABLE 5
Coronary Heart Disease Risk Factors

Negative Risk Factors

Elevated blood cholesterol levels ($\geq$ 200 mg/dl)

Age ($\geq$ 55 years in females or premature menopause without estrogen replacement, $\geq$ 45 years in males)

Family history of premature heart disease (> 65 years in female and > 55 years in male first degree relative)

Current cigarette smoking

Hypertension (high blood pressure)

Low high-density lipoprotein (HDL) cholesterol levels (< 35 mg/dl)

Diabetes mellitus

Other identified risk factors include low levels of physical activity and central obesity (apple shape vs. pear shape).

Positive Risk Factor

HDL cholesterol levels ($\geq$ 60 mg/dl)

BLOOD LIPIDS (LIPOPROTEINS)

The formation of lipoprotein particles is the mechanism by which the body accommodates the unique nature of fat and facilitates transport through the aqueous environment of the body. There are six types of lipoprotein particles: chylomicrons, very low-density lipoprotein (VLDL), intermediate density lipoprotein (IDL), low density lipoprotein (LDL), HDL, and lipoprotein a [Lp(a)]. Associated with each lipoprotein particle are one or more protein(s), frequently referred to as apolipoproteins. These lipoprotein-associated apoprotein(s) determine how the particle is handled in plasma and whether it remains in the blood stream or is internalized and used by various cells in the body. Clinically, total cholesterol and LDL cholesterol are the best predictors of cardiovascular disease risk (Table 6A, B). Individuals with elevated LDL cholesterol levels are at increased risk for developing cardiovascular disease. Individuals with high levels of HDL cholesterol seem to be protected from development of cardiovascular disease. Levels of these lipids have both strong genetic determinants as well as environmental modulators. In women after menopause, LDL levels tend to increase while HDL levels tend to remain unchanged. The postmenopausal increase in LDL cholesterol levels has been attributed to the decrease in circulating estrogen levels. Therefore, after menopause, it becomes important for health care providers to monitor women's lipoprotein profiles and, if LDL is elevated, for the women to make dietary modifications to lower it. This is especially critical because menopause is also associated with an increased prevalence of other major cardiovascular disease risk factors, including sedentariness, increased visceral fat deposition, and impairment of glucose homeostasis, which, when combined with an altered lipid profile, may markedly elevate risk of vascular disease. Estrogen replacement therapy has been associated with an improved lipid profile and a lower risk of cardiovascular events in this population, as discussed more fully in Chapter 15.

TABLE 6A
Classification System Based on Total Cholesterol Levels

	mg/dl	mmol/L
Desirable	< 200	< 5.2
Borderline high risk	200–240	5.2–6.2
High risk	> 240	> 6.2

TABLE 6B
Classification Based on Low Density Lipoprotein (LDL) Cholesterol Levels

Primary Prevention in Adults Without Evidence of Coronary Heart Disease

Lipoprotein Analysis after Fasting 9–12 Hours

Desirable LDL Cholesterol (< 130 mg/dl [3.4 mmol/L])
- provide education on Step 1 diet, physical activity, and risk factor reduction
- repeat total and HDL cholesterol within 5 years

Borderline-High Risk LDL Cholesterol (130 to 159 mg/dl [3.4 to 4.1 mmol/L])
Fewer than 2 risk factors
- provide education on Step 1 diet and physical activity
- reevaluate patient status annually, repeat lipoprotein analysis, reinforce nutrition and physical activity education

2 or more risk factors
- do clinical evaluation (history, physical examination, and laboratory tests)
- evaluate secondary causes and familial disorders (when indicated)
- initiate Step 1 diet; if inadequate response achieved, initiate Step 2 diet

High Risk LDL Cholesterol (> 160 mg/dl [4.1 mmol/L])
- do clinical evaluation (history, physical examination, and laboratory tests)
- evaluate secondary causes and familial disorders (when indicated)
- initiate Step 1 diet; if inadequate response achieved, initiate Step 2 diet

When there is compliance with a Step 2 diet, the LDL levels may be expected to fall by 10 to 15%, although individual responsiveness is highly variable. For unresponsive individuals, those with current evidence of atherosclerotic disease or several other CHD risk factors, or severe familial forms of hyperlipidemia, drug therapy is indicated in addition to attempts at dietary modulation. When obesity is present, particularly central obesity, simply altering the amount or type of fat in the diet without restricting total energy intake to reduce adiposity is unlikely to have an adequate effect on lipid profiles.

CANCER

Cross-cultural epidemiological evidence suggests that women in societies in which a high fat diet is habitually eaten are at higher risk of developing breast cancer than women in societies in which a low fat diet is habitually eaten. Migration studies have suggested that when a woman migrates from a culture where the fat content of the diet is low to a culture where the fat content of the diet is high and adopts those habits, her risk of developing breast cancer increases. There does not appear to be as clear a relationship between fat intake and risk of developing breast cancer within a single population. One factor contributing to the discrepancy between cross-cultural and intra-cultural studies may be the relatively narrow range of fat intake within a single population, which makes the relationships difficult to identify. An additional complicating factor is a potential relationship of breast cancer with habitual or early life patterns of low levels of physical activity and high body weight. Since high fat diets, obesity, and lack of physical activity are often seen in the same women, it may be difficult to separate which of these interrelated factors are causally linked to the excess cancer risk. These issues are the topic of considerable scientific inquiry at the present time.

Similar observations relating fat intake (and physical activity levels) and risk of developing colon cancer have been made. Interestingly, evidence derived from intra-cultural studies seems to be somewhat stronger for colon cancer; these relationships also hold for prostate cancer. The possible mechanisms underlying such observations are discussed in Chapter 11.

OBESITY

Some individuals go through life without thinking about what, where, and how much they eat and maintain a constant weight. Others find balancing food intake and exercise to maintain a constant body weight difficult and at times a losing battle. There are many approaches to weight maintenance as discussed in Chapter 17. However, one concept that does resurface with respect to dietary fat is caloric density and satiety. Evidence to suggest that decreasing the caloric density of the diet (i.e., decreasing fat intake) helps promote weight loss or maintenance is plentiful, but so is evidence suggesting no relationship. There is some suggestion that, for example, fat calories are more likely to be deposited as adipose tissue rather than oxidized for fuel, compared to carbohydrate calories. Consensus on this issue has not been reached. Although decreasing the fat content of the diet can be helpful in leading to the long-term reduction in caloric intake, other factors need to be factored into any dietary plan to obtain the desired result. Prime examples of such factors include increased exercise and behavior modification. There is some evidence in this regard that exercise combined with hypocaloric dieting leads to higher compliance rates with respect to the dietary recommendations, compared to dieting alone. Therefore, the combined intervention has been shown to produce higher weight loss success rates in a population, even if the average weight loss for an individual is not greatly enhanced compared to dieting alone. Without permanent changes in one's energy balance, what goes in and what gets expended (exercise), a vicious cycle of weight loss and gain frequently ensues. This can undermine one's self confidence and potentially cause unfavorable changes in body composition (loss of bone and muscle during periods of weight loss, which are not adequately regained in subsequent cycles).

With respect to satiety, early work suggested that meals high in fat took longer to be processed by the gastrointestinal system and thus delayed the signal to start eating again. Later work suggested that other factors may also be involved in these feedback mechanisms, such as prior knowledge of the fat or caloric content of the food or sensory signals (including the mouth feel of foods with different fat contents). Clearly the area is unsettled. However, decreasing the fat content of the diet will reduce the caloric density, and therefore usually the total caloric intake as well, whether through differences in the volume of food which must be consumed, or alterations in satiety, or both. This may help weight loss or maintenance when coupled with other changes such as increased physical activity, so that the sum result is a favorable shift in energy balance.

COUNSELING REGARDING DIETARY FAT INTAKE

There are a number of points that should be factored in when considering counseling regarding dietary fat intake. First, "know your numbers." The blood lipid profile should be measured in a reliable laboratory under standard conditions. This is especially important around the time of menopause and about one year later. Minor changes in plasma cholesterol levels are normal; a constant trend upward should be followed-up, particularly when levels are in the borderline or elevated range, using the risk guidelines shown in Tables 6A, B as indications for further treatment.

Second, if there is a personal or family history of diseases related to obesity, cholesterol, or dietary fat intake (e.g., breast cancer, colon cancer, diabetes mellitus, stroke, cardiovascular disease), then modification of the diet assumes more critical importance. It is important to note that although lipid-lowering medications are likely to have more of an impact on optimizing blood lipid levels than diet, they cannot address the other risk factors associated with visceral adiposity (hyperinsulinemia, glucose intolerance, hypertension), and so when used in individuals with both central obesity and hyperlipidemia, they should always be coupled with attempts to achieve and maintain an ideal body weight as well.

Third, it is important to have a good estimate of total and saturated fat, and cholesterol intake to accurately assess whether or not dietary modification is appropriate and if so, how much. A 3- to 7-day food diary will help to determine general patterns of intake, as long as intake is not intentionally altered during the monitoring period, which is often the case. If body weight is appropriate and fat intake is already at or below 30% of caloric intake, and is mainly unsaturated, it is unlikely that major reductions in LDL levels will be possible with further dietary fat restriction. However, if excess calories are being consumed in relation to energy needs, then focusing on a reduction in the total number of calories, rather than just the fat content, may have important benefits. It should be noted here that there is a certain degree of misperception in the public that fat-free is synonymous with reduced calorie. Fat-free foods may have similar caloric content as their full fat counterparts; therefore, it is important to check labels before making purchasing decisions.

Fourth, assessment of current weight, history of weight gain, and increasing abdominal girth is important, as discussed more fully in Chapters 17 and 23. With increasing age, even if body weight stays constant, there is a shift in body composition, such that typically fat mass increases and lean muscle mass decreases, particularly after the menopause in women. Hypocaloric dieting and weight cycling exacerbate age-related losses of muscle and bone in women. Therefore, maintenance of body weight through the lifecycle with attention to the energy content of the diet, coupled with muscle and bone building resistive exercises, are the best approaches to maintaining a desirable body composition in late life.

On the basis of these and perhaps other factors, and a comparison of where the individual woman is with respect to current guidelines, an assessment can be made about the need to modify the diet and/or intervene with cholesterol-lowering medications.

IMPLEMENTING CHANGES

REDUCING FAT INTAKE

There are many approaches or plans to reduce the fat content of the diet, if so indicated for an individual, some of which are discussed in detail in Chapters 17 and 24. The variety of sources and formats suggests the individual nature of diet and approaches to altering it. No one approach is best or works for everyone. The points detailed below are general guidelines that can either stand by themselves or complement others.

A simple way to reduce the fat content of the diet is to first make a critical and honest assessment of current eating patterns (types of foods, amounts, time of day, and location). As indicated above, this should include both the total and saturated fat content, which can be obtained by consulting nutrient labels now available on all packaged food in the United States, or one of the many books or computer programs on the nutrient content of foods that are widely available.

There are a number of different strategies that can be used either individually or in combination to achieve the desired goals. Any change that is instituted should be one that can be sustained in the long term. Some simple suggestions for substituting high saturated fat and cholesterol foods for lower fat choices in the diet are given in Table 7. Remember, these changes are, for the most part, going to be lifelong changes so advising slow, stepwise implementation of a plan is more likely to be met with success than drastic attempts at dietary and other behavioral modification. Often, eating certain foods is more a matter of habit and environmental cues rather than hunger or other needs, and can therefore often be modified without inordinately sacrificing taste or pleasure. Examples of typical problem situations and suggested solutions are outlined in Table 8.

TABLE 7
Examples of Simple Substitutions to Reduce the Saturated Fat and Cholesterol Content of the Diet

Less Desirable Choice	More Desirable Choice
French fries	Baked potato
White cake with icing	Angle food cake with fruit
Luncheon meat (bologna, salami)	Deli sliced turkey
Fried shrimp	Broiled flounder
Sour cream	Yogurt (low fat or fat free)
Ritz-type crackers	Saltine, matzo
Vanilla sandwich cookies	Graham crackers, fig bars
Potato chips	Pretzels, unbuttered popcorn, baked potato chips
Commercial muffin	Bagel, English muffin
Cream-type soup	Broth-based soups
Butter	Soft diet margarine

TABLE 8
Reducing Fat and Cholesterol Intake

Problem Situation or Behavior	Suggested Solutions
Ordering foods prepared with high fat condiments such as dressings	Ask for dressing to be put on the side or substitute fat-free dressing
Using margarine on toast each morning	Switch to diet margarine or jam
Having a cheeseburger and potato chips for lunch 3 days a week	Keep the potato chips, but substitute soup or salad for the cheeseburger or drop the chips and burger and substitute pasta salad
Unwillingness to give up butter on toast or baked potatoes	Eliminate meat and cheese intake on those days and switch to margarine
Inability to substitute fat-free ice milk for premium ice cream	Cut serving size of regular ice cream in half
Using sour cream and butter on food items only when eating out	Avoid ordering foods to which these toppings can be added; if eating out often, eat out less

REDUCING SATURATED FAT AND CHOLESTEROL

The key to reducing the saturated fat content of the diet is to know from where the major sources of saturated fat come (see Table 4). As a general rule of thumb, the major sources of saturated fat are found in foods of animal origin and tropical oils (coconut, palm, palm kernel). Foods of animal origin include both dairy (milk and any products made of milk) and meat. Fortunately, there are now low-fat or fat-free versions of most dairy products. With respect to meat, cuts are now available which are lower in fat than ever before. Simple tricks like removing the skin from poultry before eating it can make a big difference. Cook stews and soup containing meat using lean cuts and prepare ahead of time so that they can be refrigerated; the fat that rises to the top can be removed before reheating.

Fat Substitutes

In general, fat substitutes are foods that provide the sensation of eating fat without the caloric density of fat. A number of such products have recently been approved for human consumption. Some have the properties of fat when used in cooking and feel like fat in the mouth, yet behave differently than fat once they reach the lower gastrointestinal system. If not digested or absorbed, they do not contribute energy or calories. One consequence is that they tend to take along fat-soluble vitamins when eliminated from the body. Therefore, the United States Food and Drug Administration has required that any food prepared with non-absorbable fat substitutes have fat soluble vitamins (A, D, E, and K) included in the formulation of the product. Fat substitutes based on different principles use different limitations and have potential nutritional concerns. It is beyond the scope of this chapter to deal with them. Non-caloric fat may seem like a panacea; however, it is important to note that, as stated above, fat-free does not mean calorie free. Ultimately, in order to maintain body weight and body composition throughout a lifetime, caloric intake must be balanced with routine exercise. That is, although reduced fat foods, low fat products, and now fat substitutes seem like the way to finally have one's cake and eat it too, this is unlikely to be the case. The introduction of sugar substitutes into the U.S. food supply in massive quantities over the past several decades has not been associated with a decreased prevalence of obesity; in fact, quite the opposite has happened. Ultimately, total calorie intake and energy output will determine body weight.

REFERENCES

Clarke, R., Frost, C., Collins, R., Appleby, P., and Peto, R., Dietary lipids and blood cholesterol: quantitative meta-analysis of metabolic ward studies, *BMJ*, 314, 112–117, 1997.

Denke, M. A., Cholesterol-lowering diets. A review of the evidence, *Arch. Inter. Med.*, 155, 17–26, 1995.

Denke, M. A., Review of human studies evaluating individual dietary responsiveness in patients with hypercholesterolemia, *Am. J. Clin. Nutr.*, 62, 471S–477S, 1995.

Expert Panel High Blood Cholesterol in Adults, Summary of the second report of the National Cholesterol Education Program (NCEP) Expert Panel on Detection, Evaluation, and Treatment of High Blood Cholesterol in Adults (Adult Treatment Panel II), *JAMA*, 269, 3015–3023, 1993.

Ginsberg, H. N., Kris-Etherton, P., Dennis, B., Elmer, P. J., Ershow, A., Lefevre, M., Pearson, T., Rohein, P., Pamakrishnan, R., Reed, R., Stewart, K., Stewart, P., Phillips, K., and Anderson, N., Effects of reducing dietary saturated fatty acids on plasma lipids and lipoproteins in healthy subjects, the DELTA Study, protocol 1. *Arthero. Throm. Vasc. Biol.*, 18, 441–449, 1998.

Gould, K. L., Ornish, D., Kirkeeide, R., Brown, S., Stuart, Y., Buchi, M., Billings, J., Armstrong, W., Ports, T., and Scherwitz, L., Improved stenosis geometry by quantitative coronary arteriography after vigorous risk factor modification, *Am. J. Cardiol.*, 69, 845–853, 1992.

Grundy, S. M. and Denke, M. A., Dietary influences on serum lipids and lipoproteins, *J. Lipid Res.*, 31, 1149–1172, 1990.

Hegsted, D. M., Ausman, L. M., Johnson, J. A., and Dallal, G. E., Dietary fat and serum lipids: an evaluation of the experimental data, *Am. J. Clin. Nutr.*, 57, 875–883, 1993.

Home, I., Cholesterol reduction and its impact on coronary artery disease and total mortality, *Am. J. Cardiol.*, 76, 10C–17C, 1995.

Hopkins, P. N., Effects of dietary cholesterol on serum cholesterol: A meta-analysis and review, *Am. J. Clin. Nutr.*, 55, 1060–1070, 1992.

Jenkins, D. J. A., Wolever, T. M. S., Rao, A. V., Hegele, R. A., Mitchell, S. J., Ransom, T. P. P., Boctor, D. L., Spadafora, P. J., Jenkins, A. L., Mehling, C., Relle, L. K., Connelly, P. W., Story, J. A., Furumoto, E. J., Corey, P., and Wursch, P., Effect on blood lipids of very high intakes of fiber in diets low in saturated fat and cholesterol, *N. Engl. J. Med.*, 329, 21–26, 1993.

Johnson, C. L., Rifkind, B. M., Sempos, C. T., Carroll, M. D., Bachorisk, P. S., Briefel, R. R., Gordon, D. J., Burt, V. L., Brown, C. D., Lippel, K., and Cleeman, J. I., Declining serum total cholesterol levels among U.S. adults, *JAMA*, 269, 3002–3008, 1993.

Keys, A., Menotti, A., Karvonen, M. J., Aravanis, C., Blackburn, H., Buzina, R., Djordjevic, B. S., Contas, A. S., Fidanza, F., Keys, M. H., Kromhout, D., Nedeljkovic, S., Punsar, S., Seccareccia, F., and Toshmia, H., The diet and 15-year death rate in the Seven Countries Study, *Am. J. Epidemiol.*, 124, 903–915, 1987.

Krauss, R. M., Deckelbaum, R. J., Ernst, N., Fisher, E., Howard, B. V., Knopp, R. H., Kotchen, T., Lichtenstein, A. H., McGill, H. C., Pearson, T. A., Prewitt, E., Stone, N. J., Van Horn, L., and Weinberg, R., Dietary guidelines for healthy American adults, *Circulation*, 94, 1795–1800, 1996.

Kromhout, D., Bosschieter, E. B., De Lezenne, and Coulander, C., The inverse relation between fish consumption and 20-year mortality from coronary heart disease, *N. Engl. J. Med.*, 312, 1205–1209, 1985.

Kushi, L. H., Lew, R. A., Stare, R. J., Ellison, C. R., Lozy, M. E., Bourke, G., Daly, L., Graham, I., Hickey, N., Mulcahy, R., and Kevaney, J., Diet and 20-year mortality from coronary heart disease, *N. Engl. J. Med.*, 312, 811–818, 1985.

Lichtenstein, A. H., Ausman, L. M., Carrasco, W., Jenner, J. L., Ordovas, J. M., and Schaefer, E. J., Short term consumption of a low fat diet has a positive impact on plasma lipid concentrations only when accompanied by weight loss, *Arterio. Thromb.*, 14, 1751–1760, 1994.

Lichtenstein, A. H., *Trans* fatty acids, plasma lipid levels, and risk of developing cardiovascular disease. A statement for healthcare professionals from the American Heart Association, *Circulation*, 95, 2588–2580, 1997.

Lichtenstein, A. H. and Van Horn, L., Very low fat diets. A statement for healthcare professionals from the American Heart Association, *Circulation*, 98, 935–939, 1998.

Lichtenstein, A. H., *Trans* fatty acids: blood lipid levels, cholesterol metabolism and susceptibility to oxidation—A review, *J. Nutr. Biochem.*, 9, 244–248, 1998.

Luc, G. and Fruchart, J.-C., Oxidation of lipoproteins and atherosclerosis, *Am. J. Clin. Nutr.*, 53, 206S–209S, 1991.

Mensink, R. P. and Katan, M. B., Effect of dietary *trans* fatty acids on high-density and low-density lipoprotein cholesterol levels in healthy subjects, *N. Engl. J. Med.*, 323, 439–445, 1990.

Mensink, R. P. and Katan, M. B., Effect of dietary fatty acids on serum lipids and lipoproteins: A meta-analysis of 27 trials, *Arterio. Thromb.*, 12, 911–919, 1992.

Meydani, S. N., Lichtenstein, A. H., Cornwall, S., Meydani, M., Goldin, B. R., Rasmussen, H., Dinarello, C. A., and Schaefer, E. J., Immunological effects of National Cholesterol Education Panel Step-2 diets with and without fish-derived n-3 fatty acid enrichment, *J. Clin. Invest.*, 92, 105–113, 1993.

Neaton, J. D. and Wentworth, D., Serum cholesterol, blood pressure, cigarette smoking, and death from coronary heart disease, *Arch. Intern. Med.*, 152, 56–64, 1992.

Phillipson, B. E., Rothrock, D. W., Connor, W. E., Harris, W. S., and Illingworth, D. R., Reduction of plasma lipids, lipoproteins, and apoproteins by dietary fish oils in patients with hypertriglyceridemia, *N. Engl. J. Med.*, 312, 1210–1216, 1985.

Rimm, E. B., Stampfer, M. J., Ascherio, A., Giovannucci, E., Colditz, G. A., and Willett, W. C., Vitamin E consumption and the risk of coronary heart disease in men, *N. Engl. J. Med.*, 328, 1450–1458, 1993.

Rossouw, J. E., Lipid-lowering interventions in angiographic trials, *Am. J. Cardiol.*, 76, 86C–92C, 1995.

Schaefer, E. J., Lamon-Fava, S., Ausman, L. M., Ordovas, J. M., Clevidence, B. A., Judd, J. T., Goldin, B. R., Woods, M., Gorbach, S., and Lichtenstein, A. H., Individual variability in lipoprotein cholesterol response to National Cholesterol Education Program Step 2 Diets, *Am. J. Clin. Nutr.*, 65, 823–830, 1997.

Schaefer, E. J., Lichtenstein, A. H., Lamon-Fava, S., Contois, J. H., Li, Z., Goldin, B. R., Rasmussen, H., McNamara, J. R., and Ordovas, J., Comparative effects of National Cholesterol Education Program Step 2 diets relatively high or relatively low in fish-derived fatty acids on plasma lipoproteins in middle aged and elderly subjects, *Am. J. Clin. Nutri.*, 63, 234–241, 1996.

Stampfer, M. J., Hennekens, C. H., Manson, J. E., Colditz, G. A., Rosner, B., and Willett, W. C., Vitamin E consumption and the risk of coronary disease in women, *N. Engl. J. Med.*, 328, 1444–1449, 1993.

Sytkowski, P. A., Kannel, W. B., and D'Agostino, R. B., Changes in risk factors and the decline in mortality from cardiovascular disease, *N. Engl. J. Med.*, 322, 1635–1641, 1990.

Tang, J. L., Armitage, J. M., Lancaster, T., Silagy, C. A., Fowler, G. H., and Neil, H. A., Systematic review of dietary intervention trials to lower blood total cholesterol in free-living subjects, *BMJ*, 16, 1213–1220, 1998.

Thompson, G. R., Progression and regression of coronary artery disease, *Current Opin. Lipidol.*, 3, 263–267, 1992.

Tran, Z. V. and Weltman, A., Differential effects of exercise on serum lipid and lipoprotein levels seen with changes in body weight: a meta analysis, *JAMA*, 254, 919–924, 1985.

Tyroler, H. A., Review of lipid-lowering clinical trials in relation to observational epidemiologic studies, *Circulation*, 76, 515–522, 1987.

8 Calcium and Vitamin D

Elizabeth Krall

CONTENTS

The metabolic functions and nutritional status of calcium and vitamin D are closely dependent on one another, and a single group of foods, the dairy group, is the most common source of both nutrients. This chapter will summarize why older women need calcium and vitamin D, how much they should have in their diet each day, and how to assist them in the selection of foods to meet those recommendations.

CALCIUM

We tend to think of calcium primarily as a component of bones and teeth. In fact, more than 98% of the approximately 3 pounds of calcium in the body is incorporated into the skeleton where it provides strength and hardness. But this mineral is also essential for the transmission of nerve impulses, contraction of muscle fibers, clotting of blood, and activation of digestive enzymes. Because these functions are critical for life, the body employs several mechanisms in order to keep the blood supply of calcium within strict limits, and vitamin D is involved in each. First, the amount of calcium that is absorbed from the diet will increase or decrease as the need for calcium fluctuates. In addition, the skeleton can act as a reservoir for calcium, releasing the mineral when the blood level drops too low or storing excess calcium for future needs. Also, the body can conserve calcium to some extent by cutting back on the amount that is lost through the urine. Even so, a small amount of calcium will be inescapably lost in urine and sweat every day and must be replaced, either from the diet or from the bones. The exchange of calcium between the bloodstream and the bones is a normal process for the regulation of blood calcium levels. However, if the diet constantly contains too little calcium, the slow but steady drain on the skeleton may eventually compromise the strength of the bones. A habitually low calcium intake has been implicated in the development of osteoporosis, a thinning of the bones that greatly increases the chance of fracture (Holbrook et al., 1988).

Calcium absorption and excretion are influenced by a number of factors, including age, usual calcium intake level, other nutrients in the foods we eat, and medications. Absorption efficiency is greatest during periods of bone growth such as childhood, adolescence, and pregnancy and lactation when the demand for calcium is very high. However, absorption efficiency begins to decrease in middle age, and in women, a sharp drop is seen around the time of the menopause (Heaney et al., 1989). Although a greater percentage is absorbed when habitual calcium intake is low, the increase in absorption fraction cannot totally compensate for a diet that is inadequate. Other nutrients can enhance or inhibit the calcium absorption. Lactose, the sugar found in milk products, improves absorption. Oxalate and phytate, which are found in some vegetables and grains, reduce calcium availability. On balance, these nutrient interactions will not significantly affect calcium nutrition as long as the diet contains a wide variety of foods, each consumed in moderation. High dietary levels of protein, sodium, and caffeine can increase urinary calcium excretion (Kerstetter and Allen, 1990; Dawson-Hughes et al., 1996; Massey and Whiting, 1993) and some of these nutrients may have their most adverse effects when calcium intake is low.

On average, we absorb less than a third of the calcium contained in foods, so the diet must contain at least several times the amount actually required for calcium balance (Figure 1). The Recommended Dietary Allowance (RDA) for calcium for adults over age 50 is 800 milligrams per day (National Research Council, 1989). The RDAs are safe and adequate levels that reduce the risk of nutritional deficiency in the majority of the population, and are also the values used to calculate the percent of daily intake you see on food labels. More recently, the National Institutes of Health issued a set of optimal intakes that are geared toward maximizing bone mass in young adulthood and minimizing bone loss in later years (NIH Consensus Statement, 1994). The optimal intakes for calcium for postmenopausal women under age 65 are 1000 milligrams/day (if taking hormone replacement therapy), or 1500 milligrams/day (if not taking hormones). Women over age 65 are encouraged to consume 1500 milligrams/day.

FIGURE 1   The range of desirable calcium intake (white area) throughout a woman's lifecycle. After age 50, the width of the desirable range reflects the different needs of women who do not use hormone replacement therapy (upper end of range) and those who do (lower end of range). The range was constructed by combining recommendations from the RDAs (National Research Council, 1989) and the National Institutes of Health (NIH Consensus Statement, 1994). Intakes up to 2000 mg/day (gray area) are safe for most individuals.

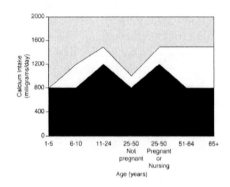

Dairy foods are the most common dietary sources of calcium. Fruits, vegetables, and grains contribute smaller amounts. In Table 1, a list of the most common food sources for calcium in the U.S. diet is presented. The table also presents a point system from which current intake can be evaluated and food selections made to optimize intake. Examples of how this can be done on a daily basis are presented in the footnote to the table. Low fat dairy foods contain as much calcium as regular fat varieties, or slightly more, so even if it is desirable to limit the fat content of the diet, the calcium content need not be compromised.

TABLE 1
Common Food Sources of Calcium in the U.S. Diet

Food Item	Serving Size	Amount of Calcium Per Serving (mg)[a]	Calcium Points Per Serving[b]
Milk			
Whole (3.5% fat)	8 fl oz	280	3
Low fat (1% fat)	8 fl oz	287	3
Yogurt			
Plain or flavored	8 fl oz	274	3
Pizza	2 slices	288	3
Cheese			
Swiss	1 oz	272	3
Cheddar	1 oz	204	2
Mozzarella, part skim	1 oz	195	2
Ricotta, part skim	$^1/_3$ cup	225	2
American	1 oz	174	2
Ice milk	1 cup	190	2
Pudding, custard	$^3/_4$ cup	216	2
Greens (collard, turnip, kale, dandelion), cooked	$^3/_4$ cup	230	2
Broccoli	$^3/_4$ cup	90	1
Calcium-fortified fruit juices[c]	1 cup	300	3

Note: Many women may find that during a typical day they have 1 glass of milk and either a container of yogurt or an ounce of cheese (plain or in sandwiches or cooking). As seen, this would provide 5 calcium points per day. Since each point represents approximately 100 mg, total intake would be approximately 500 mg daily, which is average for adult women in the U.S. Advice can be given using this table about how to get 3 additional points by adding just a few calcium-rich foods to the diet, such as: on one day, an extra glass of milk or a mug of cocoa (both are good sources of vitamin D, too); the next day, 1 serving of broccoli and 1 cup of ice milk; the next day, 2 slices of pizza; the next day, add kale or other greens to soup and top off with 1 oz of grated cheese; the next day, use $^1/_3$ C of ricotta cheese instead of cream cheese on your toast or bagel, and have a serving of pudding for dessert.

[a] Nutrient contents taken from Pennington, J. A. T. and Church, H. N., *Feed Values of Portions Commonly Used*, 14th ed., Harper & Row, New York, 1980. (With permission.)

[b] To meet the RDA of 800 mg/day for women aged 50 and older, daily calcium points must total 8; to meet a goal of 1000 mg/day, points must total 10; and to meet a goal of 1500 mg/day, points must total 15.

[c] Not all fruit juices and drinks are fortified with calcium, and the amount of calcium per 8 oz may vary. Check labels for exact amounts.

It is best to get calcium from foods rather than supplements because foods contain a greater variety of essential vitamins and minerals than is found in supplements. Some people may have difficulty relying totally on foods for their calcium, however. About one out of every five adults in the U.S. has some degree of lactose intolerance and experiences intestinal discomfort after consuming dairy products. Lactose intolerance is more common among people of Black or Asian backgrounds, and regardless of ethnicity, it becomes more frequent with age. Allergy to the proteins found in dairy foods is less common, but also limits calcium intake. Others may find it difficult to consume the calories and volume of liquid needed to meet the calcium recommendations with food sources only, especially if their goal lies in the range of 1000 to 1500 milligrams per day.

Calcium supplements can complement dietary sources. Although a number of different types of calcium supplements can be found on the market, the most common type is calcium carbonate. All are fairly similar when it comes to solubility and absorption. Look on the supplement label for the amount of elemental calcium in each tablet; this is the amount to be compared to the daily intake goal of 800, 1000, or 1500 milligrams.

VITAMIN D

The primary functions of Vitamin D are to aid the absorption of calcium from the intestinal tract, regulate urinary calcium excretion from the kidney, and control the rate at which calcium moves between the bloodstream and the bones. Vitamin D is an unique vitamin; we can manufacture our own supply and do not have to rely only on dietary sources. The body makes vitamin D from a cholesterol-like compound found in the lower layers of the skin. When the skin is exposed to ultraviolet light (for example, sunlight), this compound undergoes a series of chemical reactions to become a form of vitamin D which then enters the bloodstream. Further chemical reactions that occur in the liver are required to transform it into 25-hydroxyvitamin D, which is a useful serum marker of vitamin D status, and finally into the metabolically active form of vitamin D (1,25 dihydroxyvitamin D) after kidney hydroxylation.

Several factors are known to limit the amount of vitamin D that is made in the skin. At northern latitudes, vitamin D synthesis occurs only during part of the year. In Boston, for example, production is highest in the summer and fall months, while exposure to the sun between the months of November and April fails to produce any measurable vitamin D (Webb et al., 1988). The use of sunscreens to block ultraviolet rays also decreases the efficiency with which the body can make its own vitamin D (Matsuoka et al., 1988). Fortunately, vitamin D is stored in the body's fat cells and released when natural synthesis tapers off. The elderly tend to produce vitamin D less effectively than younger adults, and individuals with darkly pigmented skin synthesize less than whites (Matsuoka et al., 1991). Despite these factors that influence endogenous vitamin production, the ordinary daily activities of most individuals expose them to enough sunlight to make adequate amounts of vitamin D. This is often not the case, however, for homebound or institutionalized frail elders, who may never get adequate exposure to sunlight, even in the summer months. For these individuals, reliance on skin production of vitamin D is likely to result in clinical or sub-clinical deficiency states.

The RDA for vitamin D is 200 International Units (IU) daily, although intakes as high as 800 IU have been shown to be safe (Dawson-Hughes et al., 1991; Dawson-Hughes et al., 1997). Compared to many other nutrients, vitamin D is found in a limited number of foods. In the U.S., all fluid and dried milk sold commercially must be fortified with vitamin D to a level of 100 IU per eight ounce cup. Many other countries do not supplement the milk supply in this way, including the United Kingdom and Australia. It should be remembered that dairy products other than milk, such as yogurt and ice cream are not fortified, and therefore cannot be substituted for milk for the purpose of vitamin D repletion, although they can serve as excellent sources of calcium. Vitamin D is found naturally in several other foods, and certain types of fish are very rich sources (Table 2). Most multivitamin tablets and some brands of calcium supplements contain vitamin D. Table 2 also provides examples of how to reach the RDA of 200 IU daily with foods using a point system similar to that for calcium.

TABLE 2
Common Food Sources of Vitamin D in the U.S. Diet

Food Item	Serving Size	Amount of Vitamin D Per Serving (IU)[a]	Vitamin D Points Per Serving[b]
Milk			
Whole (3.5% fat)	8 fl oz	100	4
Low fat (1% fat)	8 fl oz	100	4
Chocolate candy	1.5 oz	30	1
Egg	1 medium	27	1
Margarine	2 tsp	32	1
Fish			
Salmon, canned	1 oz	143	4
Herring	1 oz	257	8
Mackerel	1 oz	200	8
Sardines	1 oz	83	4
Fortified breakfast cereals[c]	1 serving	40–200	2–8

[a] Nutrient contents taken from Pennington, J. A. T. and Church, H. N., *Feed Values of Portions Commonly Used*, 14th ed., Harper & Row, New York, 1980. (With permission.)

[b] To meet the RDA of 200 IU/day for women aged 50 and older, daily vitamin D points must total 8.

[c] Not all breakfast cereals are fortified with vitamin D and serving sizes and amount of vitamin vary. Check labels for exact amounts.

A deficiency of vitamin D will result in abnormal calcification of the bones. When it occurs in children, this condition is called rickets; the adult form is known as osteomalacia. Rickets is rare in the U.S. today because of milk fortification and because we now understand the role of sunlight. There are some segments of the population, however, who are at increased risk of vitamin D deficiency because they avoid or do not have access to these common sources of vitamin D. Elderly persons confined to nursing homes, for example, may have poor vitamin D status. Although frank vitamin D deficiency is not common in the free-living population, it has been suggested that women whose dietary levels are suboptimal, around 100 IU/day or less, experience more rapid bone loss after the menopause than those with higher vitamin D intakes (Dawson-Hughes et al., 1991).

Because excess vitamin D is stored in the body, intakes that are more than five or six times higher than the RDA should be avoided unless prescribed by a physician. Very high intakes of vitamin D over an extended period of time can result in nausea, vomiting, mineral imbalances in the bloodstream (hypercalcemia), and kidney damage. It is difficult to obtain dangerously high amounts of vitamin D from food sources alone. Most cases of vitamin D intoxication result from overuse of vitamin supplements.

USE OF CALCIUM AND VITAMIN D SUPPLEMENTATION FOR AGE-RELATED BONE LOSS IN WOMEN

Women have lower total bone mass or total body calcium than men at all ages. Over a lifetime, women lose about 40% of their skeletal calcium and of this, approximately one half occurs in the first five years after menopause and the remainder occurs at a slower rate thereafter. During the first several years following ovarian failure, calcium supplementation alone will not completely prevent bone loss. In general, however, postmenopausal women benefit significantly at the femoral neck, spine, and radius from calcium supplementation (Cumming and Nevitt, 1997). It should be recognized that calcium needs are relative, dependent upon the levels of other dietary constituents. Thus, a Western diet that is typically high in both sodium and protein, markedly increases urinary calcium losses, and may contribute to difficulty achieving calcium homeostasis and maintaining bone mass in older women in westernized societies. Rates of osteoporosis are much lower in some eastern cultures despite the near absence of dairy products in adult life, and this has been attributed in part to the much lower protein and sodium content in oriental diets, in addition to genetic differences on rates of bone loss.

Inadequate vitamin D intake can also lead to bone loss and increased risk of osteoporosis. In addition to the general finding of seasonal variation in 25-hydroxy-vitamin D, levels of this metabolite decline with age due to declining intake, decreased sun exposure, and perhaps most important, less efficient skin synthesis of vitamin D, as noted above. Treatment of an older population consuming low levels of vitamin D in the diet (less than 220 IU/day) with a 400 IU vitamin D supplement has been shown to prevent significant seasonal variation in either 25-hydroxyvitamin D or parathyroid hormone and, more important, significantly reduces wintertime bone loss from the spine.

Older women exhibiting seasonal bone changes (increases in summer/fall, decreases in winter/spring) also have seasonal changes of similar magnitude in lean tissue mass. Even such moderate changes in body composition can have a significant impact on level of function in the elderly, who may be much closer to the threshold at which muscle strength is directly related to mobility and functional tasks such as walking, stairclimbing, rising from a chair, and lifting objects. Much is to be learned about why bone, lean, and also fat tissue fluctuate with the seasons. Potential contributors to these circannual changes include seasonal changes in exercise, nutrition, and in blood levels of hormones that are known to affect the metabolism of these three tissue compartments. It is known that osteomalacia is associated with a proximal myopathy, manifested by pain, weakness, and atrophy. Whether or not milder seasonal fluctuations in vitamin D stores are responsible for the loss of lean tissue during these months remains to be proven, but is suggested by the patterns observed.

Although calcium alone has been shown to lower the risk of vertebral fractures in postmenopausal women, and vitamin D alone has reduced fractures in the arm, several other trials of isolated supplementation have failed to reduce fracture rates. Dawson-Hughes has reported that a combination of calcium (500 mg) and vitamin D (700 IU) supplementation daily resulted in a 60% reduction in non-vertebral osteoporotic fracture risk at 3 years in older men and women. Small improvements in bone density occurred, but it is unclear if they were of sufficient magnitude to reduce fracture risk. Since fracture rates between groups in this trial diverged early and progressively over the three years, despite a leveling off of bone density benefits after the first year of treatment, it is possible that calcium and vitamin D supplementation affected other factors related to injurious falls which remain to be identified.

Similarly, women at very high risk for hip fracture (elderly women aged 69 to 106 years living in nursing homes or elderly apartments) have been shown by Chapuy and colleagues to benefit substantially from vitamin D (800 IU/day) plus calcium supplementation, exhibiting increased bone density, and reduced rates of hip and other non-vertebral fracture over the course of 18 months. The magnitude of reduction in hip fracture risk in this trial (43%) has only been seen in one other intervention in the elderly which employed hip pad protectors. The finding that fracture rates began to change by 2 months of treatment, and bone density improvements were quite modest, suggests that the mechanism of effect was possibly through a reduction in fall rates (responsible for 99% of the fractures in this study), rather than an amelioration of low bone density itself. Bone density was likely still far below the fracture threshold after supplementation, given the mean age of 84 years in this study, and the mechanism responsible for the protective effect of nutrient supplementation requires further investigation. However, the potency demonstrated in these two trials is quite convincing evidence for ensuring adequate calcium and vitamin D status in women at risk for osteoporotic fracture.

SUMMARY

In the older woman, the importance of vitamin D and calcium status relates primarily to bone and muscle integrity and the prevention of osteoporotic fracture, since bone mass will always be sacrificed to maintain the metabolic and neuromuscular functions of calcium. The clinical sequelae of osteopenia (pain, deformity, osteoporotic fracture) are some of the most prevalent, burdensome, and costly syndromes in geriatric health care. The nutritional approach to osteoporosis must recognize it as a lifelong process with many points to intervene along the pathway, and opportunities to practice preventive medicine even in the last decade of life.

Attainment of peak bone mass requires adequate intake of calcium and intake or endogenous production of vitamin D in childhood and early adulthood. High levels of sodium and protein in the diet will impede the establishment of calcium balance from food sources alone. Since natural sources of vitamin D in the diet are sparse, fortification of common foods (e.g., milk) is often necessary. When it is not a national policy to fortify the food supply in this way, vitamin D deficiency in the population can be quite prevalent, particularly in northern latitudes where sunlight exposure adequate to synthesize vitamin D from precursors in the skin is limited for much of the year (as in Great Britain). It should be remembered that while calcium supplementation has now been added to some non-dairy products in the U.S. (e.g., orange juice, bread, cereal) to increase the population's exposure to this mineral, vitamin D is primarily present only in dairy foods that have been fortified with it. In addition to calcium and vitamin D, excess alcohol, protein, and sodium can lead to lower than expected peak bone mass. Low levels of physical activity which load the weight-bearing joints as well as smoking can lead to lower than normal bone density in mid-life and beyond, and are independent risk factors for osteoporotic fracture in some studies.

After menopause, the loss of bone can be slowed by attention to both calcium and vitamin D intake, which may lower the risk of spinal and appendicular fractures in women. In most cases, hip fractures result from an injurious fall of a person with osteopenia. Therefore, prevention of hip fracture requires attention to both fall-related risk factors as well as bone density. Nutritional factors that have been associated with traumatic hip fracture include protein calorie malnutrition, alcohol abuse, osteomalacia, low body mass index, low muscle mass and strength, low levels of body fat, and low amounts of soft tissue padding over the greater trochanteric region. For some of these factors, the association may be due to both increased fall risk (e.g., muscle weakness from vitamin D deficiency, loss of balance from alcohol intoxication) as well as direct effects on skeletal integrity. More work is needed to identify gait and balance disorders associated with both vitamin D deficiency as well as protein calorie malnutrition, so that these factors are considered in the mainstream of both prevention and treatment of recurrent hip fracture in the aged. The interelationship of all of these factors mandates that the recommendations for calcium and vitamin D intake and/or supplementation are best formulated in the context of a multifactorial approach to muscle and bone health and mobility in older women.

REFERENCES

Chapuy, M. C., Arlor, M. E., Duboeuf, F., Brun, J., Crouzet, B., Arnaud, S., Delmas, P., and Meunier, P. J., Vitamin D2 and calcium to prevent hip fracture in elderly women, *N. Engl. J. Med.*, 327, 1637–1642, 1992.

Cumming, R. G. and Nevitt, M. C., Calcium for prevention of osteoporotic fractures in postmenopausal women, *J. Bone Mineral Res.*, 12(9), 1321–9, 1997.

Dawson-Hughes, B., Dallal, G. E., Krall, E. A., Harris, S., Sokoll, L. J., and Falconer, G., Effect of vitamin D supplementation on wintertime and overall bone loss in healthy postmenopausal women, *Ann. Intern. Med.*, 115, 505–512, 1991.

Dawson-Hughes, B., Fowler, S. E., Dalsky, G., and Gallagher, C., Sodium excretion influences calcium homeostasis in elderly men and women, *J. Nutr.*, 126(9), 2107–12, 1996.

Dawson-Hughes, B., Harris, S. S., Krall, E. A., and Dallal, G. E., Effect of calcium and vitamin D supplementation on bone density in men and women 65 years of age or older, *N. Engl. J. Med.*, 337, 670–676, 1997.

Heaney, R. P., Recker, R. R., Stegman, M. R., and Moy, A. J., Calcium absorption in women, relationships to calcium intake, estrogen status, and age, *J. Bone Mineral Res.*, 4(4), 469–75, 1989.

Holbrook, T. L., Barrett-Connor, E., and Wingard, D. L., Dietary calcium and risk of hip fracture, 14-year prospective population study, *Lancet*, 2(8619), 1046–9, 1988.

Kerstetter, J. E. and Allen, L. H., Dietary protein increases urinary calcium, *J. Nutr.*, 120(1), 134–6, 1990.

Massey, L. K. and Whiting, S. J., Caffeine, urinary calcium, calcium metabolism and bone, *J. Nutr.*, 123(9), 1611–4, 1993.

Matsuoka, L. Y., Wortsman, J., Haddad, J. G., Kolm, P., and Hollis, B. W., Racial pigmentation and the cutaneous synthesis of vitamin D, *Arch Dermatol.*, 127(4), 536–8, 1991.

Matsuoka, L. Y., Wortsman, J., Hanifan, N., and Holick, M. F., Chronic sunscreen use decreases circulating concentrations of 25-hydroxyvitamin D. A preliminary study. *Arch. Dermatol.*, 124(12), 1802–4, 1988.

National Research Council, Subcommittee on the tenth edition of the Recommended Dietary Allowances, 10th ed., National Academy Press, Washington, D.C., 1989.

Optimal Calcium Intake, NIH Consensus Statement, 12(4), 1–31, 1994.

Pennington, J. A. T. and Church, H. N., Food values of portions commonly used, 14th ed., Harper & Row, New York, 1980.

Webb, A. R., Kline, L., and Holick, M. F., Influence of season and latitude on the cutaneous synthesis of vitamin D3: exposure to winter sunlight in Boston and Edmonton will not promote vitamin D3 synthesis in human skin, *J. Clin. Endocrinol. Metab.*, 67(2), 373–8, 1988.

9 Antioxidants and Immune Response*

Simin Nikbin Meydani, Timothy S. McElreavy,
and Mohsen Meydani

CONTENTS

INTRODUCTION

The influence of nutrition on the immune response has been intensely studied in recent years, yet the effects of diet on health, in general, and the immune system, in particular, of the older woman have not been traditionally emphasized as a preventive measure against such diseases as cancer, cardiovascular disease, and arthritis. Recent research has suggested that supplementation above the established recommended levels of certain nutrients, including dietary antioxidants, may positively affect the immune response. Indeed, many recent studies have indicated that antioxidant vitamins are highly effective in maintaining the function of the body's immune system despite the changes that may occur with aging.

According to the final 1994 data released by the National Center for Health Statistics, life expectancy at birth in the United States for all races and both sexes is 76 years.[1] Future projections indicate that increases in the population sector of

* Studies by the authors described in this chapter have been funded at least in part with Federal funds from the United States Department of Agriculture, Agricultural Research Service, under contract number 53-K06-01. The contents of this publication do not necessarily reflect the views or policies of the U.S. Department of Agriculture, nor does mention of trade names, commercial products, or organizations imply endorsement by the U.S. Government.

individuals age 65 years and over will continue into the second millennium. Age-associated changes in physiologic, psychological, social, and economic factors may adversely affect the nutritional and immunological status of older individuals; these changes are often reflected in poor health and reduced quality of life. Incidence of infections and diseases such as cancer, atherosclerosis, and autoimmunity has been shown to increase with age.

Correction of nutritional deficiencies can restore compromised immune function and aid in the maintenance of health during aging. In addition, supplementation of some micronutrients may boost the immune responses of healthy elderly and aid in the establishment of optimal health and extension of a youthful, more vigorous lifestyle.

Of course, one of the best ways of abating the dysfunction associated with aging is to maintain an active healthy lifestyle that includes a balanced diet with adequate nutrient intake. The connection between a healthy lifestyle and successful aging is as much a subject of common sense as it is of scientific inquiry; however, research is constantly revealing complex connections between nutrient intake and bodily mechanisms that can maintain and even improve health. This chapter will discuss recent evidence regarding antioxidant vitamins and immune function and their relationship to the aging woman.

ANTIOXIDANT VITAMINS

WHAT ARE THEY AND HOW DO THEY WORK?

Dietary antioxidants—vitamins E and C and β-carotene among others—are components of the average American diet and are found in a variety of foods. These substances are vital to the body in a number of ways, but perhaps most important, they offer protection against the harmful effects of oxygen to cells and bodily chemicals. These effects, in controlled amounts, are necessary for the function and survival of several cell types, organisms, and biological mechanisms. However, similar to the way that metal rusts or tarnishes or some foods turn rancid upon exposure to air, bodily tissues also suffer from prolonged exposure to oxidizing agents known as oxygen free radicals that occur naturally as part of the metabolic process of living, but are also caused by such pollutants as cigarette smoke, smog, pesticides, and many types of drugs. The effects of oxygen free radicals and oxidation initiate a highly injurious chain reaction leading to widespread damage to cell systems. When cells are injured by oxidative stress, the vital functions they perform and the complex systems they construct begin to degrade, leaving the body vulnerable to opportunistic infection and the "dys"function associated with many diseases of aging. By attacking these free radicals directly, antioxidants sacrifice themselves to maintain the integrity and function of cells and cell systems.

Among the dietary antioxidants, vitamins C and E and β-carotene are the most commonly studied micronutrients for their general health effects as well as their specific free radical-fighting properties. Vitamin C (ascorbic acid) is a water-soluble nutrient, whereas vitamin E (α-tocopherol) and β-carotene are fat soluble. Water-soluble vitamins are absorbed directly into the circulatory system but are not stored in the body. Concentrations of water-soluble vitamins in excess of those required by the body are simply excreted through the urine, rendering the purported benefits of megadoses of vitamin C virtually useless. Fat-soluble vitamins, however, are absorbed by the body in the presence of fat or in conditions that favor the absorption of fat. The body stores fat-soluble vitamins in fat cells, using these stores when necessary. Because of this storage method, certain types of fat-soluble vitamins can reach toxic levels that lead to harmful effects; therefore, individuals should consult their physicians before taking megadoses of fat-soluble vitamins, particularly those with known side effects such as vitamins A and D.

Vitamins E and C are essential nutrients that participate in numerous physiologic processes. β-carotene is a nutrient that acts as a source of vitamin A in addition to its own antioxidant properties. Despite the levels of consumption recommended for vitamins E and C, many studies indicate that higher doses of each vitamin may have health benefits. There is currently no recommended dietary allowance for β-carotene, and recent research has thrown the potential benefits of β-carotene supplementation into question, however, it should always be remembered that the body only uses what is needed. Thus, the body absorbs a lower proportion of the total amount of each of these vitamins as intake increases, either through diet or supplementation.

Table 1 provides a sampling of foods with high concentrations of β-carotene (and other carotenoids), vitamin C, and vitamin E. For the sake of comparison, Table 2 lists some of the major sources of carotenes (including β-carotene), vitamin C, and vitamin E in the American diet and the percentage of total dietary intake for each nutrient from the food listed.[2]

TABLE 1
Names, Recommended Levels, and Sources of Antioxidant Vitamins

Vitamin Names and RDA for Healthy Adults	Significant Sources
Vitamin A (retinol, retinal, retinoic acid) Precursor is provitamin A Carotenoids such as β-carotene RDA of vitamin A for women: 800 mg RE (retinal equivalents) No RDA for β-carotene	Vitamin A (retinal): fortified milk, cheese, cream, butter, fortified margarine, eggs, liver β-carotene: spinach and other dark leafy greens, broccoli, and deep orange fruits and vegetables (i.e., apricots, peaches, cantaloupe, squash, carrots, sweet potatoes, pumpkin)

Vitamin E (α-tocopherol and various other tocopherols and tocotrienols)
RDA for women:
  8 mg α-TE (α-tocopherol equivalents)
RDA for men:
  10 mg α-TE (α-tocopherol equivalents)
	Plant oils (i.e., margarine, salad dressings, shortenings), green and leafy vegetables, wheat germ, whole grain products, shrimp, butter, liver, egg yolk, milk fat, nuts, seeds

Vitamin C (ascorbic acid) RDA for men and women: 60 mg	Citrus fruits, cabbage, dark green vegetables, cantaloupe, strawberries, peppers, lettuce, tomatoes, potatoes, papayas, mangos, rosehips

TABLE 2
Major Sources of Carotenes, Vitamin C, and Vitamin E in the American Diet[a]

Carotenes		Vitamin C		Vitamin E	
Food	**Cumulative %[b]**	**Food**	**Cumulative %[b]**	**Food**	**Cumulative %[b]**
Carrots	37.8	Orange Juice	26.5	Mayonnaise	14.6
Tomatoes	51.0	Grapefruit (and juice)	33.7	Potato chips	18.8
Sweet potatoes	56.7	Tomatoes (and juice)	39.9	Apples	22.9
Yellow squash	62.3	Fortified fruit drinks	45.7	Nuts	27.0
Spinach (cooked)	67.9	Oranges	50.6	Peanut butter	30.9
Cantaloupe	71.7	Potatoes (not fried)	54.8	Oil and vinegar	34.2
Mixed vegetables	75.4	Potatoes (fried)	58.9	Tomatoes	37.4
Romaine lettuce	78.3	Green salad	62.4	Margarine	40.5
Broccoli	80.6	Other fruit juices	65.2	Sweet roll	43.2
Spinach (raw)	83.0	Broccoli	67.2	Tomato sauce	45.9
Tomato sauce	84.4	Coleslaw/ cabbage	69.1	Sweet potatoes	48.3
Margarine	85.7	Spaghetti and sauce	71.0	Eggs	50.4
Orange juice	87.0	Orange juice substitute	72.8	Cold cereal	52.5
Iceberg lettuce	88.1	Cold cereal	74.6	Shrimp	54.6
Pizza	89.1	Hot dogs/lunch meat	76.3	Cake	56.6
Cheese	90.1	Cantaloupe	77.9	Cabbage	58.5
String beans	91.0	Whole milk	79.4	Iceberg lettuce	60.3
Peas	91.9	Greens	80.8	Tuna	62.2
Oranges	92.6	Strawberries	82.1	Cheese	63.9
Whole milk	93.4	Fortified cold cereal	83.0	Whole milk	65.1

[a] Adapted from Byers and Perry, *Ann. Nutr. Rev.*, 12, 39–153, 1992. With permission.
[b] The cumulative percent of total nutrient intake in the diet provided by the listed foods.

Abundantly available in citrus fruits, broccoli, spinach, and melon, vitamin C is perhaps the most well-known vitamin to the general public, due in large part to its fabled prodigious effects. Vitamin C is necessary for various chemical reactions required for proper metabolism and for collagen formation, an important process for the maintenance of connective tissues, bone, and teeth. Though vitamin C itself was not officially discovered until 1912, citrus fruits were widely prescribed for hundreds of years to combat scurvy, a disease caused by severe vitamin C deficiency. Scurvy historically affected sailors who did not have adequate access to fresh food, and more recently has plagued undernourished children in impoverished areas of the world. Today, scurvy and lesser states of vitamin C deficiency are rare in the U.S. because of widespread availability of its sources, and one might conjecture, the public's belief in the myriad claims of its health benefits. Perhaps the most famous (and still widely believed) claim for vitamin C was Nobel laureate Linus Pauling's assertion that megadoses of the vitamin could reduce the incidence of the common cold. Scientific studies and clinical trials do not support this claim; however, there is increasing evidence that vitamin C supplementation can reduce the duration and severity of the symptoms of the common cold.

But how much vitamin C and how often? The Recommended Dietary Allowance (RDA) for vitamin C is 60 mg daily, yet it is not uncommon for people to take as much as 1,000 to 2,000 mg per day. An adequate supply is readily available in a well-balanced diet and can often be obtained from a single serving of citrus fruit (i.e., a medium-sized orange or grapefruit). There are no known major risks for taking megadoses of vitamin C; however, reports indicate that watery stool or diarrhea and intestinal discomfort may be side effects. Researchers have recommended that smokers increase their vitamin C intake because of the oxidizing effect of cigarette smoke in the body which effectively neutralizes vitamin C, offsetting the oxidant/antioxidant balance. This balance, discussed below, is important to maintain for adequate defense against oxidative stress and free radicals. Vitamin C offers the first line of defense against oxidative stress, but it also regenerates vitamin E molecules that have been reduced in effectiveness after encountering free radicals. Thus, vitamin C offers a twofold protection against oxidation and the body's subsequent susceptibility to disease, actively engaging the free radical itself and regenerating vitamin E so that it may continue battling oxidative stress.

Vitamin E (α-tocopherol as well as other tocopherols and tocotrienols) is perhaps the most widely studied antioxidant nutrient. Major sources of vitamin E in the American diet include vegetable oils, nuts, fish, shellfish, and green leafy vegetables such as spinach, kale, collard greens, and cabbage. Since many foods high in vitamin E are also high in fat (for example, nuts and fried foods are significant sources of this nutrient), people should be encouraged to eat more seafood and vegetables to maintain their vitamin E status. While researchers are still trying to define the multiple roles that this vitamin plays in the body, much evidence is accumulating that, like vitamin C, it significantly enhances the immune system. Vitamin E deficiency is rare, occurring most often in premature infants, children, and adults who have genetic defects in fat absorption (i.e., cystic fibrosis, choleostasis, and celiac disease). Symptoms of deficiency include neurological disorders, anemia, impaired function of platelets and white blood cells, reproductive or sexual dysfunction, and dysfunction of the retina. Though the current RDA for vitamin E is 8 to 10 IU per day, supplementation above the RDA has been shown to be beneficial to immuno- logic vigor.[3–5] This effect may be due in large part to the vitamin's antioxidant properties, which according to current scientific opinion are its chief function in the body. There are no known major risks for taking higher than recommended levels of vitamin E, except in those individuals who are deficient in vitamin K and are taking anti-coagulant drugs, in which case hemmorhagic side effects are possible.[6,7] Other purported effects of vitamin E, such as protection from harmful ultraviolet radiation from the sun, have not yet been established.

Antioxidants have not been shown to prevent further degeneration of the central nervous system in Parkinson's disease, as had been speculated. However, there is one trial of α-tocopherol supplementation at 2000 IU/day for 2 years in patients with moderately advanced Alzheimer's disease in which there was a significant reduction in a combined outcome which included death, time to institutionalization, and functional decline, in comparison with placebo or selegiline therapy. The mech- anism of this improved outcome for this clearly pharmacologic dose of α-tocopheral is not at all clear, and further studies of Vitamin E's role in neurologic diseases are required before conclusions can be drawn.

Antioxidant properties and prevention of lipid peroxidation of polyunsaturated fatty acids (PUFA), substances found abundantly in the diet in the form of fish oils and vegetable oils like corn oil, are the most widely accepted biological functions of vitamin E. It is the most effective chain-breaking, lipid-soluble antioxidant in the biological membrane, where it protects critical cellular structures against damage from reactive oxygen species (ROS) and other free radicals. In normal cellular metabolism, most of the oxygen in the body is consumed through general metabolic functions; however, a small amount of oxygen can escape this process to produce free radicals. These products can cause membrane lipid peroxidation and the loss of membrane integrity. The continuous and increased production of free radicals and their reactions with other critical cellular components such as DNA have been suggested to contribute to the aging process and to the pathogenesis of chronic diseases such as cancer.[8]

β-carotene, a nutrient found in many fruits and vegetables, acts as both a pre- cursor for vitamin A and as an antioxidant in its own right. The body stores β-carotene, converting it to vitamin A as needed. While these two compounds, β-carotene and vitamin A, are related structurally, they have very different functions. Vitamin A can be made from β-carotene, but the reverse is not true. The current recommendation for vitamin A is 5000 IU per day for adults. This is total for vitamin A equivalents, which can be derived from provitamin A carotenoids or from pre-formed vitamin A. When planning a diet, it is important to understand the difference between β-carotene and vitamin A. Intake of too much ready-made vita- min A may be harmful because it is stored in the body and may lead to neurological disorders in extreme cases, while β-carotene can be tolerated without side effects at higher doses and is converted into vitamin A as the body needs it. However, β-carotene in high doses can cause skin yellowing and some gastrointestinal symp- toms. It is not clear if there are other, more serious adverse effects, although some recent studies have indicated that intake of some β-carotene preparations for a long period of time increases the incidence of lung cancer in heavy smokers.[9] Of course, more research must be done to prove conclusively that there is a link between β-carotene supplementation and lung cancer in smokers. However, this does not mean that consumption of fruits and vegetables containing β-carotene and other carotenoids increases lung cancer. Several studies have shown that the incidence of cancer is lower with a higher intake of fruits and vegetables. In the meantime, the best way for smokers to significantly reduce their risk for cancer is to stop smoking.

A number of studies show that people who eat fruits and vegetables, which can be high in β-carotene, have lower risks of heart disease and cancer. Several recent experimental trials that administered either β-carotene or a placebo to subjects did not show any benefits from β-carotene in lowering the chance of heart disease or cancer, indicating that other components or a combination of components in fruits and vegetables contribute to this reduction in cancer incidence. As with other antioxidants, it has been suggested that β-carotene protects DNA from oxygen damage, possibly preventing one of the many steps that occur as normal cells turn into cancer cells. Despite the ease and availability of supplements, eating lots of fruits and vegetables, which has consistently been linked to lower rates of heart disease and cancer, is still the best approach. This type of varied diet provides not only β-carotene, but a number of other important nutrients including vitamins C and E. Furthermore, recent clinical and epidemiological evidence indicates that supplementation with β-carotene may be harmful rather than beneficial by exacerbating risk factors for cancer or heart disease already present in an individual.[10,11] Most people can get enough vitamin A and β-carotene from a balanced diet which, unlike supplementation, has been consistently linked to reduced risk for cancer and heart disease. This beneficial effect of a balanced diet is likely due to various nutrients and other natural chemicals working in concert.

Limited data are available on the effects of aging on the metabolism of vitamins E and C and β-carotene. Several reports in humans have suggested that concentrations of vitamin E in the blood do not change with aging;[12,13] however, others have indicated that there is an age-associated decrease in vitamin E concentrations found in platelets.[14] In addition, the cells of the immune system have been shown to have higher concentrations of vitamin E than other cells,[15,16] but data examining the effect of aging on vitamin E concentrations in these cells are lacking. In laboratory mice, however, scientists have observed that the vitamin E content of the cells of the spleen do not differ significantly between the young and old.

MAINTAINING THE OXIDANT/ANTIOXIDANT BALANCE

The oxidant/antioxidant balance is an important determinant of immune cell function. Cells of the immune system are particularly sensitive to changes in this delicate balance because of the high level of PUFA in their membranes or exterior boundaries. Since these substances are easily oxidizable, a proper balance of antioxidant nutrients and PUFA is needed to thwart the damaging effects of oxidizing agents in the body.

The RDAs of vitamin E for men and women are 10 and 8 mg, respectively.[17] The present RDA for vitamin E is based primarily on customary intake of this vitamin from U.S. food sources and appears to be adequate to maintain normal physiologic functions and protect the polyunsaturated fatty acids of tissue from lipid peroxidation; however, the daily requirement for this vitamin increases with a high intake of PUFA and increasing unsaturated fatty acids in the diet. Even though foods that are high in PUFA often contain high levels of vitamin E, this may not always be the case. Vegetable oils and margarine are relatively rich in γ-tocopherol which has 1/10 the biological activity of α-tocopherol, the most common form of vitamin E; therefore, increasing PUFA in the diet from these sources may not provide enough vitamin E to maintain a proper balance. A ratio of > 0.4 mg vitamin E/gram of PUFA is desirable to maintain the oxidant/antioxidant balance;[18] however, this ratio may vary significantly depending on the types of food consumed (for example, the ratio for walnuts is more than double that for olive oil because of olive oil's high PUFA content).

Several surveys and recent clinical studies have indicated that intake of vitamin E at levels more than several times the RDA is necessary to reduce the risk of cardiovascular disease and certain cancers as well as to increase immune function, especially among the elderly.[3,4] However, a recent study published in the *New England Journal of Medicine* has shown that vitamin E supplementation in post-menopausal women did not reduce their risk of death from coronary heart disease;[19] rather, results from this study indicated that risk of death was reduced with the consumption of a well-balanced diet, high in a variety of nutrients. Evidence such as that presented in this study underscores the importance of consuming adequate levels of all nutrients, not just particular ones that may be associated with specific health effects. Unfortunately, this is generally not the case in the United States. For example, according to the Second National Health and Nutrition Examination Survey (NHANES II), the vitamin E content in the diets of the majority of the U.S. population is slightly below the RDA (69% of men and 80% of women), and the diets of 20% of American men and 32% of American women contain less than 50% of the RDA.[20] This survey also reported that 23% of men and 15% of women showed a ratio of vitamin E/gram of PUFA of < 0.4, which is below the accepted level for maintenance of the oxidant/antioxidant balance.[20]

IMMUNE FUNCTION

The influence of nutrition on immune response has been studied intensely in recent years. It has long been accepted that deficiencies of many macro- and micronutrients have a negative impact on the ability of an individual to mount an adequate immune response to a pathogenic challenge. More recent research has suggested that supplementation above the accepted requirements of certain nutrients, depending on age, gender, and health status, may positively affect immunity. An optimal level of antioxidants is needed for maintenance of the immune response across all age groups. This need may be more critical, however, in the aged in general and the older woman in particular. The age-associated dysregulation of the immune response has been well documented.[21,22] The age-related increase in free radical formation and lipid peroxidation contributes, at least in part, to this phenomenon,[23,24] predisposing older women to a higher incidence of infectious, neoplastic, autoimmune, and inflammatory diseases.[25]

The alterations in bodily function affected by aging are myriad, and their causes are not easily discerned and may be the products of a combination of factors and conditions; thus, it is important to understand the complexity of what constitutes aging. Physiologic changes associated with aging may produce outcomes that alter the nutritional and immune status of older individuals. Increases in illness and chronic diseases result in physical weakness, dependence on others, decreased mobility, and isolation. These physical changes and impediments can, in turn, result in psychological repercussions such as lowered self-esteem and a sense of worthlessness as well as depression, due at least in part to the loss of independence. Increased financial burdens as a result of lowered income in retirement years and concomitant increases in health care costs add to feelings of distress. Together, these age-associated changes in physiologic, psychological, social, and economic conditions contribute to reducing quality of the diet of many older individuals, which can have quantifiable repercussions on their immune and health status.

On the other hand, immune dysregulation due to environmental factors or aging itself may be found at the root of physical ailments that contribute to a reduction in the quality of diet among older individuals. Dysregulation of immune function may be a result of reduction in beneficial immune responses, such as innate and acquired immunity, or increases in harmful immune responses, such as the production of antibodies against one's own body.

THE IMMUNE SYSTEM

The human body's ability to combat and clear foreign invaders or non-self antigens is an important part of health maintenance and contributes to decreased incidences of infection and illness. Healthy immune function has also been linked to greater life spans. There are two main branches of immunity: innate or natural immunity and acquired immunity.[26] Innate immunity involves immune surveillance and killing mechanisms which do not require a previous encounter with a foreign substance by immune cells. Examples of innate immunity include phagocytosis by neutrophils and macrophages (Mf), and the tumoricidal and virucidal activities of natural killer cells (NK). On the other hand, acquired immunity necessitates the encounter of an antigen for the priming of a specific immune response. Acquired immunity involves Mf, T-cells, and B-cells and includes cell-mediated functions and humoral immunity or antibody production.

The immune system is a complex structure in which the several types of cells mentioned above perform highly individualized functions to recognize and react to invading substances called antigens. Antigens may be in the form of a virus, bacteria, or other type of molecule that is not indigenous to the body. Of the various types of immune cells, lymphocytes and phagocytes are often the most dramatically affected by nutritional status and the oxidant/antioxidant balance.

Lymphocytes specialize the recognition of the "foreignness" of a particular antigen, setting the stage for the phagocytes to inactivate, destroy, and remove the foreign compound or substance. Lymphocytes respond to specific antigens using surface receptors that will recognize the particular shape or characteristics of a single molecule. Each lymphocyte may have hundreds of thousands of receptors, but all are identical; thus, each cell can identify only one type of antigen. Therefore, the immune system comprises a huge number of lymphocytes that can recognize between 10 and 100 million different antigens. An antigen may encounter millions of lymphocytes before finding the one with the receptors to which it can bind. This process is similar to finding the right key for a lock. Once found, the antigen binds to the lymphocyte, causing it to proliferate or create clones of itself. When enough lymphocyte clones are produced, the body is able to fight the antigen. Once the antigen is recognized, the cloned cells differentiate and secrete proteins that stimulate the attack and destruction of the antigen. Some of these cloned lymphocytes will remain in the body as memory cells once the antigen has been disposed, thereby creating immunity to that particular invader. Memory cells are easily reactivated and will mount a faster response to subsequent antigen invasions. If an individual is immune to a particular antigen, such as a virus, he or she has had a previous encounter with it—through actual illness, vaccination, or contact with that antigen which did not lead to illness.

There are two main types of lymphocytes that come into play once the immune system is prepared to attack an antigen, B- and T-cells. B-cells produce antibodies that are vital to neutralizing bacteria and toxins like tetanus toxin in the blood. If a particular antigen has infiltrated the body at the cellular level, T-cells, specifically killer T-cells, will be required to get rid of it. There are four classes of T-cells: inducer T-cells, helper T-cells, killer T-cells, and suppressor T-cells. Upon recognition of an antigen, the inducer T-cells secrete proteins that activate other T-cells and attract a type of phagocyte known as a macrophage to the area where the antigen has been recognized. Helper T-cells release proteins that activate B-cells and the generation of antibodies. Once these cells have been activated and made their "call to arms," macrophages will ingest the antigen, breaking it down into smaller parts and presenting these fragments to oncoming T-cells. Killer T-cells will then destroy any cell bearing a foreign antigen, thus neutralizing the invader. This simultaneous attack by both the macrophages and killer T-cells is so effective that neighboring cells are often damaged in the process of ridding the body of the virus, infection, or foreign antigen.

Suppressor T-cells do not play a direct role in this battlefield; instead, they oppose the helper and inducer T-cells to keep the immune system balanced. This is particularly important for maintaining general health considering the devastation that can be caused by impaired immune function. For example, people suffering from systemic lupus erythematosus make antibodies to their own DNA, while people with rheumatoid arthritis make antibodies to combat antibodies. The AIDS virus is exceptionally damaging because it reproduces or replicates itself within the genetic make-up of helper and inducer T-cells, becoming reactivated when the T-cell encounters an antigen and killing off the lymphocyte. Scientists have not yet pinpointed the exact mechanism for this destruction of helper and inducer cells, but the result of this widespread cell death is devastatingly clear in the context of the simplified summary of immune function given above.

Dysregulation of immune function with aging has been well-established[27,28] and contributes to higher incidence as well as morbidity and mortality from cancer and infectious, autoimmune, and neoplastic diseases. A decrease in T-cell-mediated function, including thymus involution and *in vivo* decreases in the delayed-type hypersensitivity (DTH) skin response; the graft-versus-host reaction; resistance to tumors, viruses, and parasites; T-cell-dependent primary and secondary antibody responses; the proportion of T-cell subsets with naïve cell surface markers encompasses a large part of the overall decline.[29] In addition, *in vitro* mitogen-stimulated lymphocyte proliferation, interleukin (IL) -2 production, and responsiveness to IL-2 have also been shown to decline with age. It appears that decreases and dysfunctions in cell function occur largely as a result of the aging cell's decreased ability to receive and respond to cell signals.[30–34] Some decline is also seen in humoral immune function, particularly in the loss of high-affinity cell surface receptors for antigen and for cytokines. Proliferation of B-cells is fairly well-maintained; however, old animals show impaired response to antigens that stimulate CD5⁻ B-cells (foreign antigen). On the other hand, the ability of CD5⁺ B-cells to respond to autoantigens remains intact.[35] Thus, while the ability to respond to foreign antigens declines with age, autoantibody formation increases with age, which may contribute to autoimmune disease.[36–38] This dysregulated immune response is also observed in T-cells in which production of Th_1 cytokines is decreased while production of Th_2 cytokines is reported to be increased with age.[39] Furthermore, increased production of suppressive factors such as prostaglandin (PG) E_2 by Mf has been reported to contribute to the dysregulation of T-cell function;[23,40] however, there is no clear consensus on age-related changes in NK activity. Reviews on research in NK activity[41,42] summarize reports of decreases, stasis, and increases in NK activity with aging. Differences in sample size, criteria used for the inclusion of healthy elderly, and age range, as well as contamination by other cell types are possible contributing factors to these wide-ranging results.[43]

THE EFFECTS OF VITAMIN E, VITAMIN C, AND β-CAROTENE ON IMMUNE RESPONSE IN THE AGING WOMAN

As evident in the extreme cases of autoimmune diseases, it is vital to maintain a healthy and balanced immune system. For example, while phagocytes produce substances through oxidation that can neutralize bacteria, oxidation and the formation of free radicals can also pose a serious threat to immune function by destroying the immune cells that produce them. The oxidant/antioxidant balance is an important determinant of immune cell function, not only for maintaining the integrity and functionality of membrane lipids, cellular proteins, and nucleic acids, but for controlling the receipt of signals that activate gene expression, turning certain genes on and off, in immune cells. The cells of the immune system are particularly sensitive to changes in the oxidant/antioxidant balance because of the relatively higher percentage of polyunsaturated fatty acids (PUFA) in their membranes. They are also frequently exposed to changes in this balance because a high level of oxidation products is produced as part of their normal function. Signaling and gene expression, events sensitive to oxidative stress, are critical in maintaining normal function of immune cells and their ability to defend against the wide range of foreign antigens to which they are exposed. It is, therefore, not surprising to note that the cells of the immune system have, in general, higher concentrations of antioxidant nutrients compared to other cells[15,16] and that severe or marginal deficiency of several antioxidants, including vitamins C and E among others, adversely affect the immune response.

It is interesting to note that upon exposure to pathogens, e.g., influenza virus, tissue concentrations of several antioxidant nutrients decrease significantly. One study[44] reported a significant decrease in lung and liver concentrations of vitamin E in mice infected with influenza virus. A nonsignificant increase in vitamin C was also observed. Furthermore, Beck and colleagues[45] noted that certain strains of influenza become more virulent or aggressive upon exposure to oxidants.

Vitamin E

We have proposed that the antioxidant nutrient intake of the elderly, by virtue of its influence on oxidant/antioxidant balance, is an important determinant of their immune response. The interaction of vitamin E and the immune response has been demonstrated in a variety of animal species.[46] Vitamin E supplementation has been successfully used to improve some aspects of age-related decline in laboratory animal immune function.[47] Meydani et al. showed that increasing the level of dietary vitamin E from 30 to 500 ppm significantly increases blood vitamin E levels, delayed type hypersensitivity, lymphocyte proliferation to concanavalin A (Con A), and interleukin (IL)-2 production in old mice; this effect of vitamin E was associated with a decrease in PGE_2 production. Vitamin E-supplemented animals from this study also had a lower incidence of kidney amyloidosis than control animals (fed 30 ppm vitamin E).[49] Another recent study confirmed these findings. Sakai and Moriguchi[50] reported that vitamin E supplementation (585 mg/kg diet) for 12 months significantly improved T-cell-mediated function compared with rats fed a control diet containing 50 mg vitamin E/kg. In another study, Meydani et al.[51] showed that while vitamin E supplementation did not have an effect on natural killer cell (NK) activity of unchallenged young or old mice, it was effective in preventing SRBC-induced suppression of NK activity in old mice.

Relatively few controlled clinical studies have been conducted to determine the effect of vitamin E on the immune response of elderly persons. Vitamin E supplementation has been shown to enhance immunity in elderly populations. Ziemlanski and co-workers[52] supplemented institutionalized, healthy elderly women with 100 mg vitamin E twice daily and assessed blood protein and immunoglobulin concentrations after 4 and 12 months. Vitamin E increased total blood protein, with the principal effects being achieved at 4 months. No significant effects were noted in the levels in the other immune parameters studied after 12 months, although there was a significant increase in blood protein concentrations. However, another group that was supplemented with vitamin C along with vitamin E displayed significant increases in other immune parameters such as IgG and complement C3 levels.

Harman and Miller[53] supplemented 103 elderly patients from a chronic care facility with 200 or 400 mg daily α-tocopherol acetate but did not see any beneficial effect on antibody development against influenza virus vaccine. Unfortunately, these researchers did not report data on the subjects' health status, medication use, antibody levels, and other relevant parameters, which renders these results inconclusive because other potential factors that may inhibit immune response cannot be evaluated.

In a double-blind, placebo-controlled study, Meydani et al.[54] supplemented 34 healthy men and women (> 60 years of age) with either a soybean oil placebo or 800 mg dl-α-tocopherol for 30 days. The study evaluated the subjects' delayed type hypersensitivity(DTH), mitogenic response, and IL-1, IL-2, and PGE_2 production. Vitamin E supplementation was associated with increases in blood vitamin E, DTH score, mitogenic response to Con A, and IL-2 production. Vitamin E supplementation was associated with decreases in PHA-stimulated PGE_2 production by peripheral blood mononuclear cells (PBMC) as well as plasma lipid peroxide levels. IL-1 production and PHA-induced proliferation of PBMC were not affected by vitamin E supplementation.

In a recent study, Meydani et al.[3] supplemented healthy elderly persons (> 65 years old) with placebo, 60 mg/day, 200 mg/day, or 800 mg/day of dl-α-tocopherol for 235 days using a double-blind, randomized design. All three vitamin E doses significantly enhanced DTH score; however, subjects consuming 200 mg/day vitamin E had the highest percent increase in DTH. Although the median percent change in the groups supplemented with 60 and 800 mg/day vitamin E (41% and 49%, respectively) were similar to the 65% change observed in the 200 mg/day group, these changes did not reach statistical significance compared with those of the placebo group. There was no significant effect of supplementation with 60 mg/day in response to hepatitis B or tetanus and diphtheria vaccines; however, a significant increase in antibody response to hepatitis B was observed in subjects consuming 200 or 800 mg/day. Those consuming 200 mg/day also had a significant increase in antibody response to tetanus toxoid vaccine. These data suggest that while supplementation with 60 mg/day vitamin E might enhance DTH, it is not adequate to cause a significant increase in antibody titer against hepatitis B or tetanus toxoid. Supplementation with 200 mg/day vitamin E, however, caused a significant increase in DTH and antibody response to vaccines, and the magnitude of response for both indices was higher than those observed in the two other vitamin E groups. Thus, it was concluded that 200 mg/day represents the optimal level of vitamin E for the immune response of the elderly. The observation that the optimal response was detected in the 200 mg/day group suggests that there may be a threshold level for the immunostimulatory effect of vitamin E. Interestingly, vitamin E-supplemented subjects had 30% lower incidence of self-reported infections, indicating that the immunostimulatory effect of vitamin E might have clinical significance for the elderly.

These findings are supported by studies conducted in laboratory animals. Hayek et al.[55] fed young and old mice either 30 or 500 ppm vitamin E for 8 weeks, at which time they were infected with influenza virus. Old mice fed 30 ppm of vitamin E had higher viral titer than young mice fed 30 ppm vitamin E. Influenza lung viral titers, a measure of the degree of infection in the lungs, were lower in old mice fed 500 ppm vitamin E compared with the age-matched mice fed 30 ppm vitamin E. The authors suggested that the effect of vitamin E may be due, in part, to preservation of antioxidant status and NK-cell activity because old mice fed 500 ppm vitamin E maintained a higher antioxidant index than age-matched controls and the normal age-associated decline in NK activity was prevented by feeding old infected mice 500 ppm vitamin E. However, the mechanism for the effect of vitamin E on reducing influenza viral titer is still unclear. In a subsequent study, Han et al.[56] showed that the preventive effect of vitamin E was not observed following supplementation with other antioxidant compounds such as glutathione, melatonin, or strawberry extract. Furthermore, vitamin E prevented the weight loss associated with influenza infection while other dietary antioxidant treatments exerted no effect on weight loss.

No adverse effects on the immune indices tested due to short-term, high-dose vitamin E supplementation were observed. Recently, the safety of 4 months of supplementation with 60, 200, and 800 IU/day of dl-α-tocopherol on general health, nutrient status, liver enzyme function, thyroid hormones, creatinine levels, serum autoantibodies, killing of *Candida albicans* by neutrophils, and bleeding time in elderly subjects was assessed. Supplementation with vitamin E at these levels and for this period of time had no adverse effects on these parameters.[7]

Several epidemiologic studies have investigated the interaction between vitamin E supplementation and immune function of free-living elderly. Goodwin and Garry[57] studied a population of healthy adults (65 to 94 years old) consuming high doses of vitamin E and did not find any correlation between vitamin E intake and DTH, mitogen-stimulated lymphocyte proliferation, serum antibodies, or circulating immune complexes. In this study, subjects taking supplemental doses of vitamin E greater than 5 times the RDA had lower absolute circulating lymphocyte counts than the rest of the population. Unfortunately, the results from this study are confounded by the fact that the subjects were consuming high doses of several vitamin supplements in addition to vitamin E.

Chavance et al.[58,59] conducted a community-based survey on the relationship between nutritional and immunologic status in 100 healthy subjects over 60 years of age. They reported that plasma vitamin E levels were positively correlated with positive DTH responses to diphtheria toxoid, *C. albicans*, and trichophyton. In men only, positive correlations were also observed between vitamin E levels and the number of positive DTH responses. Subjects with tocopherol levels greater than 135 mg/L were found to have higher helper-inducer/cytotoxic-suppressor ratios. Blood vitamin E concentrations were also negatively correlated with the number of infectious disease episodes in the preceding year.

Payette et al.[60] reported a negative correlation between dietary vitamin E and *ex vivo* IL-2 production in free-living elderly Canadians. This result is suspect, however, because 70% of the presumably healthy elderly in this study had undetectable IL-2 levels. Others have reported that while IL-2 production in healthy older adults is about one-half to two-thirds that of young subjects, it is still detectable.[5,61,62] The study is further complicated because dietary vitamin E intake rather than plasma vitamin E level was used as the indicator of a subject's tocopherol status.

The mechanism behind the immunostimulatory effect of vitamin E has eluded scientists; however, there is compelling evidence suggesting that vitamin E exerts its immunoenhancing effect by either reducing prostaglandin synthesis[5,48] and/or decreasing free radical formation.[63]

Vitamin C

Many of the purported effects of vitamin C on immune function are still only speculative. The strongest link forged thus far has been in the prevention of cataracts, which are the leading cause of blindness worldwide. Cataract removal is the most frequently performed surgery among the elderly and accounts for the largest single line item in the Medicare budget. Epidemiological evidence suggests that individuals consuming less than 125 mg per day of vitamin C have a fourfold increase in risk for cataract than those consuming more than 500 mg/day.[64] This effect may be due to the high levels of ascorbic acid found in the eye lens. However, while studies have found that increased intake of vitamin C reduces the risk of cataract in older individuals, other factors such as intake of vitamin E and carotenoids as well as ultraviolet light exposure, presence of diabetes, and smoking are involved in the quantification of risk for cataract.[65]

Several hypotheses about the effect of vitamin C on other parameters of immune response have also been expressed and are currently the subject of a wide range of clinical interventions and studies in animals; for example, the effects of vitamin C on lowering blood pressure and metabolizing cholesterol are currently being examined in a variety of research trials.[66] Preliminary data suggest that intake of foods rich in vitamin C are correlated with lower rates of stomach cancer, while poor intake (i.e., below recommended levels) of vitamin C may be associated with higher risk for cervical and esophageal cancer.[66] However, the protective effect of vitamin C is usually associated with consumption of adequate to high levels of other nutrients, for example, Penn and colleagues[67] showed that immune function in the elderly was not significantly improved by vitamin C alone but by vitamin C in concert with vitamins A and E.

Kennes et al.[68] examined the effect of intramuscular injections of vitamin C (500 mg/day for 1 month) on proliferative response of lymphocytes to PHA and Con A and DTH response to tuberculosis in 20 elderly subjects over the age of 70. A significant increase in [^{3}H] thymidine incorporation stimulated by PHA and Con A was observed after 30 days of supplementation. Vitamin C-supplemented subjects also had an increase in the mean DTH response to tuberculosis relative to placebo-treated subjects. However, since vitamin C status was not determined, it is not clear whether the observed improvement was caused by correction of a vitamin C deficiency state or by a direct immunostimulatory action of injected vitamin C.

Delafuente et al.[69] studied a group of elderly patients over 65 years of age with chronic cardiovascular diseases receiving a variety of medications; the researchers examined the effect of *in vitro* and *in vivo* supplementation of vitamin C on lymphocyte proliferation and DTH to *Candida albicans* and mumps skin test antigen. They found that although *in vitro* addition of vitamin C to lymphocytes from elderly subjects increased their Con A-stimulated proliferation to levels comparable to those of young subjects, *in vivo* supplementation with 2 g/day vitamin C for 3 weeks did not significantly affect mitogenic responses or reverse anergy. These *in vivo* results are in contrast to those from Kennes et al.,[68] described above, who employed healthy elderly subjects receiving 500 mg/day of vitamin C intramuscularly with no other medication and found improvement in the immunologic parameters measured following supplementation.

Ziemlanski et al.[52] found significantly increased IgG, IgM, and complement C3 levels in 158 women over 78 years of age receiving 400 mg ascorbic acid supplements. Goodwin and Garry[57] found that healthy elderly subjects within the top 10% for plasma vitamin C concentrations had significantly fewer subjects who mounted no response to four different antigens.

Several studies have indicated that a low vitamin C intake[70] or blood levels[71,72] is associated with increased risk of death; however, in two randomized, controlled trials, vitamin C supplementation of elderly people with low blood ascorbate levels did not decrease the mortality rate.[72,73] The failure of supplementation trials to show any beneficial effect may be because irreversible damage had occurred as a result of a long-standing vitamin C deficiency, and supplementation should have started earlier in life. On the other hand, low vitamin C status may have occurred as a consequence of poor health status, which culminated in death.

The mechanism of the immunostimulatory effect of vitamin C is not known. However, the serum level of lipid peroxides rises in healthy subjects with increasing age,[74,75] suggesting that the immunostimulatory effect of vitamin C might be mediated through its antioxidant function. The concentration of certain antioxidants such as vitamin C, selenium, and superoxide dismutase decreases with advancing age.[76] Vitamin C or vitamin E supplementation of elderly women for 12 months decreased serum peroxide levels by 13 and 26%, respectively.[77] On the other hand, vitamin C has been reported to increase *in vivo* generation of cyclic GMP,[78] a signal cell for cell commitment into S phase.[79]

In summary, lower plasma and leukocyte levels of vitamin C and age-related increases in serum lipid peroxides have been reported in the elderly. Compromised vitamin C status appears to contribute to the decreased immune responsiveness observed in the elderly, although conflicting reports on the beneficial effects of high-dose supplementation with this vitamin makes unequivocal recommendation impossible.

β-Carotene

Several human trials investigating the immunological effects of β-carotene supplementation in elderly individuals have been conducted in recent years. The first documented trial was a variable dose β-carotene supplementation (0, 15, 30, 45, 60 mg/d) trial in a mixed-gender, older population (mean age = 56 years) of a very limited sample size (4 subjects per group).[80] A significant increase in the percentage of T-helper (CD4⁺) cells, NK cells (CD16⁺), and cells expressing IL-2R (CD25⁺) and TFR was reported for subjects taking 30, 45, 60 mg/d β-carotene when compared with those receiving a placebo. However, no significant changes in total T-cells or T-suppressor/cytotoxic (CD8⁺) cells were reported as a result of β-carotene supplementation. Due to the small per group sample size and the lack of measurements of immune cell function, it is difficult to evaluate the significance of the findings of this study.

Two distinct β-carotene trials of short and long duration were presented together in support of similar conclusions. The short-term effect of β-carotene (90 mg/d for 3 weeks) on T-cell-mediated immunity was assessed in a randomized, double-blind, placebo-controlled longitudinal comparison of healthy elderly women (60 to 80 years; n = 23).[81] The long-term effect of β-carotene (50 mg every other day for 10 to 12 years) on T-cell-mediated immunity was assessed in a randomized, double-blind, placebo-controlled longitudinal comparison of men (51 to 86 years; n = 59) enrolled in the Physicians' Health Study.[81] Subjects from both the short- and long-term studies who were taking β-carotene had significantly greater plasma β-carotene levels than subjects from the respective studies taking placebo. The changes in DTH responses from baseline to follow-up between β-carotene and placebo groups were not significantly different in either the short- or long-term study. In addition, no significant effects of β-carotene supplementation on various parameters of immune response (i.e., *in vitro* lymphocyte proliferation, production of IL-2 or PGE_2), immune profile (i.e., total T-cells, CD3+; T-helper cells, CD4+; T-cytotoxic/suppressor cells, CD8+; B-cells, CD19+), or immune cell populations (i.e., CD16+ NK cells or activated lymphocytes, which express IL-2 receptor, or transferrin receptor) were observed. Consistent results from these two distinct trials demonstrate that β-carotene supplementation does not have an enhancing or suppressive effect on the T-cell-mediated immunity of healthy elderly individuals.

The potential cancer-preventing effect of β-carotene is of particular importance to the elderly, whose cancer incidence is greatest. In a recent study, we investigated the effects of β-carotene supplementation in a healthy aging population. Immune cell activity among 59 (38 middle-aged, 51 to 64 years; 21 elderly, 65 to 86 years) Boston area participants in the Physicians' Health Study, a randomized, double-blind, placebo-controlled trial of β-carotene (50 mg on alternate days) for prevention of cancer and cardiovascular disease, was evaluated after 10 to 12 years of β-carotene supplementation. The elderly had significantly lower natural killer cell activity, cells which are invoked in the killing of tumors and viruses, than the middle-aged participants; however, β-carotene supplementation eliminated this age-related difference. No significant difference was seen in natural killer cell activity due to β-carotene supplementation in the middle-aged group.[82]

We also conducted a three-week β-carotene supplementation trial to investigate the short-term effect of β-carotene (90 mg per day) on the immune response of healthy elderly women, aged 60 to 80 years. β-carotene supplementation resulted in a 35% increase in the DTH response when compared to rates in unsupplemented subjects; however, there was no significant effect due to β-carotene supplementation on the function or proliferation of T-cells.[82]

Differing results obtained from the many immunological experiments involving β-carotene supplementation may depend on the species being evaluated, whether or not β-carotene is added before or after samples from subjects have been taken, the exact dosage of β-carotene, as well as the age range and health status of the subjects. Enhancement of the immune system by β-carotene remains an attractive possibility for humans with suboptimal immune response, such as patients with pre-cancerous lesions, as well as for the healthy elderly. However, two recent studies published in the *New England Journal of Medicine*[10,11] indicate that *supplementation* with β-carotene has, at best, no effect on cancer prevention, but some results indicate that *supplementation* may actually be detrimental by promoting cancer in individuals such as smokers or former smokers with a higher predisposition to cancer. The effect of β-carotene on immune function was not tested in either of these studies. Before any conclusive recommendations on β-carotene consumption, either through diet or through supplementation, can be made, more studies that take into account such parameters as intake of other antioxidant vitamins, age, general health status, gender, nutrient source, and duration of supplementation need to be implemented and stringently analyzed. In the meantime, as we have seen with several of the studies mentioned in this chapter, more and more evidence is mounting that the key to health and longevity is variety—a variety of foods containing a variety of nutrients.

CONCLUSION

Increased oxidative stress due to lower consumption of antioxidant nutrients contributes to the decline of immune function in the aged. Increased intake of some antioxidant nutrients has been shown to enhance the immune response in the aged. The evidence supporting the beneficial role of antioxidant nutrients is stronger for vitamin E compared to other antioxidant nutrients. This is due, in part, to a lack of controlled studies of other antioxidant nutrients that are needed to determine the level of antioxidant nutrients for optimal immune response, the clinical significance of increased antioxidant intake, and the mechanisms of their effect on the immune system.

To remain healthy and active, middle-aged and older women should exercise their common sense when it comes to diet and daily activity. A well-balanced diet that includes five to nine servings of fruits and vegetables daily can provide an adequate supply of most of the antioxidant nutrients needed to maintain the oxidant/antioxidant balance and the other vital functions these vitamins perform. It may, however, be difficult to obtain adequate levels of vitamin E from the diet. Careful attention should be paid to the amount of polyunsaturated fatty acids compared to antioxidant nutrients that are consumed. If women feel they need to take supplements of these or other nutrients, they should consult their physician or dietitian for adequate and safe levels, especially if they are considering changing their fat intake by consuming more PUFA in place of saturated fats. Successful aging takes common sense and attention to the changing needs of the body.

REFERENCES

1. Singh, G. K., Kochanek, K. D., and MacDorman, M. F., Advance report of final mortality statistics, 1994. Monthly vital statistics report, 45, 19, 1996.
2. Byers, T. and Perry, G., Dietary carotenes, vitamin C, and vitamin E as protective antioxidants in human cancers, *Ann. Rev. Nutr.*, 12, 139–159, 1992.
3. Meydani, S. N., Meydani, M., Blumberg, J. B., Leka, L. S., Siber, G., Loszewski, R., Thompson, C., Pedrosa, M. C., Diamond, R. D., and Stollar, B. D., Vitamin E supplementation enhances *in vivo* immune response in healthy elderly subjects: A randomized controlled trial, *JAMA*, 277, 1380–1386, 1997.

4. Meydani, S. N., Wu, D., Santos, M. S., and Hayek, M. G., Antioxidants and immune response in the aged: Overview of present evidence, *Am. J. Clin. Nutr.*, 62 (Suppl), 1462S–1476S, 1995.

5. Meydani, S. N., Barklund, M. P., Liu, S., Meydani, M., Miller, R. A., Cannon, J. G., Morrow, F. D., Rocklin, R., and Blumberg, J. B., Vitamin E supplementation enhances cell-mediated immunity in healthy elderly subjects, *Am. J. Clin. Nutr.*, 52, 557–563, 1990.

6. Meydani, S. N., Meydani, M., Rall, L., Morrow, F., and Blumberg, J. B., Assessment of the safety of high-dose, short-term supplementation with vitamin E in healthy older adults, *Am. J. Clin. Nutr.*, 60, 704–709, 1994.

7. Meydani, S. N., Meydani, M., Blumberg, J., Leka, L., Pedrosa, M., Stollar, B. D., and Diamond, R., Safety assessment of long-term vitamin E supplementation in healthy elderly, *Am. J. Clin. Nutr.*, 68, 311–318, 1998.

8. Halliwell, B., Oxidants and human disease: some new concepts, *FASEB J.*, 1, 358–364, 1987.

9. The Alpha-Tocopherol BCCPSG. The effect of vitamin E and beta carotene on the incidence of lung cancer and other cancers in male smokers, *N. Engl. J. Med.*, 330, 1029–1035, 1994.

10. Omenn, G. S., Goodman, G. E., Thornquist, M. D., Balmes, J., Cullen, M. R., Glass, A., Keogh, J. P., Meyskens, F. L., Valanis, B., Williams, J. H., Barnhart, S., and Hammer, A., Effects of a combination of β-carotene and vitamin A on lung cancer and cardiovascular disease, *N. Engl. J. Med.*, 334, 1150–55, 1996.

11. Hennekens, C. H., Buring, J. E., Mason, J. E., Stampfer, M., Rosner, B., Cook, N. R., Belanger, C., Lamotte, F., Gaziano, J. M., Ridker, P. M., Willett, W. C., and Peto, R., Lack of effect of long-term supplementation with β-carotene on the incidence of malignant neoplasms and cardiovascular disease, *N. Engl. J. Med.*, 334, 1145–1149, 1996.

12. Heseler H. and Schneider, R., Requirement and supply of vitamin C, E, and beta-carotene for elderly men and women, *Eur. J. Clin. Nutr.*, 48, 118–127, 1994.

13. Saccari, M., Garric, B., Ponteziere, C., Miocque, M., and Cals, M. J., Influence of sex on vitamin A and E status, *Age and Ageing*, 20, 413–416, 1991.

14. Vatassery, G. T., Johnson, G. J., and Krezowski, A. M., Changes in vitamin E concentrations in human plasma and platelets with age, *J. Am. Coll. Nutr.*, 4, 369–375, 1983.

15. Hatman, L. J. and Kayden, H. J., A high-performance liquid chromatographic method for the determination of tocopherol in plasma and cellular elements of the blood, *J. Lipid Res.*, 20, 639–645, 1979.

16. Coquette, A., Vray, B., and Vanderpas, J., Role of vitamin E in the protection of the resident macrophage membrane against oxidative damage, *Arch. Int. Physiol. Biochem.*, 94, 529–534, 1986.

17. National Research Council, Recommended Dietary Allowances, 10th ed., National Academy Press, Washington, D.C., 1989.

18. Lehmann, J., Martin, H. L., Lashley, E. L., Marshall, M. W., and Judd, J. T., Vitamin E in foods from high and low linoleic acid diets, *J. Am. Diet. Assoc.*, 86, 1208–1216, 1986.

19. Kushi, L. H., Folson, A. R., Prineas, R. J., Mink, P. J., Wu, Y., and Bostick, R. M., Dietary antioxidant vitamins and death from coronary heart disease in post-menopausal women, *N. Engl. J. Med.*, 334, 1156–1162, 1996.

20. Murphy, S. P., Subar, A. F., and Block, G., Vitamin E intake and sources in the United States, *Am. J. Clin. Nutr.*, 52, 361–367, 1990.

21. Miller, R. A., Aging and immune function, *Int. Rev. Cytology*, 124, 187–215, 1991.

22. Miller, R. A., Aging and immune function: Cellular and biochemical analyses, *Exp. Gerontol.*, 29, 21–35, 1994.

23. Hayek, M. G., Meydani, S. N., Meydani, M., and Blumberg, J. B., Age differences in eicosanoid production of mouse splenocytes: Effects on mitogen-induced T-cell proliferation, *J. Gerontol.*, 49, B197–B207, 1994.

24. Franklin, R. A., Arkins, S., Li, Y. M., and Kelley, K. W., Macrophages suppress lectin-induced proliferation of lymphocytes from aged rats, *Mech. Ageing Dev.*, 67, 33–46, 1993.

25. Makinodan, T., James, S. J., Inamizu, T., and Chang, M.-P., Immunologic basis for susceptibility to infection in the aged, *Gerontology*, 30, 279–289, 1984.

26. Abbas, A. K., Lichtman, A. H., and Pober, J. S., *Cellular and Molecular Immunology*, W.B. Saunders, Philadelphia, 1991.

27. Makinodan, T. and Hirokawa, K., Normal aging of the immune system, in *Relations Between Normal Aging and Disease*, Johnson, H. A., Ed., Raven Press, New York, 117–132, 1985.

28. Green-Johnson, J., Wade, A. W., and Szewczuk, M. R., The immunobiology of aging, in *Developmental Immunology*, Cooper, E. L. and Nisbet-Brown, E., Eds., Oxford University Press, New York, 426–451, 1993.

29. Miller, R. A., Cellular and biochemical changes in the aging mouse immune system, *Nutr. Rev.*, 53 (Suppl.), S14–S17, 1995.

30. Schwab, R. and Weksler, M. E., Cell biology of the impaired proliferation of T cells from elderly humans, in *Aging and the Immune Response*, Goidl, E. A., Ed., Marcel Dekker, New York, 67–80, 1987.

31. Gottesman, S. R. S., Changes is T-cell-mediated immunity with age: an update, *Rev. Biol. Res. Aging*, 3, 95–127, 1987.

32. Chopra, R. K., Mechanisms of impaired T-cell function in the elderly, *Rev. Biol. Res. Aging*, 4, 83–104, 1990.

33. Makinodan, T., Patterns of age-related immunologic changes, *Nutr. Rev.*, 53, S27–S31, 1995.

34. Miller, R. A., Garcia, G., Kirk, C. J., and Witkowski, J. M., Early activation defects in T lymphocytes from aged mice, *Immun. Rev.*, 160, 79–90, 1997.

35. Weksler, M. E., Immune senescence, Deficiency or dysregulation?, *Nutr. Rev.*, 53, S3–S7, 1995.

36. Wade, A. W. and Szewczuk, M. R., Changes in the mucosal-associated B-cell response with age, in *Aging and the Immune Response*, Goidl, E. A., Ed., Marcel Dekker, New York, 95–121, 1987.

37. Nagel, J. E. and Proust, J. J., Age-related changes in humoral immunity, complement, and polymorphonuclear leukocyte function, *Rev. Biol. Res. Aging*, 3, 147–159, 1987.

38. Ennist, D. L., Humoral immunosenescence: an update, *Rev. Biol. Res. Aging*, 4, 105–120, 1990.

39. Ernst, D. N., Weigle, O., and Hobbs, M. V., Aging and lymphokine gene expression by T cell subsets, *Nutr. Rev.*, 53 (Suppl.), S18–S25, 1995.

40. Beharka, A. A., Wu, D., Santos, M. S., and Meyydani, S. N., Increased prostaglandin production by nurine macrophages contributes to the age-associated decrease in T cell function, *FASEB J.*, 9, A754, 1996.

41. Bender, B. S., Natural killer cells in senescence: analysis of phenotypes and function, *Rev. Biol. Res. Aging*, 3, 129–138, 1987.

42. Bloom, E. T., Natural killer cells, lymphokine-associated killer cells, and cytolytic T lymphocytes, compartmentalization of age-related changes in cytolytic lymphocytes?, *J. Gerontol.*, 49, B85–B92, 1994.

43. Krishnaraj, R. and Blandford, G., Age-associated alterations in human natural killer cells: 1. Increased activity as per conventional and kinetic analysis, *Clin. Immunol. Immunopath.*, 45, 268–285, 1987.

44. Hennet, T., Peterhans, E., and Stocker, R., Alterations in antioxidant defenses in lung and liver of mice infected with influenza A virus, *J. General Virol.*, 73, 39–46, 1992.

45. Beck, M. A., Kolbeck, P. C., Rohr, L. H., Shi, W., Morris, V. C., and Levander, O. A., Increased virulence of a human enterovirus (coxsackievirus B3) in selenium-deficient mice, *J. Infect. Dis.*, 170, 351–357, 1994.

46. Meydani, S. N. and Tengerdy, R. P., Vitamin E and immune response, in *Vitamin E, Biochemical and Clinical Applications*, Packer, L. and Fuchs, J., Eds., Marcel Dekker, New York, 549–561, 1991.

47. Harman, D., Free radical theory of aging, Beneficial effect of antioxidants on the lifespan of male NZB mice, role of free radical reactions in the deterioration of the immune system with age and in the pathogenesis of systemic lupus erythematosus, *AGE*, 3, 64–73, 1980.

48. Meydani, S. N., Meydani, M., Verdon, C. P., Shapiro, A. C., Blumberg, J. B., and Hayes, K. C., Vitamin E supplementation suppresses prostaglandin E_2 synthesis and enhances the immune response of aged mice, *Mech. Ageing Dev.*, 34, 191–201, 1986.

49. Meydani, S. N., Cathcart, E. S., Hopkins, R. E., Meydani, M., Hayes, K. C., and Blumberg, J. B., Antioxidants in experimental amyloidosis of young and old mice, in *Fourth International Symposium on Amyloidosis*, Glenner, G. G., Asserman, E. P., Benditt, E. et al., Eds., Plenum Press, New York, 683–692, 1986.

50. Sakai S. and Moriguchi, S., Long-term feeding of high vitamin E diet improves the decreased mitogen response of rat splenic lymphocytes with aging, *J. Nutr. Sci. Vitaminol.*, 43, 113–122, 1997.

51. Meydani, S. N., Endres, S., Woods, M. N., Goldin, R. D., Soo, C., Morrill-Labrode, A., Dinarello, C. A., and Gorbach, S. L., Oral (n-3) fatty acid supplementation suppresses cytokine production and lymphocyte proliferation: Comparison between young and older women, *J. Nutr.*, 121, 547–555, 1991.

52. Ziemlanski, S., Wartanowicz, M., Klos, A., Raczka, A., and Klos, M., The effect of ascorbic acid and alpha-tocopherol supplementation on serum proteins and immunoglobulin concentration in the elderly, *Nutr. Int.*, 2, 1–5, 1986.

53. Harman, D. and Miller, R. W., Effect of vitamin E on the immune response to influenza virus vaccine and the incidence of infectious disease in man, *Age*, 9, 21–23, 1986.

54. Meydani, S. N., Barklund, P. M., Liu, S., Meydani, M., Miller, R. A., Cannon, J. G., Morrow, F. D., Rocklin, R., and Blumberg J. B., Vitamin E supplementation enhances cell-mediated immunity in healthy elderly subjects, *Am. J. Clin. Nutr.*, 52, 557–563, 1990.

55. Hayek, M. G., Taylor, S. F., Bender, B. S., Han, S. N., Meydani, M., Smith, D. E., Eghtesada, S., and Meydani, S. N., Vitamin E supplementation decreases lung virus titers in mice infected with influenza, *J. Infect. Dis.*, 176, 273–276, 1997.

56. Han, S. N., Wu, D., Ha, W. K., Smith, D. E., Beharka, A. A., Martin, K. R., Meydani, M., and Meydani, S. N., Vitamin E (E) supplementation increases splenocyte IL-2 and interferon-γ production of old mice infected with influenza virus, *FASEB J.*, 12, A819, 1998.

57. Goodwin, J. S. and Garry, J. P., Relationship between megadose vitamin E supplementation and immunological function in a healthy elderly population, *Clin. Exp. Immunol.*, 51, 647–653, 1983.

58. Chavance, M., Brubacher, G., Herbeth, B. et al., Immunological and nutritional status among the elderly, in *Lymphoid Cell Functions in Aging*, De Wick, A. L., Ed., Interlaken, Eurage, 231–237, 1984.

59. Chavance, M., Brubacher, G., Herbert, B., Vernhers, G., Mistacki, T., Dete, F., Founier, C., and Janot, C., Immunological nutritional status among the elderly, in *Nutritional Immunity and Illness in the Elderly*, Chandra, R. K., Ed., Pergamon Press, New York, 137–142, 1985.

60. Payette, H., Rola-Pleszczynski, M., and Ghadriran, P., Nutritional factors in realtion to cellular and regulatory immune variables in a free-living elderly population, *Am. J. Clin. Nutr.*, 33, 606–608, 1990.

61. Meydani, S. N., Meydani, M., and Blumberg, J. B., Antioxidants and the aging immune response, *Adv. Exp. Med. Biol.*, 262, 57-68, 1990.

62. Nagel, J. E., Chorpa, R. K., Chrest, F. J., McCoy, M. T., and Schneider, E. L., Decreased proliferation, interleukin 2 synthesis, and interleukin 2 receptor expression are accompanied by decreased mRNA expression in phytohemagglutin-stimulated cells from elderly donors, *J. Clin. Invest.*, 81, 1096–1102, 1988.

63. Corwin, L. M. and Shloss, J., Role of antioxidants on the stimulation the mitogen response, *J. Nutr.*, 110, 2497–2505, 1980.

64. Jacques, P. F. and Chylack, L T., Epidemiological evidence of a role for the antioxidant vitamins and carotenoids in cataract prevention, *Am. J. Clin. Nutr.*, 53, 352S–355S, 1991.

65. West, S., Does smoke get in your eyes?, *J. Am. Med. Assoc.*, 268, 989–993, 1992.

66. Sauberlich, H. E., Pharmacology of vitamin C, *Ann. Rev. Nutr.*, 14, 371–391, 1994.

67. Penn, N. D., Perkins, L., Kelleher, J., Heatley, R. V., Mascie-Taylor, B. H., and Belfield, P. W., The effect of dietary supplementation with vitamins A, C, and E on cell-mediated immune function in elderly long-stay patients: A randomized, controlled trial, *Age Ageing*, 20, 169–174, 1991.

68. Kennes, B., Dumont, I., Brohee, D., Hubert, C., and Neve, P., Effect of vitamin C supplementation on cell-mediated immunity in old people, *Gerontol.*, 29, 305–310, 1983.

69. Delafuente, J. C., Prendergast, J. M., and Modigh, A., Immunological modulation by vitamin C in the elderly, *Clin. Immunol. Immunopathol.*, 8, 205–211, 1986.

70. Hodkinson, H. M. and Exton-Smith, A. N., Factors predicting mortality in the elderly in the community, *Age Aging*, 5, 110–115, 1976.

71. Wilson, T. S., Weeks, M. M., Mukheyee, S. K., Murrell, J. S., and Andrews, C. T., A study of vitamin C levels in the aged and subsequent mortality, *Gerontol. Clin.*, 14, 17–24, 1972.

72. Wilson, T. S., Datta, S. B., Murrell, J. S., and Andrews, C. T., Relationship of vitamin C to mortality in a geriatric hospital: A study of the effect of vitamin C administration, *Age Aging*, 2, 163–171, 1973.

73. Burr, M. L., Hurley, R. J., and Sweetnam, P. M., Vitamin C supplementation of old people with low blood levels, *Gerontol. Clin.*, 17, 236–243, 1975.

74. Satoh, K., Serum lipid peroxides in cerebrovascular disorders determined by a new calorimetric method, *Clin. Chim. Acta*, 90, 37–43, 1978.

75. Svematsu, T., Kamada, T., Abe, H., Kikudzi, S., and Yagi, K., Serum lipoperoxide level in patients suffering from liver disease, *Clin. Chim. Acta*, 79, 267–271, 1977.

76. Leibovitz, B. E. and Siegel, B. V., Aspects of free radical reactions in biological systems, *Aging J. Gerontol.*, 7, 45–56, 1980.

77. Wartanowicz, M., Panczenko-Kresowska, B., Ziemlanski, S., Kowalska, M., and Okolska, G., The effect of alpha-tocopherol and ascorbic acid on the serum lipid peroxide level in elderly people, *Am. Nutr. Metab.*, 28, 186–191, 1984.

78. Atkinson, J., Kelly, J., Weiss, A., Wedner, H., and Parker, C., Enhanced intracellular cGMP concentrations and lectin-induced lymphocyte transformation, *J. Immunol.*, 121, 2282–2291, 1978.

79. Katz, S., Kierszenbaum, F., and Waksman, B., Mechanism of action of lymphocyte activating factor, III. Evidence that LAF acts on stimulated lymphocytes by raising cyclic GMP in G1, *J. Immunol.*, 126, 2386–2391, 1978.

80. Watson, R. R., Prabhala, R. H., Plezia, P. M., and Alberts, D. S., Effect of beta-carotene on lymphocyte subpopulations in elderly humans, evidence for a dose-response relationship, *Am. J. Clin. Nutr.*, 53, 90–94, 1991.

81. Santos, M. S., Leka, L. S., Ribaya-Mercado, J. D., Russell, R. M., Meydani, M., Hennekens, C. H., Gaziano, J. M., and Meydani, S. N., Short- and long-term β-carotene supplementation do not influence T cell-mediated immunity in healthy elderly, *Am. J. Clin. Nutr.*, 66, 917–924, 1997.

82. Santos, M. S., Meydani, S. N., Leka, L., Wu, D., Fotouhi, N., Meydani, M., Hennekens, C. H., and Gaziano, J. M., Elderly male natural killer cell activity (NKact) is enhanced by β-carotene supplementation, *FASEB J.*, 9, A44, 1995.

Section III

Exercise, Nutrition, and Chronic Disease

In the previous two sections of this book, guidelines for good nutrition and physical activity habits appropriate for maintaining or optimizing the health of older women have been outlined. In this next section, we present many common syndromes and chronic diseases that are relevant to older women, and for which there are substantive data defining the important roles of lifestyle modification (exercise, nutrition, or both) in either the pathogenesis and/or the management of the specific condition. We have not tried to cover every disease process, and certain diseases extremely important to the aging process have not been included, such as cognitive dysfunction, degenerative neurological conditions, chronic lung disease, or hepatic failure. These diseases represent conditions in which disuse and secondary malnutrition may certainly be present and play a role in the morbidity and mortality of the illness. As such, recommendations about adequate prevention and treatment of undernutrition and inactivity are certainly appropriate, as they are whenever chronic disease is present. However, they do not represent conditions about which our current understanding is that habitual physical activity level and nutritional intake contribute heavily to the pathogenesis of the disease itself. Therefore, they have been mentioned in the overviews of Chapters 1 and 4, but are not reviewed in detail here. For the syndromes and diseases that are represented in this section, there is a great deal of evidence that lifestyle factors contribute quite heavily to the expression and severity of each. Appropriate counseling and intervention in these domains may therefore significantly lessen the health care burden and human suffering associated with these conditions.

We present novel approaches to syndromes that are not only prevalent but associated with significant morbidity and disability in the older population (e.g., sleep disorders, depression, mobility impairment), and for which the role of exercise and nutrition has perhaps not been widely appreciated in the past. The formulation of a more complete approach to the management of such syndromes in the older woman requires more knowledge of exercise and nutritional principles than is usually provided within the curriculum of allied health care professionals. It is possible to simply refer such women to dietitians or physical therapists for assessment and intervention as needed, and this is sometimes the only possible approach. However, such a compartmentalized subspecialty approach to all exercise and nutritional care often leads to delays in treatment, miscommunication, fractured care, excess costs, and inefficient case management, resulting in dissatisfaction on the part of the consumer, and frustration on the part of the practitioner. Earlier recognition by the primary caregiver of the important positive role played by physical activity and nutritional status in these varied medical conditions and symptoms may result in prevention of some diseases, and a reduction in the ultimate burden of disability in others. Prevention of nutritional inadequacy or wasting and disuse due to inactivity is much easier than treatment of the medical sequelae of many decades of poor lifestyle choices. Therefore, this knowledge base appropriately belongs in the curriculum of all disciplines of allied health professionals and aged care planners, not just those studying nutrition or physical modalities of therapy.

10 Arthritis

K. Lea Sewell

CONTENTS

INTRODUCTION

Arthritis is a common condition associated with aging, beginning at any age and accumulating thereafter. Over 50% of all elderly (age > 70) living in the community report arthritis and over half have specific physical limitations. These limitations, particularly if one can no longer perform a basic personal function such as dressing or bathing, independently predict an increased risk for institutionalization and even death (Yelin, 1992). Arthritis by exam is present in 25% of nursing home residents and caused the nursing home move in 15% of those residents who did not have cognitive impairment (Guccione et al., 1989). Arthritis may result in significant disability and a host of problems which accompany enforced social isolation and functional limitation. Surveys in elderly persons (age > 60) living in the community show high rates of medication use (23%), appliance dependency (15%), and home health aide assistance (10%) (Taylor and Ford, 1984) in those with arthritis.

The goals in arthritis care are, therefore, to optimize pain control and to maintain independence. There are over 100 types of arthritis and these principles are pertinent in every case. Accurate diagnosis is extremely important for tailoring the medical care of each specific type of arthritis, and an evaluation by a physician with rheumatologic experience may be advisable. But at the foundation of every therapeutic plan to maintain independence are diet and exercise.

Women and Arthritis

Women are strongly overrepresented in the arthritic population. Most types of arthritis preferentially strike women and the risk for women is twice that for men. More than 30 million Americans have arthritis and over 20 million are women. The basis for this unfortunate preference is unknown, although the suggestion that hormones play some part arises from the recognition that inflammatory arthritis may wane during pregnancy and then reflare after delivery. We will discuss both types of arthritis, including the most common, degenerative arthritis (osteoarthritis). The more aggressive type, inflammatory arthritis, is also highlighted using the most common example (rheumatoid arthritis). Our considerations for diet and exercise will differ somewhat between degenerative and inflammatory problems.

Arthritis Self-Help

Arthritis self-help involves helping women become better informed and enabling them to take charge of their day-to-day arthritis care, including the areas of diet and exercise. This personal commitment to care for oneself clearly leads to an improved long-term outcome. Several general arthritis self-help books are available, including the Arthritis Foundation's self-help manual for patients with arthritis and *The Arthritis Helpbook* by Kate Lorig, R.N. and James Fries, M.D. The Arthritis Foundation sponsors self-help courses in addition to both floor-based and water-based exercise programs, which can be an excellent way to introduce clients to the principles of exercise and self-help with arthritis.

Unproven Remedies

Because there presently is no cure for arthritis, promises of quick cures and treatments may prove tempting. Unproven remedies are treatments that have not been proven safe and effective in repeated scientific tests. Researchers test the role of diet in arthritis in specific ways and accept a connection between the diet and arthritis only after a number of studies show the same results. In these tests, one group of people with arthritis will try the new diet and another group will remain on the standard or comparison diet. The researchers who are assessing the arthritis are not told about the group assignments (single-blinded trial). No other medication or arthritis care changes can be made, only the dietary change. The arthritis is assessed in a standard format for all persons and the average change for each group is compared. Other researchers repeat the study with new arthritis groups, and only if the same results are reproduced is the dietary treatment accepted as effective.

Unproven remedies may be harmless, but some are dangerous or expensive. Because there will be times when arthritis feels better and worse—due to the up and down nature of the disease—it may appear that an unproven remedy caused improvement. Indeed, the placebo effect may lead to improvement in any participant, even those receiving the standard diet or care. It is wisest to stay with prescribed treatment plans as these have been proven safe and effective in large numbers of people. In particular, a diet which completely eliminates an entire food group should be particularly suspect.

DEGENERATIVE ARTHRITIS (OSTEOARTHRITIS)

Degenerative arthritis, also called osteoarthritis, is the common type of arthritis known familiarly as "wear and tear" arthritis. The problem resides in the joint cartilage tissue, which provides a cushioning structure to reduce the mechanical forces on joints and to cover bone ends (Figure 1). In osteoarthritis the cartilage is thinned and torn, so that both its cushioning and covering functions are diminished. The primary points of attack are the small finger joints or the large, weight-bearing leg joints including the knees and hips. The latter problem is much more significant and limiting, as finger osteoarthritis can be cosmetically nocuous but otherwise does not drastically affect function. In addition, bunions develop, which represent osteoarthritis of the great toe.

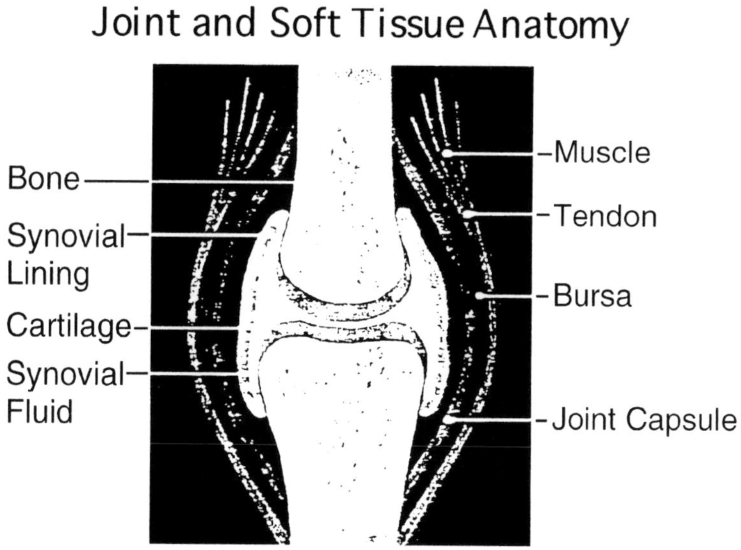

Joint and Soft Tissue Anatomy

FIGURE 1   Joint diagram of a typical joint.

Table 1 shows the higher rate of osteoarthritis in women at every age. This information comes from the National Health and Nutrition Examination Survey (NHANES) study which evaluated a large U.S. population for health problems. In hands, knees, and hips, the rate rises for women each decade and is typically one and one-half times higher than the rate for men. Indeed, Table 2 shows that severe levels of knee osteoarthritis appear to level off for men but continue to rise with age in women.

TABLE 1
Prevalence of Osteoarthritis[a]

	Hands		Knees		Hips	
Age	Men	Women	Men	Women	Men	Women
45–54	1.8	5.5	0.2	0.5	0.1	0
55–64	12.6	21.5	1	0.9	0.7	1.6
65–74	22.4	37	2	6.6	2.3	1.2

[a] Moderate/severe (rate/100 persons) NHANES study; rated by X-RAY.

From Lawrence, R. C., Hochber, M. C., Kelsey, J. L. et al., *J. Rheumatol.*, 16, 431, 1989. With permission.

TABLE 2
Radiographic Evidence of Knee Osteoarthritis from the Framingham Study

	Knee OA			Severe Knee OA		
Age	< 70	70–79	80+	< 70	70–79	80+
% of Males	30	31	33	12	18	17
% of Females	25	36	53	11	18	21

From Felson, D. T., *Semin. Arth. Rheumatol.*, 20, 44, 1990. With permission.

AGE-RELATED CHANGES IN CARTILAGE

The cartilage of the joint is composed of living cells or chondrocytes embedded in a protein matrix. With aging, the number of cells gradually declines and the amount of matrix that each one produces also declines. As a result, cartilage thickness decreases and matrix compositional changes lead to diminished resilience. Aged chondrocytes respond less well to growth factors for repair of any problem. The ability to protect the joint during heavy loading or repetitive stress is diminished; however, aged cartilage remains structurally intact and living.

Degenerative Changes in Cartilage

The earliest change in osteoarthritis is an increased water content in cartilage, a bloating or expanding of the spaces between proteins which renders the cartilage softer and less resilient (chondromalacia). Inflammation plays some part in osteoarthritis, although the extent is debatable. The inflammatory cells and stressed chondrocytes release damaging chemicals (interleukins) and enzymes capable of digesting cartilage (collagenases, metalloproteinases). As a result, breakage or clefts develop in the cartilage surface and the cartilage proteins are disarrayed (fibrillation). Unfortunately, repair is typically limited due to the blunted growth responses of aged chondrocytes. Increased pressure on the nearby cartilage leads to chondrocyte death. A secondary attempt at repair and strengthening occurs in the nearby bone, which thickens (sclerosis) or grows to form bone spurs (osteophytes) (Bullough, 1992).

Exercise and Joint Protection in Degenerative Arthritis

The goals of exercise in osteoarthritis are to prevent deconditioning of the muscles which keep the joints stable, to improve joint flexibility, and to enhance aerobic fitness, all within the guidelines of good joint protection. Muscles that are not used due to pain atrophy rapidly. A full program should therefore include stretching exercises, followed by a range-of-motion program for the joint, muscle strengthening, and aerobic exercise if possible. Range-of-motion exercises should be performed daily by those with arthritis to preserve full use of the joint and to prevent contractures.

Isometric strengthening exercises that contract muscles without moving the joint are the least likely to exacerbate arthritis pain. Extremely forceful muscle contractions do enhance intra-articular pressure and may promote cartilage damage, so multiple repetitions at a lower intensity are optimal initially to prevent flares in disease. Dynamic (isotonic) strengthening exercises that move the joint in an arc can be gently performed against gravity resistance initially and then with progressive weights added as tolerated. If joint pain prevents movement through certain ranges, the range of motion of the strengthening exercise can be limited to the pain-free zone. This zone can then be extended until the full range of motion is covered in the movement. It is desirable to exercise through as much of the range of motion as possible, as strength increases will be limited to the joint angles at which training is conducted, and the goal is to strengthen the muscle groups around the joints at all or most angles, for maximum joint stability and functional improvements. Clinically important gains in strength are only observed when the load lifted by the muscle is equal to 60% or more of its maximal capacity (McDonaugh and Davies 1984) and functional gains are higher in those exercising regularly at higher intensities, so it is important to progressively load the muscle during strengthening exercises, as described more fully in Chapter 2.

Aerobic exercise has been shown in several studies to benefit osteoarthritis as well, although the exact mechanisms for the subsequent improvements in disease control and functional status are not fully defined. Possible pathways include improvement of coexistent depressive symptoms, increases in self-efficacy, loss of body weight as well as direct effects on the affected cartilage and joint. It does not seem to operate through increases in aerobic fitness (maximal oxygen consumption), since low to moderate intensity programs that produce little physiologic adaptation may improve symptoms in osteoarthritis.

Flat walking as a modality of aerobic exercise is well tolerated in patients with mild to moderate lower extremity osteoarthritis, enhancing function and improving pain control (Lane and Buckwalter, 1993). However, in severe arthritis, this type of weight-bearing exercise is sometimes intolerable, particularly in the obese patient. In these cases, non- or partial weight-bearing aerobic exercise (biking, swimming) or seated strengthening and calisthenic exercises may need to be substituted or initiated prior to adding cardiovascular endurance activities. Resistance training exercises that stabilize the knee by increasing the strength of knee extensors and flexors, and tendons and ligaments around the joint, will often reduce pain to the extent that walking and stair climbing are again possible.

THE RELATIONSHIP BETWEEN PHYSICAL ACTIVITY AND DEGENERATIVE ARTHRITIS

Repetitive heavy activities that injure joints promote osteoarthritis. Common problems include knee arthritis in football players and hip arthritis in construction workers. The many American runners fall into a different category, as they have heavy use without heavy loading to the joint, and studies of runners with normal joints do not provide any evidence for the subsequent development of osteoarthritis. However, many cases of osteoarthritis develop in persons without a heavy "wear and tear" joint history. There is evidence from animal models that unloading of a joint for long periods is, in fact, associated with degeneration and decreased water content of the cartilage compared to normally active animals. Therefore, it would appear that as long as injury to the joint is not sustained, regular activity is not etiologic in degenerative joint disease.

Clearly, a diseased joint that no longer distributes heavy loads evenly across the entire surface area of the joint should be protected from extremes of weight. Exercises performed at an unusual angle, or bearing weight off to the side of the body, can significantly increase the stress to the joint. Once the cartilage is damaged, knee osteoarthritis may progress with running and a lower impact activity such as long-distance walking is preferable. Other non-weight-bearing exercises such as swimming and bicycling are also excellent in this situation.

DIETARY CONSIDERATIONS WITH DEGENERATIVE ARTHRITIS

No clearcut causative or therapeutic relationship appears to exist between specific dietary items and osteoarthritis. Epidemiological studies suggest that each culture may have differing rates of osteoarthritis, suggesting that a shared factor or factors combine to predict risk. Shared genes for various types and strengths of cartilage may be the predominate consideration.

A significant direct correlation exists between body weight and osteoarthritis of the knee. The Framingham study followed a specified population over decades for the development of health problems. This study unequivocally demonstrated that years of significant obesity strongly predict subsequent osteoarthritis (Felson et al., 1988).

PAIN CONTROL BY WEIGHT CONTROL

One interesting fact in osteoarthritis is that the level of pain does not correlate well with the amount of damage seen on radiographic studies. This means that other factors contribute to feeling and experiencing pain, beyond the actual joint cartilage status. Table 3 shows that pain does increase with increasing osteoarthritis severity grade, but not every patient with even advanced osteoarthritis has pain. One of the major contributing factors to the pain level at any stage of osteoarthritis is weight. Excess weight speeds up the progression of osteoarthritis and weight loss at any stage can improve joint symptoms (Felson et al., 1988). Clearly, these are two good reasons to focus on the diet in osteoarthritis.

TABLE 3
Relationship of Pain to Radiographic Stage of Arthritis

	% Symptomatic	
OA Grade	Men	Women
I (mild)	8.5	13
Ii (moderate)	9	25
III (severe)	35	43

From Felson, D. T., Naimark, A., Anderson, J. et al., *Arthritis Rheumatol.*, 20(3), 916, 1987. With permission.

A weight loss or maintenance diet (if ideal body weight has already been achieved) can be difficult with osteoarthritis due to decreased physical activity level and, therefore, caloric expenditure. The basic principles of healthful nutrition—followed by Weight Watchers™ and other weight loss plans that emphasize regular meals with normal foods—pertain. Caloric restriction should be achieved by limiting fats, eating fruits rather than concentrated sugar desserts, emphasizing fish, skin-less fowl and lean meat, avoiding alcohol, and limiting portion size. Avoid crash diets, meal skipping, or total elimination of any food group from the diet.

EXERCISE AFTER JOINT REPLACEMENT

Joint replacement surgery has been an extraordinary advance in the lives of persons with advanced osteoarthritis. Orthopedic surgeons replace damaged joints with wear-resistant plastic and metal, providing a smooth cushioning surface. The artificial knee is strong but will always be less stable than the natural knee, as tendons must be cut away to perform the surgery.

Exercise is vital both in preparation for and in recovery following joint replacement. The artificial joint is further destabilized by weak muscles surrounding the joint, creating the potential for a complicated recovery. Muscle strength allows full participation in the range-of-motion exercises following surgery and an early return to walking, with less resultant disuse muscle atrophy. Extremely active exercises such as skiing should be limited, but some surgical graduates have gradually returned to this level by strict attention to an exercise program.

INFLAMMATORY ARTHRITIS (RHEUMATOID ARTHRITIS)

Rheumatoid arthritis is experienced by one half of one percent of Americans, and two thirds of those affected are women. These numbers accumulate and nearly 5% of women over age 65 suffer this type of arthritis, as illustrated in Table 4. Wrists and knuckles are most frequently involved (Figure 2), affecting fine motor skills at work and at home, but rheumatoid arthritis can involve nearly any joint and cause a wide variety of disabilities. The cause is unknown although several genetic factors contribute to an individual's risk of developing the disease.

BASIC PRINCIPLES OF INFLAMMATION

Unlike degenerative arthritis, stiffness rather than pain may be the predominate symptom of joint inflammation. Frequent use of the joint is recommended to prevent stiffening. During inflammation and immobility, joint flexibility can be permanently lost. Independent function tends to decrease with each arthritis "flare." The goals of exercise in inflammatory arthritis are, therefore, to combat stiffness and to maintain the full flexibility and integrity of each affected joint.

TABLE 4
Prevalence of Rheumatoid Arthritis in Women

| Age | Rheumatoid Arthritis Prevalence (rate/100 persons) | |
	Men	Women
45–54	0.2	1.1
55–64	1.9	2.9
≥ 65	1.8	4.9

From Lawrence, R. C., Hochber, M. C., Kelsey, J. L. et al., *J. Rheumatol.*, 16, 432, 1989. With permission.

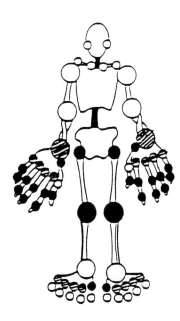

FIGURE 2   Predominate joint involvement
in osteoarthritis (black joints) vs. rheumatoid
arthritis (striped joints).

CHANGES IN THE JOINT WITH INFLAMMATORY ARTHRITIS

The problem in rheumatoid arthritis is inflammation of the joint lining (synovium). This tissue is typically microscopically thin and provides nutrition to the joint in the form of joint fluid. Once inflamed, the synovium grows visibly bulky and interferes with joint mobility. Increased blood flow to the inflamed joint results in a rise in temperature. In addition, the inflammatory cells produce chemicals and enzymes that irritate and may damage the joint structures.

EXERCISE PRINCIPLES FOR INFLAMED JOINTS

The decision to exercise or rest an inflamed joint can be a difficult one. Pain is a signal of danger and fear of injury can inhibit a person's excellent plan to exercise daily. Knowledge of the beneficial effects of regular exercise and proper methods can counterbalance this natural reluctance. Developing and practicing a full-body, home exercise plan with a physical therapist or other trained professional is optimal.

Exercise types in inflammatory arthritis are highlighted in Table 5. The 4 categories include stretching to promote flexibility and combat arthritic stiffness, special range-of-motion exercises designed for each joint group, muscle strengthening to maintain muscle strength and size and thereby joint stability, and aerobic exercise for stamina. The aerobic exercise should be selected from options which do not stress currently inflamed joints. The aerobic exercise should also enjoyable and relaxing, reducing pain and stress.

Stretching and warm-up exercises are particularly important in inflammatory arthritis to prevent undue stress to inflamed muscle tendons that can tear in their weakened state. No high-intensity or heavy-loading exercise should be attempted

TABLE 5
Exercise Types in Inflammatory Arthritis

Type	Description	Goal
Warm-up	Gentle stretch	Loosen muscles/tendons
Range of motion	Move each joint carefully through its range	Preserve joint mobility
Muscle strengthening	Resistance training of specific muscles	Strengthen and support joints
Aerobic	Exercise to increase cardiovascular endurance	Stamina

until the muscles surrounding the joint have been gently warmed with slow movements through the range of motion possible. In addition, joints should never be rapidly or ballistically stretched by bending or straightening them to their furthest degree. Joint range-of-motion exercises attempt to fully move the joint, while support is provided to the joint and the surrounding muscles. The opposite arm or leg may assist in this effort. These exercises strive to prevent joint deformity and the resultant disability and should be gently continued, if possible, through flares (Figure 3).

Muscle strengthening or resistance training is not recommended for a severely inflamed joint. However, with resolution of a flare, muscle strengthening should be immediately resumed to prevent rapid muscle atrophy around inflamed joints. In addition, all other joints should be exercised and maintained during a flare. Strong muscles provide more support to damaged joints and remove stress from the joint during use. Resistance against gravity, water, or another part of the body is often sufficient for muscle training in inflammatory arthritis when significant muscle weakness and atrophy are present. As strength is gained, however, the muscle will need to be loaded beyond gravitational forces to continue strengthening. Patients with chronic rheumatoid arthritis under control with medication have been shown to both tolerate and benefit physiologically and functionally from high-intensity progressive resistance training. Resistance training in this condition is important not only because it addresses the muscle atrophy of disuse due to pain, but also because it is the only kind of exercise that can ameliorate the muscle wasting caused by the catabolic cytokinemia that is a central part of this systemic disease.

DIET CONTROL OF INFLAMMATION: AN OVERVIEW

Weight control is also an important dietary goal for inflammatory arthritis to prevent increased mechanical stress on inflamed joints. The second major goal is to maximally optimize the functioning of the immune system through diet. This includes avoiding dietary factors which could trigger arthritis flares, or "pro-inflammatory" foods, and altering the diet to directly suppress the overactive immune system. General principles of well-balanced nutrition, complemented by appropriate rest and exercise, are also applicable to prevent the infections which can plague persons with inflammatory arthritis.

A large proportion of the local inflammatory molecules in arthritis are formed from stored fatty, or lipid, precursors. In this respect, a person directly resembles

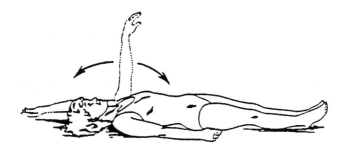

**Range-of-motion exercises keep your
joints from becoming stiff.**

FIGURE 3   Range of motion exercises.

what they eat, as their stored lipids directly reflect the dietary fats from the last few
months. Lipids are stored as fatty acids, which are then broken down in inflammation
to form potent molecules called prostaglandins and leukotrienes. Diets which are
supplemented with polyunsaturated fats alter the precise mixture and balance of
prostaglandins and leukotrienes created during an inflammatory reaction, with some
possibility of decreasing the level of arthritis pain and swelling.

FOOD ALLERGIES AND BOWEL CHANGES IN INFLAMMATORY ARTHRITIS

A small fraction of patients with inflammatory arthritis may be experiencing food
allergy. Increased immune system activity then results in a general arthritis flare.
Unique examples include food poisoning with coliform bacteria, such as *Shigella*,
that can cause flares of Reiter's arthritis, and the ingestion of wheat products in
patients with celiac sprue and associated arthritis. Arthritic reactions due to food
allergies are, however, extremely uncommon. Most patients who have observed a
connection between their arthritis and specific foods do not have this connection
confirmed by subsequent stringent testing. Skin scratch tests and RAST testing of
foods are only somewhat helpful as only 50% of the foods which definitely cause
intestinal reactions show a response (Bahna and Kanuga, 1991). The best method
for confirming allergy is a total elimination diet until the symptom subsides, with
cautious re-initiation of the suspected food and observation. Some patients have
reported improved symptoms on such individually tailored diets (Darlington et al.,
1986). Overall, true arthritis as a complication of a food allergy appears to be
extremely rare.

Another hypothesis revolves around the recognized fact that bacteria normally
reside within the large intestine. These bacteria digest food in enzymatically unique
ways, producing by-products which would not otherwise be present in humans, and
the bacteria themselves are digested intermittently by humans. The identity of the
local bacteria—which species, to what density, and with what level of activity—will
therefore influence the host human. In particular, bacteria cause local intestinal
inflammation that could change the bowel's permeability and entrance of foreign

proteins, possibly stimulating the immune system. Bacteria also synthesize unique fatty acids for their outer covering, which leads to pro-inflammatory fatty products after human digestion.

Diets alter the density, activity, and identity of the resident bowel bacteria. Decreased sugar will limit the bacterial growth, caloric limitation will alter both activity and growth, and vegetarian diets that only provide plant oils will alter the fatty acid by-products. It is possible that all of the subsequent dietary plans discussed below could affect arthritis activity indirectly, by altering bowel bacteria.

CALORIC RESTRICTION, FASTING, OR VEGETARIAN DIETS IN INFLAMMATORY ARTHRITIS

The strict limitation of calories—the body's energy source—can affect the functioning of the immune system in a multitude of ways. Importantly, a total fast or an extremely limited diet (< 500 kcal/day) cannot be safely maintained indefinitely, so these manipulations are valid only if they produce prolonged changes in arthritis activity after a normal diet is resumed.

Caloric restriction is a recognized means of prolonging life in rodents. Although no controlled study has been undertaken in humans, increased stress hormones (cortisol) are seen during caloric restriction and may be beneficial in suppressing inflammatory arthritis. Central nervous system effects, including ketosis and increased endorphins, may enhance pain control. Additional immune functions are enhanced, including the ability to form antibodies if vaccinated following a fast. Lastly, there are changes in the bacteria resident in the large intestine. These changes are not completely understood but typically converge to decrease rheumatoid arthritis activity during a fast.

Subtotal fasting for 7 to 10 days, allowing only dilute vegetable juices and broth with herbal tea (800 to 1220 kcal/day), evokes a prompt decrease in rheumatoid inflammation by the fourth or fifth day in all measures (painful joint number, inflammation blood tests, stiffness in the morning) (Hafstrom et al., 1988) (Figure 4). The effect is rapidly lost if a normal diet is resumed but may be prolonged if a new diet is begun that includes caloric restriction and leads to weight loss. One Scandinavian group followed the 10-day fast with 3 months of a strict vegetarian diet, and then an individually tailored limited diet for 9 months (Kjeldsen-Kragh et al., 1991). The first 4 months required nutritional supplements and strict monitoring. The results in comparison to a control group showed persistent arthritis improvement and weight loss throughout the year (Figure 5), as well as changes in intestinal bacteria. Clearly, some of this improvement might have been due to a placebo effect, but for those patients who can tolerate a major dietary manipulation the beneficial effect was clearly laudatory, whatever the precise basis for the improvement.

THE INFLUENCE OF DIETARY LIPID CHANGES ON THE IMMUNE SYSTEM

Polyunsaturated fatty acids from both plant and fish sources have been evaluated in rheumatoid arthritis. Evening primrose and borage seed oils are enriched in gamma-linoleic acid, which has received some scientific study and may have both

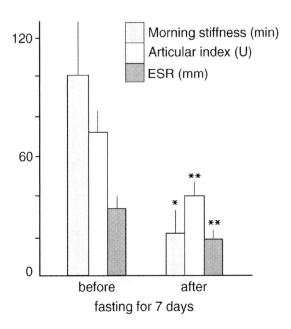

FIGURE 4   Rheumatoid arthritis after a 7-day fast: changes in duration of morning stiffness, articular index of inflammation and pain, and erythrocyte sedimentation rate blood test. * = P < 0.01; ** = P < 0.001. (From Hafstrom, I., Ringertz, B., Gyllenhammar, H. et al., *Arthritis Rheumatol.*, 31, 585–592, 1988. With permission.)

an analgesic and anti-inflammatory effect. A large amount of oil must be ingested to alter the storage profile (0.5 to 1 grams/day from 5 to 9 total capsules) and only significantly accumulates in 1 to 2 months. The gradual effect of plant oils may decrease the need for aspirin or other anti-inflammatory non-steroidal medications over 6 or more months (Callegari and Zurier, 1991). The recognized side effects are minimal, although no long-term studies have been performed, with possibly some bloating and weight increase if the calories from gamma-linoleic acid are not removed elsewhere in the diet. In summary, chronic dietary use of high-dose plant oils may mildly affect the activity of inflammatory arthritis.

Somewhat more extensive studies have been performed with fish oils in the form of eicosapentanoic acid (EPA). MaxEPA capsules provide 180 mg EPA and 90 mg docosahexaenoic acid (DHA), and most clinical studies utilize 10 to 18 capsules per day resulting in approximately 3 daily grams of EPA for the majority of such trials. Dietary EPA results in decreased leukotriene production and decreased function of immune cells termed neutrophils that produce the destructive enzymes which permanently damage joint cartilage. These effects and clinical improvement are not apparent until after 3 months of therapy, but may persist for several months after EPA cessation (Kremer et al., 1990). Safety questions remain regarding the vascular effects of fish oils, including stroke risk, and a physician's evaluation and monitoring are imperative when embarking on high-dose EPA therapy.

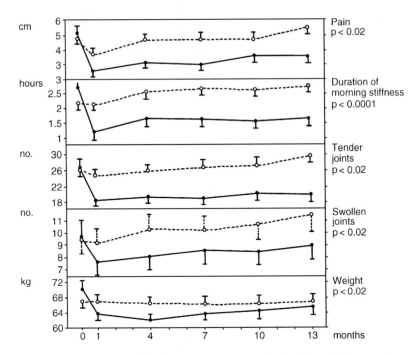

FIGURE 5   Rheumatoid arthritis changes over one year (dashed line depicts control group). P-values refer to overall group differences after one year of dietary modification vs. normal diet; solid line depicts diet group and appropriate ANOVA tests. (From Kjeldsen-Kragh, J., Haugen, M., Borchgrevink, C. F. et al., *Lancet*, 338, 900, 1991. With permission.)

ORAL TOLERANCE — THE RESEARCH FRONTIER

An exciting new frontier in dietary therapy for inflammatory arthritis capitalizes on the specialized immune system cells that line the intestines and process all food in a unique manner. Despite food proteins being entirely foreign, the gut's immune system does not reject food as would be the case with a transplanted foreign kidney or other tissue. The intestinal immune system is programmed to be tolerant or to watch without reacting as foreign molecules arrive for digestion. These immune cells circulate and carry the tolerant attitude throughout the body.

In the new methodology of oral tolerance, small amounts of proteins from the organ under inflammatory attack (in the case of the joint, the cartilage and its proteins) are fed to enhance the tolerant attitude. This change in immune balance may gradually decrease the number of reactive immune cells, replacing them with the tolerant profile. This approach is entering early study using type II collagen, the unique human collagen found primarily in joints. Other investigators are evaluating oral tolerance to myelin protein, a protein which sheaths nerves and is destroyed in the autoimmune disease multiple sclerosis (Weiner et al., 1994). To date, the results are extremely sketchy and a significant amount of research on the optimal conditions for initiating tolerance must be performed; however, a growing understanding of the uniqueness and power of the intestinal immune system supports a general enthusiasm in this field for advances against arthritis and other autoimmune diseases.

REFERENCES

Arthritis Foundation, Rheumatoid Arthritis, Arthritis information booklet, Arthritis Foundation, Atlanta, GA, 1990.

Bahna, S. L. and Kanuga, J., Food hypersensitivity, in *Nutrition and Rheumatic Diseases, Rheumatol. Clin. N. Am.,* Panush, R. S., Ed., 17, 243–249, 1991.

Bullough, P. G., The pathology of osteoarthritis, in *Osteoarthritis: Diagnosis and Medical/Surgical Management,* 2nd ed., Moskowitz, R. W., Howell, D. S., Goldberg, V. M., and Mankin, H. J., Eds., W.B. Saunders, Philadelphia, 39–69, 1992.

Callegari, P. E. and Zurier, R. B., Botanical lipids: potential role in modulation of immunologic responses and inflammatory reactions, in *Nutrition and Rheumatic Diseases, Rheumatol. Clin. N. Am.,* Panush, R. S., Ed., 17, 415–425, 1991.

Darlington, L. G., Ramsey, N. W., and Mansfield, J. R., Placebo-controlled, blind study of dietary manipulation therapy in rheumatoid arthritis, *Lancet,* I, 236–238, 1986.

Felson, D. T., The epidemiology of knee osteoarthritis: results from the Framingham Osteoarthritis Study, *Semin. Arth. Rheumatol.,* 20, 42–50, 1990.

Felson, D. T., Anderson, J. J., Naimark, A. et al., Obesity and knee osteoarthritis, The Framingham study, *Ann. Int. Med.,* 109, 18–24, 1988.

Felson, D. T., Naimark, A., Anderson, J. et al., The prevalence of knee osteoarthritis in the elderly, *Arthritis Rheumatol.,* 30, 914–918, 1987.

Guccione, A. A., Meenan, R. F., and Andersen, J. J., Arthritis in nursing home residents. A validation of its prevalence and examination of its impact on institutionalization and functional status, *Arthritis Rheumatol.,* 32, 1546–1553, 1989.

Hafstrom, I., Ringertz, B., Gyllenhammar, H. et al., Effects of fasting on disease activity, neutrophil function, fatty acid composition, and leukotriene biosynthesis in patients with rheumatoid arthritis, *Arthritis Rheumatol.,* 31, 585–592, 1988.

Kjeldsen-Kragh, J., Haugen, M., Borchgrevink, C. F. et al., Controlled trial of fasting and one-year vegetarian diet in rheumatoid arthritis, *Lancet,* 338, 899–902, 1991.

Kremer, J., Lawrence, D. L., Jubiz, W. et al., Dietary fish-oil and olive-oil supplementation in patients with rheumatoid arthritis: clinical and immunological effects, *Arthritis Rheumatol.,* 33, 810–820, 1990.

Lane, N. E. and Buckwalter, J. A., Exercise: A cause of osteoarthritis? In *Osteoarthritis. Rheumatol. Clin. N. Am.,* Moskowitz, R. W., Ed., 19, 617–633, 1993.

Lawrence, R. C., Hochber, M. C., Kelsey, J. L. et al., Estimates of the prevalence of selected arthritic and musculosketal diseases in the United States, *J. Rheumatol.,* 16, 427–441, 1989.

McDonaugh, M. J. N. and Davies, C. T. M., Adaptive response of mammalian skeletal muscle to exercise with high loads, *Eur. J. Appl. Physiol.,* 52, 139–155, 1984.

Taylor, R. and Ford, G., Arthritis/rheumatism in an elderly population: prevalence and service use, *Health Bull.,* 42, 274–281, 1984.

Weiner, H. L., Friedman, A., Miller, A. et al., Oral tolerance: Immunologic mechanisms and treatment of animal and human organ-specific autoimmune diseases by oral administration of autoantigens, *Ann. Rev. Immunol.,* 12, 809–837, 1994.

Yelin, E., The cumulative impact of a common chronic condition, *Arthritis Rheumatol.,* 35, 489–497, 1992.

11 Exercise and Nutrition in Cancer Prevention

Karen Duvall and Maria Fiatarone Singh

CONTENTS

INTRODUCTION

In the past several years, it has become increasingly apparent that lifestyle factors such as diet, level of physical activity, alcohol consumption, and cigarette smoking play a major role in the prevention and control of several cancers. During 1996, over 550,000 people died from cancer in the United States. However, strong evidence is accumulating from results of several population studies that 60 to possibly 70% of these cancer deaths could be prevented by adopting positive changes in certain lifestyle factors. Even modest shifts toward more healthy habits by the population as a whole would have a substantial impact. For example, it has been estimated that if a majority of people made at least two positive lifestyle changes, such as increased physical activity in the range of thirty minutes per day, one additional serving of dark green leafy vegetables per day, or limiting red meat consumption to once per week, both diet- and activity-related cancer mortality might be reduced by about 25%. These assumptions are supported by examining population groups who historically adhere to such practices as part of their culture. In the United States, devout Mormons (no alcohol or tobacco permitted) and Seventh-Day Adventists (largely vegetarians) have reduced risk in selected cancers largely presumed to be due to certain lifestlye patterns. Studies of recent immigrants to this country, particularly from China and Japan, also support the theory that lifestyle greatly influences cancer mortality. Unfortunately, these same studies show that immigrants tend to adopt the cancer patterns of their new country often as soon as a decade (e.g., colorectal cancer) or within two to three generations (e.g., breast cancer). Presumably, something in their new environment, such as changes in diet or exercise or environmental toxins, is responsible.

For women in the United States, the top three causes of cancer deaths, lung, breast and colorectal, are all most likely highly influenced by lifestyle factors. Tobacco is the single most lethal carcinogen, causing approximately 30% of all cancer deaths. Diet rivals tobacco as an attributable cause of cancer deaths in the U.S. Many scientists now believe that at least half of women's cancers are linked to diet alone. This chapter will attempt to sort through the often confusing and seemingly conflicting information presented in the lay media and scientific publications regarding dietary and exercise guidelines. There is an effort to clarify which recommendations are endorsed by most of the scientific community and for which there is substantial controversy. The chapter is divided into two main subheadings: (I) Nutrition and (II) Exercise. The nutrition section centers around the various dietary components such as fat and calories, fiber, fruits and vegetables, and alcohol. There is also a short discussion of selected investigational topics such as garlic and tea, for example. The exercise section centers on findings that a physically active lifestyle may reduce the risk of certain cancers. Our goal for this chapter is to show that by focusing women on a few target areas in their lifestyles, health care providers can educate them to substantially reduce their risk of developing certain cancers.

NUTRITION

INTRODUCTION

Before we discuss the specifics of dietary influences on cancer risk, it is important to remember that cancer isn't one disease but a disease process influenced by a complex set of factors. This process begins with the genetic code inherited from our parents which regulates the approximately thirty trillion cells in the body. An individual can inherit a mutant cancer-causing gene that may put them at high risk for the early development of a particular cancer. A familial form of colon cancer is a good example. Or, an individual can be exposed to a variety of environmental agents throughout her life. At some point, usually many years or even decades following the initial insult, any combinations of these agents may overwhelm normal cellular processes and initiate a program of abnormal cell growth. It is impossible to predict how a given individual's genetic make-up will interact with certain environmental exposures, be they the fat in the diet or the toxins in the air she breathes.

However, it has become increasingly clear that prevention of common cancers that routinely strike women will involve consideration of nutritional factors such as calories, fat, fiber, and micronutrients. Breast cancer, for example, is the most frequently diagnosed cancer in women and is the number two cause of cancer deaths in American women, second only to lung cancer. Known risk factors such as age, early menarche, late menopause, family history, and obesity account for only 40 to 50% of breast cancer cases. Consequently, the etiology of 50 to 60% of cases is unknown. Eighty percent of diagnosed breast cancer cases have no family history. Both epidemiological and laboratory data have strongly implicated diet as a factor in these unknowns, although the precise biological mechanism remains a matter of intense scientific debate. More conclusive data on the relationship between cancer risk and nutritional factors will be forthcoming when the National Institutes of Health concludes the Women's Health Initiative (WHI) in the year 2005. The WHI is the largest research study ever conducted on women and their health—about 160,000 postmenopausal women of various racial and ethnic backgrounds from across the United States will participate. A portion of the study will examine the relationship between cancer risk and a low-fat, high-fiber diet supplemented with calcium and vitamin D. Other dietary factors such as alcohol will be followed as well. Until these data are available, we must go with the best scientific evidence available to date.

DIETARY FAT AND CALORIES

Fat has not always been an enemy. Humans evolved in a variety of environments in which food was not always adequate to meet daily needs. Their diet was principally vegetarian, low-fat, high fiber, about 10% animal protein. To survive, early humans had to adapt by storing energy (as body fat) when their food supply was rich (high in fat and/or calorie dense) and plentiful. Large body fat stores protected our ancient ancestors from their number one nutritional problem—starvation. As a result, many people today are genetically programmed to store large quantities of body fat when they consume a high fat, calorie-dense diet. Ironically, those who tend to store body fat more easily would have historically been the ones to survive the many bouts of famine our ancestors endured. The past 100 years or so have brought an unprecedented period of excess food supply to large segments of the world's population. The outcome has produced a serious threat to the health and well-being of women today, namely, the accumulation of excess body fat.

The sources of excess body fat are primarily the total caloric content of the diet and the total fat content of the diet. While some scientific authorities have asserted that caloric content of the diet is more important than fat content, several studies have shown that the higher the proportion of fat in the diet, the more calories an individual will ingest. For example, studies done at UCLA have shown that women eating a 40% fat diet ingest 600 kcal/day more than women eating a 20 percent fat diet. Therefore, the goal for women should be to focus upon the percentage of fat in their diet as opposed to the total number of calories consumed to minimize increasing body fat stores with age.

Fat is an essential part of the diet, as discussed in Chapter 7. We need fat for energy. We need it for hormone production. We need it to absorb certain vitamins.

We need it to maintain the integrity of cell membranes. But we do not need large quantities of it. It has been estimated that for a 1250 kcal/day diet, less than one-half tablespoon of vegetable oil, which includes any oils used in processing or preparing foods, will meet the essential fatty acid requirement. Most people consume many times more than that. My colleague at UCLA likes to remark that in over 15 years of private practice, he has never seen a fatty acid deficiency in the Westside of Los Angeles.

There are three types of fat, classified according to their chemical structure. First are the saturated fats, found in meats, dark meat of poultry, eggs, dairy products made from whole or low-fat milk, nuts, and the tropical oils. These are the least desirable fats, having been associated in several scientific studies with a variety of cancers including colon, breast, lung, and prostate. Next are the polyunsaturated fats such as corn, safflower, sesame, and soybean oil, to name a few. These fats are ubiquitous in the foods we eat and certain forms have been highly implicated in specific cancers. Finally, there are the monounsaturated fats such as olive and canola oils that are considered to be the healthiest fats of the three in terms of cancer risk, just as they are in the prevention of cardiovascular disease.

Several theories have been offered to explain the relationship between fat and cancer cells. The most common of these are listed below.

1. Increased fat intake leads to increased caloric intake. Increased caloric intake leads to increased tumor cell proliferation and tumor cell growth.
2. Decreased caloric intake inhibits tumor growth in animals, possibly by decreasing insulin levels.
3. In animal studies, certain types of polyunsaturated fats (omega-6) promote mammary gland proliferation and tumor cell growth. These fatty acids also promote prostaglandin synthesis which may encourage cancer cells to proliferate.
4. Fats may reduce the ability of the immune system to supress the growth of invading tumor cells.
5. Fats may create free radicals that damage the DNA of healthy cells.
6. Fat raises estrogen levels. Estrogen has been shown to stimulate the growth of breast tumor cells in experimental studies.
7. Fat increases the secretion of bile into the intestines. Bile acids stimulate the growth of tumor cells in the colon.

It is likely that fat operates by several different mechanisms in the production of cancer, and that the mechanisms may be specific to the type of cancer that results.

The role of fat in cancer risk has been closely studied in two of the most common cancers that occur in women, namely, colon and breast. We will discuss colon cancer first since there is greater consensus regarding the importance of fat in this disease.

COLON CANCER

Several studies have found that eating a low-fat diet can reduce colon cancer risk by approximately 50%. In countries where total fat, saturated fat, and total caloric intake is high, the incidence of colon cancer is also high. In this country, studies of recent Japanese immigrants have shown that as fat intake increases from the traditional 10 to 15% of calories from fat to the typical American consumption of 34 to 37%, the rate of colon cancer increases as well. In an ongoing study of more than 88,000 U.S. nurses (the Nurses' Health Study), scientists found a clear correlation between animal fat and colon cancer. The more meats the women consumed, the higher the risk of colon cancer. Those who ate red meat every day were two to three times more likely to be diagnosed with colon cancer than those who consumed it less than once per month.

Fat is related to colon cancer in two ways. Bacterial flora that inhabit the gut interact with dietary fat, forming potentially carcinogenic compounds which can directly damage the lining of the gut and eventually lead to colon cancer. As mentioned above, fat also stimulates bile acid secretion. Increased fecal bile acid secretion has been found in patients with colon cancer and in patients with multiple polyps in the colon, who are at increased risk of developing colon cancer. In addition, certain fatty acids form a secondary type of bile acid which causes abnormal cell division and subsequent enhanced tumor formation.

Saturated fat is particularly risky. It has been estimated that a diet high in saturated fat increases the risk of colon cancer two and one-half times compared to a diet low in saturated fat. Monounsaturated fats, such as olive or canola oil, appear to cause the least damage.

To minimize the colon cancer risk, the percentage of calories from total fat in the diet should be no more than 20%. The percentage from saturated fat should be less than 7% and the remaining percentage should come primarily from the monounsaturated fats. This level of fat is actually lower than that recommended for the prevention and treatment of lipid disorders and heart disease in the majority of individuals (see Chapter 7).

BREAST CANCER

The impact of fat upon the development of breast cancer is one of the most hotly debated issues in cancer prevention. Scientists have published hundreds of studies on the association of dietary fat and breast cancer for over 50 years. Many cross-cultural analyses support the hypothesis that a low-fat diet will lower a woman's risk of developing breast cancer. Countries with high-fat diets have more breast cancer. Breast cancer rates are four to seven times higher in the U.S. than in Asia. The difference cannot be explained by genetics alone. The granddaughters and great-granddaughters of Asian women who have migrated to the U.S. are diagnosed with breast cancer at the same rate as other American women. But, study findings are inconsistent. Recently, a much-publicized analysis of those same 88,000 nurses in the Nurses' Health Study failed to find any difference in breast cancer risk between women who consumed 44% of their calories from fat and women who consumed about 32 % from fat (as opposed to the protective effect of low fat intake noted for colon cancer in this same cohort). However, to significantly lower breast cancer risk it is likely that dietary fat must be at 20%, and maybe even as low as 15%, which may explain why the American diets of these women were not protective compared to some non-Western low-fat diets, such as those traditionally consumed in Asia. These low levels of fat may be required to decrease circulating levels of estrogen. The role of estrogen in breast cancer development will be discussed in the sections that follow.

Other evidence appears conflicting. Another article widely reported in the media recently centered upon the fact that Mediterranean countries have a 50% lower rate of breast cancer than the U.S. even though more than 40% of the calories are derived from fat. Examination of the dietary fat revealed ,a high concentration of olive oil (a monounsaturated fat), leading researchers to suggest that the type of fat may be just as important as the proportion of fat. Studies examining saturated fat intake, especially from red meat, reveal a clear increase in risk with as little as 2 ounces of red meat per day.

Fat alone is not the culprit. High dietary fat tends to lead to excess body fat. Women as young as their forties and fifties with the highest amounts of body fat have double the risk of breast cancer as age-matched women with the least body fat. Endometrial and possibly ovarian cancers are also positively correlated with excess body fat. Obesity may be defined as being 20% or more over ideal body weight or alternatively as excess body fat that can occur with normal body weight in the presence of decreased lean body mass. Obesity has been repeatedly associated with more advanced breast cancer at the time of diagnosis, higher rates of recurrence, and shorter survival times. The newest health estimates in the U.S. place over 50% of the adult population in the obese range, and these percentages are even greater in older women from minority ethnic groups (Blacks, Native Americans, and Hispanics). Thus, the enormity of this problem from a public health perspective is obvious.

Body fat is believed to affect risk because increased body fat increases the amount of circulating estrogens, even in postmenopausal women. Estrogen is pro-duced in the fat cell, particularly abdominal fat cells. These cells contain an enzyme, aromatase, which metabolizes adrenal androgens into biologically active forms of estrogen. Therefore, overweight women with upper body obesity (the apple soma-totype, or those with visceral obesity) have increased levels of circulating estrogens. This is the same type of body fat distribution which is associated with metabolic derangements such as hyperlipidemia, insulin resistance, and the clinical syndromes of hypertension, diabetes, and atherosclerosis (see Chapters 12, 14, and 17). Estrogen is considered to be a *promoter* of breast cancer, not a cause. That is to say, estrogen stimulates the growth of tumor cells, but does not cause the initial insult which directly damages the DNA.

Adult weight gain increases the risk of postmenopausal breast cancer. Women who have gained more than 10 pounds since their forties have almost tripled their risk compared to what would be predicted had their weight remained stable. The increased weight no doubt reflects increased body fat (normal range for adult women is 21 to 28%). This added excess body fat in those years immediately preceding the diagnosis of breast cancer may be the critical factor in triggering breast tumor cell development.

Therefore, it is important for women in their fifties and above to maintain a healthy body composition, focusing not so much on weight per se, but on not adding excess body fat. Women often add extra pounds as they age and these extra pounds usually reflect excess body fat, as lean body mass is declining in these same years. However, just attempting to restrict calories to lose body fat can be counterproductive. Lean body mass decreases with hypocaloric dieting and the relative percent body fat may therefore actually increase. Combining resistance training with dieting can offset or prevent the loss of lean tissue, and thereby decrease percent body fat (see Chapter 2).

It is important to focus on the quality, or nutrient density of the calories consumed. Good advice for women is to limit the percentage of calories from fat to 20% and you may decrease your breast cancer risk by 50%. Replace the saturated and polyunsaturated fats with monounsaturated fats such as those in olive oil, canola oil, and avocados for maximal cancer protection.

FIBER

Research strongly suggests that dietary fiber plays a protective role in preventing certain cancers, especially colon and breast. It has been estimated that a high-fiber diet can reduce colon cancer risk by an average of 40%. Cross-sectional international studies have consistently shown that people who consume a high proportion of fiber from grains, fruits, and vegetables have a reduced risk of cancer. The most recent data from the Nurses' Health Study have failed to find an association between fiber intake and colon cancer risk in middle-aged women, however. This somewhat unexpected finding may have been due to the detail of the food frequency questionnaire used, with its ability to control for many other dietary constituents, or the prospective nature of this 16-year study, in contrast to the retrospective or case-control design of other studies. Because fiber intake tends to correlate with higher intakes of fruits and vegetables, micronutrients, phytochemicals, and other trace elements as well as lower intake of fats and meat, it is always going to be difficult to attribute reduced cancer risk to one particular component of a dietary pattern such as fiber.

Fiber is essentially the component of plant cell walls that is resistant to digestive enzymes and thereby passes through the digestive system intact. The specific types of fiber in a fruit, vegetable, or grain depend upon the age and type of plant from which it is derived. Fiber is classified as one of two types: soluble or insoluble. The fibers that readily accept and retain water are called soluble. They are only partially digestible. Oat bran, barley, fruits, and vegetables are a few examples. Insoluble fibers are more rigid, do not dissolve in water, and are largely indigestible. Wheat bran, kidney beans, and the skins of fruits and vegetables are representatives of this category. Until recently, most studies have shown a protective effect only from insoluble fibers, such as those in wheat bran. However, equal amounts of soluble and insoluble fiber have been observed to reduce colon cancer risk by nearly 50% and to be twice as effective in shrinking colon tumors in animal models than either type of fiber alone.

Fiber may theoretically protect against cancer in several ways. In the colon, fiber dilutes the concentration of carcinogens in the feces, making it less likely for these compounds to come in contact with the bowel wall. Fiber reduces the transit time for stool to pass through the colon, which also reduces contact of carcinogens with the bowel wall. Possibly mutagenic bile acids are neutralized by fiber in the colon.

Fiber binds estrogen, thereby reducing the levels of circulating estrogens which potentially promote the growth of breast tumors. There is evidence that fiber not only binds to estrogen directly, but also stimulates the production of a protein, sex hormone binding globulin, which effectively reduces the amount of metabolically available estrogen.

The role of fiber in cancer prevention is not without controversy. That often quoted Nurses' Health Study found no evidence that fiber protected against breast cancer, as was the case for colon cancer as noted above. However, fruits and vegetables were found to be highly protective against breast cancer. It is unclear, even in several clinical trials that do show a protective effect, whether it is the fiber or some other component of the foods that contain the fiber, such as antioxidants or phytochemicals, which is responsible for the effect. That is why fiber should be eaten as part of the food in a varied diet and not as a supplement. Fiber supplements are devoid of these other nutrients, and may contain only soluble or insoluble fiber, rather than the mixture of both which has been shown to be most protective in animal studies. Some of the benefits of a high-fiber diet may come from the interaction of these compounds with the fiber itself or from a complex interaction among the various components of the fiber.

Despite the controversy, it is generally agreed that the combination of a high-fiber, low-fat diet can substantially decrease the risk of cancer. The average American consumes only 11 to 14 grams of fiber per day. The amounts consumed by frail elderly adults such as nursing home residents have been found to be as low as 3 to 5 grams per day. The recommended range is 25 to 30 grams per day (including a combination of both soluble and insoluble fibers from a mixed food supply) with an upper limit of 35 grams per day. The National Research Council advises increasing fiber intake by eating five or more servings of fruits and vegetables a day and six or more helpings of legumes, whole-grain breads and cereals. Increase fiber gradually by adding a gram or two a day to minimize intestinal gas and bloating. Because fiber absorbs water, drink at least six to eight 8 ounce glasses of water a day. One caveat for women who are hypothyroid, a high-fiber diet may interfere with the metabolism of common thyroid medications causing elevated levels of TSH (thyroid-stimulating hormone).

FRUITS AND VEGETABLES: THE KEY TO CHEMOPREVENTION

Cancer develops slowly, gradually, over decades, in a carefully orchestrated process conducted at the cellular level. Chemoprevention attempts to utilize natural compounds and synthetic supplements to derail this process in the very early stages, before invasive disease begins. The evidence strongly suggests that fruits and vegetables contain a variety of substances able to accomplish just that. Population studies for the past twenty-five years have consistently found a positive association between fruit and vegetable intake and reduced cancer risk. International comparisons have shown that the 25% of the world's population who eat the most fruits and vegetables have roughly half as many cancers as the 25% who consumed the fewest.

Lung, breast, colon, and head and neck cancers are among the most responsive to fruit and vegetable consumption. Specifically, studies show that eating fruits and vegetables at least three times per week can decrease lung cancer risk by up to 70% compared to eating none at all. Risk of breast cancer was found to be 48% lower in women who ate an average of five servings of vegetables per day when compared to those who only consumed one or two servings per day. Numerous epidemiological studies have documented lower rates of colon cancer in populations whose diets are typically rich in fruits and vegetables. Animal studies have strongly supported the chemoprotective effect of fruits and vegetables; when fruits and vegetables are fed to animals prior to exposure to known carcinogens, the development of new cancers is greatly reduced.

There is general agreement among scientists that fruits and vegetables reduce cancer risk. However, there is less consensus regarding the effects of individual food constituents, such as vitamins, minerals, or any of the other hundreds, perhaps thousands, of phytochemicals found in fruits and vegetables, including the various antioxidants. Phytochemicals are simply chemicals found in plants. They are naturally ocurring substances that provide plants with their own defense system against disease. When ingested by humans in their food, these same substances may stimulate anticancer enzymes, block cell damage and/or transport carcinogens from the body. Nearly all fruits and vegetables contain a variety of phytochemicals; broccoli has at least 40, orange juice has 59; and garlic and onions have 50 that have been identified to date. Scientists have isolated many of these agents in the laboratory and shown them to protect against cancer in experimental studies.

One large class of phytochemicals includes the antioxidants. These agents act at the molecular level and are thought to protect us from cancer by inactivating free radicals, chemically reactive fragments of molecules that carry unpaired electrons which seek to combine with other charged particles. Free radicals are by-products of normal metabolic processes such as aging or they can be generated by exposure to environmental factors such as sunlight, tobacco smoke, radiation, or even exercise. They are highly unstable and can react with a gene's DNA. They can then damage and permanently mutate the gene. As such damage accumulates, the cell's normal repair mechanisms may become overwhelmed and lead to irreversible disease.

The antioxidants that have received the most attention are beta-carotene, vitamin C, and vitamin E. Beta-carotene is a pre-cursor of vitamin A and is converted to vitamin A in the body. It provides the bright, vibrant colors present in many vegetables. Beta-carotene is considered to be a highly efficient, free-radical neutralizer and has been the subject of many clinical trials that will be discussed below. Recently, attention has focused upon a relative of beta-carotene named alpha-carotene as well. Vitamin C is a water-soluble vitamin that has been credited with preventing everything from the common cold to cancer. It is a relatively weak antioxidant but is thought to help prevent cancer by enhancing the immune system, detoxifying potential carcinogens in the liver, and blocking the formation of nitrosomines (known carcinogens) in the liver. Vitamin E is a fat-soluble vitamin that is considered to be the most powerful free radical scavenger, especially in concert with the mineral selenium. Like vitamin C, vitamin E enhances the immune system and blocks the formation of nitrosamines (as discussed further in Chapter 9).

Several large, well-controlled clinical trials have been conducted to test whether or not selected antioxidants provide a protective effect on cancer risk similar to eating a diet high in antioxidant-rich fruits and vegetables. When you contrast results from the population-based studies demonstrating a relatively consistent protective effect from a diet high in fruits and vegetables with the results from some of these clinical trials, what emerges might appear to be an antioxidant paradox. For example, foods rich in beta-carotene have clearly been shown to reduce the risk of lung cancer in smokers while high doses of beta-carotene supplements seemed to increase the risk. Studies involving colon cancer have also yielded some surprising results. In spite of the fact that people who consume a diet high in fruits and vegetables consistently have lower rates of colon cancer, three large clinical trials testing the effects of beta-carotene, vitamin C, and vitamin E supplements in varying combinations have all failed to reduce the incidence of tumors in the colon. This does not mean that these antioxidants have no anticancer effect. What it does mean is that the greatest health benefit is likely to be derived from a mix of micronutrients present in a variety of foods and not in isolated micronutrients consumed as supplements.

Research is now focused upon a host of other phytochemicals that have demonstrated chemopreventive potential. The most important of these are discussed below.

1. Genistein in soy products. Population-based studies, laboratory studies, and clinical trials have strongly supported the hypothesis that soy-containing foods are highly chemopreventive. Soy has been associated with reduced rates of breast, colon, lung, and prostate cancers. Soy is extremely rich in a unique group of compounds called isoflavones. The primary isoflavone in soy is genistein, which is thought to prevent cancer through several mechanisms. Genistein, as well as the other isoflavones, competes with estrogen for available binding sites on the surfaces of cells. This effectively decreases the amount of circulating estrogen, which would then lead to a lower risk of breast cancer. Genistein also inhibits the action of a variety of key enzymes involved in the cancer process, including tyrosine kinase, an important enzyme in stimulating the growth of cancer cells. A third and perhaps most important finding is that genistein inhibits the formation of new blood vessels, a process called angiogenesis. New blood vessels are essential for the growth and spread of tumors.
2. Indoles primarily found in the so-called cruciferous vegetables such as broccoli, cabbage, cauliflower, and brussels sprouts. These substances are thought to protect against breast cancer by inhibiting the formation of biologically active estrogen.
3. Isothiocyanates: also highly concentrated in the cruciferous vegetables. These phytochemicals work by detoxifying carcinogens in the liver.

In addition to the above phytochemicals, there is a great deal of nutrition research centered around a few particular vitamins and minerals. These are

1. Folate: a B vitamin abundant in spinach, asparagus, kidney beans, lentils, whole grains, and fortified cereals. It is linked to a decreased risk of colon cancer and, possibly, cervical cancer. Animal studies have shown that even

mild depletion of folate increases the risk of colorectal tumors three- or fourfold. The Nurses' Health Study found that those who reported eating a folate-rich diet were less likely to develop colon cancer. Some observational studies have reported that low folate levels increase the risk of developing cervical dysplasia, abnormal tissue that may precede cervical cancer. Folate has a direct effect on DNA. One of folate's major functions is to transfer methyl groups to DNA. In people who have had polyps or tumors removed from the colon, even the remaining healthy tissue shows evidence of fewer methyl groups than expected. Increasing the amount of folic acid will increase the amount of methyl groups on the DNA.

However, increased amounts of folate in pharmacologic doses can mask a vitamin B-12 deficiency. Older individuals often have decreased stomach acid secretion and are therefore unable to properly digest vitamin B-12 from its protein-bound food sources. Any woman over 65 taking folic acid supplements in excess of the recommended daily allowance of 400 micrograms per day should consult with her physician about possible vitamin B-12 deficiency beforehand.

2. Calcium: a mineral, abundant not only in dairy products but in dark, green leafy vegetables, tofu, salmon, and sardines.

Calcium has received a great deal of press regarding its role in decreasing the risk of osteoporosis in women, and may be helpful for blood pressure control as well. Calcium probably plays an important role in decreasing the risk of colon cancer in addition to these established health benefits. Epidemiologic studies, including one recently done of 35,000 older women, have shown that the higher the intake of calcium-rich foods, the lower the risk of colon cancer. In experimental studies, calcium has been found to decrease cell proliferation in the lining of the colon. Calcium also binds bile acids, compounds shown to stimulate tumor growth, and decreases the levels of bile acids in the stool. One caveat when taking supplemental calcium: Calcium interferes with the absorption of zinc, a mineral essential for proper immune function and gene regulation. Nearly one half of older Americans consume only two-thirds of the recommended daily allowance for zinc (15 mg).

3. Selenium: a mineral concentrated in fish, meats, eggs, whole grain cereals, and certain nuts such as Brazil nuts.

Selenium is a powerful antioxidant, especially when combined with vitamin E and has been associated with a lower risk of breast, colon, ovarian, and lung cancers. However, it is highly toxic in large doses and total supplemental selenium should not exceed 200 micrograms per day.

People often ask whether they should eat their fruits and vegetables raw or cooked to maintain the highest nutritional quality. The answer is it depends on the nutrient. Cooked carotenoids (like beta-carotene) absorb more oxygen and lose some antioxidant effect with cooking. Foods containing water-soluble vitamins, like vitamin C, also lose some nutrients if boiled in water; but cooking also releases certain micronutrients, such as indoles in broccoli. The bottom line is that if you eat a variety of vegetables and fruits every day, the manner in which they are prepared will matter less than the actual quantity of the fruits and vegetables consumed. If boiling is used as a method of cooking, saving the cooking water to use in soups or stocks can recapture some of the lost nutrients.

CONCLUSIONS ABOUT NUTRITION AND CANCER PREVENTION

The National Cancer Institute has estimated that over 1000 of the micronutients in food may have chemopreventive properties, at least in the laboratory. However, isolated micronutrients do not work as well as the combinations found in food, and in fact most clinical trials have found them to be totally ineffective in this regard. When individual vitamins and/or minerals are removed from food, it appears that the compounding effect from the other food ingredients is lessened. That is to say, there is a synergistic relationship between the various micronutrients in food that is lost when these compounds are isolated from food.

Five to nine servings of a variety of fruits and vegetables each day will provide the appropriate mix of micronutrients as well as the fiber recommended for cancer prevention. A serving is usually one-half cup, except for leafy vegetables like spinach, which is one cup. Eating this many servings will likely replace some of the high fat or meat items in the diet, which will have additional benefits for both cancer and cardiovascular disease.

Although vitamin and mineral supplements are no substitute for a variety of foods, the absorption of certain vitamins and minerals decreases with age. Calcium and vitamin D are two examples. If a woman is unable to consume the recommended amounts of these nutrients in her food, or she is unable to consume the desired regimen of fruits and vegetables, a supplement may be indicated. A supplement should contain a balance of nutrients, usually at doses that are 100 to 200% of the recommended daily allowances (see Chapter 23). The potentially toxic vitamins A and D should be limited to 100%. For postmenopausal women not taking estrogen, calcium supplements should be 1200 to 1500 mg per day. For women over sixty who may have a decreased stomach acid secretion, the citrate form of calcium is more readily absorbed. Finally, vitamin E is one of the antioxidant micronutrients that is difficult to adequately consume in food. It is concentrated in wheat germ, nuts, and various oils, foods that are relatively high in fat or, in the case of wheat germ, not generally consumed in very large quantities. But vitamin E also has anticoagulant properties in large dosages (one of the reasons it may be useful in treating peripheral vascular disease) so dosages should be limited to 400 to 800 IU per day, or taken in consultation with physician recommendations.

ALCOHOL

Any article discussing the impact of alcohol on health is almost sure to make the evening news. Many individuals the world over were delighted to read that two or so glasses of red wine per day may decrease the risk of cardiovascular disease; however, many experts consider the health benefits of even moderate alcohol consumption to be greatly exaggerated. Alcohol has been implicated as a co-carcinogen in several cancers including breast, liver, colon, and head and neck. A co-carcinogen is simply a compound that makes other carcinogens more potent. The overwhelming number of epidemiological and clinical studies have reported an increased risk of cancer with increasing alcohol consumption. It is estimated that a lifetime average of one alcoholic beverage per day can increase a woman's breast cancer risk by 40% and that two alcoholic beverages per day may boost the risk by as much as 70%. Those 88,000 nurses in the Nurses' Health Study increased their risk of breast cancer by 30% if they imbibed three to nine drinks per week and by 60% at greater than 9 drinks per week. The author of that study is convinced there is an increased risk at even one drink a day, an intake that would be considered moderate and even beneficial (for heart disease) by almost all health care providers and consumers.

The American Cancer Society recently published their nutritional guidelines. Their report noted that mouth and throat cancers are much more prevalent in countries with high alcohol consumption. They also reported that various studies have determined an association between alcohol consumption and increased risk of breast cancer. Therefore, on balance, the potential small benefit in terms of heart disease attributed to alcohol is probably not worth the excess risk of cancer it carries, particularly in women, because of the strong link to breast cancer even at low levels of intake. There are many more healthful ways to reduce the risk of cardiovascular disease (exercise, folate, minimize fat and cholesterol, stop smoking) as outlined in Chapter 14, so that alcohol does not need to be relied on for this purpose.

Alcohol may promote cancer in several ways. Studies have shown increased estrogen levels in the blood with rising alcohol consumption. Animal studies have shown that alcohol causes a proliferation of breast cells that may lead to increased susceptibility to carcinogens. Alcohol suppresses the immune system. Alcohol allows carcinogens into the body by irritating the surface of the cells that line the mouth and throat. Alcohol may impair the body's ability to metabolize folate as well as absorb calcium, two compounds thought to reduce the risk of colon cancer.

Women are particularly susceptible to the effects of alcohol, especially as they age. Women have lower levels of an enzyme called alcohol dehydrogenase (ADH). This enzyme is responsible for oxidizing alcohol before it reaches the bloodstream. The lower the levels of ADH, the more unoxidized alcohol reaches the brain via the bloodstream and the greater the effect of the alcohol. As the efficiency of ADH declines with age, so does the ability to metabolize alcohol. In addition, women have proportionately more fat and less lean tissue (and total body water) than men, so alcohol is not as readily diluted in women, resulting in higher blood levels and exposing the body tissues to more of the toxicity prior to metabolism.

A recent study comparing drinking habits and death rates in 21 countries showed that the protective effects of alcohol on mortality from cardiovascular disease in the French, for example, are entirely eradicated by alcohol abuse that leads to premature death from cirrhosis, accidents, stroke, and other problems. It is also interesting to note that wine consumption in France has dramatically decreased in the last decade as have deaths from heart disease. Although there may be some protective association between alcohol consumption and heart disease, there is a significant increase in the risk for several cancers with alcohol. Fortunately, women have far better alternatives than alcohol to reduce their risk of heart disease: a low-fat, nutrient dense diet combined with moderate physical activity and a healthy body weight, just to name a few. If a woman does consume alcoholic beverages, she should limit them to three per week, on average.

INVESTIGATIONAL TOPICS IN NUTRITION AND CANCER

A variety of foods containing particular micronutrients are being tested in clinical trials for their chemopreventive potential. A few of current interest are

1. Tea. Several animal studies have demonstrated an inhibition of tumor cells of the breast, colon, liver, lung, and pancreas as a function of tea in the drinking water. Epidemiologial studies have been inconclusive; some showed a protective effect while others showed no effect at all. The principal chemopreventive agent is suspected to be epigallocatechin gallate, an antioxidant present in almost 50 % of the solid material in brewed green tea. Studies are suggesting similar benefits for black tea as well. The amounts used in the animal studies are equivalent to about four to six cups of tea per day, more than most Americans drink but typical for many Asian and some European cultures.
2. Garlic. Animal studies have suggested that high doses of garlic can arrest tumor development. A few observational studies have suggested a lower risk of stomach cancer. Garlic, as well as onions, leeks, chives, scallions, and shallots, contains allyl sulfides. These phytochemicals are thought to increase the production of enzymes that neutralize carcinogenic compounds. Garlic pills have not been found to confer any chemopreventive effect, however. Thus, as with fiber and antioxidants, consumption of whole foods containing these substances is the best advice.
3. Flaxseed. Also known as linseed; when processed, also known as the fabric linen. It is a high-fiber grain (two-thirds soluble) present in milled form in some breakfast cereals. Several animal studies have suggested a decreased risk of breast and colon cancers. Flaxseed contains a high concentration of the phytochemical lignin which reduces the level of circulating estrogen in postmenopausal women. Lignin may also be responsible for lower levels of colon cancer biomarkers. Flaxseed can be found in several multigrain breads and cereals and flaxseed flour can be added to muffins, cookies, and breakfast bars. Small amounts of flaxseed will provide large amounts of the desired micronutrient lignin. Freshness is essential; ground flaxseed should be used immediately or stored in the freezer.
4. Rosemary. Animal studies have demonstrated this herb can reduce the incidence of breast tumor formation in rats by as much as 74%. The phytochemical carnisol is suspected to be responsible.

PHYSICAL ACTIVITY AND CANCER

INTRODUCTION

Despite the mounting evidence of the health benefits of physical activity, a minority of Americans engages in regular exercise. In 1992, nearly 60% of the U.S. adult population reported little or no leisure-time physical activity. Yet, physical activity has been consistently associated with lowered morbidity and mortality for several chronic diseases, including certain types of cancer. The term "exercise-cancer hypothesis" which describes a role for exercise in specifically reducing cancer risk, has been proposed by some authors. Much of the evidence that physical activity protects against certain cancers can be deduced from experimental animal studies, athletes, and the occupationally and/or recreationally active individual. However, because cancer refers not just to one disease or even to one disease process, studies have often been inconsistent or difficult to interpret. Not all studies consider dietary differences between subjects and controls, or have adequate measures of body composition, for example. Subsequently, it may become impossible to adequately determine the relative effects of diet, exercise, or other healthy lifestyle traits in these individuals in cancer risk. The following section summarizes findings suggesting that a physically active lifestyle may reduce the risk of developing certain cancers.

COLON CANCER AND EXERCISE

Colon cancer is the site-specific cancer most commonly studied and the cancer for which the most persuasive data exist on the relationship to physical activity. Several studies have documented an inverse relationship between high levels of physical activity and colon cancer. In a large prospective study of male college alumni (the Harvard Alumni Study), investigators found that for those who exercised at moderate to high levels (1000 kcal/week to 2500 kcal/week in energy expenditure), there was a 25 to 50% lower incidence of colon cancer when compared to sedentary men (expending 500 kcal/week or less in physical activities). Likewise, several case-control and cohort studies suggest that exercise might reduce the risk of colon cancer in men by up to one third. Although these studies focused on men, there have been many studies on both men and women and undoubtedly these results apply to women as well. The primary mechanism for the influence of exercise centers on increased gut motility and the resultant shortened transit time. As the contractility of the intestine increases, so does the speed with which waste moves through the intestines. The greater the speed, the less contact there is between the bowel wall and any potential carcinogens or toxins present in fecal material. It is of interest that although the epidemiological data really define the benefit of aerobic activities, since that is by far the majority of exercise reported, there is now evidence that progressive resistance training increases gastrointestinal motility as well. Therefore, there would potentially be benefit for colonic protection from this modality of exercise as well, assuming that the theoretical mechanism is correct.

REPRODUCTIVE CANCERS AND EXERCISE

Exercise may change cancer risk for reproductive cancers by altering levels of sex hormones, particularly estrogen and, to a lesser degree, progesterone; physical activity may offer a means of primary prevention through its influence on estrogen levels. Of all the reproductive cancers, breast cancer has been the most thoroughly studied by far in this regard. It has been estimated that premenopausal women who have borne children and who exercise at least three and one half hours per week may decrease their risk of breast cancer by as much as 70% compared to sedentary women.

Experimental epidemiological and animal studies all indicate that breast cancer risk is influenced by exposure to endogenous estrogens. Estrogen stimulates abnormal cell growth in the breast and is therefore implicated in the induction of breast cancer. Theoretically then, any intervention which decreases a woman's lifetime exposure to estrogen, will decrease her risk of breast cancer. Experimental studies in premenopausal women have shown that vigorous exercise can change the characteristics of the menstrual cycle. Specifically, young female athletes have a delayed age at menarche as well as an increase in anovulatory cycles, both of which decrease their exposure to estrogens. For the postmenopausal woman, the influence of exercise on estrogen levels is more indirect. As women proceed into menopause, fluctuating hormone levels cause a redistribution of body fat from the typically gynoid distribution of "hips, thighs, buttocks" to the android distribution of mid and upper body. It has been well documented that women with a higher percentage of upper body fat have a significantly increased risk of breast cancer as well as a poorer prognosis at the time of diagnosis, and a higher rate of recurrence of disease. One explanation is that these women with upper body fat have elevated levels of estrogen due to the ability of fat cells in the breast and abdomen to form estrogen. These fat cells are able to do so because they contain an enzyme which converts androgens (a hormone produced throughout a woman's life) to estrogen. So the more fat cells a woman has in her upper body, the more estrogen she produces, even after menopause. Exercise, therefore, not only helps a woman maintain a desirable body weight, but decreases her central adiposity and her lifetime exposure to estrogen as well.

Several epidemiological studies have shown a decreased risk for breast cancer with increasing physical activity levels. Animal models have generally been supportive as well. There have been a few published reports of no protective effect of physical activity during adulthood for breast cancer; however, both human and animal data are much more limited for breast cancer than for colon cancer, and not all of the study designs have been scientifically sound or provided control for relevant factors. The evidence to date supports the concept that physical activity is protective for breast and possibly other reproductive cancers such as ovarian and endometrial cancers as well. More studies are needed to more fully define doses, modalities, timing, and other issues about the exercise prescription and these malignancies.

ROLE OF THE IMMUNE SYSTEM IN THE EXERCISE AND CANCER RELATIONSHIP

Much attention has been focused on the effect of physical activity on the human immune system. When tumor cells are present in the body, the immune system responds by initiating processes which will attempt to either slow the rate of the tumor's growth or destroy the abnormal cells. It has been suggested that factors which suppress immune function be considered as tumor promoters, while factors which enhance immune function be considered as tumor inhibitors. The immune system is comprised of many different cell types and cellular products, each performing a different function in regulating tumor spread. One of these cell types, called natural killer cells (NK cells), provides an important first line of defense against many types of tumor cells. It has been well documented in a large number of studies that NK-cell numbers and activity substantially increase during acute bouts of exercise. More specifically, moderate exercise has been shown to enhance the ability of NK cells to destroy breast cancer cells as well as to increase the numbers of other immune cell receptors (monocytes) in breast cancer patients. More prolonged and intensive exercise releases endorphins which may, in turn, cause an increase in the activity of NK cells. It is of note that depression, psychological stress, or bereavement results in a substantial reduction in NK cell activity, and that depression has been associated with higher rates of some cancers. It is possible that the specific benefit of exercise in psychological illness may counteract the immune system abnormalities associated with these disease states, as well as providing relief for the clinical symptoms. There are several other potential positive effects of exercise on the immune system that are currently being studied more closely.

There are also some possible negative consequences of exercise for the immune system when there is a state of over-training induced, which is associated with energy depletion, bone marrow suppression, and perhaps the production of free radicals. Such adverse consequences have only been documented in highly trained endurance athletes who may be relatively undernourished in terms of protein, energy, or micronutrients, and have no real relevance to the recreational exerciser.

HEALTHY LIFESTYLE AND CANCER PROTECTION

There are many secondary, or indirect, benefits of exercise that may be partially responsible for the observed protection against the growth of cancer cells. Physically active people tend to be those who are also interested in maintaining overall good health and engage in a variety of healthy behaviors. For example, they are more likely to eat a healthy diet and not smoke. They are less likely to be depressed. They are also more likely to maintain a desirable body weight and, for the more vigorously physically active, to possess a desirable body fat content and distribution pattern. They tend to eat more food than sedentary individuals, giving them exposure to a wider variety of micronutrients and trace elements which may provide protection. It is unclear at this time how much of a role these factors may play in the exercise–cancer relationship. Overall, the evidence is highly suggestive that exercise protects against cancer by inducing favorable changes in the function of the immune system, reducing estrogen exposure, optimizing body composition, and encouraging other healthy lifestyle behaviors such as good diet and not smoking. Thus preventive programs for cancer should clearly involve multidisciplinary efforts to encourage adoption and adherence for this range of behaviors that work independently and interactively to reduce the chance of malignancy for the older woman.

REFERENCES

Alpha-Tocopherol and Beta-Carotene Cancer Prevention Study Group, The effect of vitamin E and beta-carotene on the incidence of lung cancer and other cancers in male smokers. *N. Engl. J. Med.*, 330, 1029–1035, 1994.

American Cancer Society, Cancer Facts and Figures—1995, American Cancer Society, Atlanta, Georgia, 1995.

Boyd, N. F., Martin, L. J., Noffel, M., Lockwood, G. A., and Tritchler, D. L., A meta-analysis of studies of dietary fat and breast cancer risk, *Br. J. Cancer*, 68, 627–636, 1993.

Cao, G., Sofic, E., and Prior, R. L., Antioxidant capacity of tea and other common vegetables, *J. Agric. Food Chem.*, 44, 3426–3431, 1996.

Chapman, K. M. and Nelson, R. A., Loss of appetite: managing unwanted weight loss in the older patient, *Geriatrics*, 49(3), 54-9, 1994.

Clinton, S. K. and Giovannucci, E. L., Nutrition in the etiology and prevention of cancer, in *Cancer Medicine*, Holland, J. F. et al., Eds., 4th ed., Vol. 1, William and Wilkins, Baltimore, MD, 1997, 465–494.

Freudenheim, J. L., Marshall, J. R., Vena, J. E., and Laughlin, R., Premenopausal breast cancer risk and intake of vegetables, fruit and related nutrients, *J. Natl. Cancer Inst.*, 88, 340–348, 1996.

Fuchs, C., Giovannucci, E., Colditz, G., Hunter, D., Stampfer, M., Rosner, B., Speizer, F., and Willett, W., Dietary fiber and the risk of colorectal cancer and adenoma in women, *N. Engl. J. Med.*, 340, 169–176, 1999.

Gao, Y. T., McLaughlin, J. K., Blot, W. J., Ji, B. T., Dai, Q., and Fraumeni, J. F., Jr., Reduced risk of esophageal cancer associated with green tea consumption, *J. Natl. Cancer Inst.*, 86(11), 855–8, 1994.

Giovannucci, E. and Willett, W. C., Dietary factors and risk of colon cancer, *Ann. Med.*, 26, 443–452, 1994.

Henderson, B. E., Ross, R. K., and Pike, M. C., Toward the primary prevention of cancer, *Science*, 254, 1131–1138, 1991.

Hill, M. J., Dietary fiber and human cancer, in *Epidemiology of Diet and Cancer*, Hill, M. J., Giacosa, A., and Caygill, C. P. J., Eds., Ellis Horwood, London, 293–309, 1994.

Hunter, D. J. and Willett, W. C., Nutrition and breast cancer, *Cancer Causes Control*, 7, 56–68, 1996.

Hutchinson, F., The Fred Hutchinson Cancer Research Center Food Frequency Questionnaire, Version 01.6.88, Cancer Research Center, 1988.

Kramer, M. and Wells, C., Does physical activity reduce risk of estrogen-dependent cancer in women?, *Med. Sci. Sports Exerc.*, 28(3), 322–334, 1996.

Lakka, T. A., Venalainen, J. M., Rauramaa, R., Salonen, R., Tuomilehto, J., and Salonen, J. T., Relation of leisure-time physical activity and cardiorespiratory fitness to the risk of acute myocardial infarction, *N. Engl. J. Med.*, 330(22), 1549–54, 1994.

Le Marchand, L., Hankin, J. H., Wilkins, L. R., Kolonel, L. N., and Englyst, H. N., Dietary fiber and colorectal cancer risk, *Epidemiology*, 8, 658–665, 1997.

Li, G., Qiao, C. H., Lin, R. I., and Pinto, J. T., Antiproliferative effects of garlic constituents on cultured human breast cancer cells, *Oncol. Rep.*, 2, 787–791, 1995.

Longnecker, M. P., Alcoholic beverage consumption in relation to risk of breast cancer: meta-analysis and review, *Cancer Causes Control*, 5, 73–82, 1994.

MacDonald, P. et al., Effect of obesity on conversion of of plasma androstenedione to estrone in postmenapausal women with and without endometrial cancer, *Am. J. Obstet. Gynecol.*, 130, 448-454, 1978.

MacNeil, B. and Hoffman-Ooetz, L., Effect of exercise on natural cytotoxicity and pulmonary tumor metastases in mice, *Med. Sci. Sports Exerc.*, 25(8), 922–928, 1993.

NCI, *Cancer Prevention: Good News, Better News, Best News*, National Institutes of Health, Public Health Service, U.S. Department of Health and Human Services, U.S. Government Printing Office, Washington, D.C., 1984a.

NCI, *Diet, Nutrition, and Cancer Prevention: A Guide to Food Choices*, National Institutes of Health, Public Health Service, U.S. Department of Health and Human Services. U.S. Government Printing Office, Washington, D.C., 1984b.

NCI, *Diet, Nutrition, and Cancer Prevention: A Guide to Food Choices*, National Institutes of Health, Public Health Service, U.S. Department of Health and Human Services, U.S. Government Printing Office, Washington, D.C., 1987.

Pukkala, E., Poskiparta, M., Apter, D., and Vihko, V., Life-long physical activity and cancer risk among Finnish female teachers, *Eur. J. Cancer Prev.*, 2, 369–376, 1993.

Rose, D. P., Dietary fiber and breast cancer, *Nutr. Cancer*, 13, 1–8, 1990.

Seim, H. C. and Holtmeier, K. B., Treatment of obesity in the elderly, *Am. Fam. Phys.*, 47(5), 1183–9, 1993.

Shephard, R. J., Physical activity and reduction of health risks: how far are the benefits independent of fat loss? *J. Sports Med. Phys. Fitness*, 34(1), 91–8, 1994.

Siddiqui, R. A. and Williams, J. F., The regulation of fatty acid and branched-chain amino acid oxidation in cancer cachectic rats: a proposed role for a cytokine, eicosaniod, and hormone trilogy, *Biochem. Med. Metab. Biol.*, 42, 71–86, 1989.

Smith-Warner, S. A. et al., Alcohol and breast cancer in women: A pooled analysis of cohort studies, *JAMA*, 279, 535-540, 1998.

Sternfeld, B., Cancer and the protective effect of physical activity: the epidemiological evidence, *Med. Sci. Sports Exerc.*, 24(11), 1195–1209, 1992.

Stoll, B. A., Timing of weight gain in relation to breast cancer risk, *Ann. Oncol.*, 6(3), 245–8, 1995.

Thune, I., Brenn, T., Lund, E., and Gaard, M., Physical activity and the risk of breast cancer, *N. Engl. J. Med.*, 336, 1296–1375, 1997.

Trichopoulou, A., Katsouyanni, K., Stuver, S., Tzala, L., Gnardellis, C., Rimm, E., and Trichopoulos, D., Consumption of olive oil and specific food groups in relation to breast cancer risk in Greece, *J. Natl. Cancer Inst.* 87, 110–116, 1995.

White, S. L. and Maloney, S. K., Promoting healthy diets and active lives to hard-to-reach groups: market research study, *Public Health Reports*, 105(3), 224–31, 1990.

World Cancer Research Fund/American Institute for Cancer Research, *Food, Nutrition and the Prevention of Cancer: A Global Perspective*, BANTA Book Group, Menasha, WI, 1997.

Ziegler, R. G., Hoover, R. N., Nomura, A. M., West, D. W., Wu, A. H., Pike, M. C., Lake, A. J., Horn-Ross, P. L., Kolonel, L. N., Siiteri, P. K., and Fraumeni, J. F., Jr., Relative weight, weight change, height, and breast cancer risk in Asian-American women, *J. Nat. Cancer Inst.*, 88(10), 650–60, 1996.

12 Diabetes

Maria A. Fiatarone Singh

CONTENTS

AGE-RELATED CHANGES IN GLUCOSE HOMEOSTASIS AND DIABETES

Diabetes mellitus is diagnosed after a fasting blood glucose greater than 120 mg/dl has been obtained. The majority of diabetes (80-90%) in the elderly is Type II Diabetes, which is characterized by a reduced sensitivity to the action of insulin, and high circulating insulin levels. Some Type II diabetics will go on to require insulin when their pancreatic function is not able to secrete enough insulin to meet demands. Type I diabetics are typically diagnosed earlier in life, and have an absolute deficiency of insulin secretion from the pancreas due to islet cell failure. Better medical care and prevention or treatment of secondary complications of Type I diabetes, particularly end-stage renal disease and serious infections, have prolonged survival in these patients, so an increasing proportion of them are now surviving into old age.

Prior to the diagnosis of overt Type II diabetes, there is often an extended period of time during which the person has insulin resistance, followed by glucose intolerance (when the pancreas cannot keep up with the demands for insulin secretion imposed by the peripheral resistance to insulin action). Unless specific blood testing is done to diagnose these pre-diabetic states, they will usually go undetected and untreated. Glucose intolerant individuals have fasting glucose in the normal or high normal range, but manifest elevated and sustained hyperglycemia after an oral glucose tolerance test or meal tolerance test. This period of hyperinsulinemia is not benign, however, as the elevated post-prandial glucose levels lead to glycosylation of proteins throughout the body, resulting in end-organ damage in many systems (e.g., vascular, ocular, renal, central and peripheral nervous system). In addition, hyperinsulinemia itself is an independent risk factor for vascular disease and cardio-vascular mortality. Older adults with glucose intolerance go on to develop diabetes at an increased rate compared to the normal population, and are therefore an ideal target group for preventive medical and lifestyle changes that may prevent or delay occurrence and its associated morbidity and mortality.

The etiology of the age-related decrease in sensitivity to insulin is multifactorial, with genetic, nutritional, hormonal, and lifestyle factors playing a role. There is a clear familial clustering of Type II diabetes and glucose intolerance, such that either condition in a first-degree relative increases the risk for development of diabetes in mid or late life. Central adiposity is a major factor in resistance to insulin, whereas lower body obesity does not carry this risk by itself. The development of generalized or visceral adiposity after menopause in many women is associated with a gradual worsening of glucose homeostasis. Lean older men have much "younger" glucose and insulin profiles than normal weight or obese men. Physical activity, independent of body weight or body composition, exerts strong protective effects against the development of insulin resistance, glucose intolerance, and diabetes, even in those with a family history of this disorder. An extreme form of inactivity, complete bedrest, leads to rapid deterioration of insulin responsiveness, and may result in glucose intolerance. Muscle wasting or atrophy from any cause will exacerbate problems related to the extent and rate of the peripheral disposal of glucose into skeletal muscle, which is essential for maintenance of euglycemia in response to normal metabolism, meals, or other stressors. Certain medications, such as thiazides or particular corticosteroids or the abnormal prolonged exposure to carbohydrate during intravenous glucose infusions, total parenteral nutrition, or continuous intes-tinal tube feedings can unmask diabetes in susceptible individuals. The metabolic stress of acute infection, surgery, or other illness, with the associated elevation of insulin-antagonizing stress hormones, can lead to transient hyperglycemia in an otherwise compensated individual. Pancreatic disease may compromise insulin secretion acutely or permanently. Nutritional intake that results in an energy excess is the primary derangement which is etiologic in adult-onset diabetes, and is usually related to an excess intake of fat calories. Chromium deficiency causes glucose intolerance, as chromium is necessary for the intracellular transport of glucose for storage as glycogen, but this is only seen in individuals fed a completely chromium-deficient artificial diet. Relative degrees of chromium deficiency may exist, however, in people consuming diets devoid of unrefined flours and grains, which are rich sources of chromium. In summary, a host of factors influence genetic susceptibility to Type II diabetes, but many of these factors are also modifiable by lifestyle changes, as will be discussed below.

EPIDEMIOLOGY OF DIABETES

The incidence of diabetes in the total population in the U.S. increased from the 1986–1988 baseline of 2.9 per 1000 people to 3.1 in 1992–1994, away from the target goals set by health care agencies. Health care costs are two to three times greater for people with diabetes than the average for the total population. The American Diabetes Association estimates the total cost of diabetes in the United States to be approximately $92 billion annually.

According to estimates from the Department of Health and Human Services, an average of 1700 people are diagnosed with diabetes each day; 1000 die from its complications; 150 undergo amputations; 80 enter end-stage renal disease treatment; and 70 become blind. The prevalence of diabetes is far greater in minority populations, and increasing at a faster rate. For American Indians/Alaska Natives, for example, the prevalence was 69 per 1000 in the baseline year 1987 and increased to 73 per 1000 in 1994. For Blacks, the prevalence increased from the 1986–1988 baseline of 36 to 40 in 1992–1994.

Many reasons lie behind this increasing burden of diabetic disease, including

- a change in the definition of diabetes (120 vs. 140 mg/dL fasting glucose);
- more accurate and complete ascertainment by screening blood tests;
- the growth of the older population who are at risk for insulin resistance;
- declining levels of habitual physical activity;
- increased prevalence of generalized and central obesity;
- fewer deaths from acute complications and a correspondingly greater susceptibility to chronic complications of this illness; and
- population growth in minority communities at high risk for diabetes and associated problems, due to lifestyle and genetic, as well as socio-economic factors.

Despite the advances in the pharmacological management and early detection of diabetes, diabetes-related age-adjusted mortality is also increasing for the total U.S. population, and even more significantly for minorities, women, and the elderly. From the 1986 baseline of 38 per 100,000 people, diabetes-related deaths in the total population increased to 40 per 100,000 in 1994. Among black Americans, the 1986 baseline was 67 and the number of deaths per 100,000 in 1994 was 73, more than 80 percent higher than for the total population. Similar trends are seen for American Indians/Alaska Natives (1986 baseline, 46; 58 deaths per 100,000 in 1994) and for Mexican Americans and Puerto Ricans, the 1990 baselines were 55.7 (rising to 57.8 in 1994) and 40.7 (rising to 57.8 per 100.000 in 1994), respectively. Although some of the increased prevalence is due to differences in ethnic designations and reporting improvements, much of it represents increased disease prevalence and severity.

Diabetes is the most common cause of blindness, amputations, and end-stage renal disease in the U.S. adult population, and contributes significantly to coronary artery disease and peripheral vascular disease development. In addition to total diabetes-related mortality, it is also evident that diabetic morbidity is increasing as well. For the total population with diabetes, the rate of lower extremity amputations increased from the baseline of 8.2 per 1000 people in 1987 to 8.6 per 1000 in 1994. For Blacks with diabetes, the 1987 baseline was higher at 9, and the rate in 1994 was approximately the same at 9.1. For the total population, end-stage renal disease (ESRD) as a complication of diabetes increased to a rate of 2.4 per 1000 people with diabetes in 1993 from the baseline of 1.5 in 1987. For Blacks, the rate increased alarmingly from 2.2 per 1000 people with diabetes (1983–1986 data) to 5.7 for the period 1990–1993. ESRD as a complication of diabetes among American Indians/Alaska Natives increased similarly from a rate of 2.1 per 1000 (1983–1986 data) to 5.4 in 1992.

THE DIAGNOSIS OF DIABETES IN THE OLDER ADULT

Although the diagnostic criteria for diabetes are not different with age, the condition is often diagnosed after considerable delay in older adults. This is because the signs and symptoms may be vague and ill-defined, and overlap with many other common complaints in older adults. A high index of suspicion should be maintained, therefore, particularly in individuals at risk for diabetes. The risk factor profile which should heighten awareness includes

- history of diabetes or glucose intolerance in a first-degree relative;
- obesity (body mass index > 28 kg/m2);
- central obesity (elevated waist circumference or waist-to-hip ratio for gender);
- sedentariness or low levels of physical activity; and
- presence of hypertension, hyperlipidemia, hypertriglyceridemia (other metabolic aberrations associated with visceral adiposity).

The classical presentation of weight loss, polyuria, and polydipsia due to the hyperosmolar effects of glucose and glucosuria may be the presentation in an older adult with Type II diabetes as well. However, the changes in hypothalamic responses to hyperosmolality may reduce the perception of thirst, or eliminate this symptom entirely in the elderly. Even when blood glucose values are in the very elevated ranges of 300 to 500 mg/dl, and intravascular volume is depleted secondary to glycosuria, thirst may not be increased in older adults. Because changes in detrusor muscle function or pelvic musculature and connective tissues may have already resulted in increased urinary frequency in older women, the onset of glycosuria may not be noticed, or conversely, may result in an exacerbation or new symptom of urinary incontinence in a formerly asymptomatic or controlled bladder disorder.

One of the most common presenting symptoms at all ages is fatigue or lassitude. However, this is a common symptom in older adults with a variety of other medical and psychological disorders, and so may not provoke a metabolic work-up initially if the practitioner attributes it to other causes, or dismisses it as a consequence of aging. Other neuropsychological features may include apathy, withdrawal from activities, changes in mood, lack of concentration, changes in memory or attention, and may be confused with an episode of clinical depression or early cognitive decline. Hyperglycemia causes muscle weakness, and chronical diabetes may produce a proximal myopathy with severe wasting loss of strength. Again, however, because muscle strength tends to decline over the years in adults, this may be imperceptable to the patient or the practitioner, or may be mistakenly attributed to biological aging. Unintentional losses of body weight are rarely benign in the older adult, and may be the only sign of diabetes in these individuals, or represent other occult diseases such as malignancy, depression, or hyperthyroidism, for example. Recurrent infections, especially of the skin or urinary tract, or poor wound healing and foot ulcers are common in diabetics, and may also be the first sign of this disease. Peripheral nerve damage is rarely an early sign of diabetes, as it is usually a complication of many years of poor glucose control, but may manifest in a previously undiagnosed diabetic as paresthesias or numbness of the distal upper and lower extremities, or fecal incontinence. There is an autonomic neuropathy which accompanies diabetes as well, which will cause postural hypotension, and loss of heart rate variability. Postural hypotension may be aggravated by drugs or by intravascular volume depletion during episodes of significant hyperglycemia, and should always be looked for on examination, as it is a risk factor for falls in older adults. Visual changes may include changes in acuity, inability to see in dim light or glare, and may represent diabetic-related retinopathy or cataract formation that occurs at accelerated rates compared to non-diabetics.

In summary, a host of signs and symptoms are usually present which may be elicited with a careful history and physical exam in an older adult with diabetes who presents with vague complaints not attributable to other causes. Particularly in at-risk individuals such as those who are overweight or from non-white ethic backgrounds, a high index of suspicion should be maintained. The diagnosis of hyper-insulinemia or glucose intolerance is just as important as the diagnosis of diabetes, because these patients are in need of non-pharmacologic interventions and close follow-up that will be critical for the prevention or delay of overt diabetes in the future. Similarly, their family members who are also at risk should be screened for the presence of remediable risk factors (overweight, sedentariness) beginning in childhood if the increasing prevalence of Type II diabetes seen in national trends is to be altered in the future.

THE MANAGEMENT OF DIABETES IN THE OLDER ADULT

PUBLIC HEALTH EDUCATION

These national trends have sparked many attempts to change both patient and caregiver behavior to improve early detection, treatment, and optimal management of this condition. The National Diabetes Education Program is a broadbased effort directed toward the general public, patients, health care providers, and policy-makers.

This initiative is modeled on the experience of the successful effort to heighten public awareness about the dangers of high blood pressure and cholesterol, a campaign which has resulted in significant improvements in the detection and control of these risk factors for cardiovascular disease (see Chapter 14). There is some evidence that such public health efforts are working. The total population of people with diabetes who attend classes in the management of their condition increased from the 1983–1984 baseline of 32% to 43% in 1993. Progress was even greater for the black population, which showed an increase from 34% in 1991 to 50% in 1993. The proportion of Hispanics receiving such education is quite low, and decreased from 27% in 1991 to 26% in 1994. These figures for all demographic groups, however, are far below the desirable levels of participation in educational programs, which are considered essential for the management of this lifelong illness with its many behavioral adaptations required for optimal control.

Some of the current goals for the nation, as drafted in *Healthy People 2010*, are to develop prevention education campaigns that target Native Americans, Hispanics, Blacks, and overweight, physically inactive people, who are all at increased risk for this disorder. In addition, efforts are proposed to explore and document the connection between individual lifestyle choices, e.g., physical inactivity and obesity, and variances in the incidence and severity of chronic conditions such as diabetes. It is clear that the kinds of behavioral and education programs which will ultimately be effective in penetrating these demographic groups will have to be tailored to include ethnic food choices and preparation styles, cultural expectations and norms about body habits and activity levels for the elderly, access to and affordability of special dietary items or physical activity programs, and the increased prevalence of smoking and other health behaviors which may aggravate diabetes-associated complications.

PHARMACOLOGICAL CONTROL OF HYPERGLYCEMIA

It is now clear from experimental trials that tight contol of blood glucose levels in both Type I and Type II diabetes is important for the prevention of long-term complications of this disease. This is particularly important in the elderly, who may have glucose intolerance and then diabetes for many decades, and are therefore at extremely high risk of end-organ damage due to glycosylation of body proteins. The general pharmacological management of diabetes is reviewed in many standard textbooks and will not be detailed here. Current approaches take advantage of the improved side-effect profile of many of the newer generation of oral hypoglycemics. These newer agents have a shorter half-life compared to chlorpropamide, which is more prone to cause hypoglycemia and other side effects in older adults in particular, and therefore not recommended. Other classes of medications which decrease hepatic glucose production or enhance insulin sensitivity may be used in combination with sulphonylureas, which act primarily to enhance insulin release. Although glycemic control has been proven to be highly effective in controlling both Type I and Type II diabetes, the deleterious effects of central obesity and lack of exercise can undo the benefits of proper medical management, and tend to hasten the emergence of the disease in as yet asymptomatic, susceptible individuals with insulin resistance.

NUTRITIONAL CONSIDERATIONS IN TYPE II DIABETES

Many recent reviews of the literature regarding the nutritional management of diabetes indicate that adherence to the strict food exchange system and restriction of simple sugars in the traditional American Diabetic Association Diet is not necessary for good diabetic control in the typical Type II diabetic. Such diets were quite difficult to follow and required an enormous amount of compulsivity and compliance on the part of the patient. Although Type I insulin-dependent diabetics may need some of these dietary elements to prevent blood glucose swings, in addition to regularity in the timing of meals, medications, and physical activity sessions, Type II diabetics have a quite different set of nutritional requirements for optimal control.

In contrast to lean, young Type I diabetics, approximately 90% of Type II diabetics are obese, and this obesity is etiologic in their disease. The basic goal of the diet for the older diabetic is the achievement and maintenance of ideal body weight and body composition. There are two opposite trends in body composition which occur with aging that influence glycemic homeostasis: increase in body fat (and visceralization of fat), and decrease in muscle mass. These body composition changes are accompanied by a general increase in body weight from young adulthood to middle age, particularly after the menopause in women. The increase in weight and fat mass is attributable to decreases in energy expenditure both at rest and in physical activities, accompanied by an insufficient reduction in caloric intake, or even increases in caloric intake, thus resulting in a situation of energy surplus. Surplus energy can only be stored in the body as adipose tissue, as described further in Chapter 5. The relationship between visceral fat, insulin resistance, and lipid abnormalities is not completely understood. Visceral fat is felt to lead to insulin resistance and hyperinsulinemia because visceral adipocytes have an accelerated rate of lipolysis which is poorly inhibited by insulin, resulting in an increase in free fatty acids proportional to the fat mass. These elevated free fatty acids in the portal circulation travel to the liver, resulting in fatty infiltration of the liver and a host of metabolic alterations, including increased production of VLDL particles, triglycerides, LDL particles, and apolipoprotein-B by the liver. Skeletal muscle lipoprotein lipase, which normally catabolizes triglyceride-rich particles, is reduced in individuals with insulin resistance, further altering the lipid profile. The fatty liver does not extract insulin from the circulation normally, thus contributing to systemic hyperinsulinemia. Additionally, the excess lipid oxidation provides precursors for gluconeogenesis, elevating hepatic glucose output. Thus, the prevention or treatment of visceral obesity is central to the nutritional management of the typical insulin-resistant older diabetic and prevention of long-term atherogenic complications.

As described in more detail in Chapter 17, the primary means for weight control is limitation of fat intake, as fat is the most energy-dense component of food. In addition, it is recommended that saturated fat intake in particular be limited in diabetes, because of their predisposition to vascular disease. Limiting total fat intake to 25 to 30% of calories is the best way to achieve such weight loss. A more severe restriction in fat intake than this is generally not sustainable long term, and will lead to weight cycling which has extremely adverse consequences on body composition, metabolism, and psychological health.

Carbohydrate intake should comprise 50 to 60% of the diabetic diet. Although complex carbohydrates are desirable for their micronutrient and fiber content, as well as their relatively lower glycemic index (propensity to cause rapid rises in blood glucose), very elevated levels of carbohydrate or fiber ingestion will lead to elevations of triglycerides and lowering of HDL cholesterol ratios, thus worsening the cardiovascular risk profile related to lipids. There is little or no evidence that a high fiber diet, in the absence of weight loss will improve short- or long-term control of diabetes. In general, the adoption of a reduced fat diet will entail substitution of low fat foods such as fruits, vegetables, and grains, for high fat foods and so there will be a natural increase in complex carbohydrates and fiber in this way.

Unfortunately, many patients and even health care providers see their major nutritional goal in diabetes as the elimination of concentrated forms of sugar, or the use of artificial sugar substitutes in the diet. There is no evidence that the enormous increase in the consumption of artificial sweeteners in the U.S. population has been in any way beneficial to the epidemic of obesity and rising prevalence of Type II diabetes. Consider an individual with Type II diabetes consuming a meal of french fries, hamburger, and diet cola, for example, in contrast to a bowl of minestrone soup, whole grain bread, and non-diet cola. Although many diabetics would never consider having a real cola, they do not realize the far greater risks imposed by the typical high fat meal described. Thus, one of the major changes in behavior and understanding which must be communicated by health care practitioners is the concept that adult-onset diabetes is a disease where fat and energy intake are far more important than complex vs. simple sugar composition of the diet.

In general, protein intake recommendations in diabetics are not different than in normal healthy elderly (see Chapter 6). However, non-meat sources for at least some of the meals are recommended to avoid high intakes of saturated fat, particularly if vascular disease is present. If the diabetic has already begun to manifest diabetes-related nephropathy, then the issues become more complicated. There is evidence that the progression to chronic renal failure in diabetics and others can be slowed by compliance with a low protein diet of about 0.6 g/kg/d. However, this level of protein intake is difficult to maintain without a concurrent reduction in total energy intake. For the nonobese or quite elderly diabetic, such energy restriction may result in unwanted weight loss, and compound the failure to thrive accompanying chronic renal insufficiency. Additionally, if proximal myopathy from diabetes is also present, further losses of lean tissue will increase the associated functional deficits. Therefore, initiation of protein restriction in the diabetic, or in any patient, requires intensive dietary counseling and close follow-up for efficacy and safety. We have recently shown that the initiation of progressive resistance training in older adults with chronic renal insufficiency (secondary to diabetes) who are also on a low protein diet prevents the loss of lean tissue and muscle function seen in patients treated only with protein restriction. These kinds of integration of nutritional and exercise prescriptions are essential for the holistic management of such chronic medical conditions.

Fluid balance may be an issue in diabetes when glycosuria, fever, diarrhea, or infection is present. Avoidance of dehydration is essential for the prevention of delirium, falls, and other complications. The frequent presence of autonomic and peripheral neuropathy and visual impairment in such patients makes intravascular volume depletion particularly hazardous with respect to fall risk in the older diabetic. In general, fluid requirements outside of acute illness are similar to those in the healthy older adult (see Chapter 21).

Several micronutrients may be considered in the nutritional management of diabetes. Zinc nutrition is sometimes compromised due to the fact that diabetes is associated with impaired gastrointestinal absorption of zinc, as well as hyperzincuria compared to normals. If a diabetic patient is also prescribed chronic diuretic therapy for associated cardiovascular disease or hypertension, then zinc losses through urine will be elevated further. Zinc is absorbed more poorly in the absence of gastric acid, and therefore patients with achlorhydria or on chronic acid suppression therapy may also be at elevated risk of nutritional deficiency of this mineral. Zinc depletion will predispose to poor wound healing and increased susceptibility to infections already compromised in the presence of hypoglycemia. Serum zinc levels will not fall until tissue stores are quite depleted, and are therefore an insensitive marker for deficiency states. White blood cell zinc levels are better for early diagnosis, but may still remain normal in at-risk patients. A reasonable approach is to advise all diabetics to consume adequate amounts of zinc, either from food sources (meat, fortified cereals, oysters) or multivitamin preparations. In a diabetic, especially one on chronic diuretic or acid suppression therapy, or who presents with an active cellulitis or foot ulcer, zinc sulfate supplementation (80 mg tid) may be recommended, regardless of serum zinc levels, until recovery is complete. Higher doses of zinc are not advised, as they may cause malabsorption of copper and resultant anemia.

For the diabetic with cardiovascular disease or risk factors, all of the general nutritional recommendations for those conditions apply (see Chapter 14). Peripheral vascular disease is particularly prominent in diabetics, and consideration of vitamin E supplementation (400 to 800 IU/d) is therefore highly recommended in patients with claudication due to its benefits in coronary and peripheral vascular disease.

Chromium losses are accelerated in the face of hyperglycemia, polyuria, or exercise, and diets lacking in whole grains are most likely to contribute to low chromium balance. All of the general nutritional recommendations for diabetes in terms of increased fruit and vegetables, whole grains, and legumes will ensure a diet adequate in chromium, so that chromium supplementation (sold as glucose tolerance factor) should not be required. Replacing most or all refined flour products with their whole grain equivalents is one simple behavioral change which will bring with it a much better micronutrient and fiber content than the typical white bread and refined flour diet of many Americans. In diabetics, such a change is likely to have many positive benefits for glucose homeostasis.

Overall, the dietary recommendations for diabetes, apart from weight loss if needed, are similar to those for healthy adults, as exemplified in the Dietary Guidelines for Americans and the Food Pyramid (see Chapter 23). In addition, these recommendations will benefit individuals with obesity, heart disease, peripheral vascular disease, hypertension, and osteoarthritis. Thus, there is no need to prescribe a different diet for each diagnosis. The clustering of these diseases due to their genetic associations and relationship to visceral obesity means that many older patients will present with this pattern of chronic disease, and need coordinated management of lifestyle issues such as diet.

For diabetics on insulin, there is a need to regulate the timing of dosages and meals, as is the case in younger diabetics. However, for most older diabetics there should be no need for radically different "diabetic" foods that are typically quite expensive. The same natural foods and prescription to "eat from the bottom of the pyramid" and limit fat intake will benefit healthy adults as well as diabetics and do not require separate food items or preparation in most cases. Even concentrated sweets can be consumed in small portions, assuming that they fit within the overall energy balance requirements for the individual. Allowing such treats back in the diet is important for the prevention of feelings of depression and deprivation associated with the complete elimination of "normal" foods from the diabetic diet for life.

EXERCISE AND THE OLDER DIABETIC

There are many potential roles for exercise in the chronic management of diabetes. Cross-sectional data clearly indicate that a higher habitual level of physical activity is an important protective factor for the development of diabetes in middle and old age. Intervention trials in healthy individuals, glucose intolerant adults, and Type II diabetics demonstrate many positive effects on glucose homeostasis after both aerobic and resistance training. In the older diabetic, a complex interaction of age-related changes, pathophysiology of the disease itself, nutritional considerations, disuse syndromes, and other co-morbid conditions and medications offer a wide range of possible therapeutic roles for a physical activity prescription. These exercise benefits are reviewed in the sections that follow and are summarized in Table 1.

PREVENTION OF DIABETES

In addition to the data from the Harvard Alumni study that particpation in regular physical activity lowers the risk of adult-onset diabetes, there is also evidence that prescribing exercise to adults who already manifest glucose intolerance can reduce the incidence of overt diabetes. In a large 6-year prospective randomized trial in China, glucose intolerant adults were assigned to dietary management, aerobic exercise, both interventions combined, or usual care. Compared to the usual care group, all three intervention groups had a significant reduction in the subsequent diagnosis of diabetes. There were no significant differences among experimental treatment groups, however. This is the largest prospective study published to date, and demonstrates the clear relevance of early detection of glucose intolerance, utility of appropriate lifestyle intervention before the onset of diabetes itself, and the flexibility in approach to risk factors which can be taken. For example, some older women may be much more inclined to change exercise behavior than dietary intake, for a variety of reasons. If the same benefits can be achieved with either preventive treatment, then there is no need to impose a prescription that is very likely to fail over one that is equally beneficial and more appealing to the individual. Additionally, the establishment of these long-term behavioral changes when the person is still well will likely be more easily adopted and sustained than attempting to initiate such

TABLE 1
Use of Exercise in the Prevention and Treatment of Diabetes

Diabetic Condition	Prevention	Treatment
Glucose homeostasis, insulin resistance (increased glucose disposal rate, increased insulin sensitivity, increased glycogen storage, increased GLUT-4 receptors, decreased fasting glucose, glycosylated hemoglobin levels)	Aerobic exercise Resistance exercise	Aerobic exercise Resistance exercise
Obesity, visceral adiposity	Aerobic exercise Resistance exercise	Aerobic exercise Resistance exercise
Proximal myopathy	?	Resistance exercise
Coronary artery disease	Aerobic exercise	Aerobic exercise Resistance exercise
Peripheral vascular disease	Aerobic exercise	Aerobic exercise
Cerebrovascular disease	Aerobic exercise	Resistance exercise Balance training
Peripheral neuropathy	?	Resistance exercise Balance training[a]
Falls	Resistance exercise Balance training	Resistance exercise Balance training
Chronic renal failure	?	Aerobic exercise Resistance exercise

[a] Exercise useful to reduce gait and balance impairment secondary to neuropathy, not shown to affect the neuropathy itself.

changes in very old age or after illness has occurred. Given the familial clustering of glucose intolerance and diabetes, educating women in mid-life will also hopefully encourage similar attention to weight maintenance, diet, and physical activity in their younger family members and children, and thereby provide wider and earlier penetration into the community at risk. This issue is of particular importance in the minority communities of blacks, Native Americans, and Hispanics, whose prevalence of obesity and insulin resistance/diabetes far exceeds other demographic groups. As these demographic groups may in some cases have limited contact with health care providers, efforts at early diagnosis will require outreach efforts through schools, community centers, health fairs, churches, and other local community organizations.

IMPROVEMENTS IN GLUCOSE HOMEOSTASIS

Improvement in glucose homeostasis related to exercise is due to a variety of complementary effects on body composition and metabolism. The unique contribution of exercise, compared to pharmacological management of diabetes, is that exercise can directly change some of the metabolic derangements leading to loss of glucose homeostasis, whereas medications primarily increase the supply of available insulin, or in the case of metformin, decrease appetite and thereby overall nutritional intake. Another important distinction is that while some medications, such as sulphonylureas can only be used once fasting glucose levels are elevated, and may produce hypoglycemia if used in very mild diabetes, exercise is appropriate long before the development of overt hyerglycemia, to combat insulin resistance and glucose intolerance.

Changes in both adipose tissue and skeletal muscle occur after acute and chronic exposure to exercise and are part of the mechanism by which glucose homeostasis is improved. Acutely, even a single bout of exercise can increase glucose disposal rate, that is, the rate at which circulating glucose is transported into skeletal muscles for storage, in order to maintain euglycemia. This may be seen during glucose clamp studies, or in the glucose and insulin response to a standard mixed meal or an oral glucose tolerance test. The specific changes that have been demonstrated to be associated with improved glucose disposal rate, increased insulin sensitivity, or improved glucose tolerance include increases in GLUT-4 transporter proteins on the surface of muscle fibers which facilitate intracellular transport of glucose, as well as increased storage of glycogen in muscle tissue. This effect begins to wear off after 2 days however, and is largely gone by 4 days. Therefore, recommendations to exercise at least once every 72 hours in diabetics are usually given to take advantage of this metabolic window of improved glucose control. Chronic training, even without changes in body weight or body composition, will also result in improved glucose disposal rates and increased sensitivity to the action of insulin. Both aerobic and resistance training have been shown to improve glucose control, although at this time far more data are available on the effects of aerobic exercise. It appears, however, that resistance training may be a more potent stimulus for changes in glucose metabolism than aerobic training.

The doses and intensities of exercise needed for glucose metabolism effects are not different than those appropriate for general fitness purposes (see Chapter 2). We have shown that the metabolic response to aerobic exercise at moderate or high intensity is not different, and thus an exercise prescription for diabetes should be applicable even to very old, sedentary, or unfit individuals who cannot exercise at intensities above 50% of heart rate reserve. Resistance training at high intensity has been shown to improve glucose homeostasis; lower intensities of resistance training have not been tested for efficacy. Therefore, standard resistance training techniques are recommended, with the caveat that frequency should be once every 3 days, even though strength gains may be seen at lower frequencies than this. The fact that resistance training provides at least the same magnitude of benefit as aerobic training is important, as it broadens the population to which an exercise prescription for diabetes can be given. For example, there are many older diabetics with obesity, degenerative arthritis, peripheral vascular disease, coronary artery disease, and mobility difficulties who would find it impossible to carry out weight-bearing aerobic exercise even at 50% of heart rate reserve. However, these same patients may be quite tolerant of seated whole body resistance exercise, even at high intensity. Therefore, the exercise prescription for diabetes is flexible in terms of modality (although not in terms of frequency), and should always be tailored to the capacity and preference of the individual. This is important in light of the chronic nature of the underlying disease, which will benefit only if long-term changes in behavior are introduced.

In addition to the acute responses to exercise training, chronic training may induce very favorable changes in weight and body composition in adults with diabetes. In obese adults, aerobic exercise has been shown to increase adherence to a hypocaloric diet, which is the standard dietary prescription for most overweight Type II diabetics, so this is a potential benefit. For reasons that are not clear, however, reviews of randomized trials of diet alone vs. diet and exercise in combination have not shown that greater weight loss in diabetics results from the combined intervention than diet alone. This is similar to the result seen with the prevention of diabetics in Chinese adults with glucose intolerance described earlier, which was equivalently treated with either lifestyle change.

Apart from weight loss itself, a decrease in central adipose tissue that is mechanistic in the metabolic derangement of insulin resistance is a very important outcome related to exercise. In healthy older men and women, 3 to 4 months of either progressive resistance training or aerobic training have been shown to significantly reduce visceral adiposity (measured by MRI scans), even in the presence of only small changes in total body fat or body weight. Even in lean individuals, visceral adiposity is reduced, indicating a preferential loss of visceral fat deposits under these conditions. For example, the total body fat decrease may only be 2%, whereas visceral adipose tissue will decrease by 15 to 20% after the introduction of such exercise regimens. These kinds of studies have not yet been reported in obese elders or those with glucose intolerance or diabetes, but if similar results occur, the potential benefit would be substantial. For this reason, it is best not to follow body weight as a goal or outcome in relation to exercise prescriptions, as there is little evidence that exercise alone can meaningfully change body weight. Measurements of the waist circumference, however, as a good index of visceral adiposity measured by gold standard scanning techniques, is an excellent way to follow losses of central fat stores. Measurements should be made at the natural waist, every 4 to 6 weeks, to the nearest 0.5 cm, with a flexible anthropometric tape (see also Chapter 23). It is likely that these positive (shrinking) results will provide more encouraging reinforcement for the behavioral change than the static numbers on the scale.

Another potential benefit of exercise in diabetics is increases in the size of the muscle mass itself. Skeletal muscle is the biggest reservoir for glucose disposal, storing as glycogen that which is not immediately oxidized for use as fuel. Losses of muscle mass are common with aging, sedentary lifestyles, and diabetes itself (see below), and potentially contribute to the underlying pathology of insulin resistance. Progressive resistance training performed over many months at moderate to high intensity, will result in increases in muscle fiber size and overall muscle mass. Such adaptations would be theoretically advantageous for glucose control in the diabetic. Studies that demonstrate relationships between the changes in muscle mass and changes in diabetic control after initiation of resistance training in older diabetics are now in progress and will shed more light on the benefits of this mode of training. Aerobic exercise does not have this potential to increase muscle mass. Therefore, it may be helpful to consider the overall body composition goals when prescribing exercise. If the clinical picture is dominated by obesity rather than sarcopenia, the more extensive data on aerobic exercise and dietary behavior change may support this choice of modalities. If the picture is one of frailty and sarcopenia, resistance training may provide more benefits overall.

TREATMENT OF DIABETES-RELATED MORBIDITY

Diabetes carries with it the potential for a range of complications and associated disease states which may also be amenable to appropriate exercise interventions. The most important areas to consider are outlined below.

Vascular Disease

As mentioned above, diabetics are at increased risk for all forms of vascular disease. Therefore, the epidemiological literature on the prevention of cardiovascular, peripheral vascular, and cerebrovascular disease with aerobic exercise is of great relevance to glucose-intolerant and diabetic individuals. Once vascular disease has developed, there are again extensive data on the usefulness of aerobic exercise for these conditions (see Chapter 14), whether or not diabetes is part of the underlying etiology. In addition, resistance training has been shown to provide complementary benefits in coronary artery disease, stroke, and congestive heart failure. For patients who cannot perform aerobic exercise temporarily or permanently (e.g., arthritis, stroke, foot ulcers, claudication), resistance exercise also plays a major role in the management of these clusters of diseases.

Myopathy

Longstanding diabetes may result in a proximal myopathy manifested as weakness and wasting of the upper leg and hip muscles and shoulder girdle muscles. This may be a significant cause of functional disability and mobility impairment in the older diabetic. Progressive resistance training using standard techniques should be prescribed in such individuals identified after history and physical examination. Specific exercises for the hip extensors, hip abductors, knee flexors, knee extensors, deltoid, biceps, and triceps muscles should be included (see Chapter 2). Adequate intake of energy and protein are needed for skeletal muscle adaptation, so it is important to review dietary intake history and body weight patterns over time to coordinate nutritional and exercise recommendations for optimal benefit. Be aware, for example, of iatrogenic diatary restrictions which may have been initiated during an earlier period when obesity was prominent, but are still being followed by the much older, and now myopathic or sarcopenic diabetic.

Chronic Renal Disease

Diabetes is the most common cause of end-stage renal failure, now that hypertension (the other major etiologic factor) is treated earlier and more aggressively. As summarized in Table 2, there is a potential specific role for exercise in the prevention and treatment of various stages of renal failure in the diabetic. Prevention or delay in the onset of renal disease requires good glucose control, management of hypertension and other vascular risk factors, and aerobic exercise has been shown to be

TABLE 2
Role of Exercise at Various Stages of Chronic Renal Failure in the Diabetic

Type of Exercise	Prevention of Chronic Renal Failure	Treatment of Renal Failure before Dialysis	Treatment during Dialysis	Treatment after Renal Transplantation
Aerobic exercise	Improved metabolic control may delay onset of renal failure[a]	Adjunctive management of glucose	Improved metabolic control and treatment of cardiovascular risk factors and depression	Improved metabolic control and treatment of cardiovascular risk factors
Resistance exercise	Improved metabolic control may delay onset of renal failure[a]	Adjunctive management of glucose and prevention of wasting from low protein diet	Unknown	Treatment of steroid-induced myopathy and osteopenia Improved metabolic control

[a] No clinical trial evidence with this outcome to date.

beneficial in these areas. It is possible that resistance exercise will be shown to have preventive value as well, as it seems to induce modest decreases in blood pressure and cholesterol, but more definitive studies are required before such recommendations can be made.

Once a diagnosis of early renal disease has been made, there is evidence that dietary protein restriction can delay the progressive decline in glomerular filtration rate that may ultimately result in dialysis. During this period, we have shown that progressive resistance training can prevent the muscle wasting due to a low protein diet in patients with renal failure. This is caused by the anabolic effect of resistance training, which has been shown to improve nitrogen balance in older adults, thus reducing dietary protein requirements for balance. Once dialysis has begun, there is evidence that aerobic exercise provides substantial benefit in terms of improved cardiovascular fitness, decreased cardiovascular risk factor profile, improved depressive symptoms, and improved overall quality of life compared to usual care controls. This type of exercise has been shown to be safe in this population, despite the potential problems related to significant vascular disease, ischemia, fluid shifts with dialysis, and electrolyte abnormalities for example. There are no studies of resistance training in dialysis patients. The need for protein restriction is now gone obviously, but many of these patients who have suffered with many years of uremia and restricted activity due to illness will present at dialysis quite wasted and deconditioned. Therefore, resistance training may offer complementary benefits to those of aerobic exercise in these patients. Outcomes of clinical trials in this setting, and direct comparison of benefits of various exercise modalities are needed to develop optimal exercise treatment protocols for diabetics and others on dialysis.

Finally, there are increasing numbers of older adults who can be offered renal transplantation as an option for treatment of chronic renal failure, although most such transplants continue to be performed in those under 50 years of age. Again, this modality of treatment brings with it specific needs in terms of physical activity. All organ transplant patients will require chronic corticosteroid therapy for the prevention of rejection. In cardiac transplantation, this has been shown to result in rapid and large losses of bone density, muscle mass, and muscle strength compared to the pre-transplant condition. Such steroid myopathy and osteopenia will be super-imposed on the myopathy due to diabetes, inactivity, and protein restriction, and likely to have clinical consequences. Braith has shown that progressive resistance training three months after cardiac transplantation completely reverses the bone and muscle losses observed in controls, and increases muscle strength significantly above pre-treatment levels. Similar experiments have not yet been reported after renal transplantation, but there is no reason to suspect that similar benefits would not be found. The significant disturbance of bone metabolism in chronic renal failure would offer another potential target for both aerobic and progressive resistance training in this patient population.

Fall Risk

The older man or woman with longstanding diabetes may be at elevated risk of falling for many reasons, as shown in Table 3. Diabetic autonomic neuropathy may result in postural hypotension and orthostatic symptoms. Post-prandial hypotension is seen in a proportion of all older adults, but if present in a diabetic who also has an autonomic neuropathy related to diabetes, would increase the risk of falling after a meal. Visual impairment secondary to diabetic retinopathy or early cataract for-mation may impair gait and balance and increase the risk of injurious falls. Peripheral diabetic sensory neuropathy and loss of proprioception can contribute to poor gait, balance, and mobilty. Proximal myopathy may increase the likelihood of falls during transfers, standing, and stair climbing or descent. Dehydration during episodes of hyperglycemia, fever, or other illness may exacerbate postural hypotension. Central nervous system changes associated with poor control of glycemia either acutely or chronically may result in delirium or impaired judgment which can result in risk-taking behavior or falls from impaired neuromuscular reflexes and coordination. Amputations of the toes, foot, or leg may require special footwear, orthotics, pros-theses, or assistive devices, and result in very abnormal biomechanics of gait that increase the risk of falling. Periods of enforced bed or chair rest during treatment of active foot ulcers, cellulitis, or other conditions will result in rapid musculoskeletal deconditioning that contributes to poor gait and balance. Finally, drugs prescribed for depression, insomnia, cardiovascular disease, hypertension, or urinary inconti-nence are all common in diabetics and may impose further hazards.

The approach to such a multifactorial problem is to review all the possible etiologic factors, treat them specifically (e.g., cataract extraction, medication reduc-tion), and educate patients, family members, and other caregivers regarding safety precautions. In terms of exercise, the appropriate modality here would in most cases be a combination of resistance training and balance training (see Chapter 2). Even if the specific deficit cannot be removed (e.g., visual impairment from diabetic retinopathy), a fall may be prevented by increasing other intrinsic resources (balance, strength) that are also needed for maintenance of equilibrium in the face of a stressor.

TABLE 3
Factors Related to Increased Fall
Risk in the Older Diabetic

Amputations
Autonomic neuropathy
Cataracts
Foot ulcers
Medications producing postural hypotension
Obesity-related mobility impairment
Osmotic diuresis/volume depletion
Peripheral neuropathy
Proximal myopathy
Retinopathy
Sedentariness

Thus, a completely blind diabetic should be given, for example, the best possible chance to avoid falls by an aggressive program of strength and balance training, minimization of postural hypotension, and environmental planning. There is no demonstrated role for isolated aerobic training as a fall-prevention tool. There is evidence in healthy young and old men that aerobically trained or resistance-trained individuals are better able to withstand lower body negative pressure (an experimental model for postural blood pressure stresses) than sedentary controls. However, there is a need to test such strategies in older adults with diabetes or other diseases, or with clinical evidence of postural hypotension before definitive recommendations can be made.

INTEGRATION OF THE MANAGEMENT PLAN

Given the multitude of intersecting clinical dimensions of the prevention and treatment of morbidity and mortality in diabetics, it is clear that a holistic, multidisciplinary approach is essential. Both patient and caregiver have important roles to play in the management plan, and neither one can act alone due to the overlapping of risks and benefits in many domains. In deciding on the appropriate integration of exercise and nutritional prescriptions, all of the potential beneficial interventions should be listed for an individual based on his or her particular medical profile. Next, contraindications to specific prescriptive elements should be listed, and removed from the plan. Areas of overlap and simplification should be identified, for example, high fruit and vegetable intake for the treatment of hypertension will also contribute to the goal for increased fiber and fat restriction for the obese diabetic. Therefore, a single dietary change (eat 5 to 9 servings a day of fruits and vegetables, for example) will cover most of the nutritional goals related to diabetes, hypertension, coronary artery disease, peripheral vascular disease, and obesity). Similarly, resistance training will reduce visceral adiposity, improve insulin sensitivity, increase muscle mass, treat diabetic myopathy, reduce fall risk, and lower protein requirements in chronic renal failure. After listing overall needs and overlapping treatments, patient tolerance and preferences should then be discussed to formulate the final diet and exercise prescription. If equivalent benefit from either aerobic or resistive exercise may be derived in a middle-aged diabetic woman who is not yet frail; then choice, likelihood of compliance, and access to training facilities should dictate the mode of training ultimately recommended.

SPECIAL ISSUES IN THE OLDER DIABETIC

SEVERE VISUAL IMPAIRMENT

Visual impairment will not be uncommon in diabetes; it is the leading cause of blindness in adults. Awareness of gradual restrictions in activity that may be taking place as visual impairment increases is important in preventing disuse syndromes and substituting new forms of activity as required. For many such patients, machine-based aerobic or resistance exercise will allow full safe participation in exercise regimes, with or without a trainer present. Large print instructions or a magnifying glass over machine display boards will allow easier unsupervised use of such equipment. A guide dog who needs to be walked each day may be a very good behavioral incentive for the initiation of a regular exercise regimen in a formerly housebound diabetic with blindness or severe visual impairment. Depression is common in acquired blindness in adults, due to diabetes or other causes. Exercise is a specific and potent treatment for depression (see Chapter 22) and should be highly recommended in such patients for its multiple benefits.

In patients with chronic, treated diabetic retinopathy, exercise is not contraindicated, whereas it must be avoided at the time of acute hemorrhage, laser treatment, or any ocular surgery. There is no good data on the length of activity restriction required, but opthalmologists may suggest 2 to 6 weeks of activity restriction around these events. Activities which raise intraocular pressure (head below knees, Valsalva manuever) should be avoided in acute or chronic retinopathy or when risk of retinal detachment is present.

ABNORMALITIES OF BLOOD GLUCOSE

Exercise should not be performed during acute exacerbations of diabetes that may occur due to illness, medication changes, or other causes. Generally, if the fasting blood glucose is below 160 mg/dl, exercise will not worsen glycemic control. Hypoglycemia should be evaluated and corrected before exercising, as further symptomatic drops in glucose may occur, particularly after a prolonged or intensive bout of exercise. Sometimes it is difficult to tell if vague symptoms in older diabetics are due to poor glucose control or other causes. It is always better to avoid vigorous exercise when there is such uncertainty until definitive glucose measurements and other clinical evaluation can be made.

Exercise should never be done after taking insulin or oral hypoglycemics unless a meal has been consumed as well. Prior to exercise sessions, insulin should be injected into non-exercising limbs or the trunk if possible to avoid rapid systemic uptake from the subcutaneous depot caused by the increase in blood flow to the exercising limb. Generally, timing of exercise sessions to coincide with the post-prandial peak in blood glucose (90 to 120 minutes after a meal) in patients with glucose intolerance or Type II diabetes will be well tolerated and work to minimize the extent and duration of hyperglycemia. Particularly in insulin-dependent diabetics, ready access to a concentrated source of rapidly absorbed simple sugar is advisable during exercise sessions.

AMPUTATIONS AND FOOT ULCERS

These problems are very common in diabetics and others with peripheral vascular disease. Amputees should receive progressive resistance training for the remaining portion of the lower limbs and upper extremities to improve transfers, use of pros-theses, and independence in mobility. Even in those who cannot regain ambulation, maintenance or improvement of transfer skills with upper extremity training is extremely important. As with loss of vision, loss of a limb will be a devastating occurrence for such patients, and may result in significant clinical depression and withdrawal. Attempts at rehabilitation post-surgery will fail unless this depression is dealt with aggressively. As noted above, intensive exercise regimens may be very important to address this depression, or serve as an adjunct to pharmacological management of these symptoms. In addition to resistance training, upper extremity aerobic exercise on an ergometer is still possible, and truncal alignment and balance training may be helpful to improve wheelchair posture and comfort for those with above-the-knee amputations.

Foot ulcer prevention is essential in those with peripheral vascular and neurologic disease. Measures that should be instituted include avoidance of high impact activ-ities, prevention and treatment of fungal infections, meticulous care of toenails and skin, provision of well-fitted orthotics and footwear, use of thick socks at all times, and exercise on compliant surfaces (carpet, lawn, mattresses) if possible. Because of their associated visual impairment, diabetics may often require foot inspection by a family member or caregiver to recognize early problems.

If a foot ulcer has already developed, dependency of the extremity is to be avoided, as this will exacerbate venous pooling and edema, increase pain, and slow healing. In addition, direct pressure on the wound and surrounding skin must be avoided, which often leads to complete prohibition of weight-bearing activities involving the affected limb. Unfortunately, such treatment often produces unneces-sary immobilization of patients with resultant extensive deconditioning during many weeks of wound healing. A better approach is to switch to non-weight-bearing aerobic activities (upper ergometry, use of a seated stepper or recumbant cycle with one leg only, for example) or seated resistance training regimens on machines during which time the feet are not in contact with the ground or floor (e.g., knee extensors and flexors, upper body exercises). Thus, when the ulcer has completely healed, the patient will be more than adequately prepared for re-ambulation, compared to the patient who has undergone extensive muscle atrophy and cardiovascular decondi-tioning during the period of active ulcer treatment.

SUMMARY

Diabetes is one of the best examples of a chronic disease that is highly influenced by lifestyle choices as well as genetic susceptibility, and in which cooperation of patient and caregiver is essential for optimal management and prevention of complications. Avoidance of smoking and excess alcohol, in addition to dietary choices and regular physical activity present the best chance of reducing morbidity and mortality in this disease. Aggressive early screening and education in high risk populations is needed, as many of the early or asymptomatic signs of insulin resistance or diabetes should be treated with behavioral programs or other interventions. It is time that we move away from the model of waiting until the disease is far advanced to treat it, much as we have done in other areas of medicine. For example, vitamin D deficiency is now treated when the serum 25-OH vitamin D level is low, not after osteomalacia develops. Osteopenia is hopefully recognized and treated prior to the development of osteoporotic fracture. Hypertension should be controlled before retinopathy, cardiomyopathy, or renal failure occur. In the same way, recognition of the metabolic aberrations of visceral adiposity syndrome (hyperinsulinemia, atherogenic lipid profiles, glucose intolerance) should lead to nutritional, physical activity, and even pharmacological intervention if needed for lipids and insulin sensitivity, long before elevations of fasting glucose result in a clinical diagnosis of diabetes.

REFERENCES

ADATFNEL, American Diabetes Association Task Force on Nutrition and Exercise Exchange Lists, *Diabetes Care,* 10, 126–132, 1987.

American Dietetic Association, Diabetes Mellitus and Exercise, Position Statement, *Diabetes Care,* 13(7), 804–805, 1990.

Bassett, D. R., Skeletal muscle characteristics: relationships to cardiovascular risk factors, *Med. Sci. Sports Exerc.,* 26(8), 957–966, 1994.

Bogardus, C. et al., Effects of physical training and diet therapy on carbohydrate metabolism in patients with glucose intolerance and non-insulin-dependent diabetes mellitus, *Diabetes,* 33, 311, 1990.

Braith, R., Mills, R., Welsch, M., Keller, J., and Pollock, M., Resistance exercise training restores bone mineral density in heart transplant recipients, *J. Am. Coll. Coariol.,* 28(6), 1471–1477, 1996.

Braith, R., Welsch, M., Mills, R., Keller, J., and Pollock, M., Resistance exercise prevents glucocorticoid-induced myopathy in heart transplant recipients, *Med. Sci. Sports Exerc.,* 30, 483–489, 1998.

Brown, S., Upchurch, S., Anding, R., Winter, M., and Ramirez, G., Promoting weight loss in Type II diabetes, *Diabetes, Care,* 19, 613–24, 1996.

Buechfiel, C., Sharp, D., Curb, J., Rodriguez, B., Hwang, L., Marcus, E., and Yano, K., Physical activity and incidence of diabetes: the Honolulu heart program, *Am. J. Epidemiol.,* 141, 360–368, 1995.

Charles, M. A., Fontbonne, A., Thibult, N., Warnet, J. M., Rosselin, G. E., and Eschwege, E., Risk Factors for NIDDM in white population. Paris Prospective Study, *Diabetes,* 40, 796–799, 1991.

Colditz, G., Willett, W., Rotnitzky, A., and Manson, J., Weight gain as a risk factor for clinical diabetes mellitus in women, *Ann. Intern. Med.,* 122, 481–486, 1995.

Davidson, J.. *The effective approach and management of diabetes in blacks and other minority groups.* Report of the Secretary's Task Force on Black and Minority Health, Washington, D.C., U.S. Department of Health and Human Services, 1986.

Despres, J.-P., Body fat distribution, exercise and nutrition: Implications for prevention of atherogenic dyslipidemia, coronary heart disease, and non-insulin dependent diabetes mellitus, in *Perspectives in Exercise Science and Sports Medicine: Exercise, Nutrition and Weight Control,* Lamb, D. and Murray, R., Cooper Publishing Group, Carmel, IN, 11, 107–150, 1998.

Devlin, J. and Horton, E., Effects of prior high-intensity exercise on glucose metabolism in normal and insulin-resistant men, *Diabetes,* 34, 973, 1985.

Eriksson, K. F. and Lindgarde, F., Prevention of Type 2 (non-insulin-dependent) diabetes mellitus by diet and physical exercise. The 6-year Malmo feasibility study *Diabetologia,* 34(12), 891–8, 1991.

Ezaki, O., Higuchi, M., Nakatsuka, H., Kawanaka, K., and Itakura, H., Exercise training increases glucose transporter content in skeletal muscles more efficiently from aged obese rats than young lean rats, *Diabetes,* 41(8), 920–6, 1992.

Fluckey, J. D., Hickey, M. S., Brambrink, J. K., Hart, K. K., Alexander, K., and Craig, B. W., Effects of resistance exercise on glucose tolerance in normal and glucose-intolerant subjects, *J. Appl. Physiol.,* 77(3), 1087–92, 1994.

Gallagher-Allred, C. R. and Emley, S. J., Specific dietary interventions. Diabetes, osteoporosis, renal disease, *Primary Care: Clinics in Office Practice,* 21(1), 175–89, 1994.

Haapanen, N., Milunpain, S., Vuori, I., Oja, P., and Pasanen, M., Association of leisure time physical activity with the risk of coronary heart disease, hypertension, and diabetes in middle-aged men and women, *Int. J. Epidemiol.,* 26, 739–47, 1997.

Haffner, S. M., Stern, M. P., Hazuda, H. P., Mitchell, B. D., and Patterson, J. K., Cardiovascular risk factors in confirmed prediabetics, does the clock for coronary heart disease start ticking before the onset of clinical diabetes? *JAMA,* 263, 2893–2898, 1990.

Hanefeld, M., Fischer, S., Schmechel, H., Rothe, G., Schulze, J., Dude, H., Schwanebeck, U., and Julius, U., Diabetes Intervention Study. Multi-intervention trial in newly diagnosed NIDDM, *Diabetes Care,* 14(4), 308–17, 1991.

Harris, M. I., Hadden, W. C., Knowler, W. C., and Bennett, P. H., Prevalence of diabetes and impaired glucose tolerance and plasma glucose levels in U.S. Population Aged 20-74 yr, *Diabetes,* 36, 523–34, 1987.

Helmrich, S., Ragland, D., and Paffenbarger, R., Prevention of non-insulin-dependent diabetes mellitus with physical activity, *Med. Sci. Sports Exerc.,* 26(7), 824–830, 1994.

Helmrich, S. P., Ragland, D. R., Leung, R. W., and Paffenbarger, R. S., Physical activity and reduced occurrence of non-insulin-dependent diabetes mellitus, *N. Engl. J. Med.,* 325, 147–52, 1991.

Henry, R. et al., Effects of weight loss on mechanisms of hyperglycemia in obese non-insulin-dependent diabetes mellitus, *Diabetes,* 35, 990–998, 1986.

Higgins, M., D'Agostino, R., Kannel, W., Cobb, J., and Pinsky, J., Benefits and adverse effects of weight loss. Observations from the Framingham Study [published erratum appears in *Ann. Intern. Med.,* 1993 Nov 15, 119(10), 1055] [see comments. *Ann. Intern. Med.,* 119(7 Pt 2), 758–63, 1993.

Holbrook, T., Barrett-Connor, E., and Wingard, D., The association of lifetime weight and weight control patterns with diabetes among men and women in an adult community, *Int. J. Obes.,* 13(5), 723–729, 1989.

Holloszy, J. O., Schultz, J., Kusnierkiewicz, J., Hagberg, J. M., and Ehsani, A. A., Effects of exercise on glucose tolerance and insulin resistance, *Acta Med. Scand.*, (Suppl.) 711, 55–65, 1986.

Holman, R. R. and Turner, R. C., Insulin therapy in Type II diabetes, *Diabetes Res. Clin. Prac.*, 28(Suppl.), S179–84, 1995.

Horowitz, D., Special considerations in the dietary management of diabetes in the elderly, *Geriatric Med. Today*, 3, 41–44, 1984.

Hughes, V. A., Fiatarone, M. A., Ferrara, C. M., McNamara, J. R., Charnley, J. M., and Evans, W. J., Lipoprotein response to exercise training and a low-fat diet in older subjects with glucose intolerance, *Am. J. Clin. Nutr.*, 59(4), 820–6, 1994.

Huse, D., Oster, G., Killen, A., Lacy, M., and Colditz, G., The economic cost of non-insulin dependent diabetes mellitus, *JAMA*, 262, 2708–2713, 1989.

Inoue, T., Osteoporosis—from the view point of the orthopedic surgeon. *Nippon Ronen Igakkai Zasshi - Jap. J. Geriatr.*, 27(4), 397–403, 1990.

Ivy, J. L., Young, J. C., Craig, B. W., Kohrt, W. M., and Holloszy, J. O., Ageing, exercise and food restriction: effects on skeletal muscle glucose uptake, *Mech. Ageing Develop.*, 61(2), 123–33, 1991.

Karvonen, M. J., Determinants of cardiovascular diseases in the elderly, *Ann. Med.*, 21(1), 3–12, 1989.

Keen, H., Jarrett, R. J., and McCartney, P., The ten-year followup of the Bedford Survey (1962–1972): glucose tolerance and diabetes, *Diabetologia*, 22, 73–79, 1982.

Kohrt, W. M., Obert, K. A., and Holloszy, J. O., Exercise training improves fat distribution patterns in 60- to 70-year-old men and women, *J. Gerontol.*, 47(4), M99–105, 1992.

Kolterman, O. G., Insel, J., Saekow, M., and Olefsky, J. M., Mechanisms of insulin resistance in human obesity. Evidence for receptor and postreceptor defects, *J. Clin. Invest.*, 65, 1272–1284, 1980.

Kriska, A. M., Knowler, W. C., LaPorte, R. E., Drash, A. L., Wing, R. R., Blair, S. N., Bennett, P. H., and Kuller, L. H., Development of questionnaire to examine relationship of physical activity and diabetes in Pima Indians, *Diabetes Care*, 13(4), 401–411, 1990.

Krotkiewski, M. et al., The effects of physical training on insulin secretion and effectiveness and on glucose metabolism in obesity and Type II (non-insulin dependent) diabetes mellitus, *Diabetologia*, 28, 881, 1985.

Lee, J., Sparrow, D., Vokonas, P. S., Landsberg, L., and Weiss, S. T., Uric acid and coronary heart disease risk: evidence for a role of uric acid in the obesity-insulin resistance syndrome. The Normative Aging Study, *Am. J. Epidemiol.*, 142(3), 288–94, 1995.

Logue, E., Gilchrist, V., Bourguet, C., and Bartos, P., Recognition and management of obesity in a family practice setting, *J. Am. Bd. Family Pract.*, 6(5), 457–63, 1993.

Manson, J., Nathan, D., Krolewski, A., Stampfer, M., Willett, W., and Hennekens, C., A prospective study of exercise and incidence of diabetes among U.S. male physicians, *JAMA*, 268(1), 63–67, 1992.

Manson, J., Rimm, E., Stampfer, M., Colditz, G., Willett, W., Krolewski, A., Rosner, B., Hennekens, C., and Speizer, F., Physical activity and incidence of non-insulin-dependent diabetes mellitus in women, *Lancet*, 338, 774–778, 1991.

Martin, B. C., Warram, J. H., Krolewski, A. S., Bergman, R. N., Soeldner, J. S., and Kahn, C. R., Role of glucose and insulin resistance in development of Type-2 diabetes mellitus, results of a 25-year follow-up study, *Lancet*, 340(8825), 925–929, 1992.

Miller, M., Type II diabetes: a treatment approach for the older patient, *Geriatrics*, 51(8), 43–4, 47–9; quiz 50, 1996.

Miranda, P. and Horowitz, D., High fiber diets in the treatment of diabetes mellitus, *Ann. Intern. Med.*, 88, 482–486, 1978.

Modan, M., Harris, M. I., and Halkin, H., Evaluation of WHO and NDDG Criteria for impaired glucose tolerance, *Diabetes*, 38, 1630-1635, 1989.

Mondon, C. E., Sims, C., Dolkas, C. B., Reaven, E. P., and Reaven, G. M., The effect of exercise training on insulin resistance in sedentary year old rats, *J. Gerontol.*, 41(5), 605–10, 1986.

Morley, J. E., Mooradian, A. D., Silver, A. J., Heber, D., and Alfin-Slater, R, B., Nutrition in the elderly [clinical conference]. *Ann. Intern. Med.*, 109(11), 890–904, 1988.

Morrow, L. A. and Halter, J. B., Diabetes mellitus in the older adult, *Geriatrics*, 43(Suppl.), 57–65, 1988.

NIH, Diet and exercise in non-insulin-dependent diabetes mellitus. Consensus Development Conference Statement, Vol. 6, No. 8, 1986 December 19.

Ohlson, L., Larsson, B., Svardsudd, K., Welin, L., Eriksson, H., Wilhelmsen, L., Bjorntorp, P., and Tibblin, G., The influence of body fat distribution on the incidence of diabetes mellitus: 13.5 years of follow-up of the participants in the study of men born in 1913, *Diabetes*, 34, 1055–1058, 1984.

Raz, I., Israeli, A., Rosenblit, H., and Bar-On, H., Influence of moderate exercise on glucose homeostasis and serum testosterone in young men with low HDL-cholesterol level, *Diabetes Res.*, 9(1), 31–5, 1988.

Saxman, K. A., Barrett-Connor, E. L., and Morton, D. J., Thiazide-associated metabolic abnormalities and estrogen replacement therapy: an epidemiological analysis of post-menopausal women in Rancho Bernardo, California, *J. Clin. Endocrinol. Metab.*, 78(5), 1059–63, 1994.

Seim, H. C. and Holtmeier, K. B., Treatment of obesity in the elderly, *Am. Family Phys.*, 47(5), 1183–9, 1993.

Sjostrom, L., Larsson, B., Backman, L., Bengtsson, C., Bouchard, C., Dahlgren, S., Hallgren, P., Jonsson, E., Karlsson, J., Lapidus, L. et al., Swedish obese subjects (SOS). Recruitment for an intervention study and a selected description of the obese state, *Int. J. Obesity Relat. Metab. Disord.*, 16(6), 465–79, 1992.

Tonino, R. P., Effect of physical training on the insulin resistance of aging, *Am. J. Physiol.*, 256(3 Pt 1), E352–6, 1989.

Treuth, M., Hunter, G., Szabo, T., Weinsier, R., Goran, M., and Berland, L., Reduction in intra-abdominal adipose tissue after strength training in older women, *J. Appl. Physiol.*, 78(4), 1425–1431, 1995.

Weinsier, R. et al., Diet therapy of diabetes, description of a successful methodologic approach to gaining diet adherence, *Diabetes*, 23(8), 669–673, 1974.

White, S. L. and Maloney, S. K., Promoting healthy diets and active lives to hard-to-reach groups, market research study, *Public Health Reports*, 105(3), 224–31, 1990.

Yeater, R. A., Ullrich, I. H., Maxwell, L. P., and Goetsch, V. L., Coronary risk factors in Type II diabetes, response to low-intensity aerobic exercise, *W. V. Med. J.*, 86(7), 287–90, 1990.

Zierath, J. R. and Wallberg-Henriksson, H., Exercise training in obese diabetic patients. Special considerations, *Sports Med.*, 14(3), 171–89, 1992.

13 Falls and Balance

Justus Lehmann and Barbara de Lateur

CONTENTS

INTRODUCTION

At least one third of community-dwelling older adults have one or more falls per year, according to a random sample of enrollees 65 years and older of a large health cooperative in the Seattle area.[1] Persons who are frail, as defined below, are twice as likely to fall as those who took part in a six-month exercise training study.[2] Although some falls may be related to environmental hazards such as throw rugs and irregular paving, as well as impaired vision and medication side effects, most falls are likely to be related to impaired balance or other physiologic deficits. These impairments in balance may be subtle and not necessarily apparent to the untrained observer or even to physicians and other health caregivers, unless they have special training or equipment. Falls aggravate the fear of falling that many older adults have, and such individuals are likely to decrease their activity after falling, even if they were uninjured.[3,4] Furthermore, adults who are frail with osteoporosis or other musculoskeletal problems are, in fact, more likely to be injured if a fall occurs. Women are at an increased risk of hip fracture compared to men, a disparity that is related to differences in bone density as well as factors which contribute to musculoskeletal impairment, falls, and frailty. It is thus important to have a working concept of frailty.[5]

CONCEPT OF FRAILTY

The popular conception of frailty is a person who is thin and weak. This conception is not wrong, but it fails to include many persons whose frailty is not so readily apparent. In persons who do not exercise regularly there is a gradual loss of physiologic reserves in many, perhaps most, systems. For example, without regular exercise, there is a loss of muscle strength, local muscle endurance, and overall aerobic capacity. There will also be a gradual loss in bone mass and density, as well as muscle mass and flexibility of the muscles and connective tissues such as tendons and ligaments. In addition to these losses, there may be a gradual accumulation of fat with a resultant decrease in the strength-to-weight ratio. This ratio, which defines relative strength, is an important factor in how older adults view themselves with respect to impairment or disability. Figure 1, based upon a large HMO database,[6] shows that there is a threshold of relative strength below which older adults report themselves as impaired on the Sickness Impact Profile (SIP). Furthermore, this threshold is lower with advancing age. Thus, the relative strength that would be sufficient for a 60-year-old woman to deny any self-perceived functional loss would be insufficient for a 75-year-old woman.

Not every loss of physiologic reserve results in frailty. For example, if one is very strong and athletic in youth and early adulthood, some loss of physiologic reserve may be well tolerated. This is more likely to be the case in men than in women, however, since women generally start with lower bone and muscle mass than men. Additionally, after menopause, women are particularly susceptible to the loss of strength of bones and muscles. The useful definition of frailty of Buchner and Wagner[5] is "the state of reduced physiologic reserve associated with increased susceptibility to disability." This concept is useful because it allows one to intervene before the actual onset of disability (Figure 2). Although older adults who are disabled are usually frail, with a loss of physiologic reserve, the obverse is not necessarily true. That is, many who are frail are still (for the time being) fully functional. During the time that a woman retains the ability to exercise, it would be wise for her to take advantage of the opportunity and build up physiologic reserve in the areas of muscle strength, flexibility, bone mass, and cardiovascular functioning (aerobic capacity).

IMPORTANCE OF FITNESS AND THE PREVENTION OF FALLS

Women are known to fall more frequently than men do. Blake et al.[7] interviewed men and women aged 65 and older and found that 41.6% of women reported one or more falls over the year preceding the interview vs. only 24.3% of men. Similarly, Sattin[8] studied the rates of fall injury events for men and women aged 65–69, 70–74, 75–79, 80–84, and 85+. In every age group, women had a higher fall rate than men.

Overstall et al.[9] found that in both sexes sway increased with age but was higher (worse) in women of all ages. Sway was significantly worse in persons of both sexes who fell because of loss of balance and in women who fell because of giddiness, drop attacks, turning of the head, and rising from bed or a chair.

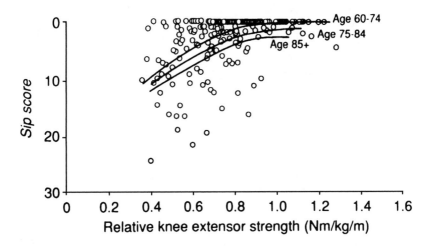

FIGURE 1   Relative knee extensor strength vs. SIP physical dimension score. Data from 434 adults aged 60+ with only every other point plotted. SIP scale is oriented so that higher scores, which reflect poorer function, are at the bottom. Curves derived from polynomial regression. (From Buchner, D. M. and de Lateur, B. J., *Ann. Behav. Med.*, 13, 91–98, 1991. With permission.)

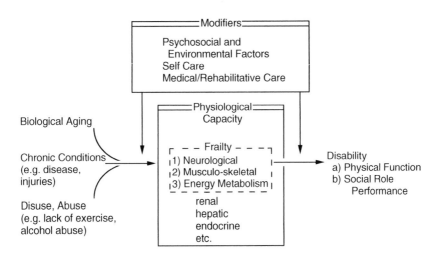

FIGURE 2   Conceptual model of frailty and disability. (From Buchner, D. M, and Wagner, E. H., *Clin. Geriatric Med.*, 8, 1–17, 1992. With permission.)

Lack of strength, especially around the ankle, has been also used as a measure of likelihood of balance problems, particularly likelihood of falls in the elderly.[10] In the Seattle portion of the FICSIT (Frailty and Injuries: Cooperative Studies of Intervention Techniques), Buchner and co-workers hypothesized that ankle weakness would be associated with poor balance. They measured postural sway, with a force platform, on 104 adults aged 68 to 85, and studied these persons in comfortable stance, narrow stance, and tandem stances with eyes open and eyes closed. Dynamic balance was measured by the ability to balance on a tilt board and hemisphere dome as well as the ability to walk on balance beams. Ankle plantar flexion strength was measured with an isokinetic dynamometer. Consistent with the hypothesis, the investigators found that stronger adults had better dynamic balance. However, contrary to the hypothesis, stronger adults showed more postural sway rather than less. The authors interpret this to mean that in difficult (dynamic) balance tasks such as walking the balance beam, compensatory movements were insufficient to overcome the lack of ankle strength in the weaker subjects.

MEASUREMENT OF BALANCE:
FUNCTIONAL MEASURES

Various methods have been used to identify balance problems specifically as they are related to falls. These methods have included simple functional measurements such as measuring the time a woman is able to stand on one foot or on two feet in narrow stance or tandem (the heel of one foot touching the toe of the other) stance positions. Other measures include tandem walking (similar to that used by police to assess intoxication) or balancing on tilt boards and walking on wide and narrow balance beams.

A useful indicator of functional mobility in older women is the timed "Up & Go" test[11] which measures, in seconds, the time taken by a person to stand up from a seated position in a standard arm chair, walk a distance of 3 meters, turn, walk back to the chair, and sit down again.

CONCEPT OF MEASUREMENT OF BALANCE:
QUANTITATIVE MEASURES

More high-tech measures requiring special equipment have also been used to assess balance. These tests allow a little more insight into the sources of the difficulty maintaining balance; these tests may thus be also helpful in designing an individualized treatment program for the patient. Such tests include the assessment of sway, determined by standing on a force platform. By combining a force platform with various conditions of stance, such as wide stance, narrow stance, tandem stance, etc.,[12] one can gradually increase the difficulty of task, and one can also determine the role of visual feedback by repeating certain measures with the subject's eyes closed. Additional difficulties occur in the presence of certain neurologic lesions such as stroke involving the right hemisphere[13] (left body weakness); disturbances of visual orientation in such cases may lead to falls even when a subject is standing quietly on a street corner watching cars go by. Disturbances of proprioception seen in some neurologic conditions or even relative weakness (decreased strength-to-weight ratio) of the ankle muscles can result in excessive sway measurable when a foam mat is placed on the force platform.

All of the aforementioned tests involve a stable platform. Nashner[14] has described a platform that can move forward and backward or tilt in any direction to allow assessment of a subject's response to such a disturbance.

MEASURES TO IMPROVE FITNESS AND BALANCE

The fundamental principle underlying any exercise program to improve performance or status in any area is the overload principle. In broad terms, the overload principle states that muscle must be taxed beyond its ordinary activity to improve performance or condition. With respect to strength training, overload is best accomplished by actually increasing the load carried through a distance by a muscle operating across a joint. There are other ways of overloading a muscle other than actually increasing the load, i.e., the amount of weight lifted. These would include increasing the number of repetitions per set, increasing the number of sets, increasing the number of days exercised or even the number of times exercised per day, i.e., sessions per day. While keeping any or all constant, one can also increase the load by increasing the speed of contraction of the muscle. For example, a woman can lift a weight up and down to increasingly faster metronome settings (provided the lifting speed is reduced to zero, or complete rest, between contractions). With progressive rate training, as this type of program is called,[15] it is important to avoid swinging the weight (by use of a backstop or foam rubber mat on the floor) so that each lifting of the weight requires new energy and a new muscle contraction, rather than using stored energy as the weight returns to the starting position. Aerobic conditioning exercise can be progressively increased by increasing either the intensity or the duration of the exercise or both. With respect to dynamic balance training, the difficulty of the maneuvers may be increased as an effective way of "overloading" the individual.

Although track-bound activities such as training on exercise machines like the weight-stack resistance machines or a stationary bicycle can and do improve one's muscle strength and aerobic capacity, respectively, this type of exercise will have only a modest effect, if any, on the improvement of one's balance. This is not to say that such devices are without value. Track-bound devices that exercise the arms, legs, and trunk simultaneously, such as stationary bicycles with movable arm levers or rowing machines, can accomplish a lot in a short time with respect to improving one's general fitness including aerobic capacity, strength, and, to some extent, flexibility. Such devices, especially the stationary cycle, take up relatively little space in the home and thus can be conveniently located for daily use, an important consideration as one attempts to develop lifelong habits. Many people complain that such track-bound activity is boring, and thus it would be well to vary the routine or to listen to music or news or watch television while exercising. In addition to alleviating boredom, adding variety to the routine may have a beneficial effect on balance, especially if the activities are weight bearing and involve single stance support, i.e., standing and balancing on one leg. In this regard, dynamic balance activities such as T'ai Chi have been shown to be of value.[2] Although it has not been proven, some types of dancing may be of value if they involve one-legged support. Figure 3 illustrates some T'ai Chi positions. Such activities are frequently carried

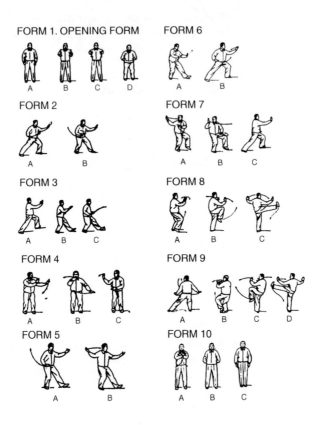

FIGURE 3   Ten forms of T'ai Chi, reduced from 108. These forms are meant to incorporate elements of movement limitation commonly depicted as part of the aging process. (From Wolf, S. L., Coogler, C. E., Green, R. C., and Xu, T., *Arch. Phys. Med. Rehabil.*, 78, 889, 1997. With permission.)

out in groups led by a T'ai Chi master. They are enjoyable and social and more likely to be continued for this reason.

TYPES OF EXERCISE FOR FITNESS AND BALANCE

The following types of activities are intended to be representative, not exhaustive. Each type of activity has advantages and disadvantages, and no one activity possesses all the advantages with no disadvantages. These activities may use equipment available in the home or may require highly specialized equipment generally found only in research laboratories or physical therapy clinics; alternatively, they may use no equipment but require the skill of an instructor, and thus may typically be done in groups.

Balance Training Devices

Some forms of balance training involve feedback devices generally available in therapy clinics or research laboratories. These usually involve a balance platform, which gives the trainee visual feedback of the position and changes in position of her center of gravity, depending upon the software used. The subject may be asked to adjust her posture to reposition her center of gravity to match a target. This has been shown in the Atlanta FICSIT study[2,16] to have only limited effectiveness in reducing falls. Furthermore, the lack of low cost availability makes this type of exercise inappropriate for a lifelong program.

T'ai Chi

T'ai Chi is an example of dynamic balance training. Steven Wolf and co-workers,[12] in the Atlanta FICSIT study describe T'ai Chi as incorporating 108 stances which could be and were reduced to 10 forms (Figure 3). The authors identified seven therapeutic elements in T'ai Chi including continuous movement, performed slowly; small to large degrees of motion; knee flexion and weight shifting; straight and extended head and trunk; combined rotation of head, trunk, and extremities; asymmetrical diagonal arm and leg movements about the waist; and unilateral weight bearing with constant shifting. It seems intuitive that these movements contribute importantly to the process of balance, i.e., correction for perturbations of the center of gravity as well as the limbs, head, and trunk. T'ai Chi is generally taught in groups, which may provide a pleasant social experience that reinforces the activity; however, it is appropriate for solo practice as well once the form is learned. It is apparent that any activity that is pleasurable is more likely to be continued as a lifelong pattern or life skill. The same would apply to aerobic dance. There may well be some expense associated with T'ai Chi or aerobic dance classes, but the expense might be minimized if one contacts a local senior center or YWCA.

Treadmill

Treadmills, found in many health clubs, have several advantages. They allow one to quantify and grade one's activity. Depending upon one's initial condition, treadmill activity may not only increase aerobic capacity but may increase lower limb strength as well. This is particularly true of older women who have been sedentary most of their lives. Treadmill training is not usually thought of as a strength training activity, but can be effective in this regard if one has not been accustomed to doing lower body weight training. There is a learning curve and a safety factor involved. Walking on a treadmill seems different initially from free walking. Fear and the learning process will initially prompt the user to grasp the safety rails. There will still be an aerobic benefit to such an activity, but balance training will be minimal. To be effective for improving balance, one should spend some of the treadmill time in walking without holding on to the rails. This should be done relatively early in the session before fatigue sets in, since it will predispose the user to stumble or trip and fall, which must be avoided at all costs. It is inappropriate for older women to run on a treadmill without holding on to the rails unless one has done this for a very long period of time and thus is only continuing a long-acquired skill.

RESISTANCE TRAINING

Muscle strength and power (force × velocity) are necessary for the corrective movements that allow maintenance of an erect posture and quick responses to perturbation. Therefore, increases in muscle strength may improve balance. This has been observed in intervention studies in both community-dwelling and institutionalized elders after strength training interventions of 8 to 52 weeks in duration. The responses in balance are variable, however, depending upon the baseline deficits in strength and balance that are present.

Although machine-based resistance training has been shown in some studies to improve balance modestly, the lack of standing postures in this mode of training probably limits the extent of balance improvements achievable. Another approach to this problem, therefore, is to use free weights (dumbbells and ankle weights) with which to train. Postures that emphasize one-legged standing (plantar flexion, hip flexion, hip extension, hip abduction, and knee flexion) and movement of the lower limb away from the center of mass may be particularly useful for the stresses they place on the balance system during strength training. In addition, these postures can be modified to gradually reduce upper limb support from holding onto a chair with two hands, one hand, one fingertip, no hands, and finally no hands with eyes closed. This gradual progression, if done under supervision, will safely and continuously increase the balance-enhancing potential of such resistive exercises without adding any more time, equipment, or routines to the exercise session itself.

Measurable improvements in gait quality (less gait variability, improved velocity and cadence, shorter stance phase, less double support time) after exercise interventions of any sort appear to be related to the robustness of the physiologic adaptation induced by the training program. Individuals with minimal physiologic adaptation (perhaps due to low intensity training or poor adherence) exhibit little if any improvements in gait or balance. Thus, adherence to general principles of exercise training as outlined in Chapter 2 are important for gait and balance outcomes just as they are for other domains.

BALANCE AND NUTRITIONAL STATUS

Nutrition is important in regard to balance and fall risk in several ways. One is the adequacy of protein, calcium, and vitamins to support the development and maintenance of muscle and bone and to prevent peripheral neuropathies. Peripheral neuropathies and even spinal deterioration associated with B_{12} deficiency will result in loss of proprioception, i.e., the ability to tell where one's limbs are in space, and secondary muscle weakness. Lack of iron, folic acid, and/or vitamin B_{12} will result in anemia, which makes exercise very difficult.

Another important reason for proper nutrition is the prevention of obesity, which has been associated with impairments of mobility. Although it may seem counterintuitive to suggest that obese persons are *mal*-nourished, such is the case. Improving the strength-to-weight ratio can occur by increasing the numerator, i.e., increasing strength, or decreasing the denominator, i.e., decreasing weight. Dietary restriction alone is not a good method for weight reduction since some protein, i.e., muscle, is always lost with weight loss due to dietary restriction alone. Only concurrent exercise allows weight reduction with preferential loss of fat, i.e., less loss of muscle protein.[17] Although some studies have shown that hypocaloric dieting in association with resistance training can result in actual increases in lean tissue, other studies have shown losses of lean tissue in this setting. Overall, the consensus of the literature at this point would be that exercise mitigates the adverse effects of dieting on body composition, but does not prevent them altogether.

At the other end of the clinical spectrum, Vellas and others have identified undernutrition as a risk factor for falling in the elderly in the Toulouse Aging Study. Undernutrition has been associated with muscle atrophy and poor balance, and these factors likely contribute to this elevated fall risk. In addition, low body mass index, muscle atrophy, low bone density, and musculoskeletal function abnormalities are associated with hip fracture risk in elderly men and women. This risk of hip fracture is due to a combination of factors that cause the fall itself (poor balance, muscle weakness) as well as factors that increase the likelihood of fracture (low bone density, minimal soft tissue padding over the greater trochanter) once a fall has occurred. Thus, attempts to identify and intervene in individuals who are undernourished are important for the prevention of injurious falls.

REFERENCES

1. Wagner, E. H., LaCroix, A. Z., Grothaus, L., Leveille, S. G., Hecht, J. A., Artz, K., Odle, K., and Buchner, D. M., Preventing disability and falls in older adults: a population-based randomized trial, *Am. J. Public Health,* 84(11), 1800–1806, 1994.
2. Province, M. A., Hadley, E. C., Hornbrook, M. C., Lipsitz, L. A., Miller, J. P., Mulrow, C. D., Ory, M. G., Sattin, R. W., Tinetti, M. E., and Wolf, S. L., The effects of exercise on falls in elderly patients: a preplanned meta-analysis of the FICSIT trials, *JAMA,* 273(17), 1341–1347, 1995.
3. Tinetti, M. E. and Speechley, M., Prevention of falls among the elderly, *N. Engl. J. Med.,* 320(16), 1055-1059, 1989.
4. Vellas B., Cayla F., Bocquet H. et al., Prospective study of restriction of activity in old people after falls, *Age Ageing,* 16(3), 189–193, 1987.
5. Buchner, D. M. and Wagner, E. H., Preventing frail health, *Clin. Geriatr. Med.,* 8(1), 1–17, 1992.
6. Buchner, D. M. and de Lateur, B. J., The importance of skeletal muscle strength to physical function in older adults, *Ann. Behav. Med.,* 13, 91–8, 1991.
7. Blake, A. J., Morgan, K., Bendall, M. J., Dallosso, H., Ebrahim, S. B. J., Arie, T. H. D., Fentem, P. H., and Bassey, E. J., Falls by elderly people at home: prevalence and associated factors, *Age Ageing,* 17, 365–7, 1988.
8. Smith, R. W., Falls among older persons: a public health perspective, *Ann. Rev. Publ. Health,* 13, 489–50, 1992.
9. Overstall, P. W., Exton-Smith, A. N., Imms, F. J., and Johnson, A. L., Falls in the elderly related to postural in balance, *Brit. Med. J.,* 1, 261–264, 1977.

10. Buchner, D. M., Price, R., de Lateur, B. J., Cress, M. E., and Wagner, E. H., Is leg weakness a cause of poor balance? *Gerontologist*, 32 (special issue III), 78 (abstract), 1992.
11. Podsiadlo, D. and Richardson, S., The timed "Up & Go": A test of basic functional mobility for frail elderly persons, *J. Am. Geriatr. Soc.*, 39(2), 142–148, 1991.
12. Lehmann, J. F., Boswell, S., Price, R., Burleigh, A., de Lateur, B. J., Jaffe, K., and Hertling, D., Quantitative evaluation of sway as an indicator of functional balance in post-traumatic brain injury, *Arch. Phys. Med. Rehabil.*, 71(12), 955–962, 1990.
13. Peszczynski, M., Prevention of falls in the hemiplegic patient, *Geriatrics*, 11, 306–311, 1956.
14. Nashner, L. M., A model describing vestibular detection of body sway motion, *ACTA Otolaryngologica*, 72(6), 429–436, 1971.
15. Hellebrandt, F. A. and Houtz, S. J., Mechanisms of muscle training in man: experimental demonstration of the overload principle, *Phys. Ther. Rev.*, 36, 371–8, 1956.
16. Wolf, S. L., Kutner, N. G., Green, R. C., and McNeely, E., The Atlanta FICSIT study: two exercise interventions to reduce frailty in elders, *J. Am. Geriatr. Soc.*, 41(3), 329–332, 1993.
17. Gwinup, G., Weight loss without dietary restriction: efficacy of different forms of aerobic exercise, *Am. J. Sports Med.*, 15, 275–7, 1987.

14 Cardiovascular Disease and Hypertension

Maria A. Fiatarone Singh and Jeanne Y. Wei

CONTENTS

SCOPE OF THE PROBLEM

Heart disease is the leading cause of death and a common cause of morbidity in the United States. According to NHANES III data, approximately 14 million Americans have coronary heart disease (CHD) based on interviews in 1988–1994, about 4 million have cerebrovascular disease, and about 2 million have peripheral vascular disease (Adams, 1995). Annually, about 1.1 million people in the United States experience a heart attack (750,000 of them are over the age of 65), and about 500,000 individuals die from CHD. The annual economic burden of cardiovascular disease in the United States is staggering, in excess of $135 billion. Approximately $100 of the $135 billion is expended for coronary artery disease and its prevention and treatment.

Patients with established CHD, clinical atherosclerotic disease of the aorta or peripheral arteries, or clinical cerebrovascular disease are at five- to seven-fold higher risk for subsequent myocardial infarction or CHD death than the general population (National Heart Lung and Blood Institute, 1996; Criqui, 1992; Pekkanen, 1990; Salonen, 1991). It is particularly important to focus within this high-risk patient group on women, African Americans, and the elderly, as these sub-populations have longer reported delays in seeking care in response to acute myocardial infarction symptoms. Such delays are often lethal, as the advent of effective thrombolytic therapy now clearly ties survival to the lag time between symptom onset and specific treatment (Kuller, 1975; Dracup, 1995).

GENERAL TRENDS

Death rates from CHD rose throughout the twentieth century to their peak in about 1960, and have been declining in all demographic groups, although at different rates, since that time. They began to decline earlier in women (1950s) than in men (1960s). Coronary heart disease deaths have fallen from 135 per 100,000 in 1985 to 108 per 100,000 in 1995 (20% decline), and are currently close to the *Healthy People 2000* target that was set by the Department of Health and Human Services at 104 per 100,000.

While the age-adjusted death rate for CHD continues to decline each year, declines in the unadjusted death rate and in absolute numbers of deaths have slowed because of an increase in the numbers of older Americans, who have higher rates of CHD than younger cohorts. This trend is expected to continue, particularly as the population over the age of 85, the fastest growing demographic group, continues to expand. This is an overwhelmingly female population, meaning that CHD in the very old is primarily a disease of women.

AFRICAN AMERICANS

Since 1915, the heart disease mortality rate has been consistently higher in the African American population than in the white population. The rates of decline are currently steeper in white males than in African-American males and the death rate is now substantially higher in African Americans than in whites. In 1995, the age-adjusted death rate for heart disease was 42% higher in African American males than in white males, and 65% higher in African American females than white females.

Although remaining substantially higher than in whites, coronary heart disease among African Americans has also declined during the past decade (by about 12%) from 168 per 100,000 in 1985 to 147 per 100,000 in 1995. Between 1980 and 1995, the percentage declines were least for African-American females, among all race-gender groups. Mortality from coronary heart disease remains far above the target of 115 deaths per 100,000 for the year 2000. Thus African Americans, and in particular women, should be targeted for prevention, access to care, physician education, and treatment strategies if these figures are to improve in the next several decades.

Older Adults

Although there have been recent declines in death due to cardiovascular disease, heart disease continues to be the single most common cause of death in older individuals, accounting for a major portion of the health care costs in this age group (Wei, 1992). Clinically evident heart disease is present in nearly 50% of older persons. Each year over half of all individuals aged 75 years and older who go to a doctor's office see a physician for diagnosis or treatment of coronary artery disease. Heart disease is the number one cause of mortality in women over the age of 65, as it is of older men. Death due to heart disease rises from 41% of all deaths in those aged 65 to 74 years to 48% in the over-85 group. Between 80 to 85% of the heart disease-related deaths are due to coronary artery disease. Unfortunately, much of the evidence for the protective effect and therapeutic benefits of exercise and other lifestyle modifications such as diet and smoking cessation has been derived from studies in middle-aged and older men, and there is a great need for further investigation in this area in the high risk population of older women.

The annual incidence of congestive heart failure rises nearly exponentially with increasing age beginning in the fifth decade, doubling every ten years in men and every seven in women (Wei, 1995; Odiet, 1996). Older women and men develop congestive heart failure (CHF) six times more commonly than younger persons. Congestive heart failure without coronary artery disease rises by nearly three-fold from age 65 to 85, to a prevalence of approximately 16% in those aged 85 years and older. The prevalence of heart failure rises more steeply with age in women, doubling at one and one-half times the rate in men.

Postmenopausal Women

Heart disease is the leading cause of death in postmenopausal women. More than 240,000 women die of heart attacks each year, which is approximately one-half of the 500,000 coronary deaths recorded annually (American Heart Association, 1995). There is a tendency still to think of coronary heart disease as a male disorder, however, which unfortunately may result in delays in diagnosis and undertreatment of this condition and its risk factors in older women. Much of the epidemiological evidence of risk factor reduction and even treatment benefits have been gathered in primarily male populations, and there is a need for more research in women to identify gender-specific risk factor weighting and responsiveness to current therapies.

Among the draft objectives to be finalized as part of *Healthy People 2010* in relation to heart disease and stroke (Department of Health and Human Services, 1999) are several goals related specifically to women as shown below in the 16 focus areas of this forthcoming report:

1. Coronary heart disease deaths
2. Female deaths after heart attack
3. Knowledge of early warning symptoms of heart attack
4. Provider counseling about early warning symptoms of heart attack
5. Females aware of heart disease as the leading cause of death
6. High blood pressure
7. Controlled high blood pressure
8. Action to help control blood pressure
9. Blood pressure monitoring
10. Serum cholesterol levels
11. Blood cholesterol levels
12. Blood cholesterol screening
13. Treatment of LDL cholesterol
14. Stroke deaths
15. Knowledge of early warning symptoms of stroke
16. Provider counseling about early warning symptoms of stroke

One of the goals proposed for the year 2010 by the Department of Health and Human Services is to reduce coronary heart disease deaths to no more than 51 per 100,000 population, which is a large reduction, particularly for older African Americans. The overall goal is to "enhance the cardiovascular health and quality of life of all Americans through improvement of medical management, prevention and control of risk factors, and promotion of healthy lifestyle behaviors." In light of this policy focus for the nation, this chapter provides an overview of the ways in which prevention and treatment of these conditions can be optimized in older women, particularly by a multidisciplinary approach of the health care team.

AGE-RELATED CHANGES IN THE HEART

Until relatively recently, it was thought that congestive heart failure in older persons developed as a result of an impairment in the heart's contractile capacity. It is now established that impaired heart muscle relaxation (diastolic dysfunction), not impaired heart muscle contraction (systolic dysfunction), is the major cause of congestive heart failure in the older person, especially in women over the age of 75 years. This is because with advancing age, the heart can contract as forcefully, but it takes longer for the older heart to relax. The heart muscle is able to pump blood as well in the old as it does in the young, but it is not able to relax as rapidly, so the heart chamber is not able to fill as efficiently in the old. This is the major change in cardiac function documented at rest in normal older persons. It has been shown that diastolic filling can be improved both at rest and during exercise after a period of endurance training in young and older healthy men. Therefore, as with many other physiologic changes in cardiovascular and other systems, there is some doubt as to whether this is a true biological change of aging, or yet another manifestation of disuse or underuse of the system. Augmentation of diastolic function after training has not yet been observed in older women, and it is not yet known if they retain this same capacity for improvement in diastolic relaxation.

Contrary to long-prevailing thought, more oxygen and energy are required for relaxation than for contraction. It is therefore not surprising that the development of relaxation abnormalities often precedes that of contraction abnormalities. When the left ventricle is not able to relax completely, it will not be able to contract as strongly during the next cycle. The rate of filling of the heart also declines with age, so that by age 70, it is only about half of that which it was at age 30. In addition, ventricular filling becomes increasingly dependent upon the atrial contraction with advancing age, which may supply one-half of the total volume of blood filling the ventricle.

Normally, when the heart rate rises, diastole becomes shortened. Thus, the problem of prolonged diastole (decreased rate of filling) becomes further exacerbated during tachycardia (e.g., fever, dehydration, illness, physical activity). In young persons, a rapid heart rate is well tolerated. In older people, however, even minor exertion can lead to shortness of breath and fatigue. About 50% of older persons experience congestive heart failure that is caused primarily by impaired relaxation, a condition known as diastolic dysfunction. Because the heart in an older person has reduced early diastolic ventricular filling and depends so heavily upon the atrial contraction during late diastole for over half of the ventricular filling, a shortened diastole due to increased heart rate may compromise cardiac output substantially more in the older compared to the younger person. Similarly, a loss of regular atrial contraction, such as occurs during atrial fibrillation or atrial tachycardia, could also reduce cardiac output much more in the older than the younger heart.

There are a number of reasons why diastolic dysfunction develops in older adults. First, the blood vessels become stiffer with age, so the older heart is required to pump against a greater systemic resistance, or afterload. This consequently places a greater workload on the heart, which in turn causes progressive cell loss of heart myocytes and compensatory hypertrophy in the remaining heart muscle cells. The myocyte loss is associated with increased cardiac connective tissue formation and collagen deposition. There is also increased cross-linking of collagen fibers as well as calcium and amyloid protein deposition between cells within the heart wall. The increased size of heart cells together with the increased connective tissue in which the heart cells are embedded make the heart muscle stiffer and therefore more resistant to changes in shape. More energy is then required for the stiffer heart to dilate.

In addition to the above structural changes, intracellular metabolic alterations characterized by impaired calcium handling and decreased energy turnover also cause prolongation of relaxation time. Cardiac relaxation depends on the dissociation of ionized calcium from the myofilaments and the uptake of the ionized calcium from the cytoplasm into storage sites. The rate of calcium uptake by the storage sites slows with age. As a consequence, there is a decreased rate as well as capacity for intracellular ionized calcium handling. Finally, the decrease in catecholamine content in the heart, the decline in capillary density and reserve blood supply to the heart, and the reduced blood oxygen content all further serve to make the heart more vulnerable to stress-induced decompensation.

What causes the heart to lose some of its ability to adapt? The answer may lie partly in the heart muscle's DNA and in the regulation of gene expression. The induction of certain immediate early genes (*c-fos, c-jun*) in the heart is reduced with age. Because the myocytes do not usually undergo proliferation after early postnatal life, they are lifelong in their terminally differentiated state. As such, each heart myocyte cell is a living record of cumulative events that have occurred to the individual in general and the heart in particular. If some inefficient cellular repair mechanism occurs as a result of the age-associated accumulation of changes due to exposure to a variety of chemicals, that problem could eventually become physiologically significant.

It is also possible that various signaling pathways from the cell surface to the nucleus might be altered with age, and might contribute to the observed heart muscle changes. The heart cells' mitochondria—intracellular bodies that aid in energy synthesis—are more susceptible to oxidative damage than other parts of the cell. Research is being done to see how signaling changes or damage to mitochondria might contribute to the development of age-related heart disease.

AGE-RELATED CHANGES IN THE VASCULATURE

The most important finding here is that arteries tend to stiffen with age. The intimal and medial layers of the walls of the senescent arteries tend to thicken throughout the body. There are increasing accumulations of scar tissue, tightly cross-linked collagen, and calcium deposits within the arterial walls. In these media, the smooth muscle cells tend to undergo hypertrophy and proliferation, adding substantially to the vessel wall thickness and rigidity.

The age-associated arterial stiffening has important physiologic implications. The central blood vessels (aorta and large arteries) in younger adults are highly elastic, a property that confers efficient pumping advantages. These large central arteries in young adults distend to accept a bolus of blood from the contracting ventricle (converting kinetic to potential energy) and then the arteries locally recoil during diastole (converting potential to kinetic energy); blood is thereby moved (pulsated) by the central arteries into the periphery. In contrast, arteries lose their elasticity with age. The heart in the older person must therefore supply all the force that is needed to push blood into the periphery. In addition, more work is required to push blood through the stiff, inelastic, nondistensible arteries. With these typical age-changes in the arteries, arterial pulse pressures widen. Systolic pressures increase as blood traverses the rigid arteries and diastolic pressures fall since the rigid senescent arteries lack the elasticity needed to maintain the intravascular pressures during diastole. These changes result in the age-associated increase in systolic blood pressure that is so commonly observed. The increased arterial rigidity is further compounded by the tendency of pulse waves to reflect from the rigid peripheral arterial walls and bifurcations back into the central vasculature. The central arterial impedance rises disproportionately to the increases in peripheral arterial pressure. Even normotensive elderly adults have significantly elevated aortic impedance, resulting in substantial increases in the physiologic burden on the heart. Consequently, left ventricular hypertrophy often develops in older persons, even those with normal blood pressures.

There is also an altered morphology of the vascular endothelium, in addition to changes in media. The endothelial cells in young adults are homogeneous in size and alignment. In contrast, endothelium in older persons is progressively more heterogeneous in size, shape, and orientation. Consequently, the blood flow becomes less laminar and more turbulent. The vessel walls become more vulnerable to subendothelial dissection and lipid deposition, and atherosclerosis becomes accelerated.

Aging is also associated with intrinsically altered endothelial cell-mediated vasodilatory functional characteristics. The endothelium usually plays a key role in the ability of the vessels to respond to physiologic demands. In young adults, endothelial cell-mediated dilation of the large arteries during physiologic stresses (such as exercise) results in important afterload reduction, facilitating the needed increases in cardiac output and ejection fraction. Similarly, coronary artery dilation increases blood flow in response to higher cardiac work demands. Such endothelial cell-mediated vasodilation is significantly diminished in older persons, in both the large central arteries as well as coronary arteries. The associated susceptibility to myocardial ischemia due to insufficient afterload reduction and insufficient vasodilation is therefore increased in older adults. As with diastolic dysfunction of the myocardium, there is some evidence that habitual cardiovascular exercise can mitigate arterial stiffening with age, suggesting again that disuse interacts with chronological aging to exacerbate these "typical" findings. Comparing 63-year-old trained, endurance athletes to age-matched sedentary men, investigators have demonstrated a larger peak cardiac index in the athletes that was mediated entirely by a greater stroke volume index, as peak heart rates were virtually identical. At exhaustion, athletes demonstrated a lower systemic vascular resistance than controls, despite a higher value at rest. Athletes also showed a greater reduction in systemic vascular resistance from rest to maximal workload than untrained controls. Whether preservation of "youthful" systemic vascular resistance profiles occurs in highly trained women or with lower levels of physical activity remains to be demonstrated.

Finally, compensatory blood pressure and heart rate response mechanisms in the elderly are often delayed or insufficient. These changes explain why fainting is common in older women and men during normal daily activities such as arising from a bed, eating a meal, or going to the toilet. These changes also explain why modest decreases in intravascular fluid volume, such as that which occur during heat prostration, viral illness, diarrhea, or decreased oral fluid intake, can often result in large drops in blood pressure that can cause falls or fainting in the elderly.

HYPERTENSION AND BLOOD PRESSURE REGULATION

Approximately 50 million adult Americans have high blood pressure. There are both age-related and racial influences on the prevalence of hypertension. The prevalence of hypertension is nearly 40% greater in African Americans than in whites (an estimated 6.4 million African Americans have the disease), and its long-term effects are more frequent and severe. Hypertension is the major cardiovascular disease of older persons. The prevalence of hypertension (defined as systolic pressure greater than 160 mmHg and diastolic pressure greater than 95 mmHg) rises with age. Data from NHANES III show that in all Americans, aged 60 and over, elevated blood pressure is found in 60% of non-Hispanic whites, 71% of non-Hispanic African Americans, and 61% of Mexican Americans (Department of Health and Human Services, 1999).

Hypertension is a major risk factor not only for coronary heart disease, but also for stroke, congestive heart failure, renal failure, and peripheral vascular disease. Systolic pressure is better than diastolic pressure as a predictor of heart attack and stroke. Isolated systolic hypertension is the most common form of hypertension in older Americans.

Awareness, treatment, and control of hypertension have increased in the past decade in response to major public health campaigns and many new drug choices. However, good control is achieved in only a minority of patients with chronic hypertension. For example, the number of persons with high blood pressure controlled to below 140/90 mmHg increased from 10% in the NHANES II to 29% in the NHANES III survey. Minority groups and the elderly have the highest prevalence of undetected and uncontrolled hypertension and its sequelae such as end-stage renal disease, blindness, stroke, and congestive heart failure.

Concerted efforts to prevent and control high blood pressure will therefore not only reduce heart disease and stroke rates, but also will reduce the incidence of end-stage renal disease and heart failure. Fortunately, there are a number of antihypertensive medications that have been shown to be effective in reducing the complications of hypertension. In addition, there are also available a number of non-pharmacologic therapies that have been demonstrated to be effective for this condition. Engaging in healthy lifestyle behaviors offers the potential for preventing hypertension, has been shown to be effective in lowering blood pressure, and can reduce other cardiovascular risk factors at little cost and with minimum risk. Patients should be encouraged to adopt lifestyle modifications such as losing weight, if overweight; eating a diet rich in fruits and vegetables and any products lower in fat, saturated fat, cholesterol, and sodium; drinking alcohol in moderation if they drink alcohol; and increasing their regular physical activity participation rates.

Goals for hypertension that have been proposed for the U.S. adult population for year 2010 include

1. a reduction of hypertension prevalence from current levels (e.g., 23% in whites, 34% in African American women), to 16% overall;
2. an increase of hypertension control from current levels (e.g., 24% overall, 19% in males, 17% in Mexican American women) to at least 50% of the hypertensive population;
3. an increase of those taking lifestyle and medical action to control their blood pressure from 71 to 95% of the hypertensive population.

HYPERLIPIDEMIA

Hyperlipidemia is discussed more fully in Chapter 7, but will be reviewed briefly here because of its role as a risk factor for cardiovascular and cerebrovascular disease. Mean cholesterol levels and the prevalence of high blood cholesterol have been decreasing in the United States over the past 30 years. From 1960 to 1994, many changes in nutritional, lifestyle, and medical therapeutic factors may have affected blood cholesterol. This is especially true for the 1980s, a period when extensive nutrition education, health promotion and disease prevention activities, decreased consumption of high-fat foods, increased use of lipid-lowering diets and drugs, increased use of postmenopausal estrogen replacement therapy, and development of lower-dose oral contraceptives could have contributed to reductions in blood cholesterol levels. Despite these reductions, it is well understood that increased blood cholesterol levels, especially high LDL-cholesterol, increase the risk for CHD. Conversely, lowering total cholesterol and LDL-cholesterol levels reduces CHD risk. Thus, two approaches have been taken to lower blood cholesterol levels in the American population. One is a clinical approach that identifies individuals at high risk who need intensive intervention efforts. The second is a public health approach that aims to shift the distribution of cholesterol levels in the entire population to a lower range through dietary change. The two approaches are complementary and together represent a coordinated strategy for reducing coronary risk.

Treatment of elevated LDL-cholesterol in patients with prior CHD is important since a substantial proportion of new CHD events occur in patients with established CHD, and it appears that many CHD patients, both men and women, may not be getting the aggressive cholesterol-lowering therapy that is warranted. Elevated blood cholesterol levels increase the risk of CHD in women, and this is primarily a problem of the postmenopausal years. Despite the magnitude of heart disease in women and the conclusive evidence that women with CHD will benefit from cholesterol lowering, the proportion of women with heart disease who are meeting the LDL treatment goals published by the National Cholesterol Education Program (NCEP) in 1993 is low. This is also the case for men with CHD. The incorporation of these treatment recommendations into general practice must be increased through further dissemination of the treatment recommendations and by additional efforts at educating the medical community and patients about their implementation.

WHY ARE HEART DISEASE AND HYPERTENSION SO COMMON IN OLDER PERSONS?

To better understand why heart disease and hypertension as well as their complications are so common among older adults, two interrelated concepts will be reviewed: (1) age-related changes in circulation and the heart, and (2) susceptibility to ischemia.

TYPICAL AGE-ASSOCIATED CARDIOVASCULAR CHANGES

With typical aging, a number of cardiovascular changes are commonly observed. Changes occur in the vasculature, the heart, and systemic neurohormonal activity (see below). These changes tend to compound one another so as to reduce overall cardiovascular reserve and lower the threshold of vulnerability.

The combined effects of arterial wall and heart muscle stiffening and impaired intracellular calcium handling are substantial. In young adults, most ventricular diastolic filling occurs early in diastole: blood is literally "pulled" from the atria into the ventricular chambers as the ventricles relax and dilate. In an older person, however, ventricular relaxation usually occurs much more slowly and sometimes incompletely, while at the same time the ventricles become stiff and nondistensible as a result of hypertrophy and fibrosis.

The number of pacemaker cells in the heart decreases progressively with age while the amount of fibrosis around the heart's sinus node and conduction pathways progressively increases. As a result, older persons are more susceptible to atrial and ventricular arrhythmias. Progressive atrial dilatation and left ventricular hypertrophy with aging further increase the propensity for these arrhythmias. The incidence of atrial fibrillation rises significantly with advancing age.

Neurohormonal changes include alterations in adrenergic activity which tend to affect cardiovascular performance among older persons. There is a progressive reduction in beta adrenergic responsiveness (both agonistic and antagonistic) with age. Manifestations include reduced maximal heart rate, diminished inotropy, increased maximal end-systolic volumes, and attenuated adrenergically mediated vasodilation. One implication of such neurohormonal changes is that the peripheral vascular tone may be slightly higher in older persons. This amplifies the physiologic burden on the heart of the older person, which is already forced to cope with stiffened arteries and elevated central vascular impedance. The age-associated adrenergic changes also tend to lower maximal cardiac output in older persons, since maximum heart rates decline and minimal end-systolic volumes rise, resulting in lesser increases of heart rate and stroke volume during adrenergic stimulation. As mentioned in Chapter 1, it is possible to restore some of the ability to augment the stroke volume ejection fraction during exercise in older men after aerobic training, whereas the reduction in maximal heart rate is not modifiable.

It is clear that even with a history of good health and/or no cardiovascular risk factors, aging itself represents a risk for cardiovascular disease. There appears to be a continuum between typical aging and the development of disease that becomes more difficult to distinguish as one reaches advanced age. The relatively sedentary lifestyle of many older persons and lifelong dietary habits (including high sodium and fat intake) typical of Western societies may further exacerbate the age-related changes that increase the risk of heart disease and stroke.

SUSCEPTIBILITY TO ISCHEMIA

Ischemia means a relative lack of blood supply for the metabolic needs of the cells. The combined effects of blood vessel and heart muscle changes render the older person particularly susceptible to the development of heart ischemia. In contrast to necrosis, which implies cell death, ischemia can be reversible if the ischemic cells receive a prompt return of the needed blood supply.

Heart ischemia is often conceptualized as an arterial blockage that prevents adequate blood flow to meet normal cellular needs. However, ischemia can also occur when metabolic demands are higher than what the maximum blood flow through the open arteries can meet. Age-related vascular and myocardial changes predispose the older person to the development of such insufficient oxygenation, or supply-demand mismatch. In older persons the stiff coronary arteries have limited dilating capacity, reducing their potential for increased coronary flow during periods of increased metabolic demand. In addition, the aorta and major arteries stiffen with age, which translates into higher afterload pressures. Consequently, cardiac metabolic requirements for adequate pumping tend to be substantially increased with age.

The age-related changes in the vascular endothelial cells further predispose the older person to a high incidence as well as acceleration of atherosclerosis. Again, a continuum may be seen between typical aging and coronary heart disease: coronary arteries in older persons are more prone to develop blockages (stenotic lesions). In addition to increased metabolic demand with age and the susceptibility to develop demand ischemia, maximum blood supply to the older person's heart is also commonly reduced, further exacerbating the supply–demand mismatch.

Ischemia in hearts of older persons may be further increased because the heart muscle is commonly hypertrophied. Perfusion of blood from the outside heart wall, or epicardial coronary arteries, to the inner myocardial regions, or endocardium, depends on the blood traversing the thickness of the heart wall during diastole. As the heart myocytes undergo hypertrophy in response to increased afterload pressures, blood must travel a greater distance through the thickened heart muscle to reach the endocardium. Ventricular hypertrophy in young adults is usually associated with cardiac microvasculature proliferation that serves to maintain perfusion through the thickened walls. In older persons, however, there is much less microcapillary proliferation around the hypertrophied myocytes. This leaves the endocardial myocytes in older persons more vulnerable to the development of inadequate perfusion, i.e., ischemia.

Another factor that predisposes the older heart to develop ischemia is the prolonged relaxation time. Perfusion of the heart usually occurs during diastole, when the heart muscle is sufficiently relaxed for blood to travel through the heart muscle. Age-related delay in myocellular relaxation and increased myocardial stiffness interfere with such diastolic perfusion. Tachyarrhythmias can further exacerbate relative ventricular underperfusion. This is because as heart rate increases, the shortened R–R interval causes the diastolic interval to be shortened disproportionately; this could result in incomplete ventricular relaxation and insufficient diastolic time for adequate perfusion.

Ischemia of the heart due to insufficient perfusion is often associated with further impaired relaxation, because it is energy dependent, and that creates a vicious cycle. Subsequent perfusion of blood across the heart wall is hampered by the already incomplete heart relaxation. Ischemia progressively worsens, with escalating myocardial stiffness. Furthermore, the acutely stiffened ischemic heart not only exacerbates diastolic perfusion abnormalities, but it also causes the heart to become evermore resistant to diastolic filling. Blood cannot enter a stiff and nondistensible chamber. Cardiac output further deteriorates as there is insufficient blood in the ventricular chamber to pump forward to the periphery, and acute hemodynamic compromise ensues.

DISEASES OF THE HEART

CORONARY ARTERY DISEASE

Coronary atherosclerosis progresses in severity with advancing age, typically with the disease in men leading that in women by about 15 years until after menopause. After menopause, the disease accelerates in women and the severity becomes nearly equal for women and men after age 75 years. Symptoms of angina pectoris (chest discomfort, palpitations) exist in about 10% of the elderly and are often the first clinical sign of coronary artery disease.

CONGENITAL HEART DISEASE

A number of heart abnormalities that occur as birth defects do not always preclude survival to old age. The classic diagnostic clinical findings associated with congenital heart lesions may be obscured or confounded in older patients by concomitant age-related changes or other diseases. Valvular disease affecting the very old are often initially mild congenital lesions, lesions that develop in late life due to age-related processes, or a combination of these factors. As primary care internists and cardiologists become increasingly aware of the safety, usefulness, and availability of recently developed noninvasive cardiac imaging techniques, the identification of congenital heart disease will probably increase in frequency in older patients.

CARDIOMYOPATHY

Cardiomyopathy is defined as a diffuse or generalized disorder of the heart without a clear underlying etiology. Patients who are so diagnosed have idiopathic or primary involvement of the heart muscle. However, valvular, hypertensive, or coronary artery disease often coexists with primary cardiomyopathy. There are three main types of ventricular dysfunction (which may overlap). Dilated or congestive cardiomyopathy is characterized by impaired systolic function with dilatation (sometimes mild) of the heart chambers and increased muscle mass without a significant increase in wall thickness. Hypertrophic cardiomyopathy is characterized by a normal or small left ventricular chamber size, increased wall thickness, hyperdynamic systolic ejection, and impaired diastolic filling. In restrictive infiltrative cardiomyopathy, the heart muscle shows increased stiffness secondary to infiltrative pathology; systolic function is impaired and the atria become dilated in the late stages.

CONGESTIVE HEART FAILURE

Congestive heart failure (CHF) is the only cardiac diagnosis which is continuing to increase in prevalence the United States, due to the prolonged survival of those with hypertension and ischemic heart disease, as well as improved average lifespan of the population. From 1979 to 1995, heart failure deaths increased 115.7%. CHF is the most common cause for acute hospitalization in the elderly (present in 30% of admissions in this age group), and accounts for over 40% of all deaths over the age of 65. In people diagnosed with heart failure, sudden cardiac death occurs at 6 to 9 times the rate seen among the general population. The clinical hallmark of the disease is exercise intolerance, manifested as fatigue and dyspnea during increasingly minimal activities.

CHF may result from compromise of either contraction (systolic) or relaxation (diastolic) function or both, resulting in elevated ventricular end-diastolic pressures. Congestion of blood vessels in the lungs or other parts of the body and the organs they drain are the associated features. Between 50 and 60% of older persons with congestive heart failure have normal or only slightly reduced contraction function. Those older persons with impaired relaxation (diastolic) function who are erroneously treated for systolic heart failure with high doses of certain medications such as digitalis and diuretics may experience further compromise. It is important, therefore, to be aware of this potential problem and to plan the appropriate therapy and dosage with care.

While coronary artery disease is common in older persons with congestive heart failure, up to one half of older persons dying of congestive heart failure have been found at autopsy to have no significant coronary artery disease. Therefore, congestive heart failure should not be equated with coronary artery disease.

Hypertension is a common cause of congestive heart failure among older persons as systolic function usually deteriorates in end-stage hypertensive cardiomyopathy. Other frequent causes of systolic impairment in older persons include valvular heart disease, diabetes mellitus, other cardiomyopathies, and thyroid disease.

When the systolic performance of the heart deteriorates in older persons, congestive heart failure symptoms may develop slowly. Gradually worsening exercise tolerance and weakness occur from reduced cardiac output and diminished peripheral muscle function. The decreased peripheral muscle function in most elderly heart failure patients tends to be exacerbated by the typically sedentary lifestyles of most older adults as well as the peripheral muscle deconditioning with which sedentary lifestyles are associated. Progressive peripheral fluid accumulation and hypoxia are also common congestive heart failure sequelae among older adults.

It is important to remember that heart disease rarely occurs in isolation among older adults. A series of age-related changes in other vital organs add to the vulnerability of the elderly to develop heart failure. The aging kidney, for example, has fewer nephrons, reduced renal blood flow, and decreased glomerular filtration. Therefore, older adults are less able to mobilize excess intravascular or extravascular fluid, and this further exacerbates their susceptibility to the development of congestive heart failure.

The degree of exercise intolerance in CHF correlates strongly with both mortality and quality of life (Wilson, 1995), and yet current medical therapies often fail to specifically address many of the potential mechanisms which underlie these symptoms. Mounting evidence exists that peripheral skeletal muscle abnormalities figure prominently in the exercise intolerance associated with CHF, while central hemodynamic parameters such as ejection fraction are far less predictive of clinical symptoms. These peripheral abnormalities include a myopathy characterized by preferential loss and atrophy of Type I (slow, oxidative) fibers, decreased oxidative enzyme capacity and mitochondrial volume density, early activation of glycolytic pathways of ATP generation during work, and reduced muscle endurance, strength, power, and overall exercise tolerance. The selective loss of oxidative fibers distinguishes this condition from the Type II fiber selectivity common to aging and disuse syndromes, and suggests that a different pathogenetic mechanism may be operative. CHF is associated with chronic elevations of cytokines, including tumor necrosis factor, interleukin-1 and -6. These cytokines, which are known to cause muscle wasting and vasocontriction, are thought to play a major role in the development of the peripheral myopathy of CHF.

Hypertension, diabetes mellitus, and coronary artery disease are common disease states among the elderly that are associated with increased risk for heart attack, congestive heart failure, and stroke. Some researchers now describe such disease states as advanced points in the continuum of normal aging, which leave the older person's heart ever-more susceptible to failure. Similarly, thyroid disease, infections, and valvular heart disease are common conditions among older persons that increase the risk for congestive heart failure.

DISEASE PREVENTION OF HEART ATTACK, CONGESTIVE HEART FAILURE, AND STROKE

GENERAL CONSIDERATIONS

One challenge for geriatrics and cardiovascular research is to differentiate the irreversible changes of aging from those that are modifiable and preventable. Hypertension and resultant heart hypertrophy can be avoided and perhaps partly reversed in many cases, by appropriate exercise, lifestyle and dietary changes, as well as medication. Likewise, coronary artery disease can also be modified and/or partly reversed by efforts at exercise, diet, and cholesterol lowering in early and mid adulthood. Some of the changes so commonly seen with aging that predispose the older person to the development of heart attack, congestive heart failure, or stroke may be delayed and/or avoided by a healthy lifestyle that begins when a person is still relatively young.

Disorders of the heart increase in prevalence, morbidity, and mortality with advancing age. As more of the older population continue to survive to older ages, our efforts at improving the prevention and treatment of heart disease in the elderly become increasingly important. Education programs in health promotion and disease prevention will be continually more critical to these goals. Increased physical activity and increased dietary intake of fruits and vegetables together with cessation of smoking and decreased dietary intake of fat, excess calories, sugar, sodium, and alcohol are vitally important to promoting healthful aging in older persons.

As a preventive maneuver, anti-hypertensive treatment reduces the major risk factor for heart disease and stroke in the elderly, two of the three most frequent causes of death and major contributors to morbidity in older adults. Aside from hypertension, other preventive measures are directed toward the other major alterable risk factors for cardiovascular and cerebrovascular disease, when present: smoking and high blood cholesterol. In addition, increased physical activity, reduction of weight and of sodium, fat, and alcohol intake, as well as stress management are essential.

Recent clinical trials of anti-hypertensive medication treatment in older adults suggest that appropriate treatment of hypertension likely lowers the risk of developing left ventricular hypertrophy, congestive heart failure, acute myocardial infarction, and stroke. Medications that have been successfully used in these studies include a diuretic (chlorthalidone or other), a central adrenergic inhibitor (alpha-methyldopa), beta blockers (propranolol, metroprolol or atenolol), calcium channel blockers (diltiazem, verapamil, nifedipine, or telodipine), and angiotensin converting enzyme (ACE) inhibitors (captopril, enalapril, lisinopril).

There are many anti-hypertensive agents that are effective in reducing blood pressure. The choice of medication often involves selecting the agent with the least risk of side effects for a particular patient. For example, in a diabetic patient, one may wish to avoid masking the adrenergic signs and symptoms of hypoglycemia, making a beta blocker such as propranolol a second choice in that case. In choosing to use a calcium channel blocker, care should be exercised to avoid orthostatic hypertension, a side effect to which age-related changes in baroreceptor sensitivity may predispose older adults. In an older hypertensive patient whose electrocardiogram shows no significant conduction defects and who is not in severe congestive heart failure, diltiazem might be a reasonable choice among the calcium channel-blocking agents.

Chemoprophylaxis to prevent ischemic heart disease and stroke is another consideration. Advanced age (over 75 years), female gender, and hypertension are indications for primary prevention with aspirin or other antiplatelet medication such as ticlopidine. Anticoagulation with warfarin is indicated if there is left ventricular dysfunction, history of a prior stroke or atrial fibrillation. If on examination the patient had a carotid bruit, even if there were no symptoms, she/he would likely benefit from further evaluation of the carotid lesion; surgical therapy would be indicated if the carotid stenosis were shown to be 60% or greater.

Diet and exercise are also very important for cardiovascular disease prevention. Administration of exogenous estrogen may be important for preventing coronary artery disease as well as osteoporosis and hip fracture. Before deciding about estrogen therapy, careful inquiry should be made about potential contraindications to estrogen replacement such as breast cancer and/or a family history of breast cancer or endometrial cancer. Likewise, one should be informed about the possible risks of endometrial cancer (low absolute risk), breast cancer (potential risk), and vaginal bleeding (often absent at low doses), as described further in Chapter 15.

CORONARY ARTERY DISEASE

Medical Therapy

In recent years, immense strides have been made in the identification and treatment of a patient with a heart attack with the development of an armamentarium of powerful technologies and drugs. Thrombolytic agents, angioplasty, and coronary stenting, and coronary artery bypass surgery can reestablish blood flow to limit infarct size, mortality, and morbidity (GUSTO IIb, 1997; Grines et al., 1993; Ziljstra et al., 1993; Gibbons et al., 1993; Every and Weaver, 1995). Because of the importance of early treatment for acute myocardial infarction, there is growing interest in detection of the earliest warning symptoms of acute coronary syndromes (including unstable angina as well as acute myocardial infection), in order to minimize treatment delays for such patients.

As therapies have become increasingly more effective, delays in treatment initiation and lack of implementation of these therapies pose major barriers to effective management. Thus far, efforts to provide appropriate access to timely and optimal care to patients presenting with acute coronary syndromes are generally not organized into a unified, cohesive system in communities across the United States. Women, African Americans, and elderly patients are less likely to receive life-saving treatments in time to provide maximal benefit. The reasons for this disparity include insufficient education of health care providers about the prevalence of CHD in women and atypical presentations in the very old, inadequate education of patients about the early warning signs of myocardial infarction and the need for urgent diagnosis and treatment, and lack of access health care and sophisticated medical technology for some low income and minority populations. For example, a recent survey by the American Heart Association reported that only 31% of women correctly identified cardiovascular disease (heart disease and stroke) as the leading cause of death for all females in the U.S. Until the level of awareness is raised sufficiently among this at-risk group, there will be little impetus for older women to alter lifestyles or seek early, potentially life-saving treatment for cardiovascular symptoms.

Women in general have poorer outcomes after a myocardial infarction than men. In 1995, 44% of women who had a myocardial infarction died within one year compared to 27% of men. At older ages, women who have heart attacks are twice as likely as men to die from them within a few weeks. Some, but not all of these gender differences in mortality are explained by co-morbidity such as diabetes or other chronic conditions, but much of it is not understood. Current national goals are to reduce to 25% the proportion of females who die within 1 year after having a heart attack. Additional research is needed to identify differential treatment strategies which may reduce the excess mortality currently seen in older women.

Exercise

Exercise has been extensively studied in patients with known coronary artery disease, and has been shown to result in a host of adaptations which are beneficial within the cardiovascular system as well as the peripheral musculature. These adaptations to aerobic training are summarized in Table 1. The clinical benefits associated with such cardiac rehabilitation programs and aerobic exercise in coronary disease patients include reductions in secondary myocardial infarction, angina, and use of medications, as well as improved exercise tolerance, functional status, adherence to diets and smoking cessation, depressive symptoms, self-efficacy, and quality of life. Thus cardiac rehabilitation addresses a multitude of risk factors important in the pathogenesis of atherosclerotic disease, as well as enhancing fitness, which drug therapy cannot do. Although most of the data on the efficacy of cardiac rehabilitation has been gathered in men, there is evidence that women benefit as well in these domains.

Unfortunately, cardiac rehabilitation is often applied less rigorously to the elderly, who may have the most to gain from the functional benefits it provides. In addition, many of the adaptations do not persist unless training is continued long term. There is a need for better transition programs to maintain exercise behavior after the supervised period of cardiac rehabilitation is over if treatment outcomes are to be optimized.

TABLE 1
Outcomes Associated with Aerobic Training
in Patients with Coronary Artery Disease

Decreased blood pressure
Decreased body fat, visceral adiposity
Decreased body weight
Decreased fibrinogen
Decreased frequency and severity of angina
Decreased mortality
Decreased use of anti-anginal medications
Higher adherence to diet, smoking cessation programs
Improved aerobic capacity
Improved insulin sensitivity
Improved lipid levels
Improved mood, self-efficacy, quality of life
Increased capillary density
Increased oxidative enzyme capacity
Prevention of secondary myocardial infarction

In recent years, there has also been a growing interest in the safety and benefits of resistance training in cardiac patients. There is now evidence that the initiation of standard high-intensity progressive resistance training in cardiac rehabilitation programs, in addition to aerobic training, provides additional benefits, and is well tolerated. The benefits associated with this modality of training are outlined in Table 2. The optimal approach to this disease may be a combination of the two exercise modalities, as the benefits they provide are complementary, but not identical. In particular, the increases in strength may be important for the older, frailer patient, and many older women would likely fall into this category. Since both forms of exercise provide benefit, however, it may be appropriate to choose one over the other in some individuals. For example, there may be an increased ability to tolerate resistive exercise in older men or women who have difficulty with weight-bearing aerobic exercise due to arthritis, gait and balance disorders, hypoxia from chronic lung disease, neurological disease, or claudication.

Additional information on the cardiovascular responses to acute resistive and aerobic exercise is provided in Chapter 2. Training regimens in cardiac patients are identical to those in healthy individuals, with the exception that workloads should be kept below the threshold at which angina or significant electrocardiogram abnormalities or arrhythmias have been documented, if any. This may necessitate deviating from the normal perceived exertion rating prescription. In patients who are

---

TABLE 2

Outcomes Associated with Progressive Resistance Training in Patients with Coronary Artery Disease

Decreased blood pressure[a]
Decreased body fat, visceral adiposity[a]
Decreased frequency of angina and arrhythmias
Improved insulin sensitivity[a]
Improved lipid levels[a]
Improved self-efficacy, mood, quality of life
Increased aerobic capacity
Increased joint range of motion
Increased muscle strength and endurance

[a] Demonstrated in healthy elderly.

---

not beta-blocked or paced, the heart rate during a stress test prior to the development of chest pain or ST segment depressions will be a good indicator of the desired workload. As in healthy adults, the absolute workload able to be performed at the target heart rate will gradually improve with training. For patients in whom heart rate cannot be followed, observations of symptoms and perceived exertion are critical to safe and progressive training. Unstable angina, critical stenosis of the left main coronary artery, ventricular tachycardia, falls in blood pressure or pulse with exercise, and decompensated congestive heart failure would contraindicate exercise training of either type. Substantial changes in body fat, hypertension, lipid levels, and glucose control usually require the combination of a hypocaloric or other dietary modification with such exercise regimens. Therefore, in patients in whom these risk factors are of concern, a multiple lifestyle intervention program is most beneficial. The behavioral approaches that predict success in such programs are outlined in Chapter 26.

Nutritional Considerations

The associations between dietary fat, cholesterol, and heart disease are widely recognized and highly relevant to the age-related changes in the vascular system. Atherosclerotic cardiovascular disease and dietary fat are closely related, as reviewed in Chapter 7, as are cardiovascular disease and obesity (see Chapter 17). Therefore, these are the primary nutritional targets in the patient with cardiovascular disease, with achievement and maintenance of ideal body weight via a reduction in total calories, fat, and saturated fat being the goals of nutritional treatment in most individuals. Even in people who are not morbidly obese, there may be a substantial amount of visceral adiposity present which is contributing to cardiovascular risk factors of hyperinsulinemia and hyperlipidemia. Changes in visceral adiposity are better followed by sequential measurements of waist circumference rather than body weight, as detailed in Chapter 23.

One relatively new entry into the spectrum of nutritional relationships with vascular disease and aging is homocysteine. Very high levels of homocysteine, a nonprotein-forming sulfur amino acid, result from a rare congenital defect. This disorder is associated with premature vascular disease and mental retardation. More recent studies indicate that moderate elevations in homocysteine associated with aging and nutritional status also increase risk of vascular disease (Graham et al., 1997). Homocysteine is a risk factor for cardiovascular and cerebrovascular disease in both women and men. There is also evidence in women that homocysteinemia is a potent predictor of premature, peripheral, occlusive vascular disease. The reasons why high circulating levels of homocysteine in the blood result in cardiovascular disease are not fully understood, but it does appear that there are effects on both thrombogenesis and on the vascular wall itself. The lower risk of vascular disease among premenopausal vs. postmenopausal women correlates with the age-related rise in homocysteine levels. The lower homocysteine levels among premenopausal women may be due to estrogens, as other studies show a reduced homocysteine level during pregnancy, when estrogens are notably elevated.

Homocysteine metabolism is also regulated by vitamins, including folate, vitamin B_6, and vitamin B_{12}. Homocysteine levels respond to folate therapy in elderly men and postmenopausal women, suggesting that the higher homocysteine levels may be due, in part, to subclinical vitamin deficiency. Twenty percent of the elderly cohort of the Framingham Heart Study (age 69–96) have elevated homocysteine levels and these levels are associated with low circulating levels of folate, vitamin B_{12}, or vitamin B_6, and low dietary intake of folate. Elevated homocysteine is an independent predictor of carotid artery disease diagnosed by ultrasound. Lowered vitamin B_{12} status, with resulting higher homocysteine levels, may also result from atrophic gastritis, which is present in approximately 35% of women by age 80 years. Achlorhydria secondary to atrophic gastritis impairs the intestinal absorption of vitamin B_{12} by decreasing gastric acidity, required for the cleavage of B_{12} from its dietary protein sources to allow facilitated absorption via intrinsic factor binding. In light of the extensive epidemiological data linking homocysteine to vascular disease, it is reasonable to look for B vitamin deficencies in high risk populations. This would include those with previous gastric surgery for peptic ulcer disease, chronic acid suppression therapy, chronic dilatin therapy, and low intake of fruits and vegetables. Depressed patient populations have also been found to have a very high prevalence of folate deficiency, for reasons that are not clear.

There is no clinical trial data yet to show that lowering of homocysteine or correction of low B vitamin intake alters the progression or symptomotology of vascular disease. However, in the absence of such evidence, provision of at least the recommended daily allowances of these vitamins is advisable. Based on the newer epidemiological evidence linking folate and homocysteine to vascular and other diseases (anemia, depression, delirium, neural tube defects, colorectal cancer), the new Dietary Reference Intakes (see Chapter 23) will recommend 400 μg of folate per day for adults. Good dietary sources include fortified breakfast cereals, lentils, chickpeas, beans, green leafy vegetables, beef liver, and orange juice, and should be recommended to all those at risk for vascular disease.

In addition to the roles of dietary fat, cholesterol, and B vitamins in the pathogenesis of atherosclerotic disease, antioxidants have recently been recognized as other nutritional factors with preventive as well as therapeutic potential. Vitamin E is the body's primary defense against lipid peroxidation in cell membranes. In the Nurse's Health Study, Harvard investigators found that women whose total intake of vitamin E was 100 IU or more per day had a 36% lower risk of heart attack than women with an intake less than 30 IU per day. Dietary supplementation with vitamin E, rather than food sources, accounted for much of the intake in the protected high-intake group. In a secondary prevention trial a benefit of vitamin E supplementation and reduced mortality from ischemic heart disease has been reported in the Cambridge Heart Antioxidant Study (Stevens et al., 1996). In this CHAOS study, supplementation with alpha tocopherol (400 or 800 IU/day) significantly reduced the occurrence of non-fatal myocardial infarction, but not fatal cardiovascular or total deaths over 510 days of follow-up in older patients with proven coronary disease at baseline. Given the other potential benefits of vitamin E for immune dysfunction (Meydani et al., 1997) and possibly Alzheimer's disease (Sand et al., 1997), treatment of high risk groups, such as frail older patients with cognitive impairment and previous coronary disease may be warranted in conjunction with other therapies.

Beta carotene may also have a beneficial effect in lowering risk of atherosclerotic heart disease, by preventing the oxidation of LDL cholesterol particles. Several lines of evidence support the role of beta carotene in CHD. A reduced incidence of myocardial infarction was observed in patients with higher serum levels of beta carotene in a case-controlled study at Johns Hopkins. Supplemental beta carotene (30 mg every other day) has been found to reduce anginal symptoms in survivors of myocardial infarction in the Physician's Health Study. In the Nurse's Health Study (Willett et al., 1995), women who consumed more than 15 to 20 mg of beta carotene a day (primarily from supplements) had a 40% lower risk of stroke and 22% lower risk of heart attack compared to those whose intake was less than 6 mg of beta carotene per day.

Thus, in contrast to the literature on antioxidant supplementation of the diet with beta carotene, vitamin A, or vitamin C for the prevention of cancer, which has so far proven disappointing, it appears that in the case of atherosclerosis and vitamin E and beta-carotene, there is epidemiological evidence of a strong relationship, biological plausibility of the interaction (prevention of LDL particle oxidation), and a limited number of intervention trials demonstrating benefit of pharmacologic administration of the isolated antioxidant nutrient. Additional primary or secondary prevention trials of vitamin E for cardiovascular or cerebrovascular disease remain to be completed before final recommendations on the use of vitamin E or other antioxidants, and dosage requirements, for these conditions can be made. In the meantime, with the exception of vitamin E, all of the other nutrients can be obtained in adequate amounts in diets rich in fruits, vegetables, and whole grains. This dietary pattern is also low in fat and saturated fat and high in fiber, all of which are desirable features as well for the patient with vascular disease and hypertension.

CONGESTIVE HEART FAILURE

Medical Therapy

Clinical trials show that therapeutic interventions can improve symptoms, reduce mortality, reduce the number of rehospitalizations, and improve the quality of life for older adults with heart failure. Despite recent clinical practice guidelines and advocation of these interventions (Stafford et al., 1997; Konstam et al., 1994), physician practice shows underutilization of the therapy recommended by both the American College of Cardiology and the American Heart Association. In fact, current clinical practice guidelines indicate that patients with heart failure due to left ventricular systolic dysfunction (i.e., an ejection fraction less than 35 to 40%) should be given a trial of angiotensin-converting enzyme (ACE) inhibitors unless specific contraindications exist. Contraindications include a history of intolerance or adverse reactions to these agents, serum potassium greater than 5.5 mEq/L that cannot be reduced, or symptomatic hypotension. The incorporation of these guidelines into clinical practice must be increased through professional education of the medical community because the number of older adults with heart failure is expected to double within the next 40 years.

Exercise

Even if clinical practice guidelines were uniformly applied to the elderly, there is evidence that quality of life would still be reduced in this condition, however. This is because the primary symptoms of CHF, fatigue and dyspnea with exertion, are present even after euvolemia and reduced afterload have been achieved with optimal medication management, and present a difficult dilemma for clinicians and patients alike. Reduced blood flow to the extremities, at rest and with exercise, are also present despite treatment, and contribute to the early muscular fatigue observed. CHF has also been associated with elevations in cytokines, in particular, tumor necrosis factor-alpha (TNF) and interleukins-1 and -6 (IL-1 and IL-6). TNF correlates with reduced blood flow to the periphery as well as lower muscle mass in patients with CHF. TNF has been shown to impair vasodilation via its effects on endothelial cells, and could thus be causally implicated in blood flow impairment. In addition, cytokines are known mediators of catabolism, and may be directly related to muscle atrophy in CHF as they are in other diseases such as rheumatoid arthritis, chronic infection, and cancer. Improved clinical status after treatment with angiotensin-converting enzyme inhibitors has been shown to be associated with lower circulating levels of TNF.

In addition to the above factors directly related to CHF, there is also a reduction in habitual physical activity levels in this disease, which further exacerbates muscle atrophy and weakness. Finally, undernutrition of calories, protein, and micronutrients is often present, due to a combination of factors including anorexia associated with cytokines and/or digoxin, excess energy expenditure due to an elevated resting metabolic rate mediated by cytokines and elevated circulating catecholamines as well as diuretic-induced losses of potassium, magnesium, calcium, and zinc. Protein calorie undernutrition is associated with reductions in insulin-like growth factor 1 (IGF-1) which will also contribute to reduced protein synthesis rates and losses of muscle tissue. Overall, these factors shift the hormonal milieu toward catabolism, with marked muscle wasting and exercise intolerance in evidence in the later stages (cardiac cachexia). For example, in comparison to 80 older women selected for functional impairment of mean age 75, we have found that women (mean age 77 years) with CHF had similar maximal oxygen consumption (15 vs. 17 ml/kg/min) but markedly reduced leg muscle strength (1292 vs. 1993 psi, p <0.0001) adjusted for age and other diseases, pointing to the relative importance of skeletal muscle dysfunction to the exercise intolerance of CHF. Thus, efforts to alleviate symptoms in CHF must be directed not only at the cardiopulmonary system, but also at the musculoskeletal system, if clinical benefit is to be optimized.

The evidence above has led to the investigation of exercise as a specific adjunctive treatment for patients with CHF. There is now evidence from at least ten randomized controlled trials that physical activity is an appropriate modality of treatment in CHF. Aerobic exercise interventions have been shown to be tolerable in middle-aged and young-old patients with stable CHF, and to result in improved endurance capacity without improving central hemodynamic features (contractility, stroke volume, ejection fraction, chamber diameter, filling times) of the disease. Physiological and clinical outcomes associated with cardiovascular training in patients with CHF are presented in Table 3. These findings suggest that aerobic exercise provides benefit by improving oxygen extraction by skeletal muscle, via observed changes in capillary density, mitochondrial function, and oxidative enzyme capacity.

TABLE 3
Adaptations to Aerobic Exercise in Congestive Heart Failure

Decreased sympathetic tone
Improved functional capacity
Improved heart rate variability
Improved quality of life
Increased aerobic capacity
Increased baroreceptor sensitivity
Increased capillary density
Increased mitochondrial volume density
Increased muscle endurance
Increased oxidative enzyme capacity
Increased vasodilatory capacity

Despite this benefit, there are several limitations to the potential use of aerobic exercise to improve exercise capacity in older patients with CHF. First, although both muscle mass and cardiac output contribute to exercise capacity (maximal oxygen consumption), the relationship to muscle mass is much stronger in CHF than in normals. The combination of CHF myopathy and age-related sarcopenia, therefore, places the elderly at highest risk for this mechanism of exercise intolerance. Second, aerobic exercise does not alter the striking muscle atrophy in CHF (Shephard, 1997). Third, effective aerobic exercise causes increases in heart rate which may be difficult to tolerate in CHF as this increases myocardial oxygen demand and reduces diastolic filling times further than may be tolerable in those with impaired diastolic relaxation, as described earlier. It is notable that even after our most aggressive medical treatment of cardiac failure, successful transplantation of a young healthy heart, such patients continue to have marked exercise intolerance, including difficulty standing up from a chair, which is minimally responsive to aerobic exercise training. This intolerance is likely attributable to the severe atrophy of skeletal muscles in such patients which is not corrected by cardiac transplantation or nonresistive exercise.

Given this important role of skeletal muscle, therefore, and the known specificity of exercise adaptations, it is critically important to design exercise strategies that can optimally influence musculoskeletal adaptation, and are clinically feasible. In this regard, resistive exercise, which is known to increase muscle fiber size, oxidative enzyme capacity, and performance in normal and frail elderly, may be more conceptually suited to address the exercise intolerance of CHF than other modalities of training.

Because of the increasingly strong evidence presented above for the role of the periphery in clinical symptoms of CHF, and the likelihood that aerobic training would not be able to reverse this peripheral myopathy, we recently conducted the first randomized, controlled trial of progressive resistance training (PRT) in 16 older women (mean age 77 ± 2 years) with CHF (New York Heart Association Class 2.2 ± 0.2; ejection fraction $36 \pm 1.5\%$). The PRT group increased muscle strength by an average of $43.4 \pm 8.8\%$ compared to $-1.7 \pm 2.8\%$ in the controls ($p = 0.001$) and muscle endurance increased by $299 \pm 66\%$ compared to $1 \pm 3\%$ in the controls ($p = 0.001$). PRT was associated with an increase in a 6-minute walk distance of 49 ± 14 m (13%), $p = 0.036$, and treadmill time ($+47 \pm 34$ s vs. -41 ± 20 s, $p = 0.06$). There was a trend toward increased cross-sectional area of $9\% \pm 16\%$ in Type I fibers, and $14\% + 10\%$ in Type II fibers, vs. changes of $-6 + 9\%$ and $0 + 11\%$, respectively, in controls ($p = 0.39$). Citrate synthase activity (CS), an oxidative enzyme, and total body muscle mass also tended to improve in exercisers, with no change in controls. In a stepwise regression model, only changes in Type I fiber area and CS were independently predictive of an increased 6-minute walk distance ($r = 0.882$, $p = 0.0024$), suggesting that improvements in musculoskeletal morphology and metabolism led to better overall functional performance. The adaptation to resistance training in CHF is summarized in Table 4.

Although not yet proven in clinical trials, it is likely that altering muscle morphology and function in older patients with CHF, if it is robust, will have significant functional impact. For example, in our study of 80 women over the age of 70 selected for functional impairment, leg muscle power and habitual activity level were the only two factors independently predictive of functional status ($r^2 = .39$ $p < 0.0001$). By contrast, age, burden of disease, medication use, BMI, psychological function, cognitive status, and aerobic capacity did not contribute independently to the variance in this model. This suggests that in community-dwelling individuals, much disability is treatable even if the underlying disease cannot be cured, with attention to accompanying disuse.

Nutrition

Although the prevention of CHF will inevitably be linked to the prevention of obesity and hypertension, the nutritional considerations in established congestive failure are often quite different. Salt restriction continues to be an important consideration, particularly in systolic dysfunction and in the presence of hypertension, and will

---

TABLE 4
Adaptations to Resistance Training in Congestive Heart Failure

Increased aerobic capacity
Increased bone density[a]
Increased muscle size
Increased muscle strength, muscle endurance
Increased oxidative enzyme capacity
Increased performance-based tests of functional status

[a] In cardiac-transplantation patients.

---

minimize the dosages of diuretic needed. Chronic diuretic therapy, however, brings with it urinary losses of calcium (with loop diuretics), potassium, magnesium, and zinc. Potassium-sparing diuretics will also spare magnesium. Magnesium and potassium balance is of particular concern in patients taking digoxin, and those predisposed to arrhythmias, as these mineral deficiencies will increase the risk of toxicity and arrthythmias. Diabetics have decreased absorption of zinc and hyperzincuria, even without diuretics. Therefore, zinc supplementation may be required in these patients, particularly if they are malnourished, have evidence of poor wound healing, peripheral vascular ulcers, or cellulitis. It should be noted that serum levels of magnesium and zinc are poorly reflective of tissue stores, and should not be relied upon to diagnose deficiency states. Rather, high risk patients should be supplemented if history and clinical features suggest potential of nutritional risk.

Although early in the development of CHF, obesity and its treatment still predominate as a nutritional problem; as time goes on, patients with CHF undergo muscle wasting as a result of the myopathy of the disease itself, disuse, and poor nutritional intake (see above). Unfortunately, it is not uncommon to find older, frail patients with cardiac cachexia still rigidly adhering to the low fat, low cholesterol, calorie-restricted diets prescribed many years earlier when obesity and not sarcopenia dominated their clinical picture. At this stage, judicious supplementation of calories and protein may be required to optimize their cardiac and peripheral skeletal muscle function as an adjunct to medical therapy.

In summary, despite the wealth of evidence that skeletal muscle abnormalities contribute to symptoms in CHF, medical interventions have not been designed with anabolism in mind, and thus the full potential of exercise and nutrition as treatment modalities in this condition has likely not yet been defined. The relative contributions of cardiac function, burden of other diseases, nutritional state, habitual physical activity level, and psychological factors to overall quality of life and function, as well as mortality need to be considered in individuals in clinical practice. A multifactorial approach to prevention and treatment of CHF is likely to be the most successful, as it is in many other geriatric syndromes such as falls, dementia, osteoporosis, depression, frailty, and incontinence. Such an approach is particularly attractive in this disease, due to the potential reversibility of all of these peripheral contributions to dysfunction in CHF.

PERIPHERAL VASCULAR DISEASE

Peripheral vascular disease shares all of the risk factors of coronary artery disease: obesity, hypertension, hyperlipidemia, sedentariness, smoking, diabetes, and older age. Therefore, much of the approach to treatment prior to surgical re-vascularization revolves around risk factor management as well. There are a few additional considerations with peripheral vascular disease however. Vitamin E has been shown to reduce symptoms in patients with claudication in several randomized controlled trials. Given its potential benefit in coronary artery disease as well (Stevens, 1996), patients with this combination of diagnoses should be treated with 400–800 IU per day pending further delineation of exact dosages required.

Patients with peripheral vascular disease also respond well to progressive aerobic training interventions with significant improvements in the time to claudication and mechanical efficiciency, meaning that they have greater tolerance for aerobic work. After only 4 months of training, such patients lower heart rate and oxygen consumption during similar submaximal workloads, increase maximal walking times and time to the onset of claudication by approximately 100%, reduce the drop in ankle pressure post-exercise usually seen in peripheral vascular disease, and increase peak aerobic capacity. Such changes may have dramatic effects on function in older adults. Not only is the limitation of activities which cause claudication markedly reduced and the total capacity for work increased, but since walking is more efficient (carries a lower oxygen cost and therefore lower heart rate), it may fall below the threshold which produces angina, thus eliminating another potential barrier to activity.

There is one difference in training technique which appears to be critical to improvement in this condition. Patients should be instructed to continue walking when claudication symptoms begin, until they have reached near-maximal tolerance of the pain, and then stop and rest. When the pain has subsided, they should resume exercise and continue again until symptoms prevent them from going further. Exercise sessions should be extended in this way so that 15 to 30 minutes of exercise (with rest periods as needed) are completed at least 3 days per week, at about 60 to 70% of maximal work capacity. Once the total time can be completed without stopping, than the workload should be advanced as well (for example, adding stairs or hills) to keep the intensity at this moderately difficult level. This method of training is different than that used in angina, in which it is recommended that exercise intensity be kept *below* the level which produces ischemic symptoms. In patients who have both coronary artery disease and peripheral occlusive disease, it may be that angina limits exercise tolerance until definitive intervention, such as coronary bypass surgery, at which time claudication dominates the clinical picture. This unmasking of peripheral symptoms is important to ascertain in the history, as the prescription should be then tailored to the specific treatment of this condition as above. It is not unusual for appropriately trained patients to double or triple the distances they can walk prior to claudication, which may substantially improve their function and quality of life.

Some patients with peripheral vascular disease may have ischemic ulcers, or near-complete intolerance to aerobic activity. If they are not candidates for peripheral revascularization, or are awaiting surgery, it is important not to let disuse atrophy occur and worsen functional status. It is therefore recommended that such patients perform seated resistance training for the legs and other muscle groups. The resistance training is usually tolerable without inducing ischemic pain, and will allow function, mobility, and strength to be preserved in the face of restrictions to ambulation. There are as yet no studies on the efficacy of progressive resistance training in peripheral vascular disease as a specific treatment, so it is currently unknown what the benefits would be in comparison to aerobic training.

HEALTH PROMOTION FOR HEART DISEASE AND HYPERTENSION

PREVENTION OF CORONARY HEART DISEASE

Between 1972 and 1992 the coronary heart disease death rate declined about 49% and stroke death rate declined about 58%. Prevention—lifestyle improvements and better control of the risk factors for cardiovascular disease—has been a major factor in these declines according to the Department of Health and Human Services.

Key to this success has been the focus on science-based strategies in which research findings are translated and applied to clinical and public health practice. Modifying risk factors, such as lowering high blood pressure, lowering high blood cholesterol, stopping cigarette smoking, reducing overweight and obesity, increasing physical activity, and controlling diabetes, has been shown to reduce heart disease risk. The high prevalence of such risk factors in older women, particularly obesity, hypertension, and inactivity, makes such a preventive strategy of key importance in the achievement of substantive reductions in cardiovascular disease morbidity and mortality.

The potential role of physical activity in preventing coronary heart disease is of particular importance given that this disease is the leading cause of death and disability in the United States. Physically inactive people are almost twice as likely to develop coronary heart disease as people who engage in regular physical activity This risk is almost as high as risk factors such as cigarette smoking, high blood pressure, and high blood cholesterol. Physical inactivity, though, is far more prevalent than any one of these other risk factors, and therefore the public health impact of changing physical activity levels in a substantial portion of the at risk population would be enormous.

There are many indicators that the strategy of risk factor reduction has met with success in U.S. adults in general, as shown in the examples below:

	1976–80	1988–91
Awareness of hypertension	51%	73%
Treatment of hypertension	31%	55%
Control of hypertension	10%	24%
Cholesterol >240 mg/dl	26%	20%
Mean cholesterol mg/dl (males)	211	205
Mean cholesterol mg/dl (females)	215	205

However, for some demographic groups, and some risk factors, the progress toward national objectives has been less than optimal. Women, minority groups, and the elderly have shown the least evidence of risk factor improvement. Smoking remains among the chief preventable causes of cardiovascular diseases, with a prevalence of about 25%, and is not declining in minority groups. Most important, in contrast to the trends for hypertension and cholesterol control, the risk factors of overweight and inactivity have both increased over the past decade. One third of the U.S. adult population is currently overweight, and in some minority groups, particularly among women, nearly one-half are overweight.

These trends taken together suggest that it is the advent of newer and more potent medications that are primarily providing control of blood pressure and lipids, rather than modifications in lifestyles such as diet and activity level. There is clearly a need to involve individuals and communities in the design of programs relevant to women, minorities, and the elderly if behavioral approaches to the prevention of cardiovascular disease are to become effective in the future. Attempts to increase consumer-friendly food labeling (see Chapter 24) and emphasize the benefits of lifestyle integration of physical activity (see Chapter 26) have tried to address these problems in recent years, but there is still much room for improvement. Persons of low socioeconomic status are of special concern, as their access to good preventive programs and health information is more limited, and yet their burden of heart disease, stroke, and chronic renal failure remain higher than the overall population.

DESIGNING A HEALTH PROMOTION PROGRAM FOR HEART DISEASE AND HYPERTENSION

A program of health promotion should include increased physical activity and exercise, proper nutrition, reduced use of tobacco and alcohol, and efforts at improving mental health and reducing adverse effects of stress and mental disorders. General principles are outlined below:

- Physical activity increases healthful lifespan. It is critical for maintaining functional independence and quality of life. It prevents falls and major diseases while building muscle strength, endurance, and self-confidence. The physical activity should be habitual, light or moderate in intensity, and last a minimum of about 20–30 minutes a day. Walking is an excellent form of exercise. Advanced age, even in the presence of cardiopulmonary and musculoskeletal disease and disability, is no absolute barrier to improving endurance and strength.
- Nutrition and dietary habits. Nutrition and dietary habits are often related to patterns of physical activity. Excesses or imbalances of food components should be avoided. Consumption of a variety of foods and a diet low in fat and cholesterol is very desirable. The diet should be high in fruit and vegetables, legumes and grains, modest in sugar and salt (sodium), and low in alcohol. Caloric intake should be adjusted to maintain a healthy body weight. Dietary fat intake should be less than 30% of the total calories. Salt should be used in moderation, and restricted in those with hypertension

or congestive heart failure. The recommended target intakes of fat, cholesterol, fiber, folate, sodium, magnesium, and calcium need to be considered.

- Use of tobacco is the most important single preventable cause of death in developed countries around the world. Because of the health risks associated with passive smoking, tobacco-free environments are beneficial to everyone. Restrictions on smoking in public places are being strengthened and enforced. More prevention education and smoking cessation programs should be offered to patients, particularly the very young and the elderly, who may not be aware of the continued benefit of smoking cessation at advanced ages.

- Alcohol. Alcohol excess is associated with well-known health problems and diseases. A limit of alcohol intake to less than the equivalent of one small glass of wine per day is desirable, and may even have beneficial effects on HDL cholesterol and heart disease risk. Excess alcohol intake is a preventable or remediable cause of falls and accidental injury, osteoporosis, nutritional deficiencies, pancreatic and liver disease, rectal cancer, gastrointestinal bleeding, anemia, cardiac arrhythmias, cardiomyopathy, stroke, urinary incontinence, peripheral neuropathy, gait and balance disorders, and dementia and delirium. Educational programs to reduce alcohol and other drug consumption, together with raising awareness of the harmful effects of addictive substances, are important. There should be increased access to treatment programs for drug dependence and social support programs.

NEED FOR FUTURE RESEARCH

In some areas, there is a great need for further research on the benefits of prevention or treatment of established risk factors. For example, it is widely believed that regular physical activity is effective as a preventive measure or an adjunctive treatment for hypertension. The epidemiological observation that physical activity reduces the risk for hypertension has only been seen in white males who self-reported hypertension. In the large prospective Atherosclerosis Risk in Communities Study (ARIC), 7, 459 black and white Americans aged 45–65 were examined clinically for the development of hypertension over 6 years and assessed for habitual physical activity levels and other risk factors. White men who were the most active had a 34% lower risk of incident hypertension, but no such relationships were seen in women or blacks. Similarly, meta-analysis of controlled experimental trials reveals that exercise by itself, without associated dietary change or weight loss, produces small changes in systolic and diastolic pressure in hypertensive or normotensive men (3 to 4 mm reduction in pressures in most trials). In women, there are currently no randomized controlled trials of aerobic exercise in women with hypertension. A recent meta-analysis of the published controlled trials in normotensive women included 732 women of mean age 53 years from 10 different randomized trials in the literature. Overall small reductions of 1 to 2 mmHg in systolic and diastolic pressures were observed after training programs up to one year in length. Of note, no women over 70 were studied, and the greatest reductions were seen in those less than 50 years of age. It is not known if the epidemiological gender differences in association between physical activity and hypertension are related to hormonal factors, intensity of exercise performed, or other factors. Importantly, there are no data on efficacy in older adults or women with hypertension.

Thus, there is a great need for studies of hypertensives, elderly individuals, women, and minorities before public health recommendations about the value of physical activity for the prevention or treatment of hypertension should be extended to these groups. On the other hand, there is much misinformation about the danger of resistance training in adults in relation to blood pressure (see also Chapter 2). There is no evidence that progressive resistance training causes sustained elevations in blood pressure in the elderly. There is, in fact, some evidence that resistance training can produce small reductions in blood pressure in men, such as those seen with aerobic training interventions. Improvements in other cardiovascular risk factors, such as elevated total and LDL cholesterol, have also been seen with progressive resistance training in men and women.

There is also a need for better translation of important findings from clinical trials into effective implementation programs. For example, in the area of nutritional control of hypertension, there is now evidence for the efficacy of salt reduction, potassium supplementation, increased consumption of fruits and vegetables in conjunction with reduced saturated and total fat, and sodium reduction and weight loss for the overweight older person. For example, in the TONE study of 975 hypertensive adults aged 60 to 80 years (Whelton, 1998), there was a reduction of hypertension and/or antihypertensive use by 53% after 29 months of follow-up in obese subjects treated with weight loss (via diet and physical activity advice) and sodium restriction compared to usual care patients. This was the first trial of sufficient size and duration to provide convincing evidence regarding the feasibility, efficacy, and safety of nutrition-related lifestyle interventions as a means to control hypertension in the elderly. The health benefits of TONE were seen in the context of reductions of only 3.5 kg of body weight and/or decreases of 40 mmol/d sodium intake, which are realistic behavioral goals. The combination of salt restriction and weight loss was more powerful than either intervention alone. The nutritional intervention effects on blood pressure in this study were about same order of magnitude (3 to 4 mmHg systolic, 1 to 2 mmHg diastolic) as have been observed in exercise intervention trials in middle-aged men. It is not clear whether the weight loss in the TONE study group was more closely related to changes in dietary intake or activity level, although other literature would suggest that energy restriction is far more powerful for weight loss. Direct comparisons of the efficacy and adherence to diet vs. physical activity for blood pressure control in the elderly have not been published, and would be of interest. The translation of all of these dietary and physical activity recommendations into clinical practice will however require implementation of specific progams that come directly from the primary health care provider who is in a position to modify pharmacologic treatment as behavioral goals are reached.

In summary, there is a wealth of evidence that exercise and nutrition play major roles in both the prevention and treatment of cardiovascular disease and the risk factors for this condition (obesity, hypertension, hyperlipidemia, insulin resistance). An overview of the integration of these lifestyle factors into the clinical management of older patients is presented in Table 5. The overlapping benefits are obvious for many of these modifications, so that a patient with multiple manifestations of vascular disease does not usually require a multitude of prescriptions. The most important factor is the need for long-term adherence if substantial health benefits are to be gained, and the complementary nature of these interventions with the many medical and surgical options now available.

TABLE 5
Exercise and Nutritional Approaches to the Prevention and Treatment of Cardiac and Vascular Disease

Disease State	Nutritional Approaches to Prevention	Nutritional Approaches to Treatment	Exercise Approaches to Prevention	Exercise Approaches to Treatment
Hypertension	Maintenance of ideal body weight Prevention of visceral adiposity Moderate salt intake Increased potassium, magnesium, calcium, fiber intake Low fat/saturated fat intake Moderate alcohol intake	Achievement and maintenance of ideal body weight Reduction of visceral adiposity Sodium restriction Increased potassium, magnesium, calcium, fiber, and fruit and vegetable intake Low fat/saturated fat intake Reduced alcohol intake	Aerobic exercise at least 3 days per week at moderate intensity	Aerobic exercise at least 3 days per week at moderate intensity; dose sufficient to aid in weight loss if needed
Coronary artery disease	Low fat, saturated fat, cholesterol intake Energy balance or deficit to maintain or achieve ideal body weight Prevention of visceral obesity Increased intake of fruits and vegetables, fiber Increased intake of vitamin E Adequate intake of folate Increased intake of β-carotene Control of glucose, hyperinsulinemia	Low fat, saturated fat, cholesterol intake Energy balance or deficit to maintain or achieve ideal body weight Prevention of visceral obesity Increased intake of fruits and vegetables, fiber[a] Vitamin E 400–800 IU/day Adequate intake of folate[a] Increased intake of β-carotene Control of glucose, hyperinsulinemia	Aerobic exercise to expend about 2000 kcal/week	Aerobic exercise for 20–30 minutes at least 3 days per week at moderate intensity; keep workload below the threshold for angina Progressive resistance training 2–3 days per week at moderate to high intensity

Congestive heart failure	All factors above related to the prevention of CAD and HTN	Fluid balance to prevent dehydration Sodium restriction Replacement of diuretic-induced losses of magnesium, potassium, calcium, zinc Maintenance of lean tissue with adequate energy and protein intake	As for prevention of CAD and HTN	As above for treatment of CAD May specifically target Type I myopathy of CHF with slow, moderate to high intensity resistance/endurance skeletal muscle training using increased number of repetitions or sets
Peripheral vascular disease	As above for prevention of CAD and HTN Control of diabetes and hyperinsulinemia	As above for treatment of CAD Vitamin E 400–800 IU/day	As above for prevention of CAD, HTN	Aerobic exercise, 15–30 min, 3 days per week, walking to the limits of pain tolerance each time
Stroke	As above for the prevention of HTN	As above for the treatment of HTN Prevention/treatment of undernutrition due to swallowing difficulties, functional decline, cognitive impairment, depression Minimal or no alcohol intake	As above for prevention of CAD, HTN	High intensity progressive resistance training 3 days per week Muscle power training to increase velocity of peak force generation Balance training to improve mobility, prevent falls Flexibility training to prevent/treat contractures

[a] No clinical trial evidence yet for benefit in treatment of established disease.

REFERENCES

ACC/AHA Task Force. Guidelines for the evaluation and management of heart failure: Report of the American College of Cardiology/American Heart Association Task Force on practice guidelines (committee on evaluation and management of heart failure), *J. Am. Coll. Cardiol.*, 26, 1376–1398, 1995.

Adamopoulos, S., Coats, A. J., Brunotte, F., Arnolda, L., Meyer, T., Thompson, C. H., Dunn, J. F., Stratton, J., Kemp, G. J., Radda, G. K., and Rajagopalan, B., Physical training improves skeletal muscle metabolism in patients with chronic heart failure, *J. Am. Coll. Cardiol.*, 21(5), 1101–1106, 1993.

Adams, P. F. and Marano, M. A., Current estimates from the National Health Interview Survey, 1994, National Center for Health Statistics, *Vital Health Statistics*, 10, 193, 1995.

AIMS Trial Study Group. Effect of intravenous APSAC on mortality after acute myocardial infarction: Preliminary report of a placebo-controlled clinical trial, *Lancet*, 1(8585), 545–549, 1988.

Ambrosioni, E., Borghi, C., and Magnani, B., The effect of the angiotensin-converting-enzyme inhibitor zofenopril on mortality and morbidity after anterior myocardial infarction. The Survival of Myocardial Infarction Long-Term Evaluation (SMILE) Study Investigators, *N. Engl. J. Med.*, 332, 80–5, 1995.

American Heart Association, Heart and Stroke Facts: 1995 Statistical Supplement, American Heart Association, 1995.

Angioplasty Substudy Investigators, The Global Use of Strategies to Open Occluded Coronary Arteries in Acute Coronary Syndrome's (GUSTO IIb) A clinical trial comparing primary coronary angioplasty with tissue plasminogen activator for acute myocardial infarction, *N. Engl. J. Med.*, 336, 1621–1628, 1997.

Anker, S., Swan, J., Volterrani, M., Chua, T., Clark, A., Poole-Wilson, P., and Coats, A., The influence of muscle mass, strength, fatigability and blood flow on exercise capacity in cachectic and non-cachectic patients with chronic heart failure, *Eur. Heart J.*, 18(2), 259–269, 1997.

Anker, S., Volterrani, M., Egerer, K., Felton, C., Kox, W., Poole-Wilson, P., and Coats, A., Tumor necrosis factor alpha as a predictor of impaired peak leg blood flow in patients with chronic heart failure, *Q. J. Med.*, 91(3), 199–203, 1998.

Appel, L., Moore, T., Obarzanek, E., Vollmer, W., Svetkey, L., Sacks, F., Bray, G., Vogt, T., Cutler, J., Windhauser, M., Lin, P.-H., Karanja, N., and DCR Group, A clinical trial of the effects of dietary patterns on blood pressure, *N. Engl. J. Med.*, 336(16), 1117–1124, 1997.

Beniamini, Y., Rubenstein, J., Faigenbaum, A., Lichtenstein, A., and Crim, M., High-intensity strength training of patients enrolled in an outpatient cardiac rehabilitation program, *J. Cardiopulmon. Rehabil.*, 19, 8–17, 1999.

Benn, S., McCartney, N., and McKelvie, R., Circulatory responses to weight lifting, walking and stair climbing in older males, *J. Am. Geriatr. Soc.*, 44, 121–125, 1996.

Blair, S., Cooper, K., Gibbons, L., Gettman, L., Lewis, S., and Goodyear, N., Changes in coronary heart disease risk factors associated with increased treadmill time in 753 men, *Am. J. Epidemiol.*, 118, 352–359, 1983.

Blair, S., Shaten, J., and Brownell, K., Body weight change, all-cause mortality in the multiple risk factor intervention trial, *Ann. Intern. Med.*, 119, 749–757, 1993.

Blair, S. N., Kohl, H., Barlow, C., Paffenbarger, R. S., Gibbons, L., and Macera, C., Changes in physical fitness and all-cause mortality: A prospective study of healthy and unhealthy men, *JAMA*, 273(14), 1093–1098, 1995.

Braith, R., Welsch, M., Mills, R., Keller, J., and Pollock, M., Resistance exercise prevents glucocorticoid-induced myopathy in heart transplant recipients, *Med. Sci. Sports Exerc.*, 30, 483–489, 1998.

Brandon, L., Sharon, B., and Boyette, L., Effects of a four-month strength training program on blood pressure in older adults, *J. Nutr. Health Aging*, 1(2), 98–102, 1997.

Chati, Z., Zannad, F., Robin, B., and Mertes, P., Skeletal muscle phosphate abnormalities in experimental heart failure may be present at an early stage of the disease, *Int. J. Cardiol.*, 14, 338S, 1993.

Clark, A., Poole-Willson, P., and Coats, A., Exercise limitation in chronic heart failure: central role of the periphery, *J. Am. Coll. Cardiol.*, 28(5), 1092–1102, 1996.

Coats, A. J., Adamopoulos, S., Meyer, T. E., Conway, J., and Sleight, P., Effects of physical training in chronic heart failure, *Lancet*, 335, 63–66, 1990.

Coats, A. J., Adamopoulos, S., Radaelli, A., McCance, A., Meyer, T. E., Bernardi, L., Solda, P. L., Davey, P., Ormerod, O., Forfar, C., Conway, J., and Sleight, P., Controlled trial of physical training in chronic heart failure, *Circulation*, 85(6), 2119–2131, 1992.

Coats, A. J., Clark, A. L., Peipoli, M., Volterrani, M., and Poole-Wilson, P. A., Symptoms and quality of life in heart failure: the muscle hypothesis, *Br. Heart J.*, 72, s36–s39, 1994.

Coats, A. J. S., Exercise rehabilitation in chronic heart failure, *J. Am. Coll. Cardiol.*, 2 (Supplement 4), 172A–7A, 1993.

Cohn, J. N., *Drug Treatment of Heart Failure*, Advanced Therapeutics Communications International, Secaucus, NJ, 1988.

Cohn, J. N. and Rector, T. S., Prognosis of congestive heart failure and predictors of mortality, *Am. J. Cardiol.*, 62(Suppl.), 25A–30A, 1988.

Criqui, M. H., Langer, R. D., Fronek, A., Feigelson, H. S., Klauber, M. R., McCann, T. J. et al., Mortality over a period of 10 years in patients with peripheral arterial disease, *N. Engl. J. Med.*, 326(6), 381–386, 1992.

Department of Health and Human Services, Draft report of *Healthy People 2010* for public comment available at www.HealthyPeople.com. 1999.

Dastur, D., Manghani, D., Osuntokun, B., Sonrander, P., and Kondo, K., Neuromuscular and related changes in malnutrition: A review, *J. Neurol. Sci.*, 55, 207–30, 1982.

Davies, S. W., Jordan, S. L., and Lipkin, D. P., Use of limb movement sensors as indicators of the level of everyday physical activity in chronic congestive heart failure, *Am. J. Cardiol.*, 69, 1581–1586, 1992.

Davey, P., Meyer, T., Coats, A., Adamopoulos, S., Casadei, B., Conway, J., and Sleight, P., Ventilation in chronic heart failure: effects of physical training, *Br. Heart J.*, 68, 473–7, 1992.

de Bono, D. P., The European Cooperative Study Group trial of intravenous recombinant tissue-type plasminogen activator (rt-PA) and conservative therapy versus rt-PA and immediate coronary angioplasty, *J. Am. Coll. Cardiol.*, 12(6 Suppl. A), 20A–23A, 1988.

Douard, H., Patel, P., and Broustet, J. P., Exercise training in patients with chronic heart failure, *Heart Failure*, 10(2), 80–87, 1994.

Dracup, K., Baker, D. W., Dunbar, S. B., Dacey, R. A., Brooks, N. H., Johnson, J. C., Oken, C., and Massie, B. M., Management of heart failure: II counseling, education and lifestyle modifications, *JAMA*, 272(18), 1442–1446, 1994.

Dracup, K., Moser, D. K., Eisenberg, M., Meischke, H., Alonzo, A. A., and Braslow, A., Causes of delay in seeking treatment for heart attack symptoms, *Soc. Sci. Med.*, 40, 379–392, 1995.

Drexler, H., Riede, U., Munzel, T., Konig, H., Funke, E., and Just, H., Alterations in skeletal muscle in chronic heart failure, *Circulation*, 85(5), 1751–1759, 1992.

Every, N. R. and Weaver, W. D., Prehospital treatment of myocardial infarction, *Curr. Probl. Cardiol.*, January (1), 7–50, 1995.

Feinstein, A. R., Fisher, M., and Pigeon, J., Changes in dyspnea-fatigue ratings as indicators of quality of life in the treatment of congestive heart failure, *Am. J. Cardiol.*, 64, 50–55, 1989.

Fiatarone, M. A., O'Neill, E. F., Ryan, N. D., Clements, K. M., Solares, G. R., Nelson, M. E., Roberts, S. R., Kehayias, J. K., Lipsitz, L. A., and Evans, W. J., Exercise training and nutritional supplementation for physical frailty in very elderly people, *N. Engl. J. Med.*, 330, 1769–1775, 1994.

Fiatarone Singh, M., Pu, C., Johnson, M., Forman, D., Hausdorff, J., Roubenoff, R., and Fielding, R., The effects of progressive resistance training on skeletal muscle and exercise performance in older women with heart failure. Presented at the Australasian Society for Geriatric Medicine Annual Meeting, Perth, Australia, 1999.

Fleg, J. L., Schulman, S. P., O'Connor, F. C., Gerstenblith, G., Becker, L. C., Fortney, S., Goldberg, A. P., and Lakatta, E. G., Cardiovascular responses to exhaustive upright cycle exercise in highly trained older men, *J. Appl. Physiol.*, 77(3), 1500–6, 1994.

Foldvari, M., Clark, M., Laviolette, L., Bernstein, M., Castaneda, C., Pu, C., Hausdorff, J., Fielding, R., and Fiatarone Singh, M., Assocation of muscle power with functional status in community dwelling elderly women, *J. Gerontol. (Biol. and Med. Sci.)*, in press, 2000.

Forman, D., Manning, W., Hauser, R., Gervino, E., Evans, W., and Wei, J., Enhanced left ventricular diastolic filling associated with long-term endurance training, *J. Gerontol.*, 47, M56–58, 1992.

Franciosa, J., Park, M., and Levine, T., Lack of correlation between exercise capacity and indexes of resting left ventricular performance in heart failure, *Am. J. Cardiol.*, 47, 33–9, 1981.

Freeman, L. M. and Roubenoff, R., The nutrition implications of cardiac cachexia, *Nutr. Rev.*, 52(10), 340–347, 1994.

Gaasch, W. H., Diagnosis and treatment of heart failure based on left ventricular systolic or diastolic dysfunction, *JAMA*, 271(16), 1276–1280, 1994.

Garg, R., Packer, M., Pitt, B., and Yusuf, S., Heart failure in the 1990s: Evolution of a major public health problem in cardiovascular medicine, *J. Am. Coll. Cardiol.*, 22 (Supplement 4), 3A–5A, 1993.

Ghali, J. K., Cooper, R., and Ford, E., Trends in hospitalization rates for heart failure in the United States: Evidence for increasing population prevalence, *Arch. Intern. Med.*, 150, 769–773, 1990.

Gibbons, R. J., Holmes, D. R., Reeder, G. S., Bailey, K. R., Hopfenspirger, M. R., and Gersh, B. J., Immediate angioplasty compared with the administration of a thrombolytic agent followed by conservative treatment for myocardial infarction, *N. Engl. J. Med.*, 328, 685–691, 1993.

Gordon, A. and Voipio-Pulkki, L., Crosstalk of the heart and periphery: skeletal and cardiac muscle as therapeutic targets in heart failure, *Ann. Med.*, 29(4), 327–331, 1997.

Graham, I. M., Daly, L. E., Refsum, H. M., Robinson, K., Brattstrom, L. E., Ueland, P. M., Palma-Reis, R. J., Boers, G. H. J., Sheahan, R. G., Israelsson, B., Uitenwaal, C. S. et al., Plasma homocysteine as a risk factor for vascular disease: The European Concerted Action Project, *JAMA*, 277, 1775–1781, 1997.

Grines, C. L., Browne, K. F., Marco, J. et al., A comparison of immediate angioplasty with thrombolytic therapy for acute myocardial infarction, *N. Engl. J. Med.*, 328, 673–679, 1993.

Gruppo Italiano per lo Studio della Streptochinasi nell'Infarto Miocardico (GISSI). Long-term effects of intravenous thrombolysis in acute myocardial infarction: Final report of the GISSI study, *Lancet*, 2(8564), 871–874, 1987.

Guadagnoli, E., Hauptman, P. J., Ayanian, J. Z., Pashos, C. L., McNeil, B. J., and Cleary, P. D., Variation in the use of cardiac procedures after acute myocardial infarction, *N. Engl. J. Med.*, 333, 573–8, 1995.

Haapanen, N., Milunpain, S., Vuori, I., Oja, P., and Pasanen, M., Association of leisure time physical activity with the risk of coronary heart disease, hypertension, and diabetes in middle-aged men and women, *Int. J. Epidemiol.*, 26, 739–47, 1997.

Hackworthy, R. A., Sorensen, S. G., Fitzpatrick, P. G. et al., Effect of reperfusion on electrocardiographic and enzymatic infarct size: Results of a randomized multicenter study of intravenous anisoylated plasminogen streptokinase activator complex (APSAC) versus intracoronary streptokinase in acute myocardial infarction, *Am. Heart J.*, 116, 903–914, 1988.

Harrington, D., Anker, S., Chua, T., Webb-Peploe, K., and Ponikowski, P., Skeletal muscle function and its relation to exercise tolerance in chronic heart failure, *J. Am. Coll. Cardiol.*, 30(7), 1758–1764, 1997.

Harrington, D. and Coats, A., Skeletal muscle abnormalities and evidence for their role in symptom generation in chronic heart failure, *Eur. Heart J.*, 18(12), 1865–1872, 1997.

Ho, K. K., Pinsky, J. L., Kannel, W. B., and Levy, D., The epidemiology of heart failure: the Framingham Study, *Am. J. Cardiol.*, 22 (Supplement A4), 6A–13A, 1993.

Hurley, B., Hagberg, J., Goldberg, A., Seals, D., Ehsani, A., Brennan, R., and Holloszy, J., Resistive training can reduce coronary risk factors without altering VO_2max or percent body fat, *Med. Sci. Sports Exerc.*, 20(2), 150–154, 1988.

Jondeau, G., Abnormalities of vascular response to exercise in patients with congestive heart failure, *Heart Failure*, 10(2), 72–78, 1994.

Kannel, W. B. and Schatzkin, A., Sudden death: Lessons from subsets in population studies, *J. Am. Coll. Cardiol.*, 5(6 Suppl.), 141–149B, 1985.

Kelley, G., Aerobic exercise and resting blood pressure among women: A meta analysis, *Prev. Med.*, 28, 264–275, 1999.

Kelley, G. and McClellan, P., Antihypertensive effects of aerobic exercise: a brief meta-analytic review of controlled clinical trials, *Am. J. Hyperten.*, 7, 115–9, 1994.

Kobashigawa, J., Leaf, D., Lee, N., Gleeson, M., HongHu, L., Hamilton, M., Moriguchi, J., Kawata, N., Einhorn, K., Herlihy, W., and Lakas, H., A controlled trial of exercise rehabilitation after heart transplantation, *N. Engl. J. Med.*, 340, 272–277, 1999.

Konstam, M. A., Dracup, K., Baker, D. W., Bottorf, M. B., Brooks, N. H., Dacey, R. A. et al., Heart failure evaluation and care of patients with left-ventricular systolic dysfunction. Clinical Practice Guideline No. 11. DHHS publication no. (AHCPR) 94–0612. Rockville, MD: Agency for Health Care Policy and Research, 1994.

Krumholz, H. M., Forman, D. E., Kuntz, R., Baim, D., and Wei, J. Y., Coronary revascularization after myocardial infarction in the very elderly: Outcomes and long-term follow-up, *Ann. Int. Med.*, 119, 1084–90, 1993.

Kuller, L., Perper, J., and Cooper, M., Demographic characteristics and trends in arteriosclerotic heart disease mortality: Sudden death and myocardial infarction, *Circulation*, 51 (suppl.), III-1–15, 1975.

Lanzi, R. and Pontiroli, A., Growth hormone treatment for the elderly?, *Aging Clin. Exp. Res.*, 4(3), 179–181, 1992.

Leier, C. V., Regional blood flow in human congestive heart failure, *Am. Heart J.*, 124(3), 726–738, 1992.

Leithe, M. E., Morgorien, R. D., Hermiller, J. B., Unverferth, D. V., and Leier, C. V., Relationship between central hemodynamics and regional blood flow in normal subjects and in patients with congestive heart failure, *Circulation,* 69(1), 57–64, 1984.

Levine, B., Kalman, J., Mayer, L., Fillit, H. M., and Packer, M., Elevated circulating levels of tumor necrosis factor in severe chronic heart failure, *N. Engl. J. Med.,* 323(4), 236–41, 1990.

Levy, W. C., Cerqueira, M. D., Abrass, I. B., Schwartz, R. S., and Stratton, J. R., Endurance exercise training augments diastolic filling at rest and during exercise in healthy young and older men, *Circulation,* 88(1), 116–126, 1993.

Lexell, J., Henriksson-Larsen, K., Wimblod, B., and Sjostrom, M., Distribution of different fiber types in human skeletal muscles: Effects of aging studied in whole muscle cross sections, *Muscle Nerve,* 6, 588–595, 1983.

Lipkin, D. P., Jones, D. A., Round, J. M., and Poole-Wilson, P. A., Abnormalities of skeletal muscle in patients with chronic heart failure, *Int. J. Cardiol.,* 18, 187–195, 1988.

Magnusson, G., Isberg, B., Karlberg, K.-E., and Sylven, C., Skeletal Muscle Strength and Endurance in Chronic Congestive Heart Failure Secondary to Idiopathic Dilated Cardiomyopathy, *Am. J. Cardiol.,* 73, 307–309, 1994.

Malone, M. L., Sial, S. H., Battiola, R. J., Nachodsky, J. P., Solomon, D. J., and Goodwin, J. S., Age-related differences in the utilization of therapies post acute myocardial infarction, *J. Am. Geriatr. Soc.,* 43, 627–33, 1995.

Mancini, D. M., Coyle, E., Coggan, A., Beltz, J., Ferraro, N., Montain, S., and Wilson, J. R., Contribution of intrinsic skeletal muscle changes to 31P-NMR skeletal muscle metabolic abnormalities in patients with chronic heart failure, *Circulation,* 80(5), 1338–1346, 1989.

Mancini, D. M., Ferraro, N., Tuchler, M., Chance, B., and Wilson, J. R., Detection of abnormal calf muscle metabolism in patients with heart failure using phosphorus-31 nuclear magnetic resonance, *Am. J. Cardiol.,* 62, 1234–1240, 1988.

Mann, D. L. and Young, J. B., Basic mechanisms in congestive heart failure: Recognizing the role of proinflammatory cytokines, *Chest,* 105(3), 897–904, 1994.

Mason, J. and Selhub, J., Disease prevention: Broadening the definition of folate nutrition, *Nutr. Clin. Care,* 2, 82–86, 1999.

McCartney, N., Acute responses to resistance training and safety, *Med. Sci. Sports Exerc.,* 31(1), 31–37, 1999.

McCartney, N., McKelvie, R., Haslam, D., and Jones, N., Usefulness of weightlifting training in improving strength and maximal power output in coronary artery disease, *Am. J. Cardiol.,* 67, 939–945, 1991.

McKelvie, R. and McCartney, N., Weightlifting training in cardiac patients: considerations, *Sports Med.,* 10, 355–64, 1990.

McMurray, J., Abdullah, I., Dargie, H., and Shapiro, D., Increased concentrations of tumor necrosis factor in cachectic patients with severe chronic heart failure, *Br. Heart J.,* 66, 356–358, 1991.

Meydani, S. N., Meydani, M., Blumberg, J. B., Leka, L. S., Siber, G., Loszewski, R., Thompson, C., Pedrosa, M. C., Diamond, R. D., and Stollar, D., Vitamin E supplementation and *in vivo* immune response in healthy elderly subjects: A randomized controlled trial, *JAMA,* 277, 1380–1386, 1997.

Minotti, J. and Massie, B., Exercise training in heart failure patients: Does reversing the peripheral abnormalities protect the heart?, *Circulation,* 85(6), 2323–2325, 1992.

Minotti, J. R., Christoph, I., Oka, R., Weiner, M. W., Wells, L., and Massie, B. M., Impaired skeletal muscle function in patients with congestive heart failure: Relationship to systemic exercise performance, *J. Clin. Invest.,* 88, 2077–2082, 1991.

Minotti, J. R., Pillay, P., Oka, R., Wells, L., Christoph, I., and Massie, B. M., Skeletal muscle size: Relationship to muscle function in heart failure, *J. Appl. Physiol.*, 75(1), 373–381, 1993.

National Heart, Lung, and Blood Institute. Morbidity and Mortality Chartbook on Cardiovascular, Lung, and Blood Diseases. Bethesda, MD: Public Health Service, National Institutes of Health, National Heart, Lung, and Blood Institute, May 1996.

National Vital Statistics System (NVSS) and Health, United States, CDC, NCHS, 1996–97.

Nelson, M., Fiatarone, M., Morganti, C., Trice, I., Greenberg, R., and Evans, W., Effects of high-intensity strength training on multiple risk factors for osteoporotic fractures, *JAMA*, 272, 1909–1914, 1994.

Odiet, J. A. and Wei, J. Y., Heart failure and the aging myocardium, *Heart Failure Rev.*, 1996.

Oldridge, N., Guyatt, G. H., Fisher, M., and Rimm, A. A., Cardiac rehabilitation after muocardial infarction: Combined experience of randomized clinical trials, *JAMA*, 260(7), 945–950, 1988.

Paffenbarger, R., Jung, D., Leung, R., and Hyde, R., Physical activity and hypertension: An epidemiological view, *Ann. Med.*, 23, 219–227, 1991.

Paffenbarger, R. S., Jr., Hyde, R. T., Wing, A. L., Lee, I. M., Jung, D. L., and Kampert, J. B., The association of changes in physical-activity level and other lifestyle characteristics with mortality among men [see comments], *N. Engl. J. Med.*, 328(8), 538–45, 1993.

Park, K. C., Forman, D. E., and Wei, J. Y., Utility of beta-blockade treatment for older post-infarction patients, *J. Am. Geriatr. Soc.*, 1995;43, 751–5.

Pate, R. R., Pratt, M., Blair, S. N., Haskell, W. L. et al., Physical activity and public health: A recommendation from the centers for disease control and prevention and the American College of Sports Medicine, *JAMA*, 273(5), 402–407, 1995.

Pekkanen, J., Linn, S., Heiss, G., Suchindran, C. M., Leon, A., Rifkind, B. M. et al., Ten-year mortality from cardiovascular disease in relation to cholesterol level among men with and without preexisting cardiovascular disease, *N. Engl. J. Med.*, 322(24), 1700–1707, 1990.

Pereira, M., Folsom, A., McGovern, P., Carpenter, M., Arnett, D., Lian, D., Szklo, M., and Hutchinson, R., Physical activity and incident hypertension in black and white adults: The Atherosclerosis Risk in Communities Study, *Prev. Med.*, 28, 304–312, 1999.

Poehlman, E. T., Scheffers, J., Gottlieb, S. S., Fisher, M. L., and Vaitekevicius, P., Increased resting metabolic rate in patients with congestive heart failure, *Ann. Int. Med.*, 121(11), 860–862, 1994.

Pu, C., Johnson, M., Forman, D., Piazza, L., and Fiatarone, M., High-intensity progressive resistance training in older women with chronic heart failure, *Med. Sci. Sports Exerc.*, 29(5), S148, 1997.

Salonen, J. T. and Salonen, R., Ultrasonographically assessed carotid morphology and the risk of coronary heart disease, *Arteriosclerosis and Thrombosis*, 11(5), 1245–1249, 1991.

Sand, M., Ernesto, C., Thomas, R. G., Klauber, M. R., Schafer, K., Grundman, M., Woodbury, P., Growdon, J., Cotman, C. W., Pfeiffer, W. E., Shneider, L. S., Thal, L. J., and the Members of the Alzheimer's Disease Cooperative Study, A controlled trial of selegiline, alpha-tocopherol, or both as treatment for Alzheimer's Disease, *N. Engl. J. Med.*, 336, 1216–22, 1997.

Schwengel, R. H., Gottlieb, S. S., and Fisher, M. L., Protein-energy malnutrition in patients with ischemic and nonischemic dilated cardiomyopathy and congestive heart failure, *Am. J. Cardiol.*, 73, 908–910, 1994.

Shephard, R., Exercise for patients with congestive heart failure, *Sports Med.*, 2(2), 75–92, 1997.

Shephard, R. and Bouchard, C., Associations between health behaviours and health related fitness, *Br. J. Sports Med.*, 30(2), 94–101, 1996.

Sparling, P., Cantwell, J., Dolan, C., and Neiderman, R., Strength training in a cardiac rehabilitation program: a six-month follow-up, *Arch. Phys. Med. Rehabil.,* 71, 148–152, 1990.

Stafford, R. S., Saglam, D., and Blumenthal, D., National patterns of angiotensin-converting
enzyme inhibitor use in congestive heart failure, *Arch. Intern. Med.,* 157, 2460–2464, 1997.

Stevens, N. G., Parsons, A., Schofield, P. M., Kelly, F., Cheeseman, K., Mitchinson, M. J.,
and Brown, M. J., Randomised controlled trial of vitamin E in patients with coronary
disease: Cambridge Heart Antioxidant Study (CHAOS), *Lancet,* 347, 781–786, 1996.

Verril, D. and Ribisl, P., Resistive-exercise training in cardiac rehabilitation: an update, *Sports
Med.,* 21, 347–385, 1996.

Wei, J. Y., Age and the cardiovascular system, *N. Engl. J. Med.,* 327, 1735–39, 1992.

Wei, J. Y., Congestive heart failure, in *Merck Manual of Geriatrics,* 2nd ed., Abrams, W. B.
and Berkow, R., Eds., 513–522, 1995.

Wenger, N. K., Froelicher, E. S., Smith, L. K., Ades, P. A., Berra, K., Blumenthal, J. A.,
Certo, C. M., Dattilo, A. M., Davis, D., DeBusk, R. F. et al., Cardiac rehabilitation as
secondary prevention. Agency for Health Care Policy and Research and National Heart,
Lung, and Blood Institute, Clinical Practice Guideline - Quick Reference Guide for
Clinicians, (17), 1–23, 1995.

Whelton, P., Appel, L., Espeland, M., Applegate, W., Ettinger, W., Kostis, J., Kumanyka, S.,
Lacy, C., Johnson, K., Folmar, S., Cutler, J., and TCR Group, Sodium reduction and
weight loss in the treatment of hypertension in older persons: A randomized controlled
trial of nonpharmacologic interventions in the elderly (TONE), *JAMA,* 279(10),
839–846, 1998.

Whelton, P., He, J., Cutler, J., Brancal, F., Appel, L., Folmann, D., and Klag, M., Effects of
oral potassium on blood pressure: Meta-analysis of randomized controlled clinical trials,
JAMA, 277, 1624–1632, 1997.

Wilcox, R. G., von der Lippe, G., Olsson, C. G., Jensen, G., Skene A. M., Hampton, J. R.
(for the ASSET Study Group). Trial of tissue plasminogen activator for mortality reduction in acute myocardial infarction: Anglo-Scandinavian Study of Early Thrombolysis
(ASSET), *Lancet,* 2(8610), 525–530, 1988.

Willett, W., Manson, J., Stampfer, M., Colditz, G., Rosner, B., Speizer, F., and
Hennekens, C., Weight, weight change, and coronary heart disease in women, *JAMA,*
273(6), 461–465, 1995.

Wilson, I. B. and Cleary, P. D., Linking clinical variables with health-related quality of life:
a conceptual model of patient outcomes, *JAMA,* 273(1), 59–65, 1995.

Womack, C., Sieminski, D., Katzel, L., Yataco, A., and Gardner, A. W., Improved walking
economy in patients with peripheral occlusive disease, *Med. Sci. Sports Exerc.,* 29(10),
1286–1290, 1997.

Ziljstra, F., de Boer, M. J., Hoorntje, J. C. A., Reiffers, S., Reiber, J. H. C., and
Suryapranata, H., A comparison of immediate coronary angioplasty with intravenous
streptokinase in acute myocardial infarction, *N. Engl. J. Med.,* 328, 680–684, 1993.

15 Sexuality in the Menopausal Years and Beyond

Fran E. Kaiser

CONTENTS

A DEFINITION OF MENOPAUSE

Menopause (which means *month stop*) can be defined as the end of menstrual periods, when hormone production by the ovaries diminishes and finally ceases. Menopause is not affected by the age at which women began to menstruate, or the age at or number of pregnancies, race, body habitus, or socioeconomic status. The average age of menopause in the U.S. is 51. This has barely altered since the beginning of the 20th century. The age at menopause is only affected by smoking (which causes an earlier than normal menopause, by at least 2 years). The lack of a menstrual period (for at least six months or more, in the absence of pregnancy) is a good indication that hormone production has ceased. However, many physicians use a 12-month absence of menses in women at the general age of menopause to make the diagnosis. Menopause is not a disease, but part of the natural events of a woman's life. In the 1990s there were more than 40 million women in the U.S. over age 50. That is an incredible number of women, of whom many still are not aware of the changes and options that menopause can bring.

Menopause generally does not happen overnight, as fewer than 10% of women have abrupt stopping of menstrual periods, but gradually over a period of time, when menstrual periods may occur too frequently, or infrequently, but are still occuring. This is known as the *perimenopause*. There is still enough hormone produced from the ovaries to cause menstrual periods, but these levels are waning. The perimenopausal era may last weeks, months, or even years before final entry into menopause. While hormone levels are dropping, it is still possible to have ovulatory (eggs capable of being fertilized) cycles, so although not common, late life pregnancy may take place.

Menopause is a fact of life—it will occur in all women. Women who have their ovaries removed or have natural menopause at age 35 or younger are considered to have premature ovarian failure, that is, earlier than one might have expected. Often this can be associated with other hormone deficiencies (if non-surgically related) such as hypothyroidism (too little thyroid hormone). Following menopause, a woman is postmenopausal.

HORMONAL CHANGES

The changes in menstrual cycles that lead to menopause begin with alterations in estrogen and progesterone which decrease in concentration, and the aging ovaries' ability to produce eggs (oocytes). Other hormones also begin to change; the relative amount of androgen (testosterone) also produced by the ovary goes down, but not to the same extent as estrogen. Regulator hormones from the hypothalamus and pituitary that oversee hormone production from many glands also reflect changes in the ovaries (feedback). The hypothalamus and pituitary produce high levels of follicle-stimulating hormone (FSH) and luteinizing hormone (LH) in an effort to respond to low hormone levels from the ovaries, but to no avail; the ovarian hormone production is impaired with age and cannot be stimulated. Inhibin is a hormone produced by ovarian cells and when its levels fall as the ovaries' ability to produce hormone (estrogen) is diminished, it provides feedback to the pituitary to regulate FSH, and may be responsible for the increase in FSH seen in menopause. Thus, the hormonal hallmarks of menopause are a low estrogen (estradiol) concentration and a marked elevation in FSH concentration.

SYMPTOMS OF MENOPAUSE

HOT FLASHES

The most classic symptom associated with menopause or perimenopause is the hot flash or flush. Approximately 10% of women will have hot flashes prior to menopause and up to 75% of menopausal women have them. While the actual physiology of the flash/flush still remains poorly understood, it is clearly related to a loss of estrogen. Over 80% of women who experience hot flashes will have them for more than a year, and in 10–20% of women they will last five years or more. Hot flashes, the feeling of intense body heat (in which an actual rise in skin temperature occurs), may be preceded by head pressure and rapid heart rate. The heart rate quickly falls to normal. Profuse sweating/perspiration may occur. Reddening of the skin may accompany a hot flash. Hot flashes are more common at night and during periods of psychological stress. Although night sweats may have other causes, when they accompany day-time hot flashes, they are the nocturnal equivalent of a hot flash. Complaints of insomnia and restless sleep can be closely associated with the occurrence of night sweats. Clearly, chronic sleep deprivation can be associated with fatigue, depression, poor motor performance, and poor concentration, among other things, and is therefore an important symptom complex to diagnose properly (see also Chapter 20). Trigger phenomena that can set off hot flashes include hot weather, caffeinated beverages, stress, and alcohol usage.

OTHER SYMPTOMS

To understand the role that estrogen and progesterone have in the body, knowing what happens when these hormones are no longer being produced by the ovaries can be helpful. Estrogen is important in maintaining vaginal lubrication, and following menopause, loss of tissue strength and lubrication can lead to burning, itching, bleeding, and even painful intercourse (dyspareunia). The vagina shrinks after menopause, without the presence of estrogen. The uterus shrinks as well, by about 80%. The pelvic floor can stretch after pregnancy, but with the loss of estrogen that is seen with menopause, the pelvic floor may be unable to retain its function as a support for the uterus, bladder, and rectum. Both bladder and the urethra (urine tube) are dependent on estrogen to maintain their integrity; loss of estrogen may be associated with frequent urination and even incontinence (loss of urine) that occurs with sneezing, bending, or coughing (stress incontinence). Breast tissue is also affected by menopause; the glandular tissue shrinks, and loss of elasticity of ligaments can be associated with drooping of the breasts.

There is little consensus regarding some other symptoms, such as depression, that may be identified at the time of menopause. In surgically menopausal women, clinical studies have shown that depression scores increased when estrogen and testosterone levels fell. However, little data exist to substantiate an increased risk of depression specifically linked to a change in hormone levels in natural menopause. Life stressors, i.e., children moving out (or moving back in), career expectations, marital discord, changes in body image, feelings of self-worth, and other factors may all contribute to changes in affective state around the time of menopause. The fatigue that can accompany hot flashes can certainly be ameliorated by estrogen; sleep quality and the length of rapid eye movement sleep time are improved with estrogen. Skin changes in postmenopausal women are primarily a function of sun exposure and aging, but skin collagen changes can be noted after menopause, and are felt to contribute to wrinkles and sagging. This decrease in skin collagen can be prevented by estrogen.

Aging has been associated with an increase in body fat and loss of body lean mass (see Chapter 1). However, this increase in body fat may start to occur as early as 30 years of age, before declines in estrogen begin. Losses of muscle mass have also been noted in cross-sectional studies on the two decades preceding menopause. In some studies, an accelerated loss of muscle mass accompanying the loss of bone mass at the time of menopause is shown, but this finding is not universal. Menopause itself may be associated with weight gain, but weight changes are inconsistently linked to hormonal levels or estrogen replacement therapy. There is as yet no solid evidence that estrogen replacement can prevent the sarcopenia of the postmenopausal woman.

HEART DISEASE AND HORMONES

It has been 100 years since Oster noted that coronary heart disease was a disease of middle-aged men, and it is only recently that recognition has been given to the fact that women are by no means immune from coronary disease. More than one-half of postmenopausal women will die from cardiovascular disease. Since heart disease in women is uncommon prior to menopause, and a tenfold increase in coronary artery disease occurs with age (comparing women ages 35 to 54 to those over 55), heart disease risk can be attributed in large part to physiologic consequences of estrogen deficiency. In fact, menopause has recently been added to the list of coronary risk factors that also includes hypertension, diabetes, smoking, elevated cholesterol levels, obesity, family history of early heart disease, and sedentary lifestyle.

Women undergo changes that directly impact on heart disease risk when menopause and loss of estrogen occur. There appears to be a direct benefit of estrogen on the heart above and beyond the changes in lipid (fat) levels that occur if estrogen is given after menopause. When estrogen goes down, HDL (high density lipoprotein) decreases, and LDL (low density lipoprotein) increases. Oral estrogen replacement therapy will increase HDL and decrease LDL levels. Estrogen can increase triglyceride levels in the blood, but this is rapidly cleared from blood and does not appear to increase the risk of heart disease. Although vaginal estrogen cream does not appear to lower cholesterol, triglycerides may rise in response to this mode of therapy. In the largest epidemiological study of postmenopausal use of estrogen (over 48,000 women were studied in the Nurses' Health Study) ever conducted in the U.S., for women who were still using estrogen, the risk of heart disease was only half of that seen in women who were not taking estrogen. Protection from heart disease was found with estrogen use even in women who had few other risk factors for heart disease. In another study by Barrett-Conners of 7610 women whose average age was 73, women who had taken estrogen had 20% lower mortality than women who had not taken estrogen. Most recently, in a report from Kaiser Permanente, women on estrogen had a 46% reduction in the rate of death from all causes, and even greater reductions in the death rates from coronary heart disease (60% reduction), and stroke (73% reduction). While hormones are not guaranteed to make anyone immortal, the epidemiological data showing cardiovascular benefit are now very strong. In should be noted, however, that these observational studies of estrogen use may be biased to some degree by the fact that women who are prescribed and compliant with postmenopausal estrogen replacement are, in general, better educated, white, more affluent, more physically active, and healthier than those who are not on estrogens. These factors may have independent effects on heart disease risk and overall mortality that cannot be completely controlled for in such non-experimental studies.

More recently, a study of women with pre-existing heart disease was conducted to see if estrogen plus progesterone made a difference in heart disease progression (the HERS trial). Depite a decrease in LDL, no difference in the rate of myocardial infarction was found, especially in the earlier years of the study which had an overall follow-up period of 4.1 years. Fewer coronary heart disease events occurred in years 4 and 5. Based on this study, secondary prevention of heart disease does not seem to occur with hormone replacement therapy. Primary prevention may occur, but prospective data are still needed to corroborate the epidemiologic data noted above. It is not unusual to find that something which can prevent a disease (e.g., aspirin and myocardial infarction) is insufficient to treat a disease or stop its progression once it has become manifest.

In women who still have a uterus, there is a need for a progestational drug to prevent changes in the uterus from unopposed estrogens that could lead to endometrial (uterine) cancer. Progestational agents tend to increase LDL cholesterol levels, in contrast to estrogens. In the PEPI trial (Postmenopausal Estrogen/Progestin Intervention study), 875 postmenopausal women aged 45 to 64 helped answer the question of whether or not the addition of progesterone to estrogen negated the positive effects of estrogen on lipids. Estrogen, with or without progesterone, improved lipid profiles in this study. Favorable effects of estrogen on cardiac disease endpoints have been attributed to lowering of LDL cholesterol and the raising of HDL cholesterol, as well as antioxidant and blood vessel dilating effects. The effects of transdermal estrogen patches may not be the same in regard to lipid alterations as taking oral estrogen. Therefore, prospective data on transdermal hormone replacement and cardiovascular disease risk are urgently needed, as this form of replacement therapy has increased in prevalence in recent years.

Nearly 30% of postmenopausal women in the U.S. take hormone replacement therapy (HRT) for some period of time. The benefits of estrogen for heart disease and osteoporosis appear to require long-term usage for sustained risk reduction. However, true long-term comparisons of HRT vs. lifestyle modifications such as weight control, exercise, and diet on the outcomes of hyperlipidemia and heart disease or osteoporosis have not been made. An accurate assessment of the total risk and benefit of the various interventions and effects on quality of life needs to be considered. For example, the long-term risk of estrogen replacement includes breast cancer, whereas a low-fat diet, prevention of excess adiposity, and regular exercise decrease the risk of breast cancer as well as heart disease. Since estrogen and exercise both lower the risk of heart disease by approximately 50%, then the risk:benefit ratio must clearly take into account the total accumulation of disease risks and benefits in this way before rational recommendations can be made. Someone at very low risk of heart disease and osteoporosis but high risk of breast cancer, for example, may not want to risk the possible side effects of long-term HRT.

OSTEOPOROSIS

Though covered elsewhere in this book (Chapter 18), it is important to note that after age 50, the lifetime risk of an osteoporotic fracture is 30 to 40%. That is a 30 to 40% risk of loss of height through vertebral fractures, 30 to 40% risk of hip fracture or wrist fractures. Osteoporosis, low bone mass with an increase in bone fragility and susceptibility to fracture, affects over 25 million people in the U.S. Over 250,000 hip fractures and 500,000 vertebral fractures occur annually, resulting not only in high hospital, nursing home, and rehabilitation costs (the combined costs of $10 billion per year), but enormous suffering and disability as well. Over 20% of patients with hip fracture are dead at 12 months, and the majority never regain their previous levels of functional independence or mobility. Among the risk factors for osteoporosis, the estrogen deficiency that occurs with menopause is a major factor for bone loss. There is a dramatic increase in osteoporosis from age 40 to 50, and bone mass decreases quickly after age 50. Rates of bone loss can vary from .5% to 3% per year. If a women undergoes surgical menopause (removal of the ovaries) or premature menopause, this bone loss starts earlier. Risk factors include Caucasian race, thin body habitus, a family history of osteoporosis, sedentary life-styles, smoking, and chronic corticosteroid use. African-American women, who in general have greater bone mass than Caucasian women, get osteoporosis, but when it occurs, it occurs about 10 years later than in Caucasians. This appears to be related to alterations in vitamin D metabolism.

Women who stay on estrogen from the menopausal years and beyond maintain the bone density they had at the time they began therapy, as estrogen is an anti-resoptive agent. However, women who are on estrogen, but then stop estrogen, begin to lose bone density rapidly, and bone protection from resorptive forces ceases. Estrogen replacement begun early after menopause can decrease the occurrence of fractures of the arm and hip by as much as 50%, and if calcium is added, can dramatically reduce the occurrence of vertebral fractures. Even if estrogen is begun in later years (> age 65), there appears to be some benefit in reducing fracture risks. However, in the recent HERS trial, there was no difference in the occurrence of hip fracture between patients on estrogen and placebo. Furthermore, in the Study of Osteoporotic Fractures (SOF) as many as one third of women on estrogen from the time of menopause were osteopenic on bone density testing of the spine, over one third were osteopenic at the hip, 14% had vertebral osteoporosis, and 4% had frank osteoporosis of the hip.

Apart from vitamin D and calcium in combination, the only medication at present with proven hip fracture reduction potential is alendronate. The addition of at least 1000 to 1500 mg of elemental (usable) calcium adds benefit, and since older individuals tend to have decreased vitamin D levels, small amounts of vitamin D should be added as well (400 to 800 IU per day). Progestational agents also have a positive impact on bone density, independent of estrogen, so here too, the com-bination of estrogen and progesterone serves to help protect bone and reduce fracture risk. Androgen replacement is also currently being considered in trials as a strategy to reduce bone fragility in postmenopausal women who are also deficient in testosterone.

WHY ARE WOMEN RELUCTANT TO TAKE HORMONE REPLACEMENT?

With all of the benefits noted above on cardiovascular protection, bone density, reduction in mortality, maintenance of urogenital support structures, maintenance of collagen in skin, and vaginal lubrication, it would seem likely that most post-menopausal women would choose permanent hormone replacement therapy (HRT). But in fact, only about 30% of postmenopausal women ever use estrogen replacement therapy and fewer than half of those (10 to 15%) will remain on therapy for over one year. Knowing that bone and heart benefits stop completely when estrogen levels go down, why does that happen?

Barriers to the use of long-term HRT exist for both the practitioners as well as older women themselves. Risks and benefits must be reviewed in the context of a woman's medical and family history, whether she has symptoms of menopause or is taking hormones because of the risk of heart disease and bone loss which occur without hormone replacement. Fears of cancer of the breast and uterus (endometrial cancer), lack of information from a health care provider, inconsistent messages on the dose and type of hormones to take, or a prescription given with no information at all, do not enhance the desire to take hormones.

Let's begin with some of the different estrogens and progesterones, and some of the different methods of administering these hormones. All women who are going to be considered for hormone replacement and who still have a uterus (have not had a hysterectomy) must take both estrogen and progesterone. The reason for this is to protect the uterus from developing overgrowth (hyperplasia) or even cancer. As we shall see later, estrogen and progesterone may actually protect women from developing cancer of the uterus, compared to women who use no hormones at all. Estrogen can be given by mouth (orally) or using a skin patch (generally applied to buttocks or abdomen). There are differences when estrogen is given by mouth instead of through the skin by a patch—only the oral form of estrogen has a positive benefit on HDL and lowers LDL. However, both the patch and oral estrogen have positive benefits on bone. Because the estrogen patch misses the first pass or initial metabolism by the liver, it may have less effect on the gall bladder (estrogen should not be used in women with active gall bladder disease), and less effect on clotting factors, and has therefore been recommended as a safer alternative to oral therapy in women with a history of gall bladder disease in the past or deep venous thrombosis or other risk factors for blood clots. Patch therapy may be better tolerated by women with migraines. However, it must be remembered that if they have a uterus, women using the estrogen patch must still take a progestational agent. If the primary purpose of prescribing estrogen is to prevent heart disease, this mode of administration is not recommended.

Estrogen and small dose progesterone (2.5 mg) can be given every day, or estrogen can be given daily, and a larger dose of progesterone (5 to 10 mg) can be given for 12 days, usually days 1 to 12. The advantage to this latter regimen (cycling) is that if bleeding occurs on days 10 to 12 or immediately after the progesterone stops, this is considered expected bleeding, and does not require medical evaluation. That is, the progesterone keeps the lining of the uterus from building up. If bleeding occurs at other times during the month, or if a woman is on daily estrogen and daily lower dose progesterone for the entire month, and bleeding occurs at any time, it is recommended that she have an endometrial biopsy to ensure that everything is normal in the uterus. It is very true that no one enjoys having their menstrual period back, but over time, even on a cycling regimen, menses associated with HRT generally diminish and cease. While women on daily estrogen and lower dose progesterone may have a lesser occurrence of menstrual bleeding, if bleeding does occur, it is not clear without an endometrial (uterine) biopsy that everything is normal.

WHO SHOULD DEFINITELY NOT TAKE A HORMONE REPLACEMENT?

Women with undiagnosed vaginal bleeding, known or suspected breast cancer, suspected or known uterine cancer or acute (recent) history of clotting problems should not take estrogen. Relative contraindications to using hormone replacement therapy include liver disease (such as adenoma or carcinoma), gall stones (here, the patch may reduce the occurrence of worsening gall bladder disease), and high levels of triglycerides (the patch will have less affect on triglycerides). Women who have had a history of endometriosis (uterine tissue outside the uterus), even if a hysterectomy has been done, should consider using both estrogen and progesterone, as the disease maybe re-activated by postmenopausal estrogen.

WHAT SHOULD BE DONE BEFORE TAKING HORMONES?

The appropriate workup prior to HRT prescription encompasses an extensive medical history including smoking, alcohol use, and type of exercise, and habitual nutritional intake should be ascertained. A physical exam including a normal pelvic exam, normal pap smear and normal mammogram are vital. Obtaining liver tests and lipid (cholesterol, HDL, and LDL) concentrations to ascertain preexisting liver disease and coronary risk factors is important. If a woman is at increased risk for osteoporosis, (see Chapter 18) or already has osteoporosis, bone densitometry should be obtained of the spine and hip so that response to therapy can be monitored over time.

WHAT ARE THE MAJOR CONCERNS ABOUT TAKING HORMONES?

Again, the greatest concerns relate to cancer risk. While it is true that estrogen, given by itself with no progesterone, will increase the risk of endometrial (uterine) cancer, up to 6.5 times greater than non-users, progesterone will actually lower the risk of uterine cancer below that of women taking no hormones at all. This is because progesterone decreases build-up of the lining of the uterus.

Whether or not estrogen actually causes breast cancer remains a topic of great controversy. Two meta-analyses have been carried out to look at this topic. In one, treating women with 0.625 mg or less per day of a conjugated estrogen, such as Premarin, did not increase the risk of breast cancer. In a second meta-analysis, the risk of breast cancer increased slightly after 15 years of hormone use. A 1989 Swedish study using a formulation of estrogen that is not used in the U.S., showed an increased risk of breast cancer. Other studies have suggested that estrogen–progesterone combinations may lower the risk of breast cancer. The lifetime risk of developing breast cancer (even with no hormone use) is estimated to be one women in nine. The risk increases with a positive family history of breast cancer. However, even with a positive family history of breast cancer, the risk of cardiovascular disease and death is 50% (1 out of two women). If you weigh the odds, the risk of heart disease outweighs the risk of breast cancer. These risks may be further reduced by careful screening, continued breast self-exams, and follow-up mammograms, which should be part of ongoing care. There may be an increased risk of breast cancer in women who use HRT for more than 15 years, though this, too, remains controversial.

However, it is often the nuisance adverse symptoms of hormone replacement such as nausea, headache, breast tenderness/enlargement, and bloating that may cause enough irritation for a woman to stop her hormones. Often these problems can be decreased or eliminated by altering dose/brands/type of replacement.

There are some alternatives for women who cannot be on hormone replacement or choose not to take hormones. Hot flashes can be ameliorated by layered clothing, fans, and clonidine (a blood pressure lowering drug) which has been cited as decreasing hot flashes. Herbal therapies, though poorly studied, have been advocated as being beneficial for hot flashes, i.e., ginseng, yerba buena, and dong quai to name a few. Some plants/herbs may contain estrogen-like substances, and if a women uses herbal therapy, but has a contraindication to estrogen (such as an estrogen responsive tumor), these may pose problems. Drugs such as tamoxifen, used as chemotherapy for breast cancer, act as "anti-estrogens" on the breast, but act as "pro-estrogens" on bone. Of course, reduction of osteoporotic risk can be enhanced by a diet high in calcium-containing foods, 400 U vitamin D per day, regular weight-bearing aerobic or resistive exercise, and not smoking. Heart disease risk can also be reduced with a heart healthy (low saturated fat) diet, smoking cessation, and exercise.

SEXUALITY

It is important to remember that there is no age at which sexual feelings end. There is more to sexuality than just hormones. A woman's emotional and physical health, life stressors, relationship strengths and weaknesses, all connect to sexuality. There is no impediment to intimacy, desire, arousal, or orgasm associated with menopause. Women who enjoyed their sex lives prior to menopause continue to enjoy and maintain their sexuality. Postmenopausal women who are not on estrogen, but are sexually active, have fewer problems with vaginal lubrication and have less painful intercourse than postmenopausal women who are not sexually active, giving rise to the "use it or lose it" phenomenon apparent in this realm as in many others. For some women, menopause means the ability to enjoy sexual feelings without pregnancy occuring, which can be liberating. The major predictors of decreasing sexual activity are ill health and the absence of a sexually functioning partner, not age itself as is sometimes thought.

Physiologically, some alterations do occur with menopause and aging. The sexual response cycle has been divided into four phases by Masters and Johnson. The excitement phase generally is accompanied by an increase in vaginal lubrication and an increase in muscle tension. During the plateau phase the outer one third of the vagina constricts and the clitoris, which has increased in size due to increase blood flow, elevates. During orgasm, the outer one third of the vagina and the uterus contract and muscle tension is released. During the resolution phase, there is a decrease in blood flow and relaxation back to the unaroused state. With menopause and the loss of estrogen, vaginal lubrication decreases, breast and clitoral enlargement due to increased blood flow is less than when younger. The uterus does not rise as much, and during orgasm, fewer contractions may be noted. Women still retain their multiorgasmic capacity, but there is increased speed of return to the unaroused state.

Vaginal dryness can cause problems in having intercourse, and without estrogen, the vaginal walls stretch less. Without estrogen the vagina actually shrinks and shortens. The amount of time taken to become aroused and lubricated may increase. Estrogen in oral tablets, transdermal (skin patch) preparations or even as estrogen cream inserted into the vagina will improve vaginal lubrication, but it does need to be remembered that vaginal estrogen is absorbed systemically and has many of the same side effects as oral/transdermal estrogen. Non-estrogenic, water-soluble lubricants are available, including Astroglide, Embrace, Slick, and vaginal suppositories such as Replens or Lubrin, can help keep vaginal tissue moist.

The occurrence of hot flashes and insomnia are going to interfere with quality of life, mood, and well-being and will not enhance anyone's desire. Alterations in libido (sexual desire) may occur when intercourse is painful. This may also be the result of relationship issues: stress, boredom, anger that may be taken out in the sexual arena. While testosterone has been linked to sex drive even in women, the use of testosterone in a woman may have adverse effects on liver (if taken by mouth), and will decrease HDL and potentially increase cardiovascular risk. There is an absolute lack of long-term data, which makes it difficult to recommend this therapy at the present time. Few data exist about the sexual activity of women alone and even less on lesbians. Sexual activities for one (masturbation and other autoerotic pleasures) are available options for many. In one study of lesbians over 60, many issues they faced were identical to those of all women—lack of a partner, lack of opportunity, and health issues were predictors of activity. Since women outlive men by 7 to 8 years on average, and most individuals over the age of 85 are widowed females, the fastest growing population in the U.S., these issues will require greater study in the future.

Another concern that must be raised is whether depression is a cause or result of sexual difficulties. In either case, recognition that depression may be present and dealing with it through appropriate therapy (see Chapter 19) should be considered.

Self-image and the alterations that age and lifestyle can inflict on body habitus—loss of skin elasticity, smaller breast size, weight changes, excess central adiposity, mobility impairment if hip fracture occurs, loss of height or kyphotic deformities of the spine from vertebral fractures, for example, may also impair sexual feelings and self-esteem. Maintaining a positive outlook is vital as is realizing that exercise, nutrition, and smoking cessation (remember, it causes extra wrinkles) can assist in minimizing these physical changes in the postmenopausal years.

An important aspect of sex is the need to remember that sexually transmitted diseases such as herpes, syphilis, gonorrhea, and AIDS are not just diseases of those in their teens and twenties. Especially if a woman is not in a monogamous long-term relationship, care must always be taken. Condom use prevents these infections and should be part of the "dress code."

Suggestions for maintaining a healthy sex life in older women include focusing on communication with one's partner, making sex a joint venture, using the best sexual organ (the brain), and seeking help for problems that arise. Appropriate therapy from a relevant health care provider (internist, gynecologist, psychologist, etc.) can go a long way toward ensuring that sex is forever for older women.

REFERENCES

Barrett, C. E. and Bush, T. L., Estrogen and coronary heart disease in women, *J. Am. Med. Assoc.,* 265, 1861, 1991.

Belchetz, P. E., Hormonal treatment of postmenopausal women, *N. Engl. J. Med.*, 330, 1062–1071, 1994.

Evan, E. P., Fleming, K. C., and Evans, J. M., Hormone replacement therapy: Management of common problems, *Mayo Clin. Proc.*, 70, 800–805, 1995.

Harriet, C., Anderson, M., Raju, S. K. et al., Estrogen replacement after oophorectomy. Comparison of patches and implants, *Br. Med. J.*, 305, 90, 1992.

Harris, R. B., Laws, A., and Reddy, V., Are women using postmenopausal estrogen? A community survey, *Am. J. Publ. Hlth.,* 80, 1266–1268, 1990.

Heinrich, J. B., The postmenopausal estrogen/breast cancer controversy, *J. Am. Med. Assoc.,* 268, 1900–1902, 1992.

Kaiser, F. E., Wilson, M. M. G., and Morley, J. E., Menopause and beyond, in *Geriatric Medicine*, 3rd Edition (in press).

Landau, C., Cyr, M. G., and Moulton, A. W., *The Complete Book of Menopause,* GP Putnam's Sons, New York, 1994.

Lenton, E. A., Sexon, L., Lee, S. et al., Progressive changes in LH and FSH and LH:FSH ratio in women throughout reproductive life, *Maturitas*, 10, 35, 1988.

Lindsay, R., Estrogens, bone mass and osteoporotic fracture, *Am. J. Med.*, 91, 105–125, 1991.

Mathews, K. A., Meilahn, E., Kuller, L. H. et al., Menopause and risk factors for coronary heart disease, *N. Engl. J. Med.*, 321, 641, 1989.

McKinaly, S. M., Brambilla, D. J., and Posner, J. G., The normal menopause transition, *Maturitas*, 14, 103, 1992.

Roughan, P. A., Kaiser, F. E., and Morley, J. E., Sexuality and the older women, *Clin. Geriatr. Med.,* 87–106, 1993.

Stampfer, M. J., Postmenopausal estrogen therapy and cardiovascular disease, *N. Engl. J. Med.*, 325, 756–762, 1991.

Utian, W. H. and Jacobowitz, R. S., *Managing Your Menopause*, Simon and Schuster, New York, 1990.

16 Minority Women's Health

Cynthia T. Henderson and
Maria A. Fiatarone Singh

CONTENTS

INTRODUCTION

Any discussion of the health of minority women in the U.S. must be tempered by the question — "What's in a name?" The term "minority" has been used to refer to groups of people who are present in the U.S. in smaller numbers than Whites, who comprise the largest population group in the country. The process used by federal, state, and local governmental agencies to count and classify the population includes our present system of racial classification. The data produced in this manner are presumably used to distribute societal resources. However, in recent years, scientists, sociologists, and public policy analysts have questioned the accuracy and appropriateness of reporting by race.[1] They point out that the intermingling of human populations over time has made racial categorization a difficult exercise. For example, there are Black and non-Black Hispanic populations, and White and nonwhite Hispanics. Birth records currently label the race or ethnicity of a child as that of the mother. This concept is challenged by a growing number of mixed race individuals who refuse to be categorized as either one race or another. As a result, ethnicity is the preferred term, as it allows for the cultural, environmental, and social factors which distinguish groups of people.[2,3]

Currently, the predominant minority population groups in the U.S. are African-Americans, Hispanics, Asian and Pacific Islander Americans, American Indians, and Alaska Natives. Even where ethnic groups are identified, the groups' names hide the tremendous diversity within those groups. Current ethnic group definitions used by federal governmental agencies are used for collecting and reporting information such as census data and birth records.[3] The use of these terms is not uniform among public agencies, researchers, and the media. It is no surprise that the terms themselves are not uniformly accepted by members of these groups. An interesting case in point involves people of Caucasian descent who were born in Africa and have immigrated to the U.S. One could argue (and some have) that these individuals are African-Americans!

The identification of health, educational, economic, and social patterns by population group is clearly important for fair distribution of society's resources. In health care, it is important for the development of effective interventions that are sensitive to the needs and concerns of the people being served. This is particularly true with regard to improving dietary, physical activity, and other health habits.

In addition to ethnic group differences, geographic factors may significantly influence dietary and health habits. For example, a sixteen-state study of fruit and vegetable consumption found that across ethnic groups, women in western states ate more fruits and vegetables than men or women in other states. People who were younger and less educated ate fewer servings of fruit and vegetables per day. The availability of fresh produce was a key factor in the states studied.[4] This same study showed that when it comes to what people eat, the influence of age, gender, and education may be more important than a person's ethnic background.

Scientists have not yet found a simple way of dealing with issues of race and ethnicity either. Many researchers simply avoid reporting results by race or ethnicity of their subjects, making it difficult to know if the results are applicable to diverse populations. Unfortunately, this omission does not serve the need for deeper knowledge of the groups of people being studied. The majority of studies that examine minority women's health, exercise, and nutrition, report data on African-American and Mexican-American women, with little data on the other ethnic population groups.

Information regarding older women in nonwhite population groups is even harder to come by. Large data sets developed by U.S. governmental agencies often do not include sufficient numbers of Hispanics, American Indians, Asian Americans, or Pacific Islanders for meaningful research on age-related changes in these populations.[1] Consequently, the scientific literature described in this chapter should be cautiously applied to older nonwhite women. Despite these limitations, this chapter will describe some of the available research data on minority women's health, and specific strategies for improving exercise and nutrition.

COMMON HEALTH PROBLEMS IN
OLDER MINORITY WOMEN

In its report, *Healthy People 2000*, the U.S. Public Health Service identified obesity as a problem for 44% of African American, 39% of Mexican American, 37% of Puerto Rican, and 34% of Cuban women over the age of 20 years.[5] Given these figures, to say that obesity is epidemic in the U.S. is not an exaggeration. Excessive fatness contributes to diabetes, hypertension, and heart disease in older women regardless of ethnicity. Obesity also contributes to osteoarthritis, and the joint pain of this condition creates a vicious cycle. In this cycle, obesity puts excess weight on the knee and hip joints, which may cause pain and limit exercise. The limitation of exercise and mobility further reduces the likelihood of weight loss. Up to 54.5% of elderly Black women report physical disability and poor health, and the role of obesity and its limitations cannot be overlooked.[6]

Diabetes and hypertension, which are also closely linked to excessive visceral adiposity, are also more common among minority women than among White women. Many studies have demonstrated that control of body weight through diet and exercise can improve blood pressure and control of diabetes. This chapter will focus on research related to obesity because of its widespread prevalence and its potential for preventing or improving the management of diabetes and hypertension, as well as hyperlipidemia and atherosclerosis.

OBESITY: DIMENSIONS OF A SOCIAL PROBLEM

The notion that "Good geriatrics starts with good pediatrics" is definitely applicable to the health problems facing older minority women. Obesity, diabetes, heart disease, and hypertension start with the eating and exercise patterns of childhood and early adulthood. In turn, these problems reflect advances in modern society. We enjoy a rich, convenient food supply, with plenty of fat. The transformation of work through technology has reduced the physical demands of work. It would not be far-fetched to say that the meaning of the term 'work' has changed to signify employment, regardless of the physical effort required.

The social dominance of television and the automobile have contributed to the obesity epidemic by reducing work-time and leisure time physical activity.[7] One interesting study compared the metabolic rates of obese and normal weight children as they watched television.[8] The researchers demonstrated that the resting metabolic rate slows in both groups of children while they watched a nonviolent, medium-paced program. In adolescents, the late effects of early onset obesity cannot be ignored. Overweight girls are at increased risk for arthritis in later life, regardless of their adult body weight.[9] Although this study of more than 500 people excluded nonwhite subjects, it demonstrates an important link between weight problems in youth and joint problems later.

As women move through the lifecycle to adulthood, there is a tendency to gain weight. A large 10-year study of race and weight change reported that Black women were more likely to gain weight than White women, but that race alone was not a risk factor for weight gain.[10] They found that women who were educated below college level, had low income, and were recently married had the greatest risk of weight gain. They also found that those women who were overweight at baseline were more likely to have a weight gain of 10 lb or more after a decade of follow-up. These findings suggest two important things. First, efforts to prevent weight gain in adult women should be aimed at those with lower education, and low income. Second, the role of major life change in weight gain should be considered. Most people will agree that marriage produces major life change, and may be a stressor, for better or for worse. Becoming married may lead to changes in dietary patterns and activity levels. Childbearing, with weight gain, may also be a contributing factor.

Very few studies have compared weight loss in overweight nonwhite women to the weight loss experience of their White counterparts. One such study compared the weight loss of White men and women to that of Black men and women. The Black women in the study were less successful in losing weight than White women on a similar weight-loss regimen.[11] The participants were involved in studies on the effects of weight reduction and dietary changes on blood pressure. Although lower educational levels are usually associated with obesity, the educational levels of the Black and White women in this study were similar.[12] Among other possible explanations, the investigators suggest that cultural differences and perceptions of obesity may be involved. For example, they point out that thinness is regarded as more desirable than plumpness late in the economic development of sociocultural groups. Indeed, many older people will recall a time when a thin person was labeled as "poor," suggesting they did not have enough to eat. Among those same people, being "poor" meant one was more likely to become ill. A woman who was "poor" was not a desirable marriage candidate and was more likely to have difficulty in fertility and childbearing. Little wonder that plumpness has been held as desirable in many non-Western and non-industrialized countries until now.

Do income and social status outweigh the influence of culture on obesity? This question was posed by researchers in Texas, who studied Mexican Americans aged 25 to 64.[13] Since Mexican-Americans' socioeconomic status has improved and many of them have become acculturated to U.S. society, the authors sought to show a decline in obesity and diabetes. They defined acculturation as occurring when individuals whose primary learning has been in one culture begin to adopt the ways of living of another culture. A series of detailed questionnaires was used to determine acculturation and socioeconomic status.

The more acculturated participants in this study had greater proficiency in English, used English with family and friends more often, and had a majority of close friends, neighbors, and coworkers who were non-Hispanic White. The more acculturated individuals tended to feel it was not important for Mexican-American children to learn Mexican history and customs, and were less likely to follow traditional family customs, such as having close relations with extended family members. They were also more likely to view brothers and sisters within a family as having equal status. The investigators found that among acculturated women there were less obesity and diabetes. Socioeconomic status was also important; the higher the status, the lower the prevalence of diabetes and obesity.

The idea that greater acculturation, education, and higher income play a role in health and nutrition may have significance for some minority women who live in isolation from the larger society, with lower income and education. Problems associated with poor health and nutrition, and inadequate exercise are unlikely to improve as these women age. Differences in physical activity between older Blacks and Whites have been shown to be largely associated with educational level.[14] Prevention of problems associated with obesity may be improved by helping women with low education and income improve their exercise and nutrition. Such efforts must be age, culture, and educational appropriate.

OSTEOPOROSIS AND HIP FRACTURE

Osteoporosis mainly affects older women, due to their generally lower bone density and longer lifespan than men. This disease is important because it increases the risk of fractures, especially hip fractures, as described more fully in Chapter 18. Women who develop osteoporosis tend to be small and thin, and have lighter skin color. Estrogen deficiency, due to surgical removal of the ovaries or menopause, is a major factor contributing to osteoporosis. Other factors include smoking, excessive alcohol intake, inadequate calcium intake, a sedentary lifestyle, and certain medical conditions and medications. In addition, osteoporotic fractures occur when risk factors for falls are superimposed on those for low bone density. Such factors include environmental hazards, malnutrition and weight loss, muscle weakness, sarcopenia, poor gait and balance, postural hypotension, and visual impairment.

Minority women, particularly Black women, are less likely to develop osteoporosis than White women. However, more than 1% of Black women over age 80 suffer a hip fracture each year. A recent study of Black women who had hip fracture revealed that that they were more likely to have a fracture if they were thin, consumed 7 or more drinks of alcohol per week, or had a previous stroke. Women who reported having difficulty walking or required a walker or a cane also had a higher risk of hip fracture.[15] The high prevalence of mobility impairment secondary to osteoarthritis, as well as the very low levels of physical activity reported by older Black women may be relevant to this "difficulty walking" risk factor. This study also showed that the risk of hip fracture was lower in heavier women, just as is the case in Whites. Obesity has a complex interaction with osteoporosis—contributing to higher bone density on the one hand via the increased weight-bearing loading of bone as well as increased conversion of adrenal androgens to estrone in the adipose tissue, but often leading to osteoarthritis, and thereby the risk factors of decreased physical activity levels, and mobility disorders on the other hand. Since even nonobese Black women have high bone densities, there is little reason to want to encourage high body weights for this purpose. Although being overweight appears to be protective overall against osteoporosis and hip fracture, this benefit definitely does not outweigh the other health risks of excessive fatness, which include cardiovascular disease, cancer, stroke, and diabetes. This constellation of diseases is, in fact, responsible for the majority of mortality in non-White as well as White populations.

BARRIERS TO GOOD NUTRITION AND
EXERCISE — COPING WITH LIFE'S LEMONS

STRESS

The role of stress in eating disorders, particularly with regard to obesity, has been of interest to researchers of minority women's health. Since stress, like beauty, is in the eye of the beholder, a universally accepted definition of stress is difficult to achieve. One study explored the relationship between stress and weight control in middle income Black women aged 25 to 75 years.[16] Interviews were conducted using a Perceived Stress Scale and a uniform set of questions. The women identified family illness/death and work as the most important life stressors. The extended family among Blacks is an important source of both support and stress, as reflected in this study. Working women who were interviewed identified other life stressors including "the difficulty of being an African-American woman in society, safety issues, career options ... and the lack of positive images in the media...". Lack of time constituted a major barrier to successful weight control for many of these women. Family responsibilities such as caring for children, elderly relatives, or both, and heavy work responsibilities made regular exercise difficult for the women in this sample. Stress eating was identified as a problem by more than 50% of the women in this study.

The idea that workplace discrimination, racism, sexism, and lack of respect in society may play a role in stress and weight control is one that some people may have difficulty accepting, especially since it is difficult to measure. Nevertheless, it should not be dismissed out of hand. This is a complex set of social realities which persist despite the acculturation achieved by many middle-class Blacks. While the above study examined these issues in Black women, the findings may have significance for other nonwhite women. One interesting finding is that most of the women in the study belonged to a professional and/or community organization. Such involvements may be important to the ability to maintain self-esteem and may provide a source of information and support for them.

THE EXTENDED FAMILY

For minority women, the extended family, with its supports and its stressors, is often an important fact of life. More Black women than White women live in or interact frequently with their extended family households.[17] Nonwhite women are also more likely to assume leadership of the extended household, including parenting of their grandchildren. In 1991, the U.S. Bureau of the Census reported that 12% of all Black children live with their grandparents, compared to 5.8% of Hispanic and 3.6% of White children.[18] The rise in children being raised by grandparents reflects societal problems including parents who are substance abusers, incarcerated parents, and births to teenage mothers. Resources among these families may be stretched, and the financial and emotional demands of raising grandchildren have sparked the formation of more than 300 support groups across the country to help grandparents cope with these challenges. Although programs such as Aid to Families with Dependent Children and foster care may provide assistance, there are often legal and eligibility barriers which limit support. The American Association of Retired Persons has developed The Grandparent Information Center. This center serves as an information resource for grandparents raising children and offers training and technical assistance to community-based grandparent support groups.[19]

The aware reader will, of course, point out that not all grandmothers are older women. One study which examined this point found that women who become grandparents at a younger age are less likely to accept this role, and may reject the title of grandmother. Where the responsibilities for grandparenting a child are concerned, the great-grandmother may step in to fill this role.[20]

CAREGIVER STRAIN

In addition to coping with the stresses of caring for younger family members, women frequently serve as caregivers to elderly relatives. In general, regardless of race or ethnicity, caregivers for aging parents tend to be daughters and daughters-in-law. A detailed study of caregiver strain among Black and White women caring for elderly parents examined this issue.[21] The author found that the Black parents being cared for were more impaired than their White counterparts; the Black daughters overall had less education and income and were more likely to report that their own health was poor. Although the Black daughters' caregiving demand was greater (due to greater impairment of their parent) the daughters reported less strain than white daughters. Where Black daughters did report caregiver strain, the most important factors were their own poor health and lack of respite. Among White daughters, conflicts between life activities, work, and caregiving demands were important stressors. In addition, for White daughters, a poor quality mother–daughter relationship also contributed. These results point out how important it is to carefully examine the caregiver role and to identify the stressors in order to ease caregiver strain.

DEPRESSION

Depression affects one quarter of all women in the U.S. at some point in their lifetime. Among lower income women, the figures are reported to be higher. Women respond to depression in a variety of ways, including stress-related eating behavior and reducing their activity level. Both of these responses increase the likelihood of weight gain, poor nutrition, and lower self-esteem. For minority women of all ages, a variety of factors may combine to make depression and low self-esteem hard to combat. These include the negative images of minority women projected by the media, stress from a wide variety of sources, transportation, financial and safety issues associated with establishing regular exercise, and the responsibilities these women assume for their extended families.

Nevertheless, the presence of depression is exactly the reason to exercise. The psychological benefits of exercise in depression cannot be overlooked,[22] as examined in detail in Chapter 19. Regular exercise promotes a sense of well-being, improves mood, provides a temporary escape from anxiety, and improves one's sense of control.

ALCOHOL

Alcohol use and abuse have been documented to contribute directly and indirectly to health problems, regardless of gender, age, or ethnicity. Studies have demonstrated that Black and White women do not differ significantly in the proportion who drink heavily.[23] However, Black women over age 60 were more likely to be non-drinkers than White women of comparable age. Heavy or frequent drinking, when it does occur in older women, may contribute to falls, resulting in hip fracture or other trauma. Heavy drinking may reduce intake of healthier foods, and may contribute to vitamin deficiencies (particularly B vitamins such as folate) which may cause irritability, personality changes, and exacerbate depression.

So how does one get from the above research on causes of poor exercise and nutrition habits to reality? The next section of this chapter may provide some useful strategies.

STRATEGIES FOR IMPROVING NUTRITION AND EXERCISE — MAKING LEMONADE

ENCOURAGING CONTACT WITH HEALTH CARE PROFESSIONALS

As women get older, they visit the doctor more often. These opportunities should always be used by the health care professional to promote healthy lifestyle approaches, regardless of the age or health status of the older woman. After ascertaining current lifestyle, relevant advice should be given, supplemented with descriptive, easy to follow directions and educational materials on ways to reduce stress, stop smoking, reduce alchohol intake, lose weight, control blood pressure, optimize diet, and increase exercise habits.

Each woman needs a plan that fits her own health profile, needs, and lifestyle. The prevalence of hypertensive and diabetic medications may require consideration of the interaction of these factors with exercise, as described in Chapter 3. If depression is present, or if alcohol intake has increased, it is important to discuss this with the woman at an early stage. Rates of suicide are highest in the oldest old, and often occur when depression has gone unrecognized or untreated, despite visits to health care professionals very close to the time of suicide. The short lifespan of Black men means that older Black women will usually be widowed, and at high risk of isolation and its related problems, including depression, malnutrition, and inactivity.

It's hard to make major lifestyle changes alone. Sometimes outside influences can be the key to success. A professionally developed approach to health and nutrition can be extremely helpful in getting started. Sometimes pointing out opportunities to participate in clinical research studies of women's health may be the first step to a permanent change in lifestyle. Since there is a great need for more research on obesity, diabetes, heart disease, and other common conditions in minority women, this is a very important way to create and support behavioral change in older women and at the same time provide valuble new scientific data. Diet and weight management studies are particularly relevant to minority women. Nutrition and exercise counseling and other services are often available as part of such projects. Researchers of women's health are making a greater effort now to include minority and older women, but the health care practitioner needs to be part of this referral mechanism to expand the benefits. One such study of Black, diabetic women used a group approach, with nutrition classes and low impact exercise. The women were 41 to 66 years old, and the 12-week course resulted in weight loss and improved diet which were sustained at one year.[24] The success of this study was attributed in part to its culturally sensitive approach to the dietary and exercise changes offered, and the supportive effect of a group of peers among whom these obese Black women did not feel inhibited, discriminated against, or inferior.

Until more studies in various ethnic minorities are conducted, we will not be able to develop appropriate behavioral interventions in these domains. For diseases which are so prevalent in non-White groups (diabetes, obesity, hypertension, osteoarthritis) this is critical. For example, the promotion of water exercises for arthritis is reasonable in upper income White women with access to aquatic facilities, but may be completely irrelevant to the needs of the urban, low income Black or Hispanic woman, and alternative effective programs which are accessible in local church or communty centers or feasible at home should be offered.

SETTING GOALS

Most overweight women have tried to lose weight in the past, usually by counting calories and keeping track of exercise as part of those efforts. It has been shown that one reason some people fail to lose weight is because they overestimate the amount of exercise they do and they underestimate the calories they eat by more than 800 kcal per day.[25] Like any other therapy, success in achieving a comfortable body weight and healthy nutritional status depends on an honest appraisal of current behavior. Open, non-threatening discussions with a health care practitioner can facilitate this process. It may be helpful to have a part-time health educator from a minority background if there is a large clientele in your practice who need similar educational efforts. This person may be able to conduct focus groups and culturally sensitive assessment and training sessions which produce more accurate tracking of behavior than can be achieved by the physician with limited time to spend on these topics during the course of a routine visit. Consider replacing the standard blood pressure check or diabetes check with a much more valuable health education and health promotion session given by such an educator. The blood glucose and blood pressure readings can still be taken, but the patient's time is not wasted, and the doctor is freed to concentrate effort where it is needed. Or turn the waiting room in the outpatient hypertension clinic into a workout room where patients can try new exercise equipment, watch videos to learn new cooking techniques, test their strength or endurance or balance; all more helpful than waiting for the doctor.

It's important to set goals, and to set meaningful goals. Calorie and weight goals are only one way to identify progress. Try setting a different kind of goal with your patient. If she is a stress eater, set a goal aimed at reducing the stresses she can identify. If she doesn't do *any* kind of exercise, start low and go slow, a behavioral method called "shaping" which works one small step at a time to reach the ultimate change desired. Advise her to find a partner and share goals with that partner so they can encourage each other. This may help to keep each of them honest. Be realistic and time-limited about behavioral goals that you set with your patients, and be clear that the goal *is* the behavior itself (the exercise sessions attended this week, the dietary changes made today), *not* the hoped for outcome (weight loss, decrease in blood sugar, reduction in blood pressure, etc.). In this way it is similar to the approach of Alcoholics Anonymous, in which the goal is simply to not drink one day at a time, not to get back one's family, find a new job, eliminate depression, or even eliminate the cravings for alcohol. Practiced long enough, the day-by-day achievement of goals in any of these realms adds up to long-term behavior change that is real and sustainable.

FIGHT PHYSIQUE ANXIETY

Self-acceptance is something older minority women often struggle with, because the larger society reveres both youth and White images. Self-confidence and self-acceptance are two sides of the same coin. To compound this problem, as women get older, they commonly experience more anxiety over their appearance and avoid settings where they may have to undress or wear tight, unflattering clothing.[26] The prevalence of leotards and spandex in most health and fitness centers is enough to send most older women running in the other direction. Instead, these women should be advised to wear comfortable, loose clothing and select a class where they can dress comfortably. Some women are more comfortable in an all-female class than in a coed class. If completely undressing in a health club locker room is too difficult psychologically, simply avoid activities (like swimming) which would require undressing. An important part of changing lifestyle is to identify the things that can be controlled and make them work for you. On the other hand, a flexible attitude goes a long way toward reducing stress, and maximizing the benefit one can get from the resources at hand.

IDENTIFY PARTNERS: START WHERE YOU STAND

Changing one's diet and exercise program requires a great deal of commitment, regardless of your age and ethnic background. Some studies have been conducted among African-Americans and Mexican-Americans to determine the best way to accomplish these lifestyle changes. One way to accomplish these changes is to link them with an ongoing activity. In Baltimore, a church-based weight loss program for Black women succeeded in helping women ages 18 to 81 years lose weight and lower their blood pressure.[27] Since many Black and Hispanic older women are members of churches, this is an ideal place to look for or start a neighborhood health program or support group. You might be surprised at how many other women are looking for a group to join, and just need the facilitation or interest of a health care professional to get started. Nurses aides in this country are very often from minority backgrounds (Black, Hispanic, and Asian-Pacific), and these young or middle-aged women may be the perfect partners for the older women in their community who need culturally palatable help to change their lifestyles. A partnership at the local community level between volunteer and paid practitioners, for-profit and non-profit organizations is needed to effectively bridge the gaps in minority health care education and delivery of services.

INTERGENERATIONAL FAMILY INVOLVEMENT

Another approach is to involve other family members in lifestyle change efforts. One study of a younger group of Mexican-American women showed that a family-oriented weight loss program could be successful in helping women lose weight. This program provided nutrition and health counseling for women and their spouses, with separate classes for preschool-aged children.[28] Although this program was aimed at younger women, inclusion of the children made it possible for them to attend the classes without having to worry about child care. In addition, it will likely have long-term effects on the rates of obesity in adulthood for these children, as body weight patterns are established very early.

The medical literature abounds with studies of group exercise and nutrition classes that are shown to benefit the participants. However, for the women who drop out of these studies, the most common problems are transportation, work schedules, and child care. If this sounds like your patient's dilemma, advise her to start where she stands and involve the kids. Turn on the radio, and have a family dance contest. Ask the children to teach mom (or grandmother) the latest steps. Challenge them to learn the dances of the older generations. Music makes any kind of exercise more fun, and ten minutes can turn into twenty minutes without much difficulty. Television exercise shows during the early morning hours can replace cartoon shows with more benefit for the whole family.

LEARNING TO COOK — AGAIN

Chances are your older female patient learned how to cook a long time ago. She learned to cook the foods that her mother, family, and community cooked and ate. Sometime during the past several decades, diet has probably changed. Perhaps she eats more fast and prepared foods now. Perhaps her teeth and digestion don't quite allow her to be as adventurous as she would like. Regardless of her ethnic background, there are ways to adapt the cuisine to a lower fat, higher fiber content and still enjoy its taste. In recent years, many cookbooks have been written to adapt time-honored recipes of traditional favorites to a lower fat, cholesterol, or salt content. Public libraries are a great place to search for these cookbooks and try them before purchasing. Consider stocking your office waiting room with these choices instead of the traditional magazines. Include notecards or a copying machine so that interesting recipes can be copied to take home immediately. As with exercise, this life change may be easier to achieve and sustain with a partner, so counseling may best be done with the whole family gathered together for a session.

ENCOURAGING LIFELONG EDUCATION AND OUTREACH

Learning something new can be a powerful stimulant to lifestyle change. Advise older women to take a class, any kind of class, even if they have never had formal education beyond grade school. This alone may help them become more active and feel in control of their lifestyle choices and take charge of their health care. Since the chronic diseases that afflict older minority women are so closely tied to lifestyle (arthritis, obesity, hypertension, hyperlipidemia, atherosclerosis, diabetes), this is critical for better management of these conditions. By learning something new, we open ourselves to new possibilities, and big lifestyle changes may not seem as overwhelming.

It may also help to advise women to take time to volunteer for something outside of home, work, or family. Shifting the focus from personal problems to helping someone else can help in many ways. It develops new skills and enlarges the social support network in a setting where we have some control over how much and when we will give. Volunteering in this way is much different than fulfilling responsibilities to one's extended family (which may not always feel voluntary). Show women how they can use the volunteer activity as a way to learn about other resources that may be available to support better health, exercise and nutrition habits. Volunteering for community activities is a win–win proposition.

Seeking Inspiration

The idea that it's never too late to start a healthy diet and regular exercise has been put to the test by many older women. Two such women are Sadie and Bessie Delany. Their father, Rev. Henry Delany, was a former slave. At the time they wrote their first book, *Having Our Say*,[29] they were 103 and 101 years old. When their second book, *The Delany Sisters' Book of Everyday Wisdom*, was published in 1994, they were 105 and 103 years old. In their *Book of Everyday Wisdom*, Sister Sadie gives us sage advice:

> "So you want to live to be 100. Well, start with this: No smoking, no drinking, no chewing. And always clean your plate.
>
> Well, you can drink a little bit, but not too much!
>
> We get up with the sun, and the first thing we do is exercise. God gave you only one body, so you better be nice to it. Exercise, because if you don't, by the time you're our age, you'll be pushing up daisies.
>
> Most folks think getting older means giving up, not trying anything new. Well, we don't agree with that. As long as you can see each day as a chance for something new to happen, something you never experienced before, you will stay young. Why, we don't feel that we're 105 and 103—we feel half that old! We've only just started."[30]

The Delany sisters began doing yoga when they were in their sixties. Forty years later, they still got up each morning and did their exercises. In addition to daily exercise, Sadie and Bessie made it a point to eat seven different vegetables each day, and to take vitamin supplements. Most of their vegetables were grown in their garden, which they tended themselves. Sadie's advice to always clean your plate reflects her low-fat, low-volume approach to eating. The plate you clean doesn't have to be full.

There are many older minority women whose success in living a long, healthy life goes uncelebrated. These women may work long hours, care for extended family members, or may have retired from a job to take up other productive activities. Despite the debilitating effects of racism, sexism, and limited opportunities, they have made a conscious decision to tend to their own well-being as they tend to others, and have succeeded. They are all around, one simply has to look for them and learn from them.

REFERENCES

1. LaVeist, T. A., Data sources for aging research on racial and ethnic groups, *The Gerontologist*, 35(3), 328–339, 1995.
2. Cooper, R., A case study in the use of race and ethnicity in public health surveillance, *Public Health Rep.*, 109(1), 7–15, 1994.
3. Hahn, R. A. and Stroup, D. F., Race and ethnicity in public health surveillance: Criteria for the scientific use of social categories, *Public Health Rep.*, 109(1), 7–15, 1994.
4. Serdula, M. K., Coates, R. J., Byers, T. et al., Fruit and vegetable intake among adults in 16 states: Results of a brief telephone survey, *Am. J. Public Health*, 85(2), 236–239, 1995.
5. U.S. Department of Health and Human Services, Public Health Service. *Healthy People 2000*: National Health Promotion and Disease Prevention Objectives, Jones and Bartlett Publishers, Boston, MA, 1992, 596–601.
6. Miles, T. P. and Bernard, M. A., Morbidity, disability, and health status of Black American elderly: A new look at the oldest-old, *J. Am. Geriatr. Soc.*, 40(10), 1047–1054, 1992.
7. Stamler, J., Epidemic obesity in the United States, *Arch. Intern. Med.*, 153 (9), 1040–1044, 1993.
8. Klesges, R. C., Shelton, M. L., and Klesges, L. M., Effects of television on metabolic rate: Potential implications for childhood obesity, *Pediatrics*, 91(2), 281–286, 1993.
9. Must, A., Jacques, P. F., Dallal, G. E. et al., Long-term morbidity and mortality of overweight adolescents. A Follow-up of the Harvard Growth Study of 1922 to 1935, *N. Engl. J. Med.*, 327(9), 1350–1355, 1992.
10. Kahn, H. S., Williamson, D. F., and Stevens, J. A., Race and weight change in U.S. women: The roles of socioeconomic and marital status, *Am. J. Public Health*, 81(3), 319–322, 1991.
11. Kumanyika, S. K., Obarzanek, E., Stevens, V. J. et al., Weight-loss experience of Black and White participants in NHLBI-sponsored trials, *Am. J. Clin. Nutr.*, 53(6S), 1631–1638S, 1991.
12. Sobal, J. and Stunkard, A. J., Socioeconomic status and obesity. A review of the literature, *Psychol. Bull.*, 105(2), 260–275, 1989.
13. Hazuda, H. P., Haffner, S. M., Stern, M. P. et al., Effects of acculturation and socioeconomic status on obesity and diabetes in Mexican Americans, *Am. J. Epidemiol.*, 128(6), 1289–1301, 1988.
14. Clark, D. O., Racial and educational differences in physical activity among older adults, *Gerontologist*, 35(4), 472–480, 1995.
15. Grisso, J. A., Kelsey, J. L., Strom, B. L. et al., Risk factors for hip fracture in Black women, *N. Engl. J. Med.*, 330(22), 1555–1559, 1994.

16. Walcott-McQuigg, J. A., The relationship between stress and weight-control behavior in African-American women, *J. Natl. Med. Assoc.*, 87(6), 427–432, 1995.

17. Beck, R. W. and Beck, S. H., The incidence of extended households among middle-aged Black and White women: Estimates from a 5-year panel study, *J. Family Issues*, 10, 147–168, 1989.

18. U.S. Bureau of the Census. Current population reports. Marital status and living arrangements: March 1990, Series P-20 No. 450, U.S. Government Printing Office, Washington, D.C.

19. Larsen, D., Unplanned parenthood, *Modern Maturity*, 32–36, 1990/1991.

20. Burton, L. M. and Bengston, V., Black grandmothers: Issues of timing and continuity of roles, in *Grandparenthood*, Bengston, V. and Robertson, J., Eds., Sage, Beverly Hills, 1985, 61–77.

21. Mui, A. C., Caregiver strain among Black and White daughter caregivers: A role theory perpsective, *Gerontologist*, 32(2), 203–212, 1992.

22. Coppel, D. B., Psychological factors and exercise, *Phys. Med. Rehabil. Clin. N. Am.*, 5(2), 377–391, 1994.

23. Lillie-Blanton, M., MacKenzie, E., and Anthony, J. C., Black-White differences in alcohol use by women: Baltimore survey findings, *Public Health Rep.*, 106(2), 124–133, 1991.

24. McNabb, W. L., Quinn, M. T., and Rosing, L., Weight loss program for inner-city black women with non-insulin dependent diabetes mellitus: PATHWAYS. *J. Am. Dietetic Assoc.*, 93(1), 75–77, 1993.

25. Lichtman, S. W., Pisarska, K., Berman, E. R. et al., Discrepancy between self-reported and actual caloric intake and exercise in obese subjects, *N. Engl. J. Med.*, 327(27), 1893–1898, 1992.

26. McAuley, E., Bane, S. M., Rudolph, D. L. et al., Physique anxiety and exercise in middle-aged adults, *J. Gerontol.*, 50B(5), P229–235, 1995.

27. Kumanyika, S. K. and Charleston, J. B., Lose weight and win: A church-based weight loss program for blood pressure control among Black women, *Patient Educ. Counseling*, 19, 19–32, 1992.

28. Cousins, J. H., Rubovits, D. S., Reeves, R. S. et al., Family versus individually oriented intervention for weight loss in Mexican American women, *Public Health Rep.*, 107(5), 549–555, 1992.

29. Delany, S., Delany, A. E., with Hearth, A. H., *Having Our Say. The Delany Sisters' First 100 Years*, New York: Kodansha International, 1993.

30. Delany, S., Delany, A. E., with Hearth, A. H., *The Delany Sisters' Book of Everyday Wisdom*, New York: Kodansha International, 1994, p. 11.

17 Obesity

Sharon Bortz and Maria A. Fiatarone Singh

CONTENTS

THE PREVALENCE OF OBESITY

Webster's Dictionary defines obesity as "a condition characterized by excessive bodily fat." Depending on the standards of classification used, 30 to 40% of adult Americans are overweight, with more women than men affected.[1] The percentage of white Americans in the 65 to 74-year-old age group who are overweight is 36.5% for women and 25.8% for men, and for black Americans these percentages rise to 60.8% in women and 26.4% in men.[2] In the U.S., obesity is a major health problem, with costs and treatments exceeding $100 billion per year.[3] Unfortunately, the prevalence is rising despite massive public health campaigns to increase awareness of the associated risks, and the fact that nearly one-third of Americans report in surveys that they are currently on a weight-loss diet at any given time.

    Factors contributing to obesity among older adults are diverse, including both genetic and environmental influences, but the storage of excess energy as adipose tissue in the body can only arise when energy intake chronically exceeds energy expenditure, however that situation occurs. If energy intake exactly matches energy requirements, then weight will remain stable. As discussed further in Chapter 5, energy needs are determined by resting metabolic rate (which is, in turn, highly related to the amount of lean body mass), the thermic effect of food and energy expenditure in physical activity, all of which are reduced with age,[4-6] although the amount of reduction may vary between individuals, depending on both lifestyle and genetic factors. A proportional reduction in energy intake is thus required with age, to offset these alterations in expenditure, or fat accretion will occur. As with many other systems in the body, the tightly controlled homeostatic mechanisms which serve to link energy intake to requirements at younger ages appear to falter with age, and the result is a gradual deposition of fat due to chronic energy imbalance. The uncoupling of intake and requirements may have its basis in both biological control mechanisms governing hunger, satiety, and oxidation of fuels, but also clearly involves environmental cues, food availability, psychosocial factors, and health status as well; all of which must be considered in the etiology and treatment of obesity in the older adult.

THE DEFINITION OF OBESITY

BODY WEIGHT FOR HEIGHT TABLES

Most methods of defining obesity have relied upon relating body weight to one's height, and identifying a range of values which are either *normative* for age and gender (i.e., the distribution observed, without relation to health risks), or *ideal* (implying no added risk of weight- or fat-related diseases are present at this level). Height–weight tables have been published for decades, and have been adjusted over the years to reflect newer studies of the relationship of body weight to disease and mortality. Examples of those which are most widely used in the U.S. are presented in Tables 1 and 2.

The 1995 edition of the Dietary Guidelines for Americans provides a height and weight table with a range of weights considered desirable (see Table 1). The main difference between this table and its predecessor of five years earlier is that it does not allow for a ten or more pound weight gain after age 35. In other words, the emphasis is on maintaining, not gaining, weight despite prevalence of such gains in the population of the U.S. and most other westernized cultures. This change in the guidelines reflects the fact that at all ages, the incidence of health risks associated with premature disability and death increases as weight goes up.

However, there is some evidence from life insurance databases that the weight associated with lowest mortality increases somewhat with age, which has led to the generation of age-adjusted height–weight tables as shown in Table 2. These age-specific weight ranges have been derived from the 1983 Metropolitan Life Insurance Company Weight-for-Height Tables.[7] The 1983 weight tables present ranges that are 2 to 13% higher than the 1959 tables. The bias involved with the life insurance database is that the individuals who participated were in relatively good health or they would not have been able to receive a life insurance policy, and people over

TABLE 1
1995 Weight Guidelines for Men and Women

Height	Recommended Weight Range
4'10"	91–119
4'11"	94–124
5'0"	97–128
5'1"	101–132
5'2"	104–137
5'3"	107–141
5'4"	111–146
5'5"	114–150
5'6"	118–155
5'7"	121–160
5'8"	125–164
5'9"	129–169
5'10"	132–174
5'11"	136–179
6'0"	140–184

Note: Height measured without shoes, weight taken without clothing.

From U.S. Department of Agriculture, U.S. Department of Health and Human Services.

TABLE 2
Height/Weight Chart Adjusted for Age

Height (ft and in)	Age		
	40–49	**50–59**	**60–69**
4'10"	99–127	107–135	115–142
4'11"	103–131	111–139	119–147
5'0"	106–135	114–143	123–152
5'1"	110–140	118–148	127–157
5'2"	113–144	122–153	131–163
5'3"	117–149	126–158	135–168
5'4"	121–154	130–163	140–173
5'5"	125–159	134–168	144–179
5'6"	129–164	138–174	148–184
5'7"	133–169	143–179	153–190
5'8"	137–174	147–184	158–196
5'9"	141–179	151–190	162–201
5'10"	145–184	156–195	167–207

From Andres, R. et al., *Ann. Intern. Med.*, 103(6) pt 2, 1030–1033, 1985. With permission.

age 59 were not included. In addition, physical activity levels of the original participants were not considered and no consideration was made for cigarette smoking. Smoking is associated with lower weight and a shorter lifespan so including smokers as part of the data skewed the ideal weights upward.

Whichever standard one uses, there is only a minimally increased risk of dying in older people with a body weight of 10 to 30% above the 1983 Weight Guidelines.[5] When compared to the more stringent 1995 Weight Guidelines (Table 1), the percentages above desirable weight associated with low mortality would be even higher. Some investigators have shown lower mortality rates with a weight gain of about 1 pound per year in midlife.[7,8] Conversely, weight loss in old age (almost always unintentional) is associated with increased mortality.

When interpreting the weight-mortality data, it is important to understand that these databases describe the lowest risk of dying, not general health and well-being. There are conditions associated with obesity in older men and women that may not increase mortality, yet adversely affect quality of life, including degenerative arthritis, mobility and functional impairment, gall bladder disease, sleep apnea, varicose veins, and low self-esteem, for example. Therefore, it is important to individualize the decision to diagnose and treat obesity in the older woman, taking into account the general guidelines provided by actuarial data and other epidemiological studies as well as her specific health profile.

Since people over the age of 70 are not, in general, newly enrolled in life insurance policies, similar mortality-based data for desirable weight in this age group is not as readily available. Therefore, the ideal weight ranges are not known with the same precision for adults older than 70 as they are for younger people. However, it appears that a little more weight in the very old may be associated with better survival, particularly compared to those who have lost weight in old age. Obesity in the very old tends to be less associated with the undesirable cardiovascular risks accompanying central adiposity in younger cohorts, perhaps because of the premature death of many individuals with the metabolically unfavorable central obesity. Additionally, having extra weight preserves lean body mass (muscle and bone), which may be beneficial in times of catabolic stress due to illness or surgery, as well as protective against hip fracture.

BODY MASS INDEX

Another method for relating weight to height is calculation of the body mass index or BMI (simply body weight in kg divided by the square of the height in meters) which provides a single range of values for all individuals, regardless of gender. A healthy range for older adults has been defined by Reubin Andres as the BMI associated with the lowest risk of mortality based on 1983 U.S. life insurance databases, and is approximately 24 to 27.1 kg/m².[7] Using this scale, overweight is defined as having a BMI of > 27.3 kg/m² and severe overweight as a BMI of >32.3 kg/m². This BMI standard is quite high in comparison to more recent analyses published by Willet et al. from the Nurses Health Study,[9] in which a BMI of 21 kg/m² was associated with the lowest risk of cardiovascular disease. The cohort used by Willett consisted of 115,818 nurses, aged 30 to 55 years old when enrolled in the study. This study did not control for physical activity levels of the participants, however, and it is likely that some of the protective value attributed to a low BMI was actually due to the exercise habits of these leaner individuals, which would serve to skew ideal BMI's downward in this study in comparison to CHD studies controlling for this factor.

In summary then, various BMI standards have been developed by different investigators in an attempt to define a level associated with minimal health risks, but all of these studies have their biases and shortcomings. Most experts would agree that a BMI above 27 kg/m² increases the risk of cardiovascular disease and death, even if this risk is attenuated somewhat with age. There is more controversy at the other end of the range, however. A consensus panel has stated that healthy weights, in terms of BMI, are 19 to 25 kg/m² for individuals 19 to 34 years of age and 21 to 27 kg/m² in those 35 years of age and older.[10]

Despite being the tool most often used to define obesity, BMI has several drawbacks, and is not considered as sensitive an indicator of risk of major diseases as methods that are able to determine the amount of body fat and its regional distribution. The BMI can increase simply because height decreases, and thus an increasing BMI with age may be a sign of osteoporosis in a woman, rather than or in addition to, increasing adiposity with age. Severely osteoporotic women may lose 3 to 5 inches in height, which would significantly increase the BMI without necessarily implying greater risk for cardiovascular disease or diabetes. Conversely, a BMI may remain unchanged with age if height and weight are stable, despite a radical shift in body composition with losses of 20 to 30% of lean tissue and gains of a similar magnitude in fat mass. This shift in body composition would then alter the risk of fat-related diseases, but would be completely masked by the unchanging BMI. Finally, being overweight by itself, without a significant amount of central adiposity and no associated risk factors (hyperlipidemia, hypertension, insulin resistance) has limited impact on the risk of cardiovascular disease and mortality, and intervention efforts in these cases should therefore be individualized, depending on the presence of other health concerns which may be weight related, such as degenerative arthritis or disability.

BODY FAT

An alternative method for defining obesity is to measure body fat, in either absolute or relative terms, which may be more closely related to health risks and functional status than body weight. A sedentary woman who appears of normal weight can actually be overfat, while a muscular person whose weight is above the weight range for height can actually have a healthy percentage of body fat. The techniques for estimating body fat can be as simple as measuring skinfold thicknesses at various sites with a pair of skinfold calipers or as sophisticated as neutron activation analysis and total body carbon measurements. The ideal body-fat range for women has not been defined in relation to mortality in the way that body weight has, due to the lack of availability of adequate measurement tools in epidemiological surveys, but has been estimated to be between 15 and 22%.[11] Estimates of percent body fat obtained via bioelectric impedance measurements are being gathered in current national nutrition surveys, however, which should provide much needed information in this area when they are available. Without access to methods such as hydrodensitometry, dual photon absorptiometry, total body water measurements, or bioelectric impedance analysis, skinfold thickness measurements provide the only index of total body fat available to many practitioners. The triceps skinfold thickness can give an approximation of the total body fat, if measured by a skilled practitioner, although the estimates are quite coarse. Triceps skinfold values which are considered to be in the normal range or indicative of obesity are listed in Table 3. It should be remembered that because aging is associated with a gradual shift in the distribution of fat from subcutaneous to visceral sites, and from appendicular to central deposition, skinfold measurements over the extremities are going to have less predictive value for total body fat than they do in younger individuals. Better estimates are, in general, provided by the use of multiple measurements, such as the sum of 7 skinfolds, including truncal as well as appendicular sites.

TABLE 3
Triceps Skinfold Values for
Older Women

Age Range (yrs)	Healthy (mm)	Overfat (mm)
55–65	25–38	>38
65–75	24–36	>36

From Frisancho, A. R., *Am. J. Clin. Nutr.,* 34, 2540–2545, 1981. With permission.

REGIONAL FAT DISTRIBUTION

Even more significant than generalized obesity, the presence and quantity of central obesity is predictive for a number of adverse health risks and is, therefore, important to diagnose and intervene when excessive. The presence of central obesity is a risk factor for cardiovascular disease and death, diabetes, hypertension, and hyperlipidemia.[12] Genetic, gender, and age effects are related to the accumulation of central obesity, in addition to dietary intake and physical activity levels. The metabolic abnormalities associated with abdominal obesity, particularly when it is predominantly visceral (intra-abdominal) as opposed to subcutaneous in distribution are listed in Table 4. Men tend to have much more abdominal adipose tissue than women prior to menopause, as well as those kinds of metabolic abnormalities which predispose them to premature cardiovascular disease and diabetes. After menopause, however, the withdrawal of estrogen in women is associated with a more masculine pattern of fat distribution as well as its associated metabolic profile and disease risk.

Central obesity may be assessed most precisely using computerized tomography or magnetic resonance imaging scans of the abdomen or estimated anthropometrically by waist circumference or the ratio of waist-to-hip circumference (WHR).[13] Studies show that the greatest incidence of cardiovascular disease for those over 50 was in

---

TABLE 4
Spectrum of Metabolic
Abnormalities Associated with
Visceral Adiposity

Decreased high density lipoprotein 2 levels
Decreased lipoprotein lipase activity
Glucose intolerance
Hypertriglyceridemia
Increased fasting plasma insulin levels
Increased hepatic triglyceride lipase activity
Increased low density lipoprotein levels
Increased very low density lipoprotein levels
Insulin resistance

---

men whose WHR was greater than 0.9 and in women greater than 0.8,[14] measured as the narrowest circumference of the torso between the lower rib and the iliac crest, divided by the widest circumference around the buttocks. Data collected from the Iowa Women's Health Study have shown higher WHR being strongly and positively associated with an increased risk of death.[15] A 12-year follow-up of a longitudinal study in Sweden of 1,462 women concluded that the WHR correlates with the 12-year incidence of myocardial infarction, stroke, and death.[16] Studies have shown that WHR is also predictive of diabetes in men[17] and CHD in both men and women.[18]

More recent studies, however, have suggested that the waist circumference alone is actually a better predictor of abdominal obesity as assessed by computerized tomography scans of the abdomen, and is a better way to follow changes in risk profile with weight gain or loss. For example, the WHR may decrease if either the waist circumference decreases *or* the hip circumference increases, and obviously only the first scenario would imply a more favorable body composition and metabolic profile have been achieved. The waist circumference which is associated with less than 100 cm^2 of abdominal fat by computerized tomography and a good cardiovascular risk profile in women over the age of 40 is 80 cm or less. Waist circumference measurements of greater than 90 cm are associated with abdominal fat areas of 150 cm^2 or more and a much higher risk of cardiovascular disease in both men and women.[12]

WEIGHT CHANGES WITH AGE IN WOMEN

TRENDS IN BODY WEIGHT

Although body composition begins to change in the 30s, such trends are accelerated at the time of menopause, when decreases in muscle and bone and increases in fat mass and body weight tend to occur simultaneously. In addition to the obvious hormonal changes in the years preceding the menopause and afterward, this is also a time when physical activity levels may decline as well, compounding the body composition shifts attributable to age and the waning influence of estrogen. After the menopause, women begin to resemble men in their increasing prevalence of the syndromes of central obesity, hypertension, hyperlipidemia, insulin resistance, and cardiovascular morbidity and mortality. Thus, even if body weight does not change greatly during the perimenopausal years, the indicators of unfavorable shifts in body composition should be screened for and steps taken as prophylaxis against these risks to health.

PREVALENCE OF OBESITY IN OLDER WOMEN

Using the definition of overweight as a BMI of greater than 27 kg/m^2, approximately 27% of women between the ages of 20 and 74 years in the U.S. are overweight.[19] If these women are divided into 10-year age groups, the prevalence increases with age, with the peak prevalence of 38.5% occurring in 65–74 year olds. Approximately one in nine women falls into the severely overweight category overall (BMI > 32.3 kg/m^2), and again the peak prevalence of about one in seven is seen in the older age bracket.

Similarly, absolute and relative body fat has been shown to increase with age in women, with values ranging from 25 to 35% in some studies.[20] However, due to the differences in methodologies used and the differential risk attributable depending on the distribution of fat, it has not been possible yet to define an *ideal* level for percent body fat at various ages which is linked to mortality. Until such data emerge, it is suggested that efforts be focused clinically on assessment and appropriate management of regional fat distribution, particularly if associated with obesity-related syndromes and metabolic profiles.

CAUSES OF OBESITY IN OLDER WOMEN

Obesity occurs when there is an imbalance of energy requirements and intake, such that dietary fat is stored in an enlarging adipose tissue pool rather than oxidized for fuel. Changes in energy requirements with age are part of the etiology. There are three main components of energy expenditure: the thermic effect of food, resting metabolic rate (RMR), and physical activity. Of these, RMR and physical activity appear to have the greatest influence on the change in energy requirements with age, and differences in physical activity levels between individuals are most closely related to differences in levels of body fat.[21,22] In women, the decline in RMR is most notable around the age of 50, at the time of menopause. This may be due in part to the elimination of the energy expenditure for menstrual function,[23] which has been estimated to reduce energy expenditure by about 15,000 to 20,000 calories per year.[24] With all other caloric intakes and outputs remaining the same, this would contribute a 4 to 6 pound weight gain over one year. However, the primary reason for the decline in RMR is the loss of fat-free weight (FFW), which in turn is partially accounted for by decreased physical activity levels as well as reduced estrogen and androgen levels after menopause. Therefore, increasing or maintaining physical activity levels in older women may play a crucial role in preserving energy expenditure directly, as well as by attenuating the decline of RMR due to loss of muscle mass.

On the other side of the energy balance equation, caloric intake may increase in older women despite declining needs for a multitude of reasons. Among older women, common psychosocial reasons given include stimulation (to give a lift or keep from slowing down) or as a way of dealing with negative emotions, such as anger and depression.[25] Another reason may be the intake of prescription drugs that can increase the appetite, such as tricyclic antidepressants, thyroid medication, insulin, and corticosteroids. Additionally, the ability to regulate food intake to match energy requirements precisely appears to be altered with age, and this mismatch may result in expansion of the adipose tissue mass.[26]

RISKS ASSOCIATED WITH OBESITY IN OLDER WOMEN

The health implications of obesity as women age are substantial. Obesity is linked to numerous chronic diseases that can lead to premature illness and death. Cardiovascular disease (CVD) remains the leading cause of death in the U.S., with almost 66 million Americans affected. There is a strong association between the prevalence of obesity and CVD risk factors. Obesity has been associated with hypertension and elevated systolic blood pressure in 50 to 75 year olds,[27] which may in turn be associated with hyperinsulinemia.[28] The National Health and Nutrition Examination Survey, which included 11,864 men and women during 1976 to 1980, found that being overweight (BMI > 28 kg/m^2) was associated with an increased risk of developing hypertension, diabetes, and hypercholesterolemia.[29] Hypertension affects almost three times as many overweight as normal weight people, and weight loss is an effective modality for reducing blood pressure if it can be sustained over time.

A number of studies have shown that the risk of developing CVD increases with the level of blood cholesterol, which increases substantially in women after menopause, particularly if their obesity is visceral, and if they are not on hormone replacement therapy. This increase in cholesterol appears to be more closely related to obesity than age, as weight loss can significantly lower lipid levels in this population.[30]

In postmenopausal women, a positive relationship has been noted between body weight and breast cancer.[31] For every pound a woman gains after age 30, her risk of breast cancer goes up more than 1%. While this may initially sound trivial, gaining ten pounds after age 30 raises breast cancer risk by 12%, 15 pounds by 19%, and 20 pounds by 26%. On the other hand, losing 10 pounds or more may drop breast cancer risk by 45%.

For women with osteoarthritis, obesity is not only etiologic in the degenerative changes of the weight-bearing joints, but it is associated with mobility impairment and functional difficulties on its own,[32] and worsens the disability of arthritis.[33] Conversely, weight loss has been shown to reduce the symptoms associated with knee osteoarthritis in women.[34]

Sleep-disordered breathing has been associated with obesity in older people, and although more common in men, increases in prevalence after the menopause in women.[35] A study by Grunstein and associates demonstrated that sleep apnea was strongly associated with a central pattern of obesity in men. It was noticed that as the severity of sleep apnea increased so did the subjects' body mass index and waist-to-hip ratio.[36] As discussed in Chapter 20, sleep apnea is a morbid condition which can cause fatal machine and traffic accidents, cardiac arrthymias, morning headaches, and daytime fatigue, among other symptoms.[37] Weight loss is one of the effective treatments for obstructive sleep apnea.

Although obesity and non-insulin-dependent diabetes mellitus (NIDDM) are not thought to be genetically linked, they clearly are related in the population. Approximately 80 to 90% of individuals with NIDDM are obese.[13] Central obesity poses a much greater risk than generalized obesity in this regard. As with many other conditions mentioned above, weight loss, particularly if it decreases visceral adipose tissue stores, is a potent tool in the treatment of NIDDM and should always be the first line of treatment.

ASSESSMENT OF THE NEED TO INTERVENE

With all of the information about obesity, weight guidelines, and other health-related risk factors, it can still be difficult to know in some cases if an older woman needs to lose weight. The series of questions in Table 5 may help assess the severity of the risk associated with her body weight and the urgency of intervention. If weight or BMI is elevated, and in addition, the answer is Yes to at least one other question in Table 5, weight loss may be beneficial. If weight and anthropometric indices of body fat are within the healthy range, yet the woman desires to lose weight for other reasons such as improved appearance or sense of well-being, the decision to lose weight should take into account the difficulty of the task as well as the potential adverse physical and psychological effects of weight loss regimens. These effects include the risk of poor nutrition (micronutrient, mineral, or protein deficiencies) and the some-times serious psychological consequences of repeated failed attempts to lose weight.

In addition, weight cycling, or the repeated loss and gain of weight which is a common syndrome in the repetitive or chronic dieter, can have a negative effect on long-term weight management. There is evidence that with each weight cycle the metabolic rate is decreased, thereby taking the dieter longer to lose weight and less time to regain weight.[38] Hypocaloric diets are associated not only with reduced basal energy expenditure, but also a reduction in the thermic effect of feeding, and often reduced energy expenditure in physical activity, and all of these effects will tend to attenuate the energy deficit meant to be introduced via caloric restriction. When the energy balance alterations due to repeated dieting are superimposed on the lowered basal metabolic rate seen with aging, as is the case in the postmenopausal woman, the rate of weight loss may be slowed down even further. The other adverse conse-quence of dieting is that weight loss is composed of both fat and lean tissue, including bone and muscle. Women in the postmenopausal years are losing lean tissue anyway, and this accelerated loss of lean tissue may increase the risk of osteoporosis, mobility impairment, and functional decline. Weight cycling is associated with mortality in women at all weight ranges, lean to obese.

TREATMENT OF OBESITY IN OLDER WOMEN

Of the Americans trying to lose weight, most are women.[39] The peak age group of women trying to lose weight is 40 to 49 years, with fewer women attempting weight

TABLE 5
Assessing the Need for Weight or Fat Loss in the Older Woman

Factor	Yes	No
Weight for height above the range of Table 1 or BMI > 27 kg/m^2		
Age < 70 years		
History of > 10 lb weight gain since reaching adult height		
Triceps skinfold above the normal range for age		
Waist-to-hip ratio more than 0.8 or waist circumference more than 80 cm		
Hypertension present (> 140/90 mm Hg)		
Elevated total cholesterol (> 240 mg/dl)		
Type II diabetes mellitus, glucose intolerance, or insulin resistance present		
Symptomatic osteoarthritis of weight-bearing joints present		
Sleep disordered breathing diagnosed		
Family history of CVD, Type II diabetes, or breast cancer		
Sedentary lifestyle		
Current smoker		

loss with increasing age. Thus, most treatments of obesity are geared toward premenopausal women, not taking into account the changing nutritional and physical needs with age. It is therefore important when designing or choosing a program that age-specific needs are addressed.

For most weight loss methods, there are few scientific studies that indicate long-term success. Success rates can be expected to vary according to initial weight, the length of the weight loss period, the magnitude of weight loss desired, and the motivation for wanting to lose weight. A fundamental principle for losing weight is the commitment to a lifelong change in lifestyle, behavioral responses, and dietary practices.

TYPES OF WEIGHT LOSS PROGRAMS

Weight loss programs vary in intensity and scientific basis from the latest do-it-yourself diet book to hospitalization, and the decision about which type of program to recommend is critical if healthful weight management is the ultimate goal. It is of utmost importance that the program chosen match appropriate weight-loss goals and that the older woman is a reasonable candidate for such a method of weight loss. The basic categories of treatment available are outlined below.

"Do-It-Yourself" Programs

This type of program includes those which individuals start on their own, including personal methods (no desserts, no alcohol), diet books and products, and community-based programs (e.g., Overeaters Anonymous™ and Take Off Pounds Sensibly™). The methods vary and are not normally tailored to individual health risks and needs. If someone is highly motivated and otherwise healthy, this method is a reasonable choice. However, as there are some diet books which, without scientific evidence, advocate imbalanced and/or unsustainable radical changes in dietary composition as a means to quick weight loss, it is a good idea to review the basic premise of such plans before supporting the woman in her choice. Be wary of programs that advertise losses of greater than one pound per week, as faster rates of loss are rarely sustainable lifestyle choices in the long term, and may result in the metabolically dangerous practice of weight cycling mentioned above.

Nonclinical Programs

These include the popular and commercially franchised programs such as Jenny Craig™, NutriSystem™, and Weight Watchers™. They often use instructional and guidance materials that are prepared by health-care professionals, yet are provided by variably trained counsellors. If someone has tried do-it-yourself programs and failed because of lack of guidance and support, this may be an appropriate choice, because of the built-in system of behavioral reinforcement based on social-cognitive theory. Some programs offer a health evaluation before enrolling participants, while others do not or include only a cursory assessment. It is a good idea to reinforce these programs with a clinical assessment of the current health profile, metabolic factors related to obesity, and risks for obesity-related diseases in the individual about to embark on such a program. In that way, the health-care professional can reinforce the goals of the weight loss program with evidence of clinical improvements accompanying changes in body weight or fat.

Clinical Programs

This type of program is conducted by a licensed professional who may or may not have received special training to treat obese patients. The programs may or may not be part of a commercial franchise. They include such services as nutrition, medical care, behavior therapy, exercise, and psychological counselling, and may utilize very-low-calorie diets, medications, inpatient treatment, and dental wiring or gastric stapling or bypass surgery in a small subset of refractory cases. If a woman is morbidly obese, or has serious health problems related to obesity (poorly controlled diabetes or coronary disease, sleep apnea associated with cardiac arrthymias, etc.) clinical status may need to be monitored during weight loss, and this type of program may be required during the initial phases of treatment.

IMPORTANT COMPONENTS OF A WEIGHT LOSS/MANAGEMENT PROGRAM

Regardless of the specific type of program chosen, there are five areas that should be addressed in any valid and reputable weight loss/management program, as indicated below.

Assessment of Physical Health and Psychological Status

Particularly if a woman is considering a do-it-yourself or nonclinical program to lose weight, she should have some basic knowledge about her overall state of health before beginning. Practitioners should, therefore, review the health history and provide a physical examination to such clients, with particular attention to conditions that may be related to obesity and age, or may be aggravated by weight loss or sudden change in diet or physical activity patterns, such as insulin or antihypertensive drug timing and dosages, bone density, or cardiopulmonary symptoms. Very rapid weight loss associated with diuresis may cause postural hypotension and falls, water-soluble drug toxicity, renal impairment, electrolyte imbalances, or mental status changes including fatigue, irritability, and delirium. Such issues as tooth or mouth problems, medication use, or being limited in the ability to shop, cook, or feed oneself independently may make it difficult for women to follow certain weight loss programs, and advice regarding the likelihood of success and safety should be given when such problems are identified during assessment. Identification and treatment of serious psychological issues such as drug and alcohol dependency, obsessive-compulsive personality disorder, depression, and eating disorders are vital as these problems may co-exist with or be a contributing factor to obesity in older women, and should be dealt with directly by health-care professionals prior to non-clinical treatment of the symptom of obesity itself.

Diet

The best diet plans are those that offer a new way of eating for a lifetime, not just during the time of weight loss. Programs that promise results without a change in energy intake and physical activity patterns will not promote long-term success. A good diet plan should have at least 1200 calories a day and contain 100% of the RDAs for vitamins and minerals. It should also contain adequate protein to limit the loss of lean body mass which accompanies hypocaloric dieting. Calorie intakes of less than 1200 calories a day may not meet micronutrient requirements of older women and a dietary supplement may be needed. Diets of less than 800 calories per day should not be used except under a doctor's supervision. Special attention should also be given to age-specific nutritional needs, such as calcium and fluid intake, as discussed in Chapters 8 and 21, respectively.

Dietary guidelines that are common to all Americans should remain as the goal of a good weight management program, within the context of creating an energy deficit by a combination of decreased energy intake and increased energy expenditure. Specifically, the guidelines, as shown in Table 6 are a combination of the recommendations by the American Heart Association[40] and the National Research Council.[41]

Ideally, adherence to these guidelines provides approximately the following dietary composition daily:

$\leq 30\%$ calories from fat;
$< 10\%$ calories from saturated fat;
up to 10% polyunsaturated fat;
< 300 mg. cholesterol;
$\geq 55\%$ calories from total carbohydrates; and
the remainder of calories from protein not to exceed twice the RDA.

TABLE 6
Dietary Guidelines During Weight Loss Programs

Dietary Component	Number of Servings per Day
Vegetables	3–5
Fruits	2–4
Cereals, breads, rice and pasta	6–11
Low-fat milk, yogurt, and cheese	2–3
Meat, poultry, fish, and legumes	≤ 6
Alcohol	< 1 Drink = 12 oz. beer, 5 oz. wine, or 1 1/2 oz. of distilled spirits (80 proof)

In addition to these guidelines being recommended by the AHA and NRC, the percentages of calories from fat and carbohydrate serve another purpose. Calorie for calorie, dietary fat may be more efficiently converted to adipose tissue than is carbohydrate during metabolism.[42,43] An emphasis on foods high in carbohydrate and low in fat will therefore assist with the goal of reducing body fat during weight loss. However, it should be kept in mind that a change in dietary composition itself, without an energy deficit leading to weight loss, will not lead to a loss of body fat, improvement in lipid levels, or better glucose regulation,[44] and therefore the primary role of dietary fat restriction, since it is the most calorically dense part of the diet, is to promote the achievement of an energy imbalance, with expenditure exceeding intake.

One pound of weight loss is theoretically produced by a 3500-calorie deficit. Therefore, a 500-calorie deficit from usual intake should produce a one pound per week weight loss, and a 1000-calorie deficit should produce a 2-lb per week weight loss. With the addition of regular exercise, the rate of weight loss would increase, due to an even larger caloric deficit. Weight loss should be limited to no more than two pounds per week, since a rate beyond this may produce a greater loss of lean mass than fat, and is largely unsustainable in the long term, leading to extremely high recidivism rates and thereby weight cycling. Rates of weight loss will be different from person to person, so calorie deficit prescriptions may need to be refined beyond these general guidelines.

Physical Activity

In a 1988 policy statement, the Council on Scientific Affairs of the American Medical Association stated that the most beneficial way to lose weight is to both increase caloric expenditure through exercise and to decrease caloric intake.[45] The Council further stated that diet, exercise, and behavior modification are interdependent and mutually supportive, and a comprehensive weight-reduction program that incorporates all three components is the most likely to lead to long-term weight control. The scientific rationale underlying these exercise recommendations is reviewed below, followed by the specifics of an exercise plan designed to treat obesity.

Rationale for the Use of Exercise in the Treatment of Obesity

Aerobic Exercise

There are, in fact, no randomized controlled trials using aerobic exercise as an isolated treatment for obesity in the elderly. Until such data are generated, studies in young and middle-aged adults must be used to derive guidelines for older women. In one of the earliest uncontrolled series, Gwinup reported[46] that 34 subjects started an exercise intervention of at least 30 minutes per day of walking and were followed for one to two years. Only 11 subjects aged 19 to 41 years (all women) were able to comply with the study requirements, and among them, weight loss averaged 22 lb with apparently no concurrent dietary restriction. The exercise regimens actually performed by 9 of these 11 women, however, were 2 to 3 hours of walking 7 d/wk. Thus, the practicality of this approach seems limited, particularly for older or frailer adults.

In a more recent study of middle-aged obese women, Despres found that aerobic exercise resulted in reductions in abdominal adipose tissue as well as the ratio of subcutaneous abdominal to thigh fat,[47] indicating preferential losses of central adiposity, just as has been seen after aerobic exercise in non-obese older adults.[48,49] Thus, the undesirable body composition changes associated with the perimenopausal and postmenopausal years are apparently amenable to changes in physical activity patterns.

In summary, there is no evidence to date from randomized clinical trials in obese elderly that aerobic exercise without dietary restriction can significantly lower body weight, percent body fat, or lipid profiles, with meta-analyses from general populations suggesting a 1 to 2 kg loss of body weight on average across all studies using exercise as the sole means of weight loss. Other reasons to advocate such exercise in this population, however, include increases in aerobic fitness[50] and insulin sensitivity[51] which may occur independently of weight loss in the elderly, as well as evidence that compliance with dietary restrictions may be better in those who are concurrently exercising.

In one such study at Stanford University, a one year exercise program was compared to a one-year diet intervention program to determine the effects of exercise or diet on weight loss and cholesterol levels in middle-aged men and women.[52] The results of the study indicated that although a significant amount of weight was lost in both groups the weight loss was greatest in the diet alone group as has been seen in many other studies. However, when the body composition data were analyzed, it was noted that the two groups lost the same amount of fat tissue. The difference was that the diet group lost a significant amount of lean body tissue and the exercise group lost no lean body tissue. In addition, both groups had significant increases in high density lipoproteins and decreases in triglyceride levels. One year follow-up data indicated the exercise group had been the most successful in not gaining back the weight that had been lost during the study.[53] This indicates that exercise is important not so much for the extra weight lost (if any) during the treatment period but for the fact that at follow-up there appears to be less weight cycling in individuals who have established exercise programs.

Resistance Training

Although aerobic exercise has been most often studied in relation to obesity, resistance training studies in the healthy elderly suggest favorable shifts in energy balance which may be important in weight loss. Campbell has reported that total energy requirements for weight maintenance are increased approximately 15% after 12 weeks of resistance training in older men and women, primarily due to increases in RMR.[54] Treuth has also described increased resting energy expenditure and fat oxidation after resistance training in postmenopausal women.[55] Over the long term, such acute adaptations may significantly affect energy balance and contribute to the maintenance of a healthful body weight while minimizing fat deposition.

There are no trials yet of resistance training as an isolated intervention to induce weight loss in obese older adults. However, tolerance to resistance training is likely significantly better than to weight-bearing endurance training in obese individuals with lower extremity arthritis because of associated pain, mobility impairment, and exacerbation of underlying joint symptoms.[56,57] The lower cardiovascular stimulation of resistance training as compared to aerobic training may also be of benefit in obese elders with many cardiovascular risk factors, overt cardiac disease, or diabetes.

Treuth and colleagues examined the effects of a total body strength training program on changes in total and regional body composition with emphasis on intra-abdominal adipose tissue in older women. There were no changes in body weight. However, there were significant reductions in intra-abdominal adipose tissue (143.9 ± 13.3 vs. 130.0 ± 12.4 cm^2) in addition to a reduction in midthigh adipose tissue (141.7 ± 11.5 vs. 133.6 ± 10.8 cm^2).[58] Thus, even without change in total body weight, resistance training has been shown to significantly improve regional fat deposition in older women, which should improve metabolic profiles associated with central obesity.

The Interaction of Exercise and Dietary Modification

Most major reviews would suggest that exercise alone exerts only modest effects on body weight and fat mass, particularly in women. For example, in a meta-analysis of 89 studies involving 1800 Type II diabetics conducted over the past 30 years, diet alone had a significantly greater effect on weight loss (9 kg) and glycosolated hemoglobin levels, compared to mean losses of 3.8 kg in exercise, diet, and behavioral interventions.[59] In another meta-analysis of 53 studies (up to 36 weeks in duration), Ballor reported that in men, aerobic exercise resulted in an average loss of 1.2 kg of body weight compared to a 1.2 kg gain in weight lifting studies.[60] Body fat decreased regardless of exercise modality, by 1.5 kg (1.7%) compared to controls. Weight training was significantly better at increasing FFM compared to walking/jogging studies. In women, only walking/jogging resulted in a decrease in body weight (0.6 kg) compared to controls, as well as significant reductions in body fat (1.3 kg, 1.7%) and no change in FFM. Weight and fat loss was greatest in those with high body fat initially and the highest exercise-related energy expenditure. The gender differences seen in these studies may relate to the higher energy cost of equivalent activities in men due to their greater body mass.[61] Overall, substantial changes in body mass would seem to require dietary modification.

However, hypocaloric dieting alone, although effective if adhered to in creating an energy deficit and therefore loss of body weight and fat, has undesirable consequences in the elderly, including exacerbation of age-related losses of lean tissue, decreased metabolic rate, and risk for micronutrient deficiencies. Reduction in resting energy expenditure secondary to dieting may be prevented or attenuated by concurrent exercise.[62] Aerobic exercise may attenuate the losses of FFM which account for 10–50% of weight lost by hypocaloric dieting.[63]

Both endurance and resistance training are associated with increased energy expenditure through the cost of activity, increased basal metabolic rate, increased thermic effect of a meal, and increased lean body mass (primarily resistance), and can induce small losses of body weight and total fat as well mobilization of fat from abdominal sites in older men and women.

It makes sense, therefore, that a combination of diet and exercise modalities in obese individuals may produce the largest losses of weight while attaining more desirable body composition ratios and metabolic profiles than either treatment alone. Additionally, the increase in aerobic fitness and/or strength itself has many physiologic and psychological consequences which cannot be achieved by dieting alone and may enhance long-term behavioral adaptations to minimize weight cycling.

Although theoretically advantageous, as noted above, the combination of diet and aerobic exercise for the purposes of weight loss in obese elderly has so far only been tested in two non-randomized studies reported in this population. Dengel[64,65] studied obese 60-year-old men who were nonrandomly assigned by preference to 10 months of hypocaloric dieting and behavioral modification, diet plus aerobic exercise, or a control group which received brief dietary instructions only. Results were presented only for those subjects who completed the study and lost at least 3 kg (in the case of experimental groups). Thus, 33% of the diet group, 62% of the diet plus exercise, and 57% of controls were analyzed. Weight loss averaged 8 to 9 kg, body fat decreased by approximately 5%, and FFM by 1 to 2 kg by underwater weighing, with no difference between treatment groups. Fat-free mass loss was directly related to the change in total body weight in both groups. There was no difference in lipid lowering effects of the interventions. Thus, no additional benefit to weight loss, body composition, lipid profile, or fat distribution was attributable to exercise. However, it should be noted from the perspective of clinical relevance that more than twice as many exercisers as dieters achieved the minimum study goal (loss of 3 kg), one of the most important findings of this study.

In the only other such study of older subjects, Fox[66] reported that 41 healthy obese women of average age 66 years were non-randomly assigned to diet groups who reduced their intake by 500 or 700 kcal/d, or a diet plus aerobic and resistive exercise group with a combined deficit of 700 kcal/d.[66] After 24 weeks, weight loss (6.5 kg), body fat, lean body mass, and fasting glucose decreased similarly over time with all treatments.

In contrast to aerobic exercise, the primary purpose of combining weight lifting and diet in obese individuals is to stimulate accretion of lean mass in the face of an energy deficit. In the first such report, Ballor randomly assigned obese young women to diet, exercise, diet plus exercise, or control groups for 8 weeks.[67] Dieting significantly decreased body weight, arm fat area, circumferences, skinfolds, and fat mass.

Resistance training significantly increased arm muscle area, strength, lean body weight, and decreased percent body fat, and the combined therapy group ended up with a better body composition profile (increased lean, decreased fat) than either isolated intervention. Importantly, strict hypocaloric dieting (1000 kcal/day) did not appear to limit the functional adaptation or hypertrophy of muscle secondary to resistance training.

This potential benefit of resistance training was directly compared to aerobic training in obese older subjects. After 11 weeks of dieting, Ballor randomly allocated 18 older subjects to moderate intensity resistance or aerobic exercise training for an additional 12 weeks.[62] Weight remained stable in the weight lifters, as the decline in fat mass was more than replaced by a gain in FFM. By contrast, the endurance training group lost fat and FFM, which combined to produce a significant drop in total body weight. Thus, knowing that weight loss is occurring may be insufficient to judge the metabolic benefit of an intervention when divergent adaptations in fat and lean tissue are occurring.

In terms of energy expenditure, resistance training but not aerobic training was associated with a tendency to increase resting energy expenditure and the thermic effect of a meal in Ballor's study.[62] Thus, overall, more favorable body composition and energy balance changes could be attributed to resistance exercise than aerobic exercise in this study. In the long-term control of body weight, these body composition and resting energy expenditure adaptations seen with resistance training may be extremely important in minimizing the tendency for weight and fat to be regained after dieting.[68]

The Exercise Prescription for Obesity

Exercise is potentially beneficial for weight loss because it increases energy expenditure. All forms of exercise increase energy expenditure, with the greatest expenditure achieved during prolonged aerobic exercise. Low intensity, greater frequency, and longer duration activities are recommended for maximizing fat loss as they tend to require more energy and to utilize fat rather than carbohydrate stores as fuel during the activity,[22] and minimize orthopedic complications as they are less traumatic to joints than high intensity and high impact activities such as running. It is recommended that obese individuals move toward an initial goal of expending at least 300 calories per workout a minimum of three times per week to promote weight loss. Examples of a range of possible activities are given in Table 7.

Energy expenditure during exercise is dependent upon the individual's body weight, the duration of the exercise, and the intensity of the exercise. For example, if a 154-pound woman exercises on a cycle for 45 minutes at 50 watts and incorporates a 5-minute warm-up and cool-down program into the exercise session, the total energy expenditure during that time is approximately 230 kcal/session. However, if a 198-pound man exercises on a cycle for 45 minutes at 75 watts and incorporates the same warm-up and cool-down session into the exercise session, he will burn approximately 300 kcal/session.

Excess caloric expenditure which results from physical activity should lead to weight loss if caloric expenditure at other times remains constant. While there is

TABLE 7
Fat Loss Benefits of Various Exercises

Exercise	Fat Loss Potential	Calories Used[a]
Aerobic dance	High	325
Basketball	Moderate	350
Biking	High	325
Brisk walking	High	275
Cross-country skiing	High	350
Jogging	High	325
Rowing	High	325
Running	Moderate	325
Strength training	Low	210
Swimming	Moderate	340
Tennis/singles	Moderate	210

[a] Total calories (basal plus activity) burned in 30 minutes of continuous exercise by a person weighing 150 pounds.

From Fitness Wellness Maps, BlueCross BlueShield Brochure, Mosby-Great Performance, Inc., 1993–1995. With permission.

good evidence for such an effect in men, there is little evidence for a similar effect in women. Potential reasons for this irregularity could be smaller body size, lower aerobic capacity, differences in body fat distribution, and under-reporting of caloric intake. Nevertheless, regular exercise in women has many positive benefits on lipids, glucose homeostasis, and bone metabolism, even if weight loss does not occur as often as with men.[61]

As noted above, the evidence to support the use of exercise as an isolated treatment for obesity in older adults, and women in particular, is not convincing, which is why exercise is always recommended as part of a total plan which includes dietary modification. Fortunately, there is evidence that overweight subjects do not increase energy intake when involved in an exercise program. In two carefully controlled in-patient studies, Woo et al.[69,70] reported that when involved in an exercise program, normal weight people increase food intake as the level of energy expenditure increases so that weight is maintained. However, obese subjects who are involved in an exercise program do not naturally increase food intake to offset the increased energy expenditure and therefore, lose weight. These studies indicate that the appetite drive that is present for normal-weight individuals on an exercise program may not be functioning normally for overweight people. This lack of appetite drive during exercise in overweight individuals may be beneficial for long-term weight loss.

The energy expenditure goals related to exercise are to expend 1,100 to 2,100 extra calories per week in exercise. This amount of energy corresponds to 220 to 420 calories expended for each exercise session if a woman exercises five days a week, for example. This may occur during discreet, planned exercise events, as shown in Table 7, or by a generalized change in the pattern of daily activities and approach to physical exertion, as suggested in Tables 8 and 9. This change in physical activity level in conjunction with decreased energy in the diet should result in a weight loss of 1 to 2 pounds per week.

The goal of a weight loss program is threefold: 1) to lose weight and ultimately attain ideal body weight; 2) to preserve lean body tissue and lose predominantly fat mass, and preferentially visceral fat during the weight loss program; and 3) most important, to maintain the weight loss for the rest of the woman's life. Particularly for the last two goals, exercise appears to be essential to the treatment of obesity in older women.

TABLE 8
Ways to Improve Adherence to an Exercise Program

Make an appointment with a partner (dogs included!)
Make it part of a daily schedule
Make a commitment to a program or enroll in a club
Sign up for an event that requires training
Remember the good feeling that accompanies the completion of an exercise session
Set up environmental cues: alarm clock, walking shoes at the front door, tennis racket in the car, etc.
Set up rewards for meeting exercise goals: a massage, new walking shoes, etc.
Subscribe to a fitness magazine
Vary the exercise routine: try different forms of exercise, walk a new route, exercise at a different time of day

---

TABLE 9
Progressive Ways to Incorporate Physical Activity into Daily Routines

Sit instead of lying down
Stand instead of sitting
Walk instead of standing
Walk instead of driving short distances
Walk the dog, or volunteer to walk a friend's or neighbor's dog
Pick up walking pace if safe or add hills and inclines
Take the stairs instead of the elevator or escalator whenever possible
Park car at the farthest point in the parking lot
Park car a few blocks from final destination and walk
Get off the bus or subway one stop early and walk the rest of the way
Visit with friends or family on a walk
Take walks after dinner
Use coffee breaks at work to walk or climb stairs
Use airplane delays for a walk through the airport
Involve yourself in active hobbies: gardening, shuffle-board, etc.
Limit TV watching time; think of active alternatives
Watch TV only if exercising (weights, stretching, stationary cycling, callisthenics, etc.) at the same time
Keep a set of weights under the desk to use during breaks from reading or working on a computer

---

Soundness and Safety

Any reputable program in which a woman is enrolled should provide detailed information about any potential risks that could occur, since risks to health from weight loss vary with the individual and the type of program. Generally, the more restrictive the diet, the greater are the risks of adverse effects associated with weight loss. Assessment of not only change in weight, but also change in related health risks such as abdominal girth, blood pressure, sleep disturbance, cardiopulmonary symptoms, joint pain and mobility impairment, lipid levels, glucose homeostasis, and medication requirements, for example, should also be closely followed during the initiation and maintenance phase of the treatment program.

Outcomes

The most important feature of a successful weight loss program is maintenance of stable weight or of reduced weight, which is a dual responsibility of the woman and the program itself. To improve chances for success, women should choose a program that focuses on long-term weight management, provides instruction in healthful eating and increasing activity, and explains thoroughly the potential health risks from weight loss. In all cases, look for evidence that the program is successful; if information is absent or consists primarily of testimonials or other anecdotal evidence, the program should be viewed with suspicion.

The program should be devoted to helping the older woman change behaviors through information, guidance, and skills training. In do-it-yourself or nonclinical programs, women should have additional support from a health care practitioner who can monitor the status of any obesity-related conditions she may have and provide additional incentives to adherence.

PREVENTION OF OBESITY IN OLDER WOMEN

As the saying goes, "an ounce of prevention is worth a pound of cure." This cannot be more true than when it comes to obesity. Many women find that their weight has been slowly creeping up since reaching menopause, without any modifications in their lifestyle. It needs to be emphasized to older women that this *lack* of change in lifestyle in the face of significant changes in hormonal status, metabolic rate, and body composition may be precisely the problem. There are really only three ways of preventing obesity in the postmenopausal years: staying active, eating a balanced diet, and taking personal responsibility for one's health.

PHYSICAL ACTIVITY

Many of the changes in muscle mass, body fat, resting metabolic rate, and psychological well-being that occur as women age can be directly offset with regular exercise. For women who are already exercising, there may be a need to look at the type of exercises being done and how conducive they are to weight loss, as shown in Table 7. Even though strength training is listed as a low-fat loss modality of exercise, it is still an important part of an exercise program designed to prevent obesity. Since strength training increases muscle mass, RMR is increased, thereby enhancing weight loss efforts. In addition, the increasing strength allows longer participation in many aerobic activities, and may lessen the chance of injury during them as well. More detailed information on the specifics of strength training can be found in Chapter 2.

If lack of time, inconvenience, laziness, old habits, decreased motivation, or boredom become a problem, Table 8 provides some advice to provide motivation and prevent relapse, which is a common problem in any long-term lifestyle change. It should be remembered that if a person can sustain a new habit continuously for 6 months or more, the chance of it becoming a permanent lifestyle change is very high. Therefore, it makes sense to put a great deal of emphasis on motivational incentives and support in this critical first 6-month period, as described in more detail in Chapter 25.

In addition to a regular exercise program, it is also important to encourage older women to increase their day-to-day activity levels. Most overweight people did not get that way from eating too much, but from moving too little, not during exercise classes themselves, but during the other 23 hours of the day. Creating a more active lifestyle pattern, as shown in Table 9, is accessible to everyone, even those who are too ill or disabled to participate in vigorous exercise. If pursued on a daily basis, it can contribute substantially to a more desirable energy balance and promote weight and fat loss. Changes suggested should be gradually introduced, using the concept of shaping behavior in small, acceptable increments, rather than risking overall failure by attempting too many modifications at once.

A Balanced Diet

A balanced diet is no longer conceptualized as a square containing 4 food groups consumed in equal quantities, but rather a pyramid of increasing caloric density as it rises toward the peak. If one eats according to the USDA guidelines, from the *bottom* of the Food Pyramid, you will be able to eat a larger volume of food, yet consume less calories since the foods on the bottom of the pyramid are either low or lacking in fat. The sample menus in Table 10, one utilizing the Food Pyramid and the other a typical American dinner, illustrate the important differences in dietary composition and energy intake resulting from each approach. Chapter 24 provides more details on the Food Pyramid guidelines that are relevant to both prevention of obesity as well as general health and well-being in the older woman.

Encouraging Personal Responsibility

A third yet often forgotten way to prevent obesity is to advocate personal responsibility for health as a woman ages, as much of what needs to be done falls outside of the realm of the current health care system's direct reach. However, practitioners can use the principles of behavioral change to assist with this process. Lifetime patterns are not easy to change, so behavior modification works by giving the dieter new patterns for life, not just during weight loss. The most important reason for employing such techniques is that it puts the responsibility for weight loss in the

TABLE 10
The Food Pyramid Meal Plan

Food Pyramid Dinner	Typical American Dinner
1 cup pasta	
2 ounces lean ground meat	8 ounce steak
$^1/_2$ cup spaghetti sauce	baked potato
1 slice french bread	1 slice french bread
2 cups romaine lettuce	$^1/_2$ cup green beans
1 carrot	
$^1/_4$ cup sliced mushrooms	
1 cup skim milk	1 cup 2% milk
2 tablespoons fat-free salad dressing	$^1/_4$ cup sour cream
1 cup chocolate frozen yogurt	1 cup chocolate ice cream

Analysis:	Calories	% Fat
Food Pyramid	815	23
Typical American	1426	50

hands of the dieter, not the program or the instructor. With guidance, the dieter makes his/her own choices for the most appropriate weight loss techniques. Methods of intervention are introduced gradually to not only increase the dieter's control, but provide the changes in easy stages. The components of behavior modification most identified with successful weight loss include self-monitoring (e.g., counting calories, keeping food and exercise diaries, charting weight loss) and regular exercise.

REFERENCES

1. Kuczmarski, R., Flegal, K., Campbell, S., and Johnson, C., Increasing prevalence of overweight among U.S. adults: national health and nutrition examination surveys, 1960 to 1991, *JAMA*, 272, 205–211, 1994.

2. Van Itallie, T., Health implications of overweight and obesity in the United States, *Ann. Intern. Med.*, 103, 983–988, 1985.

3. Institute of Medicine, Weighing the Options: Criteria for Evaluating Weight Management Programs, in Thomas, P., Ed., National Academy Press, Washington, D.C., 1995, 225.

4. Bray, G., Obesity: Part 1 - Pathogenesis, *West. J. Med.*, 149, 429–441, 1988.

5. Morley, J., Obesity, in *Geriatric Nutrition: A Comprehensive Review*, Morley, J., Glick, Z., and Rubenstein, L., Eds., Raven Press, New York, 293–306, 1990.

6. Owen, O., Resting metabolic requirements of men and women, *Mayo Clin. Proc.*, 63, 503–510, 1988.

7. Andres, R., Elahi, D., Tobin, J., Muller, D., and Brant, C., Impact of age on weight goals, *Ann. Intern. Med.*, 103, 1030–1033, 1985.

8. Andres, R., Mortality and obesity: the rationale for age-specific height-weight tables, in *Principles of Geriatric Medicine*, Andres, R., Bierman, E. L., and Hazzard, W. R., Eds., McGraw-Hill, New York, 1985.

9. Willett, W., Manson, J., Stampfer, M., Colditz, G., Rosner, B., Speizer, F. et al., Weight, weight change, and coronary heart disease in women, *JAMA*, 273, 461–465, 1995.

10. National Cancer Institute. Diet, Nutrition, and Cancer Prevention: A Guide to Food Choices, National Institutes of Health, Public Health Service, U.S. Department of Health and Human Services, U.S. Government Printing Office, Washington, D.C., 1987.

11. Nieman, D., *Body Composition Measurement. The Sports Medicine Fitness Course*, Bull Publishing, Palo Alto, CA, 1986, 107.

12. Despres, J.-P., Body fat distribution, exercise and nutrition: Implications for prevention of atherogenic dyslipidemia, coronary heart disease, and non-insulin dependent diabetes mellitus, in *Perspectives in Exercise Science and Sports Medicine: Exercise, Nutrition and Weight Control*, Vol. 11, Lamb, D. and Murray, R., Eds., Cooper Publishing Group, Carmel, IN, 107–150, 1998.

13. Kissebah, A. and Krakower, G., Regional adiposity and morbidity, *Physio. Rev.*, 74, 761–811, 1994.

14. Bray, G., Pathophysiology of obesity, *Am. J. Clin. Nutr.*, 55, 488S–494S, 1992.

15. Folsom, A., Kay, S., and Sellers, T., Body fat distribution and 5-year risk of death in older women, *JAMA*, 269, 483–487, 1993.

16. Lapidus, L., Bengtsson, C., Larsson, B., Pennert, K., Rybo, E., and Sjostrom, L., Distribution of adipose tissue and risk of cardiovascular disease and death: a 12-year follow-up of participants in the population study of women in Gothenburg, Sweden, *Br. Med. J.*, 289, 1257–1261, 1984.

17. Ohlson, L., Larsson, B., Svardsudd, K., Welin, L., Eriksson, H., Wilhelmsen, L. et al., The influence of body fat distribution on the incidence of diabetes mellitus: 13.5 years of follow-up of the participants in the study of men born in 1913, *Diabetes*, 34, 1055–1058, 1984.

18. Lapidus, L., Bengtsson, C., Hallstrom, T., and Bjorntorp, P., Obesity, adipose tissue distribution and health - results from a population study Gothenburg, Sweden, *Appetite*, 12, 25–35, 1989.

19. National Center for Health Statistics, Anthropometric Reference Data and Prevalence of Overweight, United States, 1976–80, in Office UGP, ed., Vol. 87–1688. Department of Health and Human Services, Washington, D.C., 1987.

20. Friis-Hansen, B., Hygrometry of growth and aging, *Symp. Soc. Hum. Biol.*, 7, 191–209, 1965.

21. Roberts, S. B., Fuss, P., Evans, W. J., Heyman, M. B., and Young, V. R., Energy expenditure, aging and body composition, *J. Nutr.*, 123, 474–480, 1993.

22. Melby, C., Commerford, R., and Hill, J., Exercise, macronutrient balance, and weight control, in *Perspectives in Exercise Science and Sports Medicine: Exercise, Nutrition, and Weight Control*, Vol. 11, Lamb, D. and Murray, R., Eds., Cooper Publishing Group, Carmel, IN, 1998, 1–60.

23. Heymsfield, S., Menopausal changes in body composition and energy expenditure, *Exper. Gerontol.*, 29, 377–389, 1994.

24. Ferraro, R., Lower sedentary metabolic rate in women compared to men, *Am. J. Clin. Nutr.*, 90, 780–784, 1992.

25. Guinn, B., Relationships of emotional motivators for eating and body fatness among elderly individuals living in recreational vehicle parks, *J. Am. Dietet. Assoc.*, 91, 978–979, 1991.

26. Roberts, S. B., Fuss, P., Heyman, M. B., Evans, W. J., Tsay, R., Rasmussen, H. et al., Control of food intake in older men, *JAMA*, 272, 1601–1606, 1994.

27. Garn, S. et al., Effects of skinfold levels on lipids and blood pressure in younger and older adults, *J. Gerontol.*, 43, M170–174, 1988.

28. Coon, P. J., Bleecker, E. R., Drinkwater, D. T., Meyers, D. A., and Goldberg, A. P., Effects of body composition and exercise capacity on glucose tolerance, insulin, and lipoprotein lipids in healthy older men: a cross-sectional and longitudinal intervention study, *Metabol.: Clin. Exper.*, 38, 1201–1209, 1989.

29. Najjar, M. and Rowland, M., Anthropometric Reference Data and Prevalence of Overweight: National Center for Health Statistics, 1987.

30. Tremblay, A., Normalization of the metabolic profile in obese women by exercise and a low fat diet, *Med. Sci. Sports Exerc.*, 23, 1326–1331, 1991.

31. Kissebah, A., Health risks of obesity (review), *Med. Clin. North Am.*, 73, 111–138, 1989.

32. Harris, T., Kovar, G. M., Suzman, R., Kleinman, J. C., and Feldman, J. J., Longitudinal study of physical ability in the oldest-old, *Am. J. Public Health*, 79, 698–702, 1989.

33. Morley, J. and Glick, Z., Obesity. Geriatric Nutrition: A Comprehensive Review. Raven Press, New York, 1990.

34. Felson, D., Weight loss reduces the risk of symptomatic knee osteoarthritis in women, *Ann. Int. Med.*, 116, 535–539, 1992.

35. Bliwise, D., Risk factors for sleep disordered breathing in heterogeneous geriatric population, *J. Am. Geriatr. Soc.*, 35, 132–141, 1987.

36. Grunstein, R., Wilcox, I., Yang, T., Gould, Y., and Hedner, J., Snoring and sleep apnoea in men: association with central obesity and hypertension, *Int. J. Obesity*, 17, 533–540, 1993.

37. Young, D., Haskell, W., and Jatulis, D., Association between changes in physical activity and risk factors for coronary heart disease in a community-based sample of men and women: the Stanford five-city project, *Am. J. Epidemiol.*, 138, 205–216, 1993.

38. Blackburn, G., Weight cycling: the experience of human dieters, *Am. J. Clin. Nutr.*, 49, 1989.

39. Williamson, D., Weight loss attempts in adults: goals, duration, and rate of weight loss, *Am. J. Pub. Health*, 82, 1251–1257, 1992.

40. Fletcher, G., Balady, G., Hartley, L., Haskell, W., and Pollock, M., Exercise standards. A statement for healthcare professionals from the American Heart Association, *Circulation*, 91, 580–616, 1995.

41. National Research Council. Recommended Dietary Allowances, National Academy of Sciences, Washington, D.C., 1989.

42. Danforth, E., Diet and obesity, *Am. J. Clin. Nutr.*, 41, 1132–1145, 1985.

43. Flatt, J., *Recent Advances in Obesity Research II*. The biochemistry of energy expenditure, Newman Publishing, London, 1978.

44. Hughes, V. A., Fiatarone, M. A., Ferrara, C. M., McNamara, J. R., Charnley, J. M., and Evans, W. J., Lipoprotein response to exercise training and a low-fat diet in older subjects with glucose intolerance, *Am. J. Clin. Nutr.*, 59, 820–826, 1994.

45. Council of Scientific Affairs. Treatment of obesity in adults, *JAMA*, 260, 2547–2551, 1988.

46. Gwinup, G., Effects of exercise alone on the weight of obese women, *Arch. Intern. Med.*, 135, 676–680, 1975.

47. Despres, J.-P., Pouliot, M., and Moorjani, S., Loss of abdominal fat and metabolic response to exercise training in obese women, *Am. J. Physiol.*, 24, E159–167, 1991.

48. Kohrt, W. M., Obert, K. A., and Holloszy, J. O., Exercise training improves fat distribution patterns in 60- to 70-year-old men and women, *J. Gerontology*, 47, M99–105, 1992.

49. Schwartz, R. S., Shuman, W. P., Larson, V., Cain, K. C., Fellingham, G. W., Beard, J. C. et al., The effect of intensive endurance exercise training on body fat distribution in young and older men, *Metabolism: Clin. Exper.*, 40, 545–551, 1991.

50. Ruoti, R. G., Troup, J. T., and Berger, R. A., The effects of nonswimming water exercises on older adults, *J. Orthop. Sports Phys. Ther.*, 19, 140–145, 1994.

51. Hersey, W. Cr., Graves, J. E., Pollock, M. L., Gingerich, R., Shireman, R. B., Heath, G. W. et al., Endurance exercise training improves body composition and plasma insulin responses in 70- to 79-year-old men and women, *Metabolism: Clin. Exper.*, 43, 847–854, 1994.

52. Wood, P. D., Stefanick, M., Dreon, D. M., Frey-Hewitt, B., Garay, S. C., Williams, P. T. et al., Changes in plasma lipids and lipoproteins in overweight men during weight loss through dieting as compared with exercise, *N. Engl. J. Med.*, 319, 1173–1179, 1988.

53. King, A., Frey-Hewitt, B., Dreon, D., and Wood, P., Diet vs. exercise in weight maintenance: the effects of minimal intervention strategies on long-term outcomes in men, *Arch. Intern. Med.*, 149, 2741–2746, 1989.

54. Campbell, W. W., Crim, M. C., Young, V. R., and Evans, W. J., Increased energy requirements and changes in body composition with resistance training in older adults, *Am. J. Clin. Nutr.*, 60, 167–175, 1994.

55. Treuth, M., Hunter, G., Weinsier, R., and Kell, S., Energy expenditure and substrate utilization in older women after strength training: 24-h calorimeter results, *J. Appl. Physiol.*, 78, 2140–2146, 1995.

56. Oddis, C. V., New perspectives on osteoarthritis, *Am. J. Med.*, 100, 10S-15S, 1996.

57. Mangione K. K., Axen, K., and Haas, F. Mechanical unweighting effects on treadmill exercise and pain in elderly people with osteoarthritis of the knee, *Phys. Ther.*, 76, 387–394, 1996.

58. Treuth, M., Hunter, G., Szabo, T., Weinsier, R., Goran, M., and Berland, L., Reduction in intra-abdominal adipose tissue after strength training in older women, *J. Appl. Physiol.*, 78, 1425–1431, 1995.

59. Brown, S., Upchurch, S., Anding, R., Winter, M., and Ramirez, G., Promoting weight loss in type II diabetes, *Diabetes Care*, 19, 613–624, 1996.

60. Ballor, D. and Keesey, R., A meta-analysis of the factors affecting exercise-induced changes in body mass, fat mass, and fat-free mass in males and females, *Int. J. Obesity*, 15, 717–726, 1991.

61. Gleim, G., Exercise is not an effective weight loss modality in women, *J. Am. Coll. Nutr.*, 12, 363–367, 1993.

62. Ballor, D. L., Harvey-Berino, J. R., Ades, P. A., Cryan, J., and Calles-Escandon, J., Contrasting effects of resistance and aerobic training on body composition and metabolism after diet-induced weight loss, *Metabolism: Clin. Exper.*, 45, 179–183, 1996.

63. Durrant, M., Garrow, J., Royston, P., Stalley, S., Sunkin, S., and Warwick, P., Factors influencing the composition of the weight lost by obese patients on a reducing diet, *Br. J. Nutr.*, 44, 275–285, 1980.

64. Dengel, D. R., Hagberg, J. M., Coon, P. J., Drinkwater, D. T., and Goldberg, A. P., Effects of weight loss by diet alone or combined with aerobic exercise on body composition in older obese men, *Metabolism: Clin. Exper.*, 43, 867–871, 1994.

65. Dengel, D. R., Hagberg, J. M., Coon, P. J., Drinkwater, D. T., and Goldberg, A. P., Comparable effects of diet and exercise on body composition and lipoproteins in older men, *Med. Sci. Sports Exerc.*, 26, 1307–1315, 1994.

66. Fox, A. A., Thompson, J. L., Butterfield, G. E., Gylfadottir, U., Moynihan, S., and Spiller, G., Effects of diet and exercise on common cardiovascular disease risk factors in moderately obese older women, *Am. J. Clin. Nutr.*, 63, 225–233, 1996.

67. Ballor, D. L., Katch, V. L., Becque, M. D., and Marks, C. R., Resistance weight training during caloric restriction enhances lean body weight maintenance, *Am. J. Clin. Nutr.*, 47, 19–25, 1988.

68. van Dale, D. and Saris, W., Repetitive weight loss and weight regain: effects on weight reduction, resting metabolic rate, and lipolytic activity before and after exercise and/or diet treatment, *Am. J. Clin. Nutr.*, 49, 409–416, 1989.

69. Woo, R. et al. Voluntary food intake during prolonged exercise in obese women, *Am. J. Clin. Nutr.*, 36, 478–484, 1982.

70. Woo, R., The effect of increasing physical activity on voluntary food intake and energy balance, *Int. J. Obes.*, 9, 155–160, 1985.

18 Osteoporosis

Jennifer E. Layne and Miriam E. Nelson

CONTENTS

INTRODUCTION

Osteoporosis is a disease characterized by low bone mass, excessive weakening of the bones and increased susceptibility to fractures, particularly of the hip, spine, and wrist. Osteoporosis literally means "porous bone," as pictured in Figure 1. More than 28 million Americans over the age of 65 are affected by osteoporosis; 10 million with osteoporosis and 18 million with bone loss called osteopenia. Eighty percent of those affected by osteoporosis are women.

Osteoporosis is a major public health problem with great economic and social costs. Osteoporosis is estimated to cause 1.5 million fractures annually in the United States in people aged 50 years and older. Over the age of 65 a woman has a one-in-three chance of fracturing her hip in her lifetime. Hip fractures alone cost the U.S. health care system $14 billion annually. Almost 50,000 people a year die from complications associated with hip fractures. Fear of injury is also devastating and often causes people with osteoporosis to become inactive or homebound and results in isolation from friends and family and a loss of independence.

Osteoporosis is a serious medical condition that is painful, can result in physical limitations, and is a major cause of loss of mobility, nursing home placement, and excess mortality. There are actions which can be taken at many stages of life to help decrease a woman's risk of developing osteoporosis and to prevent further deterioration of the skeleton. Prevention and treatment of osteoporosis include understanding some basic facts about bone physiology and body composition followed by meaningful lifestyle changes with respect to physical activity and nutrition, and in some cases pharmacologic intervention as well.

BONE PHYSIOLOGY

There are 206 bones that make up the skeleton of the human body. The skeleton provides the basic structure of our bodies. It serves as a framework to which our muscles are attached. When muscles contract they transmit both mechanical and electromagnetic forces to the bones to which they are directly attached by tendons. The skeleton gives us the capacity for upright locomotion, as well as protecting internal organs including the heart, lungs, stomach, and brain.

Bones are primarily made up of calcium, protein in the form of collagen fibers, and other minerals. There are two different types of bone tissue: trabecular bone and cortical bone. Approximately 80% of the skeleton is cortical bone, with the remaining 20% being made up of trabecular bone. All bones have both types of tissue; however, some bones are predominantly trabecular while others have greater amounts of cortical bone. Trabecular bone is lightweight and spongy in appearance because it is filled with red marrow and fat and is found in the vertebrae of the spine, the top part of the hips, the breast bone, and at the ends of the long bones in the arms and legs. Cortical bone, which is denser but thinner, surrounds trabecular bone and is found to a greater degree in the long bones of the arms and legs.

Bone is a living, growing tissue, with metabolic as well as structural roles. Bone cells are constantly renewing themselves much like the skin. Healthy bone is maintained through a process called "remodeling" in which old bone cells are slowly removed and replaced by the formation of new bone cells. Old bone cells which have signs of age or damage are removed by bone-removing cells called osteoclasts. This resorption process leaves tiny, microscopic holes in the bone. These holes are then filled by bone-forming cells or osteoblasts which are the beginning of the new bone cells. This process takes between one to two months to complete. Calcium, phosphorus, and other minerals are then added over the next two to three months, which gives hardness to the bones and completes the remodeling process. Calcium and other minerals that are consumed each day through the diet are the raw materials used in the bone-forming process.

In one year approximately 40% of trabecular bone goes through this remodeling process, compared to 10% of cortical bone, despite the fact that we have about four times more cortical bone than trabecular bone. It is speculated that because trabecular bone is more fragile than cortical bone it may need to be replaced more frequently to repair microfractures in the trabecular network which have been sustained by normal loading, trauma, or pathologic processes. The spongy structure of trabecular bone also provides a greater surface area for the bone-removing

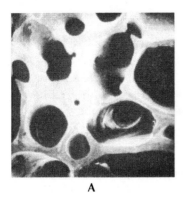 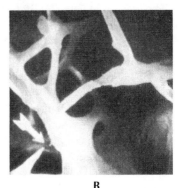

A   B

FIGURE 1 Micrographs of biopsy specimens of normal and osteoporotic bone. Panel A is from a 75-year-old normal woman. Panel B is from a 47-year-old woman who had multiple vertebral compression fractures. (From Dempster, D. W. et al., *J. Bone Min. Res.*, 1, 15–21, 1986. With permission.)

osteoclasts to attach and begin breaking down bone cells. The fragility of trabecular bone is indicated by the preponderance of osteoporotic fractures at the wrist, spine and hip, which have greater amounts of trabecular bone than the mid-sections of the appendicular bones.

Bone tissue increases throughout the early stages of life until somewhere between 25 to 35 years of age when peak bone mass is reached. After this time most women start to lose bone at the rate of approximately 0.5% each year. After menopause, the rate at which bone is lost accelerates to 1 to 2% per year for the next five years. Subsequently, the rate of bone loss gradually slows and returns to between 1/2 to 1% per year. It is not clear if this rate of loss continues indefinitely, as there is limited longitudinal data available from women over the age of 85, and there is some suggestion from cross-sectional data of a leveling off of these rates in the last decade of life. Cross-sectional data in this population may certainly be biased in that only survivors are represented, and those with lower bone densities may have died secondary to complications of hip fractures or unrelated causes. Therefore, more extensive longitudinal sampling is needed to better understand the forces acting on bone at the very end of life. These trends represent averages at different points in the lifespan, since it is clear that bone density and rates of loss are quite heterogeneous, and subject to many genetic and lifestyle factors that converge to determine bone mass in a given individual over time. The end result, in general, however, is that more bone is lost than is gained in adulthood, and this loss has serious clinical consequences.

RISK PROFILE AND DIAGNOSIS OF OSTEOPOROSIS

Many risk factors have been identified from epidemiological studies which can be used to form a profile of relative risk for this disease. The most important and clinically relevant of these are outlined in the questionnaire shown in Table 1. Some of the factors are modifiable by lifestyle changes; others are genetically determined and beyond the reach of current treatment options.

If a woman has one or more of any of the non-modifiable risk factors in Category 1, in addition to the highlighted boxes (Caucasian or Asian, over 65 years of age, postmenopausal), or if she answered yes to any of the questions in the modifiable risk factor Category 2, then she is at an increased risk for developing osteoporosis compared to women with none of these characteristics.

Bone mineral density and bone mineral content measurements allow the comparison of bone health to what is normal or expected based upon age and body size. Osteoporosis is diagnosed as 2.5 standard deviations below normal on a bone density test, or approximately 25% bone loss compared to a healthy young adult. Osteopenia refers to bone density which is between 1.0 and 2.5 standard deviations below the mean, and may precede the overt clinical syndrome by many years.

Bone densitometry is currently the gold standard for the clinical diagnosis of osteopenia and osteoporosis due to its relative precision, low radiation exposure, ease of administration, provision of a comparison with normative values at various ages, and ability to predict the risk of future fracture. This test uses a very low dose of radiation, approximately one-tenth of a traditional X-ray, and is much more sensitive to measuring the amount of bone present than ordinary X-rays.

There is currently a great deal of controversy over the use of densitometry as a screening tool. Some scientists and practitioners advocate mass screening of all newly postmenopausal women with periodic follow-up, while others advocate limiting such exams to high risk women (identified by questionnaires such as those in Table 1) or those suspected of having low bone mass based on history and physical exam findings (such as loss of stature or kyphosis). The cost of screening all women at menopause would be enormous and the public health recommendations to prevent or treat this disease in its early stages would be the same, regardless of current bone density measurement. Therefore, a rational approach may be to reserve bone measurements for those women in whom a decision regarding the institution of pharmacological therapy in addition to lifestyle changes is needed. For example, recommendations for densitometry measurements may be made in the case of

- Women who have more than three of the risk factors for osteoporosis;
- A practitioner's need to assess current bone health to make an informed decision regarding whether or not to prescribe pharmacological therapy; and/or
- The need to monitor response to a chosen pharmacological therapy.

However, such measurements may also serve an important motivational role, as do lipid measurements, by providing an incentive to either change or adhere to lifestyle and behavioral choices (such as smoking cessation or regular exercise participation).

There are several common techniques for measuring bone density which are often identified by their abbreviation as listed in Table 2. All of these tests can effectively measure bone density at different sites in the body and can be used to predict total bone mineral content. Bone mineral density describes how tightly packed the bones are and therefore how "dense" they are. Bone mineral content is

TABLE 1
Risk Profile Quiz*

Risk Profile Quiz	Check		Risk Factor Type
1. Are you...	Yes	No	Non-Modifiable
Caucasian or Asian?			
over 65 years of age?			
postmenopausal?			
someone who had early (before the age of 50) or surgical menopause?			
from a family with a history of osteoporosis?			
lactose intolerant?			
fair skinned or light haired?			
Total			
2. Do you...			Potentially Modifiable
exercise so much that you do not have regular menstrual cycles?			
live a sedentary lifestyle?			
drink more than one alcohol-containing drink per day on average?			
smoke nicotine-containing product?			
eat a low calcium and/or low vitamin D diet?			
follow a very low calorie or protein diet or have an eating disorder?			
consider yourself to be underweight, losing weight, or very thin?			
take thyroid hormone replacement or cortisone-like medication?			
Total			

* This series of questions has been adapted from the complete list of risk factors for osteoporosis and can help determine your relative risk of developing osteoporosis.

often referred to as bone mass and describes the total amount of bone in the body. The test that is used depends upon which tests are available as well as the expertise and preference of the radiologist overseeing the procedure. It is usual to measure the hip and spine bone density in addition to the total body bone mass, because these are the clinically relevant sites for osteoporotic fracture.

Currently, DXA is the most widely available and precise technique and has very little radiation associated with the test. The combination of these factors makes DXA the measurement of choice at the present time. The precision of DXA can vary markedly due to differences in the type of machine used, the software equations chosen, the skill of the technician, and day-to-day variability in machine performance. These factors make it critical that if serial measurements are taken with the purpose of monitoring response to therapy or determining that a threshold has been reached below which pharmacological agents will be initiated, then the same medical

TABLE 2
Common Bone Density Tests

Bone Density Tests	Abbreviation	Bones Examined
Dual energy X-ray absorptiometry	DXA	Hip, spine, total body
Dual photon absorptiometry	DPA	Hip, spine, total body
Quantitative computed tomography[a]	QCT	Spine
Peripheral computed tomography	pQCT	Wrist
Radiographic absorptiometry	RA	Hand
Single energy X-ray absorptiometry	SXA	Heel, wrist
Single photon absorptiometry	SPA	Wrist
Ultrasound		Heel

[a] QCT has a greater radiation dose than the other tests.

center is used and satisfactory quality assurance measures are in place, including frequent calibration checks and assessment of technician reliability. The coefficient of variation of repeated bone density measurements should be on the order of 1 to 2% in skilled hands and with well-calibrated equipment. Many effective treatments change bone density by only this amount or slightly more over the course of a year, so that inaccurate measurements could be very misleading with regard to judging the efficacy of such interventions.

Ultrasound technology, which is commonly used during pregnancy, has recently been approved by the Food and Drug Administration for bone density testing. This test measures the speed of sound in the heel to determine bone density. Because sound waves are used, there is no radiation exposure. Ultrasound is purported by some to predict hip fractures equally as well as DXA, and may become more widely used in the future if such predictions prove valid.

THE CLINICAL SYNDROME

Osteoporosis is often referred to as a silent disease. X-rays cannot clearly detect it until at least 30% of bone density is lost. Most people do not realize they have it until they break a bone. Loss of height and thoracic kyphosis (the "dowager's hump") are common visible indicators of osteoporosis. These conditions are often misperceived by family members as indicative of poor posture but actually result from a weakening and, ultimately, a compression of the vertebrae of the spine.

Pain, mobility impairment, and bone fractures as well as this loss of height are the physical symptoms of osteoporosis. A fracture is often the first sign of osteoporosis, despite the fact that osteopenia may have existed for 20 to 30 years prior to any overt clinical manifestation of the disease.

Fractures of the wrist, often called Colle's fractures, occur most frequently in women between 50 and 70 years of age. Women in this age group move faster than very old women, and if they fall, they tend to fall forward due to the forward momentum of their gait. They are also more likely to break their fall with a hand or arm and consequently break a wrist, perhaps due to better preserved neuromuscular reflexes than the older woman. This type of fracture appears to be less common in older women because they more often fall on their buttocks or greater trochanter, presumably due to differences in gait velocity and neuromuscular activation patterns, including difficulty with lateral balance movements at the time their equilibrium is challenged.

After age 60, vertebral fractures of the thoracic and upper lumbar spine are common. Vertebral "crush" fractures are a compression or flattening of both the front and back sections of a spinal vertebra. "Wedge" fractures are a compression of just the front part of the vertebra so it resembles a wedge shape. These fractures may occur spontaneously due to decreased bone density or they may be caused by trauma or an accident. Seemingly very minor trauma, particularly that which increases compressive forces on the vulnerable anterior lip of the vertebra may be all that is needed when osteopenia is advanced. Any flexion of the thoracic spine places very large compressive forces on the vertebrae, and if flexion is accompanied by the holding of a heavy mass out in front of the body, the forces will be many times higher. Examples of such mechanically disadvantageous activities for women with osteoporosis include 10-pin bowling and golf swings, which are unfortunately often favorite activities in this population. Vertebral fractures are difficult to document in time because they generally do not involve hospitalization, and are in fact usually asymptomatic. These fractures do heal but the vertebrae cannot return to their original shape as do fractures of other bones such as the arm or leg. Over time, multiple vertebral fractures become evident by a loss of height or kyphotic posture. Painful muscle spasms and feeling of self-consciousness may result from these changes in posture. In severe cases, the lower rib may appear to be resting directly on the iliac crest as several inches of thoracic height are lost, with respiratory symptoms secondary to resultant restrictive lung volumes.

Hip fractures generally occur in the later years, rising in incidence exponentially after age 70, when muscle weakness, visual impairment, orthostatic hypotension, slowed reaction time, balance impairment, cognitive impairment, and/or medication usage may all decrease the ability to respond to challenges to the maintenance of an upright posture, and increase the likelihood of falling. Decreased soft tissue (muscle or adipose) mass over the greater trochanter in this age group, when present as well, significantly increases the transmission of the kinetic energy of the fall to the underlying bone, and is thus an independent risk factor for injury should a fall occur. More than 90% of the hip fractures that occur in the United States each year are associated with osteoporosis. The National Osteoporosis Foundation estimates that nearly 50% of people suffering hip fractures subsequently lose their ability to walk independently and approximately 30% of those individuals will become totally dependent on others for care.

THE ROLE OF BODY COMPOSITION

Body composition refers to the partitioning of the body into its component parts which may be defined by tissue type (fat and lean mass), elemental analysis (such as calcium, nitrogen, or potassium content) or physiologic properties (such as the relative ability to conduct electricity). A simple approach is to divide the body into two general categories: (1) fat and (2) lean tissue (which includes bone, muscle, water, and internal organs). Body weight, size, or the relationship of weight to height (body mass index or BMI) are significant predictors of the amount of bone mass in the body. Extremes of BMI, either low (<19kg/m^2) or high (>30kg/m^2) are associated with higher mortality rates than a BMI in the middle range of 20 to 30kg/m^2. For example, a high BMI is associated with a greater chance of death from heart disease, stroke, hypertension, hyperlipidemia, and adult onset diabetes. An extremely low BMI is also a health risk and is associated with a greater instance of death from suicide and certain types of cancer.

Osteoporosis is one of the few medical conditions in which being a little heavy can be an advantage. Having greater body weight affects bone in several different ways. First, people with greater body weight tend to have greater bone density than thinner people. This may be the result of the greater "weight bearing" that occurs simply by the extra effort required to move their bodies against gravity to do everyday activities. Second, greater body fat, which generally accompanies greater body mass, is associated with greater bone density, as well as reduced risk of hip fracture after a fall. It is not known if adipose tissue is protective due to shock absorbing effects over the hip, increased weight bearing forces on bone over time due to adipose tissue mass, enhanced peripheral conversion of androgens to estrogens in women with more body fat, or increased total body stores of the fat soluble vitamin D. Third, there are direct correlations between the size and strength of muscles, the major component of lean tissue, and bone density. In particular, bone density is related to the size and force-producing capacity of muscles to which it is directly attached. For example, tennis players will exhibit differential bone mass in their dominant forearms, as well as muscle hypertrophy, compared to the nondominant arm. Such findings suggest that the effect of muscle on bone growth is largely local (associated with mechanical or electromagnetic forces) rather than systemic (via hormonal or other circulating factors). In addition, larger amounts of muscle tissue in the body and increased muscle strength are associated with a decreased risk of falling and greater ease in doing everyday activities.

Certain ethnic groups including African-Americans and Mexican-Americans tend to have body compositions that are protective against osteoporotic fractures. Studies of body composition have shown that African-Americans have greater bone and muscle mass, both of which are important factors in preventing osteoporosis and injurious falls. However, these groups have greater amounts of body fat, higher body mass index (BMI), and prevalence of obesity than Caucasian populations as well, which puts them at a higher risk for other chronic diseases, such as cardiovascular disease, diabetes, and degenerative arthritis. In addition, very obese individuals are more susceptible to falls associated with gait problems that may result in increased risk for fractures, as well as mobility impairment and functional limitations.

Thus, given the divergent effects of excess adipose tissue on health, particularly in the young old (age 50 to 70), it does not make sense to promote body fat accretion as a means to protect bones. Attempts to maintain or increase lean tissue, on the other hand, have a much higher benefit-to-risk ratio. However, it should be remembered that in the very old, undernutrition may emerge as more of a problem than obesity, and low BMI, small amounts of soft tissue over the hip, protein calorie malnutrition, and weight loss are risk factors for hip fracture in this population. In these individuals, attempts to maintain or increase body mass (both fat and lean compartments) are warranted. Although not yet studied as a primary prevention tool for osteoporotic fracture, complete nutritional supplementation has been shown to significantly improve rehabilitation outcomes after operative treatment for hip fracture.

LIFESTYLE FACTORS AND OSTEOPOROSIS

Fortunately, there are modifiable risk factors for osteoporosis and related fractures for which interventions can be recommended at every stage of life. These include lifestyle decisions such as getting the proper amounts and types of exercise, minimizing risks for falling and compressive forces on the spine, getting adequate amounts of sunlight, calcium and vitamin D, limiting alcohol, sodium and caffeine intake, and quitting smoking. The chronic nature of this disease necessitates permanent behavioral change in these areas, which will require the kinds of approaches to adoption and adherence outlined in Chapter 25. If a woman already has osteoporosis or is at high risk for this disease, then you may want to consider dietary supplements and traditional pharmacological agents such as estrogen replacement therapy or more recently approved drugs that help to maintain or increase bone density. The major therapeutic modalities are reviewed in the sections below.

EXERCISE

Exercise is known to provide a stimulus that is important for the maintenance and improvement of bone health. A sedentary lifestyle has been implicated in bone loss and its associated health problems. A comprehensive approach based on a review of numerous research studies suggests that there should be three components in an exercise program for older women who are at risk for osteoporosis and falling. These include (1) strength training, (2) balance training, and (3) aerobic training. Of these, strength training, often referred to as "weight lifting" or "resistance training" may actually be the most important for decreasing the risk of osteoporotic fractures. Both aerobic training and resistance training have direct impact upon bone tissue, and have been shown to increase the peak bone mass which is attained as well as attenuate the rates of loss in the postmenopausal years. There is some suggestion in the literature that resistance training may be more powerful in this regard, as it has been shown to increase bone density in older women in some cases. In contrast, many trials of aerobic exercise demonstrate a maintenance of bone density but no accretion. Balance training is not meant to impact upon bone health, but rather to reduce the risk of falling, and thereby reduce fracture risk independent of bone density changes. Resistance training can also improve balance to a small degree, and may thus protect against falls as well, whereas aerobic training has not been shown to affect balance in any substantive way.

These and other known effects of the various exercise modalities on osteoporotic fracture risk are summarized in Table 3. The important emphasis on resistance

TABLE 3
Exercise Modalities and the Risk of Osteoporotic Fracture

Risk Factor	Aerobic Training	Resistance Training	Balance Training[a]
Improves bone density	Yes	Yes	No
Improves balance	No	Yes	Yes
Increases muscle strength	No	Yes	No
Increases muscle mass	No	Yes	No
Increases spontaneous levels of physical activity[b]	No	Yes	No
May enable discontinuance of hazardous drugs[c]	Yes	Yes	No
May enhance rates of smoking cessation	Yes	Unknown	Unknown
Visual impairment	No	No	No

[a] Balance training refers to repetitive static and dynamic balance postures, T'ai chi, and other forms of exercise that specifically enhance balance.

[b] Sedentariness has been identified as a risk factor for osteoporosis and fracture.

[c] Antidepressants and sedative hyponotics are associated with falls and hip fractures; both aerobic and resistance training are effective treatments for clinical depression and insomnia and can potentially substitute for these classes of drugs. Certain drugs used for cardiovascular disease and hypertension may cause orthostatic hypotension and increase fall risk; aerobic exercise may reduce the need for these drugs.

training stems from its ability to influence more risk factors, as well as its more potent effect on bone accretion. However, it should be pointed out that in clinical trials to date, only exercise programs that have included balance training as an isolated or multi-faceted intervention have shown significant reductions in fall rates. Additionally, there has been no evidence published demonstrating a reduction in osteoporotic fractures prospectively in subjects randomized to any form of exercise, although such long-term trials are ongoing at present.

Strength Training

Scientific research indicates that strength training is associated with high bone mineral density in young and old adults. Progressive, high intensity strength training has significant potential in the prevention and treatment of osteoporosis. It may help to achieve the highest possible peak bone mass in premenopausal woman and may aid in maintaining or increasing bone in postmenopausal women.

Our laboratory has demonstrated potent effect from a one year study of high intensity strength training in postmenopausal women ranging from 50 and 70 years of age. The women strength-trained two times a week for approximately 40 minutes, lifting weights that were set at approximately 80% of the peak load they could lift. The women gained an average of 1% in bone mineral density of the hip and spine when compared to a group of sedentary woman who did not exercise and lost 2.5% and 1.8% at these sites, respectively. The strength-trained women also tended to maintain their total bone mineral content while the sedentary women lost 1.2% of their total bone mineral content over the year. The strength-trained women had increases in strength ranging from 35 to 76% in the various muscles of the body.

These same woman had a 2.6 pound increase in their muscle mass without a weight gain, e.g., they lost fat and gained muscle while the women in the control group lost about a pound of muscle over the year and gained the same amount of fat. Dynamic balance, measured by backward tandem walk, improved significantly by 14% in the strength-trained group. In addition, the strength-trained women were 27% more active: they started participating in activities such as walking, ballroom dancing, gardening, and canoeing. The women who did not strength train showed declines in these same parameters.

The overall findings of our study indicate that strength training in postmenopausal women, in contrast to traditional pharmacological and nutritional approaches for improving bone health, has the added benefit of influencing multiple risk factors for osteoporotic fractures including improved strength, balance, increased muscle mass, and increased participation in leisure-time activities.

There is also evidence that severe forms of osteopenia secondary to high dose corticosteroid treatment in heart transplant recipients are responsive to this form of weight lifting exercise, completely reversing this unwanted side effect of treatment. In another model, the osteopenia of the lumbar vertebrae secondary to immobilization or disuse in patients with chronic low back pain can be reversed with specific lumbar extensor muscle resistance training. These studies and others suggest that both normal age-related bone loss as well as that due to disuse, disease, or medications can be addressed with targeted progressive resistance training.

The key to successful strength training for osteoporosis is that it must be progressive and of a high intensity. Typically, many aerobic classes or health instructors advocate light hand weights and many women continue to use these after months or even years of exercising, not knowing that they are short-changing themselves from important improvements in bone health, bone density, and body composition. Since loading of the bone and muscle appears to be the single most important factor determining physiologic adaptation, the type of training system utilized (machines, free weights, compressed air or fluid, elastic tubing, etc.) is not important as long as appropriate loading at a high enough intensity can be achieved.

Improvements in bone density have been seen after training regimens of 1, 2, or 3 days per week, provided the intensity (relative load) is high. Although the exact dose of resistive exercise that is optimal for osteoporosis specifically has not been defined, the dose which produces peak changes in muscle strength is what is most often used, and is therefore recommended currently. Optimal duration of training for peak bone effects are also not known, but since discontinuance of exercise leads to atrophy of muscle and loss of strength, regular training is recommended as long as a woman's health permits.

We recommend strength training exercises that target the major muscle groups of the body, particularly those involved in gait and balance, and those attached to the bones prone to osteoporotic fractures. These muscles are the quadriceps (front of the thighs), gluteals and hamstrings (buttocks and back of thighs), abductors (sides of thighs), back extensors (along the spine and lower back), and abdominal flexors (stomach), and dorsiflexors (anterior calf). Overall upper body strength is also important and can be improved by training the shoulders and chest, upper back, and arms. Chapter 2 provides specific exercise instructions and illustrations for each of these exercises.

There are resistive exercises that should be avoided in the woman at risk for osteoporotic fracture. In particular, flexion of the spine against resistance is not recommended because of the risk of thoracic compression fractures. Ordinary functional activities such as bending over to pick up a heavy object are an example of such a movement. Bending the knees should always be encouraged for this reason when picking up objects, as well as to protect the lower back from soft tissue injury. Some abdominal machines encourage flexion of the spine as opposed to the appropriate shortening movement as the rectus abdominus muscles contract (bringing the rib cage closer to the pelvis). Similarly, sit ups that bring the trunk all the way to the knees or with the knees extended rather than flexed will place strain on the vertebral bodies, whereas a partial sit up, just lifting the head and neck a few inches toward the ceiling, and leg lifts with the upper body resting on the floor will target both the upper and lower abdominal muscles with no spine flexion involved. Also to be avoided for the woman with significant spinal osteoporosis are weight machines or free weight exercises which load the spine excessively, such as certain leg press or plantar flexor machines where the padded bars rest on the shoulders and the feet are pushed against an immobile footplate, or squats performed with the bar resting on the shoulders. Alternative ways to exercise these muscle groups without potential injury to the spine are illustrated in Chapter 2.

Balance Training

A fall results from a mismatch between external stimuli that displace the center of mass and the intrinsic capacity of an individual to withstand such perturbations, as more fully described in Chapter 13. Although older adults tend to blame falls on extrinsic factors the majority of the time, the cause in fact is more likely to be intrinsic. For example, a robust young person, when exposed to the same set of circumstances (such as a curb to navigate) would be unlikely to fall. Improving your balance is one of the best ways to reduce the risk of falling. Most osteoporotic fractures happen as the result of a fall that can occur either while standing still or moving.

A major cause of falls is tripping while walking. This may be related in part to the decreased step height that is a typical feature of the senile gait. Conscious efforts to reduce shuffling the feet may help, but this may be difficult to modify if there are neuromuscular changes (such as weakness of the hip flexors or dorsiflexors, frontal lobe apraxia of gait, or periventricular cortical infarcts) that predispose to abnormal gait characteristics.

A meta-analysis of the FICSIT trials of frailty and injury prevention techniques indicated that exercise in the elderly had a modest (approximately 10%) effect on fall prevention overall, and that only interventions which included a balance-enhancing component contributed significantly to this protective effect. More recently, research in New Zealand by Campbell et al. indicated a very significant reduction in fall rates in older community-dwelling women randomized to a combination of home-based strength and balance training compared to controls.

In our research with older adults, we are finding that static and dynamic balance training exercises are effective if they require one to

- Transfer body weight from one leg to another;
- Stand on a narrowed base of support (e.g., one leg);
- Maintain stability during dynamic movements (e.g., walking); and
- Practice transfer skills (e.g., standing up from a seated position, getting up off the floor).

Some specific balance training exercises that may be included in an exercise program for osteoporosis are chair stands, toe stands, heel stands, tandem stand and tandem walk. These exercises require the maintenance of balance under both static and dynamic conditions. Balance training should always be done slowly, cautiously, safely, and near a wall or sturdy table for support if needed. As with strength training, it is important that balance exercises are progressive and that the individual is challenged with a greater level of difficulty as they become easier to do. Health clubs and adult education centers also offer classes in T'ai Chi and yoga, which are Eastern forms of exercise that emphasize balance, posture, and flexibility. Yoga has not yet been formally studied as a fall prevention technique, but may certainly have this capability. T'ai Chi has been shown to significantly reduce the rate of falls in a relatively healthy, older, community-dwelling population. The feasibility and efficacy of this mode of training remain to be demonstrated in frail elders with significant risk factors for falls, but such trials are currently in progress. Balance training of any kind is most likely to be successful as an isolated intervention if other major contributants to falling such as severe orthostasis, visual impairment, strokes, muscle weakness, etc. are not prominent in the clinical picture.

Based on the principles discussed above, a simple home-based balance training regimen is outlined below. There is as yet no definite data from clinical trials on the precise dose of balance exercises needed to effectively modify this parameter. Investigators have used protocols ranging from 1 to 7 days per week with success. Developed from research in our laboratory, practical and effective recommendations for a balance training program are

- Five exercises;
- Two to three times per week;
- Two sets of eight repetitions; and
- Work safely toward the highest level of difficulty.

Each of the five exercises and the progressive levels of difficulty within each exercise are detailed in the sections which follow. For each exercise, the individual should be instructed to start with Level 1 and proceed to the successive levels as soon as the exercise can be completed without danger of falling.

1. Chair Stands

   Level 1. Place the back of a chair against the wall, then sit toward the middle of the seat with your feet flat on the ground. Stand up very slowly from the chair using your hands to help you up to a three second count of 1-2-3. Hold when fully standing and return very slowly to the seated position to the count of 1-2-3. Perform 8 times. Rest and repeat.

   Level 2. Sit with your arms crossed over your chest. Stand up very slowly from the chair without using your hands to the count of 1-2-3. Hold when fully standing and return very slowly to the seated position to the count of 1-2-3. Perform 8 times. Rest and repeat.

   Level 3. Stand up very slowly from a low chair or couch to the count of 1-2-3. Use your hands to help you up initially, then graduate to not using your hands. Hold when fully standing and return very slowly to the seated position to the count of 1-2-3. Perform 8 times. Rest and repeat.

   Level 4. Sit with your arms crossed over your chest and cross one leg over the other. Stand up very slowly from the chair using only one leg for support to the count of 1-2-3. Hold when fully standing and return very slowly to the seated position to the count of 1-2-3. Perform 8 times. Rest and repeat.

2. Toe Stands

   Level 1. Stand approximately 8 to 12 inches from the wall and place the fingertips of both hands on the wall for support. Raise up on your toes to the count of 1-2-3. Hold for the count of 1-2-3. Slowly lower your feet back down to the floor to the count of 1-2-3. Perform 8 times. Rest and repeat.

   Level 2. Place the fingertips of both hands on the wall for support. Stand on one leg. Slowly raise up on the toes of that foot so that your heel is lifted off the ground to the count of 1-2-3. Hold for the count of 1-2-3. Slowly lower your foot back down to the floor to the count of 1-2-3. Perform 8 times with each leg, alternating between right and left legs. Rest and repeat.

   Level 3. Perform toe stand exercise as described in Level 2. Perform all 8 repetitions on your right leg continuously, followed by 8 repetitions with your left leg. Rest and repeat.

   Level 4. Perform toe stand exercise as described in Level 3, except place only one fingertip on the wall, and when you are able, remove this fingertip support as well.

3. Heel Stands

   Level 1. Stand with your back and buttocks leaning on the wall with the palms of both hands touching the wall. The heels of your feet should be 6 to 8 inches away from the wall and hip width apart. Lift the toes of both feet off the floor to the count of 1-2-3 so that you are balancing on your heels. Hold this position (balancing on your heels with the toes of both feet off the floor) for one second, then return your toes back to the floor to the count of 1-2-3. Perform 8 times. Rest and repeat.

Level 2. Perform heel stands as described in Level 1, holding toes off the floor for a count of 1-2-3-4-5-6-7-8. Rest and repeat.

Level 3. Stand with your back 2 to 3 inches away from the wall with your hands poised near wall for support. Raise toes of both feet off the ground so that you are balancing on your heels. Hold heel stand for 8 seconds trying not to let your back or hands touch the wall. Rest and repeat.

4. Tandem Stand

Level 1. Stand about one and a half feet away from a table or counter with both hands on the table for support. Place one foot directly in front of the other foot so that the heel of one foot is touching the toes of the other foot. Both feet in tandem should form a straight line. Hold this position for 10 seconds without moving your feet around to maintain balance. Rest and repeat 8 times, alternating right and left feet positions.

Level 2. As you feel more comfortable, perform the tandem stand as described in Level 1 holding onto the table with just one hand. Rest and repeat 8 times, alternating right and left feet positions.

Level 3. Perform the tandem stand without holding onto the table. Keep your hands poised near the table for safety. Rest and repeat 8 times, alternating right and left feet positions.

Level 4. Lift one leg completely off the floor and stand on just one leg for 10 seconds. Rest and repeat 8 times, alternating right and left legs on the floor. As you are able, withdraw hand support from two hands to one, to none.

5. Tandem Walk

Level 1. Stand with your side and shoulder near an unobstructed length of wall or hallway and place your hand on the wall for support. Walk by placing one foot in front of the other so that the heel of one foot is touching the toes of the other foot. Walk toe to heel in tandem style for approximately 20 steps with the hand closest to the wall touching it for support. Turn around carefully and repeat tandem walk back to the starting point. Rest and repeat.

Level 2. Perform tandem walk without touching the wall.

Level 3. Backward tandem walk by placing the toe of one foot in line with the heel of the foot behind it for approximately 20 steps. Initially, your hand should touch the wall for support, then graduate to not holding onto the wall but keeping your hand poised near it for support. Turn around and repeat backward tandem walk back to the starting point. Rest and repeat.

Level 4. As in Level 3 but with eyes closed and hand poised near wall for support if needed.

Aerobic Exercise

Aerobic exercise is any activity in which you use the large muscle groups of the body, is rhythmic in nature, and causes your heart and breathing rate to increase. There are many different kinds of activity that fit into this general category, and individual preference, feasibility, and access will play a role in determining what type of aerobic activity is recommended for optimal bone health. However, in contrast to other health benefits associated with aerobic activity, such as prevention of heart disease, stroke, or diabetes, only certain types of aerobic exercise confer substantial benefit in osteoporosis prevention and treatment. The key factor appears to be mechanical loading of the skeleton, and higher impact loading (such as occurs during stepping or jogging) appears to be more effective than lower impact loading (such as walking). Partially or completely unloaded aerobic activity (such as bike riding or swimming) have not been shown to have positive impact on bone density in older women, and therefore are not recommended as the primary mode of exercise if this is a major or important goal of the exercise prescription.

Because higher impact activities may be intolerable or undesirable in a woman with concurrent arthritis of the foot, ankle, knee, or hip, the aim is to load the skeleton without trauma as much as possible. This can be accomplished by weighting the torso with a lead vest or loaded backpack (assuring that an erect rather than flexed posture is maintained throughout) while walking or hiking or climbing stairs. Stepping up and down from a platform or aerobics step has also been used to load the skeleton, although this activity has been associated with many ankle injuries, especially if done in a ballistic fashion, and may be a risk for falls in women with impaired balance.

Walking and related activities (hiking, stair-climbing) may offer the best benefit-to-risk ratio in terms of bone health as they provide loading with minimal joint trauma. Some forms of walking, such as treadmill walking, are probably not the best choice for an osteopenic woman with poor balance, as the risk of injury may be greater, and the benefit no different than ordinary walking. Walking outdoors, however, has its dangers as well in the form of rough terrain, inclement weather, humidity, and darkness, and thus mall walking offers a safe alternative if available. The dose of exercise needed for bone maintenance is not precisely known, but positive results have been achieved with programs of 3 to 4 days per week, at a moderate intensity, and durations consistent with those that confer cardiovascular and other health benefits. Therefore, we would recommend the following goals for an aerobic exercise program designed to have favorable impact on bone health:

- Three to five times per week;
- Twenty to sixty minutes per time; and
- Moderate intensity (slightly difficult and you are able to maintain a conversation).

Summary of Exercise Guidelines for Reducing the Risk of Developing Osteoporosis

Ideally an exercise program for osteoporosis should include strength, balance, and aerobic training activities. This combination targets both bone tissue as well as fall risk, and therefore represents the most comprehensive approach to the prevention of osteoporotic fractures in terms of physical activity patterns. Strength and balance training can be easily combined and done in one training session, with aerobic training on alternate days, as outlined in Table 4.

As illustrated in the sample weekly training schedules in Table 5, these general goals can be operationalized depending upon the commitment and capacity of the individual woman. It is important to include at least one day of rest between strength and balance training sessions to give skeletal muscle time to repair damage to muscle fibers and adapt to the loading via synthesis of new myofibrillar proteins.

Some individuals will not be able to comply with all three forms of exercise. In addition, certain medical conditions (such as claudication, a low threshold for desaturation or ischemia, severe degenerative arthritis, etc.) may make aerobic exercise itself impossible or unsafe, at least initially. In these cases, resistive exercises, including standing postures with gradually reduced hand support (as illustrated in Chapter 2) will effectively address the risk factors listed in Table 3, and represent an efficient and feasible compromise for the frailer woman with osteoporosis.

TABLE 4
The Exercise Prescription for Osteoporosis

Modality	Frequency	Duration
Strength and balance training	2–3 times per week	45 minutes per session
Aerobic exercise	3–5 times per week	20–60 minutes per session

TABLE 5
The Weekly Exercise Schedule

Day	Beginning Program	Advanced Program
Monday	Strength and balance training	Strength and balance training Aerobic exercise (20–30 min. walk)
Tuesday	Aerobic exercise (10–20 min. walk)	Aerobic exercise (30 min. walk)
Wednesday	Aerobic exercise (10–20 min. walk)	Strength and balance training
Thursday	Strength and balance training	Aerobic exercise (30 min. walk)
Friday	Day off	Strength and balance training
Saturday	Aerobic exercise (10–20 min. walk)	Aerobic exercise (30 min. walk)
Sunday	Day off	Day off

NUTRITION

Vitamin D

Our current knowledge of the role of nutrition and understanding of the specific functions of the nutrients in vegetables and dairy products has been refined through scientific research over the past few decades. Calcium and vitamin D have been identified as the two key nutrients in the prevention and treatment of osteoporosis. For a complete discussion of these nutrients in the diet please refer to Chapter 8.

Our bodies can also make vitamin D, which is required for calcium absorption, through exposure to sunlight and subsequent processing in the liver and kidney. This process depends upon geographic location, time of year, the use of sunscreen lotions, and age. Vitamin D is made in the skin through interaction with the sun's ultraviolet rays. Fifteen minutes of midday sun exposure to the arms, hands, and face helps people meet the daily requirement for vitamin D year-round in warm climates and between the months of March through October in northern climates. The angle and decreased intensity of the sun during the winter do not allow individuals living in northern climates to manufacture vitamin D in the skin. Therefore, vitamin D needs must be met either through adipose tissue stores or diet if one lives in a northern climate during the winter. Sunscreens with a sun protection factor (SPF) greater than 8 will prevent the skin from making vitamin D by blocking out the sun's ultraviolet rays. The risk of skin cancer from overexposure to the sun's rays is minimal with 15 minutes a day exposure. There is evidence that the ability to manufacture vitamin D in the skin and hydroxlylate it to its active form in the kidney decreases with increasing age. All of these influences on vitamin D status highlight the importance of ensuring adequate dietary intake for older adults.

Other Dietary Recommendations

For good bone health, caffeine, sodium, and protein should be consumed in moderation. This is of particular importance for older women because too much of these things can increase the elimination of calcium in the urine leading to accelerated bone loss. Some scientists believe that the calcium requirement on a western diet which is high in these nutrients is greatly exaggerated because of these losses, and can therefore only be realistically met with dairy products or supplements.

Exceeding more than 1,000 milligrams of caffeine a day, or the amount of three cups of caffeinated coffee, soda, or tea, may adversely affect calcium retention through its diuretic effect. Women who consume more than this amount should be advised to replace caffeinated beverages with calcium-containing beverages. This will help to prevent dehydration and lower caffeine intake at the same time.

Alcohol is toxic to the osteoblast cells which build bone. Moderate alcohol consumption is defined as one to two drinks a day (one drink is 12 ounces of beer, a five-ounce glass of wine, or one ounce of hard liquor) for women. Amounts greater than this or excessive alcohol use are linked with an increased risk for bone loss, falling, malnutrition, and liver disease, all of which increase the risk and severity of complications related to osteoporosis, in addition to other health problems.

Over the years there has been controversy regarding whether or not high amounts of protein in the diet lead to increased loss of calcium in the urine. While this is still a controversial issue, excess dietary protein does increase calciuria, and will thus increase calcium requirements for homeostasis. This is primarily an issue if one were to take protein or amino acid supplements on a chronic basis. For the majority of older women, there is no need to take these supplements, as most people get more than enough protein from their diet alone. Exceptions would include those who are undernourished or losing protein because of a catabolic illness, for example. Adequate protein intake for most women ranges between four to six ounces per day of meat or fish. (A piece of cooked chicken the size of the palm of your hand is approximately two to three ounces.) Dairy products are important sources of both protein and calcium; therefore, it is important not to cut back on these as a way to minimize protein intake.

Phosphorus is a mineral that is a major component of bone, much like calcium. Phosphorus does not affect calcium absorption as initially thought. However, excess phosphorus may indirectly lead to low bone density by increasing parathyroid hormone, which in turn increases bone resorption. Phosphorus is found in red meat and is commonly added to soft drinks and processed foods. The recommended dietary allowance (RDA) for phosphorus is the same as calcium; however, the problem lies in the fact that most people consume phosphorus in amounts far in excess (two to three times) of their calcium intake, and this imbalance is problematic. Food labels of processed foods should be checked to determine their phosphorus content. A particularly dangerous trend, especially in young women, is the substitution of sodas (high in phosphorus and devoid of calcium) for milk products as beverages (which have a balanced ratio of calcium to phosphorus). If this trend begins in the pre-teen years and continues through adulthood, significant adverse consequences are likely in terms of postmenopausal bone health. It is not simply the absence of calcium and vitamin D that is a concern, but its replacement with the phosphorus-rich substance which is so damaging. Until further research is done to better understand the effect of phosphorus on bone health, it is recommended that women of all ages limit the amount of phosphorus containing foods in their diet.

SMOKING

Nicotine from cigarettes lowers estrogen levels in the body. This, in turn, decreases calcium absorption and can cause bone resorption in an attempt to maintain calcium homeostasis. Numerous research studies have shown that bone density is lower in women who smoke than those who don't and that women who smoke lose bone at a faster rate. Increased risk for osteoporosis in combination with known health risks such as lung and breast cancer are just some of the many reasons for emphasizing abstinence from cigarettes in women.

MEDICATIONS ACCELERATING BONE LOSS AND FRACTURE RISK

Glucocorticoids are the most commonly prescribed drugs that can increase the risk of developing osteoporosis. Glucocorticoidss directly affect bone by increasing the activity of the osteoclasts (the cells that remove bone) and decreasing the activity of the osteoblasts (the bone-forming cells). In addition, these drugs interfere with vitamin D and calcium metabolism and thus both decrease calcium absorption in the gut and increase calcium losses in the urine. These effects on multiple pathways explain the large and rapid losses of bone seen with high doses of these drugs. Examples of drugs in this pharmacological class include cortisone, hydrocortisone, prednisone, prednisolone, triamcinolone, methylprednisolone, dexamethasone, betamethasone, flunisolide, and beclomethasone dipropionate. Short courses of topical corticosteroids do not pose a hazard for bones, in contrast to drugs used chronically and systemically.

An additional risk of chronic glucocorticoid therapy is a proximal myopathy characterized by muscle weakness and atrophy, particularly of the hip and thigh muscles. Such weakness may pose a risk for falling, which, when superimposed on an osteopenic skeleton, considerably heightens the chance of fracture.

Other drugs associated with bone loss and the medical condition they are commonly used to treat are listed in Table 6. Fortunately, not all of the drugs used to treat these medical conditions have a negative impact on bone, and less toxic substitutions may be possible in some cases, or adjustments in dose made when no therapeutic alternative is available. The general dictum of using the lowest possible dose for the shortest period of time will help minimize adverse impacts on bone. Supplements of calcium and vitamin D at levels exceeding the RDA should be prescribed to attempt to offset drug–bone interactions, but may not be completely effective in this regard. Additionally, it should be noted that resistance training has been shown to counteract steroid-induced myopathy and bone loss, and should be prescribed whenever long-term moderate to high-dose systemic corticosteroid therapy is required.

Other medications may not affect bone, but may increase the risk of falling and thus also be related to osteoporotic fractures. Long-acting sedative–hypnotics, antidepressants, muscle relaxants, and some antihypertensive and antianginal medication can cause orthostatic hypotension, neuromuscular coordination difficulties, or mental status changes that may contribute to loss of balance and increased risk of falling. A combination of alcohol, dehydration, acute febrile illnesses, and these types of medications is particularly hazardous for the older woman.

PHARMACOLOGICAL TREATMENT FOR OSTEOPOROSIS

In addition to the lifestyle modifications for prevention and treatment outlined above, some women at high risk for osteoporosis will require additional therapy. There is currently some controversy regarding which subset of women fall into this category. All medical treatment carries with it potential benefits and health risks, and the decision to use pharmacological therapy for osteoporosis requires careful

TABLE 6
Medications Related to Osteopenia

Medication	Condition Treated
Glucocorticoids	Rheumatoid arthritis, osteoarthritis, asthma, lupus, multiple sclerosis, hepatitis, glaucoma, Crohn's disease, allergic reactions
Thyroid hormones	Underactive thyroid
Phenytoin and barbiturate anticonvulsants	Epilepsy, head injury, cardiac irregularities
Aluminum-containing antacids	Stomach upset, heartburn
Methotrexate	Cancer, psoriasis, arthritis
Cyclosporine A	Organ transplant, immune system diseases
Gonadotropin-releasing hormone analogs	Endometriosis
Heparin	Cardiac conditions, prevent blood clotting
Cholestyramine	High cholesterol
Furosemide	Congestive heart failure, edema

consideration of this balance in each individual woman, taking into account her health profile, potential for side effects, likelihood of benefit, and preferences. The major categories of pharmacological treatment are outlined below.

Estrogen Replacement Therapy (ERT)

Estrogen helps the body to absorb calcium and to maintain bone mineral density by protecting against the bone-resorbing effects of parathyroid hormone, as discussed more fully in Chapter 15. It has been shown in epidemiological studies and randomized trials to reduce the risk of both vertebral and hip fractures in postmenopausal women compared to those without a history of hormone replacement therapy. A recent study of surgically postmenopausal women found that those who strength trained and were receiving ERT were able to increase their bone density at several sites in the body, while the women who received ERT but did not exercise simply maintained their bone density. This study clearly demonstrates the benefits of strength training on the skeleton and has important implications for women receiving hormone replacement therapy to improve bone density. In general, estrogen slows the rate of bone loss, but does not cause bone accretion. The use of estrogen in the very old has not been demonstrated to have benefit in terms of fracture prevention. Other benefits of estrogen on cardiovascular disease, lipid profiles, and possibly cognitive function should be weighed in the therapeutic decision as well.

Bisphosphonates

Alendronate is the first non-hormonal treatment for postmenopausal women with established osteoporosis that has been approved by the Food and Drug Administration (FDA). Alendronate sodium comes from a class of drugs called bisphosphonates which have been used for the past two decades to treat other bone diseases. This drug helps to slow bone removal, as does estrogen, but in addition reverses some bone loss by building healthy new bone. Several long-term clinical trials have shown that this drug can lead to progressive increases in bone density of the spine and hip and reduces the occurrence of vertebral and appendicular fractures. Additional advantages of this drug are that it is relatively inexpensive and has few side effects.

CALCITONIN

Calcitonin is a naturally occurring hormone in both men and women that protects bones by inhibiting bone resorption and slowing the bone remodeling cycle. Women have lower levels of calcitonin than men and these levels decrease with age, particularly after menopause, possibly due to decreased estrogen production.

Calcitonin is an FDA-approved treatment of osteoporosis which may increase bone mass in the lumbar spine. Calcitonin can be taken by injections or nasal sprays. It may reduce bone fracture and pain and has been shown to increase bone density when combined with calcium and vitamin D supplements. Side effects with calcitonin are generally minimal, particularly with nasal spray calcitonin, but can include nausea, vomiting, abdominal pain, diarrhea, facial flushing, and tingling of the hands, and it may be more costly than other treatments.

SELECTIVE ESTROGEN RECEPTOR MODULATORS (SERMs)

SERMs (such as raloxifene) are a class of compounds that provide the benefits of estrogen on bone and blood cholesterol without the negative effects on the breast or uterus. SERMs offer promise for the prevention of postmenopausal osteoporosis by decreasing bone loss. Unlike ERT, SERMs do not result in menstrual-type bleeding and breast tenderness and do not increase the risk of breast or uterine cancer. Side effects are uncommon but may include leg cramps and, in rare cases, blood clots.

NEW TREATMENTS UNDER INVESTIGATION

New treatments being explored include other forms of bisphosphonates, parathyroid hormone, sodium fluoride, estrogen and vitamin D analogs, and combination regimens. As with the treatment of hypertension, hyperlipidemia, obesity, diabetes, or heart disease, pharmacological management of osteoporosis should complement, but not precede or replace the foundation of diet, exercise, and smoking cessation.

There is still much room for investigation of combinations of exercise, drugs, and nutritional modulation in this disease. It should be remembered that an osteoporotic appendicular fracture usually combines a fall with an individual with bone density near or below the fracture threshold. With the possible exception of vitamin D, none of the pharmacological agents discussed above has an impact on muscle strength, muscle mass, orthostasis, or balance. Therefore, they are most likely to be clinically relevant in women in whom bone still retains enough integrity so that halting its loss or increasing it slightly means the difference between fracturing and not fracturing after a fall. In the extremely old, bone density is likely to be so low that current treatment modalities that might increase it by 1 to 4% would be unlikely to prevent fracture anyway. In such women, measures to prevent falls or lessen their impact, as discussed here and in Chapter 13, are more likely to be efficacious. Hopefully, new combinations of exercise and bone-modifying agents with maximum potency due to their combined effects on fall risk and bone health will be developed in the future for this population.

REFERENCES

Adinoff, A. and Hollister, J., Steroid-induced fractures and bone loss in patients with asthma, *N. Engl. J. Med.,* 309, 265–268, 1983.

Aloia, J., Cohn, S., Ostuni, J., Cane, R., and Ellis, K., Prevention of involutional bone loss by exercise, *Ann. Intern. Med.,* 89, 356–358, 1978.

Bevier, W. C., Wiswell, R. A., Pyka, G., Kozak, K. C., Newhall, K. M., and Marcus, R., Relationship of body composition, muscle strength, and aerobic capacity to bone mineral density in older men and women, *J. Bone Min. Res.,* 4, 421–432, 1989.

Campbell, A. J., Robertson, M. C., Gardner, M. M., Norton, R. N., Tilyard, M. W., and Buchner, D. M., Randomized controlled trial of a general practice programme of home based exercise to prevent falls in elderly women, *Br. Med. J.,* 315, 1065–1069, 1997.

Chow, R., Harrison, J. E., and Notarius, C., Effect of two randomised exercise programes on bone mass of healthy postmenopausal women, *Br. Med. J.,* 295, 1441–1444, 1987.

Cummings, S. et al., Epidemiology of osteoporosis and osteoporotic fractures, *Epidemiol., Rev.,* 7, 178–208, 1985.

Dalsky, G., Stocke, K., Ehsani, A., Slatopolsky, E., Lee, W., and Birge, S., Weight-bearing exercise training and lumbar bone mineral content in postmenopausal women, *Ann. Intern. Med.,* 108, 824–828, 1988.

Drinkwater, B., Grimson, S., Cullen-Raab, D., and Harter-Snow, C., ACSM position stand on osteoporosis and exercise, *Med. Sci. Sports Exerc.,* 27, i–vii, 1995.

Edelstein, S. L. and Barrett-Connor, E., Relation between body size and bone mineral density in elderly men and women, *Am. J. Epidemiol.,* 138, 160–169, 1993.

Fallon, M. et al., Exogenous hyperthyroidism with osteoporosis, *Arch. Intern. Med.,* 143, 442–444, 1983.

Felson, D. T., Zhang, Y., Hannan, M. T., Kiel, D. P., Wilson, P. W., and Anderson, J. J., The effect of postmenopausal estrogen therapy on bone density in elderly women [see comments], *N. Engl. J. Med.,* 329, 1141–1146, 1993.

Garton, M., Reid, I., Loveridge, N., Robins, S., Murchison, L., Beckett, G. et al., Bone mineral density and metabolism in premenopausal women taking L-thyroxine replacement therapy, *Clin. Endocrinol.,* 41, 747–755, 1994.

Halle, J. S., Smidt, G. L., O'Dwyer, K. D., and Lin, S.-Y., Relationship between trunk muscle torque and bone mineral content of the lumbar spine and hip in healthy postmenopausal women, *Phys. Ther.,* 70, 690–699, 1990.

Huddleston, A. L., Rockwell, D., and Kulund, D. N., Bone mass in lifetime tennis players, *JAMA,* 244, 1107–1109, 1980.

Hughes, D. B., Nutrition, exercise, and lifestyle factors that affect bone health, in *Nutrition in the 90's: Current Controversies and Analysis,* Vol. 2, Kotsonis, F. and Mackey, M. A., Eds., Marcel Dekker, New York, 170, 1994.

Kohrt, W. M., Snead, D. B., Slatopolsky, E., and Birge, S. J., Jr., Additive effects of weight-bearing exercise and estrogen on bone mineral density in older women, *J. Bone Min. Res.,* 10, 1303–1311, 1995.

Krall, E. A. and Dawson-Hughes, B., Walking is related to bone density and rates of bone loss, *Am. J. Med.,* 96, 20–26, 1994.

Lau, E. M. and Cooper, C. The epidemiology of osteoporosis. The oriental perspective in a world context, *Clin. Orthop. Rel. Res.*, 65–74, 1996.

Marcus, R., Ed., *Osteoporosis*, Blackwell Scientific Publications, Boston, 1994.

May, H., Murphy, S., and Khaw, K. T., Alcohol consumption and bone mineral density in older men, *Gerontology*, 41, 152–158, 1995.

Mazess, R. and Whedon, G., Immobilization and bone, *Calcif. Tissue Int.*, 35, 265–267, 1983.

McCartney, N., Hicks, A., Martin, J., and Webber, C., Long-term resistance training in the elderly: effects on dynamic strength, exercise capacity, muscle, and bone, *J. Gerontol.*, 50A:B97–B104, 1995.

Meyer, H. E., Henriksen, C., Falch, J. A., Pedersen, J. I., and Tverdal, A., Risk factors for hip fracture in a high incidence area: a case-control study from Oslo, Norway, *Osteopor. Int.*, 5, 239–246, 1995.

Nelson, M., Fisher, E., Dilmanian, F., Dallal, G., and Evans, W., A 1–y walking program and increased dietary calcium in postmenopausal women: effects on bone, *Am. J. Clin. Nutr.*, 53, 1394–1411, 1991.

Nelson, M. E., Fiatarone, M. A., Morganti, C. M., Trice, I., Greenberg, R. A., and Evans, W. J., Effects of high intensity strength training on multiple risk factors for osteoporotic fractures, *JAMA*, 272 (24):1909–1914, 1994.

Nguyen, T. V., Kelly, P. J., Sambrook, P. N., Gilbert, C., Pocock, N. A., and Eisman, J. A., Lifestyle factors and bone density in the elderly: implications for osteoporosis prevention, *J. Bone Min. Res.*, 9, 1339–1346, 1994.

Notelovitz, M. and Tonnessen, D., *Menopause & Midlife Health*, St. Martin's Press, New York, 1993.

Notelovitz, M., Martin, D., Tesar, R., Khan, F. Y., Probart, C., Fields, C. et al., Estrogen and variable-resistance weight training increase bone mineral in surgically menopausal women, *J. Bone Min. Res.*, 6, 583–590, 1991.

Peck, W. and Avioli, L., *Osteoporosis: The Silent Thief*, Foresman and Co., Glenview, IL, 1988.

Pocock, N., Eisman, J., Gwinn, T., Sambrook, P., Kelly, P., Friuend, J. et al., Muscle strength, physical fitness and weight but not age predict femoral neck bone mass, *J. Bone Min. Res.*, 1989.

Riggs, B., Wahner, H., Melton, L., Richelson, L., Judd, H., and Offord, K., Rates of bone loss in appendicular and axial skeletons of women: evidence of substantial vertebral bone loss before menopause, *J. Clin. Invest.*, 77, 1487–1491, 1986.

Riis, B. J., Biochemical markers of bone turnover. II: Diagnosis, prophylaxis, and treatment of osteoporosis, *Am. J. Med.*, 95, 17S–21S, 1993.

Sinaki, M., McPhee, M. C., and Hodgson, S. F., Relathionship between bone mineral density of spine and strength of back extensors in healthy postmenopausal women, *Mayo Clin. Proc.*, 61, 116–122, 1986.

Swissa-Sivan, A., Azoury, R., Statter, M., Leichter, I., Nyska, A., Nyska M. et al., The effect of swimming on bone modeling and composition in young adult rats, *Calcified Tissue Int.*, 47, 173–177, 1990.

Trotter, M. et al., Densities of bones of white and negro skeletons, *J. Bone Joint Surg. (Am.)*, 42A, 50–58, 1960.

van der Wiel, H. E., Lips, P., Graafmans, W. C., Danielsen, C. C., Nauta J., van Lingen, A. et al., Additional weight-bearing during exercise is more important than duration of exercise for anabolic stimulus of bone: a study of running exercise in female rats, *Bone*, 16, 73–80, 1995.

19 Depression in the Older Woman

Nalin A. Singh

CONTENTS

INTRODUCTION

It is largely our perception of ourselves and our circumstances in life that determines our quality of life. It is commonplace to see people in similar health and social circumstances with very different perceptions of their quality of life. Happiness and contentment in life are primarily related to one's attitude. Herein lies the hidden importance of depression. Nothing affects one's attitude and, consequently, quality of life more negatively than depression.

The recognition of the role depression plays in people's lives and their health is only beginning to be appreciated. It is estimated to be a major world-wide health problem, causing increased morbidity, mortality, health care usage, functional decline, and institutionalization.[1-3] Its presence impedes rehabilitation, compliance with medications, and treatment of disease and leads to suicide. In this chapter a framework for health professionals to identify and understand depression in the older woman with an emphasis on the non-pharmacological management of depression will be provided.

DEFINITIONS

GENERAL PRINCIPLES

Defining depression is difficult, as the term has been variably used to describe a symptom, a syndrome, or a disease. When does a normal human experience or emotion become a disease or a problem requiring treatment? Depressive symptoms span a continuum from transient sadness to psychotic suicidal depression. At the extremes of this continuum there are few problems in identification, but where along the onset of clinical disease begins is not clear. This is especially true in the elderly.

There is no diagnostic test for depression and, therefore, it is diagnosed by clinical interview. There are two principal approaches for defining depression: (1) depressive symptoms and (2) more specific disorders defined in terms of duration and constellation of symptoms. Most health professionals use the first concept while psychiatrists use the second. The *Diagnostic and Statistical Manual for Mental Disorders* (DSM-IV)[4] is a manual used by psychiatrists that outlines the various constellations of symptoms required to allow classification into various psychiatric diagnoses. It was designed so that when psychiatrists discuss patients and interpret treatment effects they can be certain they are talking about similar people. In their definition, *depression* is a collective term referring to a group of disorders in which the central features are lowering of mood and reduced ability to enjoy or take interest in one's usual activities. There is a spectrum of depressive disorders including major depression, minor depression, dysthymia, and depressive disorder not otherwise specified.

Major and minor depression comprise the majority of depressive disorders seen in clinical practice. For diagnosis these require the presence of <u>one</u> of two core symptoms of depression.

(1) Dysphoric mood characterized by symptoms such as feeling sad or blue, or
(2) Loss of interest or pleasure in almost all usual activities and pastimes.

Disturbance in mood is prominent and persistent, but not necessarily the most dominant symptom; other symptoms are listed in Table 1. Major depression differs from minor depression in the required number (less than four for minor, vs. five or more for major) but not duration, severity, or type of symptoms. In general, increasing severity, duration, and number of symptoms of depression differentiate a clinical depression (one requiring treatment) from the less serious mood disturbances transiently experienced by all of us. Two weeks of continuous symptoms interfering with normal social or occupational functioning are necessary for a diagnosis of clinical depression.

Unfortunately, DSM-IV makes no specific provision for age- or gender-related changes in the way depression presents. The alternative approach of using depressive symptoms and a measure of the suffering it is causing in a person's life rather than a specific constellation of symptoms may well be as valid an approach to identify and decide if depression requires treatment in the elderly.

How Age Affects the Recognition of Depression

The failure to recognize depression is common in the elderly because there are always plausible alternative explanations other than depression for their symptoms. In young people these are rarely issues. With age the combination of increasing prevalence of disease, and functional and cognitive declines complicate the diagnosis. Aging usually means increases in disability and chronic illness, and this illness burden often leads both medical staff and patients to focus on physical issues rather than depressive symptoms. Health workers' expectations and assessments of capacity are often lowered in illness and retirement, with impairment in function being attributed to age and disease rather than depression. The constellation of symptoms may also differ, as the older person may tend to complain of somatic symptoms rather than mood change.[5] The difficulty for clinicians is that the standard DSM criteria used to diagnose clinical depression include somatic symptoms such as sleep disturbance, appetite and weight change, psychomotor retardation and fatigue, which are common in the physically ill older person as well. There is still considerable stigma attached to being psychiatrically unwell or unable to cope. Men tend not to admit to sadness or other psychological symptoms but to just complain of fatigue and lack of interest. Cognitive impairment also gives rise to many of the diagnostic criteria of depression such as diminished ability to concen-

TABLE 1
Criteria for Major Depressive Episode

Five (or more) of the following symptoms have been present during the same two-week period and represent a change from previous functioning; and at least one of the symptoms is either (1) depressed mood or (2) loss of interest or pleasure.

1. Depressed mood most of the day, nearly every day, as indicated by either subjective report (e.g., feels sad or empty) or observation made by others (e.g., appears tearful).
2. Markedly diminished interest or pleasure in all, or almost all, activities most of the day, nearly everyday (as indicated by either subjective account or observations made by others).
3. Significant weight loss when not dieting or weight gain (e.g., a change of more than 5% of body weight in a month), or decrease or increase in appetite nearly every day.
4. Insomnia or hypersomnia nearly every day.
5. Psychomotor agitation or retardation nearly every day (observable by others, not merely subjective feelings of restlessness or being slowed down).
6. Fatigue or loss of energy nearly every day.
7. Feelings of worthlessness or excessive or inappropriate guilt (which may be delusional) nearly every day (not merely self-reproach or guilt about being sick).
8. Diminished ability to think or concentrate, or indecisiveness, nearly every day (either by subjective account or as observed by others).
9. Recurrent thoughts of death (not just fear of dying), recurrent suicidal ideation without a specific plan, or a suicide attempt or a specific plan for committing suicide.

The symptoms do not meet criteria for a Mixed episode.

The symptoms cause clinically significant distress or impairment in social, occupational, or other important areas of functioning.

The symptoms are due/not due to the direct physiologic effects of a substance (e.g., a drug of abuse, a medication) or a general medical condition (e.g., hypothyroidism).

The symptoms are not better accounted for by bereavement, i.e., after the loss of a loved one; the symptoms persist for longer than 2 months or are characterized by marked functional impairment, morbid preoccupation with worthlessness, suicidal ideation, psychotic symptoms, or psychomotor retardation.

From *Diagnostic and Statistical Manual of Mental Disorders, 4th ed.*, American Psychiatric Association, Washington, D.C., 1994. With permission.

trate, indecisiveness, and loss of interest. Therefore, the combination of disease, social changes, and societal expectations associated with aging complicates the recognition of depression.[6]

PREVALENCE

The association between aging and depression has aroused much interest recently with community-based studies being carried out across the world; however, reported rates of depression vary widely in the elderly. Epidemiological studies that use the standard diagnostic criteria or a constellation of symptoms to identify clinical depression show a decrease in the prevalence of depression with age.[7] Clinical studies and epidemiological studies using symptom scales, on the other hand, find that symptoms of mood disturbance are *more* common in older adults.[8]

It appears that the major depressive disorders defined and measured according to rigorous research diagnostic criteria are relatively rare among the elderly. Their prevalence seems to decrease from around 5% in middle age to about 2% in the elderly. This decrease may be because older people with major depression, who are the population under study, leave the community due to excess mortality, institutionalization, or dementia.

The rates of serious depression vary widely depending upon residential setting, with rates as low as 5% in primary care clinics of community-dwelling elderly up to 15–25% in the nursing home.[9] There is a 13% annual incidence of new episodes of depression among aged long-term care residents, who therefore represent a high-risk group.

In summary, when depression is viewed along a continuum, there appears to be an increased number of elderly below the cutoff for formal psychiatrically defined major depression but an increase in categories such as minor depression or subsyndromal depression. It has been argued that the criteria for major depression were derived from clinical experience with younger patients and that they are not adequate in the elderly.[5] Instead, the level of suffering and impairment that is related to depressive symptomatology should be the decisive factor in whether or not treatment is indicated. Using these sorts of definitions, it is estimated that 15 to 20% of community-dwelling elders have a type and degree of depression warranting clinical and public health attention.[7]

RISK FACTORS

Family studies consistently show that major depression is highly familial with a two- to threefold increase in major depression in first-degree relatives of probands with major depression.[10] Cross-national epidemiological studies have consistently shown that the rate of depression is higher in women[11] than in men.

The major medical, social, and demographic risk factors for the development of depression are similar to those in younger age groups, including chronic illness, disability, unmarried or widowed status, stressful life events, and lack of a supportive social network.[12] The impact of risk factors is largely independent of age; however, the rate of exposure to risk factors dramatically increases with age. This is particularly true for the risk factors such as illness, functional impairment, and loss of significant others.

NATURAL HISTORY OF DEPRESSION

There appears to be increasing recognition that the majority of major depressive episodes are recurrent in nature, that the course is lifelong, and appropriate treatment is for a chronic disease.[3] The natural history of untreated major depression is roughly as follows: one-third will recover, one third will stay the same, and one third will worsen over a one-year period. Older persons are more likely to have lengthy episodes and a higher rate of relapse.[13]

The natural history of minor depression is poorly studied by comparison. It has been estimated that 25% of minor depression will evolve into major depression within two years.[14] Whether or not early intervention may reduce the pool of milder depressives who would go on to develop major depression is unknown.

SUICIDE

The rate for completed suicide is highest among elderly white males. The 85 and older age group have a suicide rate that is six times that of the general population. Women outnumber men in suicide attempts, but men exceed women in suicide completion. The gender disparity in suicide completion increases with age, such that over the age of 85, the rate of suicide is 12-fold higher in men. The method of suicide attempt seems to vary between the genders, with 40% of women overdosing on prescription drugs vs. only 6.4% of men.[15]

The most common risk factor in the aged for suicidal behavior is mental illness, of which depression is the major category. Rates of contact with medical personnel in the month prior to suicide vary but appear to be about 60% in the last month of life, 20 to 30% in the week prior, and 10 to 20% on the actual day of suicide. Of the elderly suicide completers at least 70% were recognized as depressed by a health care professional prior to death. Most had a first time episode of major depression that was only moderately severe, yet symptoms went unrecognized and/or untreated.

In dealing with the depressed elderly, risk of suicide must be assessed in each individual, including the strength of the suicidal ideation and plans to complete an attempt. When an elderly patient refuses to eat or requests withdrawal of all medical support, a thorough assessment of the presence of potentially treatable depressive symptoms should be undertaken to guide medical decision-making.

TRADITIONAL APPROACHES TO TREATMENT OF DEPRESSION

Once a diagnosis of clinical depression has been made, treatment traditionally has included one or more of the following: psychological approaches such as psychotherapy (cognitive, behavioral, brief dynamic therapy), family and social therapies, or biological approaches such as pharmacotherapy, electroconvulsive therapy, and correction of medical illness. In the management of clinical depression, a combination of these treatment approaches is typically used for maximal efficacy.

MEDICAL ILLNESS

Depression may be the direct physiologic consequence of a general medical condition or its treatment such as hypothyroidism, vitamin B_{12} deficiency, substance abuse, or the prescription of a centrally acting medication such as alpha-methyldopa for hypertension. In the elderly, where drug side effects are not well studied prior to marketing, all centrally acting drugs should be viewed with suspicion. In these instances correction of the deficit or removal of the drug significantly improves the depression.

Psychotherapy

There are many forms of psychotherapy, each involving in varying degree listening and speaking by a therapist. A comprehensive review of these techniques is beyond the scope of this chapter but they are all utilized to some degree in the treatment of the depressed person. These therapies may range from re-parenting in personality disorders to just being supportive and allowing the expression of emotions in counseling. Interpersonal psychotherapy is a systematic and standardized treatment approach to relationships and life problems while cognitive therapy is directed toward changing the patient's way of thinking about these problems to a more positive way.

Pharmacotherapy

A variety of chemical classes of medications are available to treat depression including tricyclics, monoamine oxidase inhibitors (MAOI), heterocyclics, and selective serotonin reuptake inhibitors (SSRIs). The majority of these drugs work on the principle of increasing post-synaptic neurotransmitter availability in the brain. These drugs vary in their postulated actions and side-effect profiles, with the more recent (selective serotonin reuptake inhibitors) demonstrating an improved side-effect profile. No single antidepressant is clearly more effective than another. They all have similar response rates (around 60% of patients clinically improve during treatment of an index episode), but many retain significant residual symptomatology.

The data for effectiveness of antidepressants in the very old (over 80 years of age) is minimal and is largely based on extrapolation from younger subjects.[16] It is clear that response depends on adequate length of treatment, and requires at least 6 to 12 weeks, with the majority responding by 8 weeks. However, response occurs later in older patients, so more prolonged periods of treatment may be required to prevent relapse. The use of antidepressant drugs has now been documented to be effective in both dysthymia and major depression. Their clinical use is now being extended to milder forms of depression, where evidence of efficacy is currently under study.

Electroconvulsive Therapy (ECT)

Electroconvulsive therapy is the passing of an electrical current through the brain to induce seizure activity under general anesthesia. In those with severe melancholic depression who are not eating, are catatonic, delusional, have previously responded to ECT or are unable to participate in any other treatments, it is the preferred option. In a hospital setting, 6 to 9 sessions are usually required and the response rate approaches 90%. The side effect risks include those of a general anaesthetic and a seizure as well as amnestic syndromes, delirium, and possible permanent cognitive impairment. The extent of possible permanent cognitive changes characteristics of patients at higher risk for such side effects, and the lowered risk of unilateral ECT in this regard are still matters of debate.

OTHER THERAPIES

There is a range of other therapies used in the treatment of depression which are poorly studied including homeopathy, hypnotherapy, massage therapy, acupuncture, music therapy, dance and movement therapy.[17] The most promising of these is a herbal medication known as St. John's Wort (*Hypericum perforatum*; for a review, please see Reference 18).

TREATMENT DECISIONS AND INDICATIONS FOR HOSPITALIZATION

The management of a patient with moderate to severe depression requires a decision regarding the setting in which she would be optimally treated. The answer to this question depends on the severity of the disorder and the quality of the patient's social resources.

In judging severity, an assessment of the risk of suicide and any failure to eat or drink that may endanger the patient's life are crucial. Provided that these risks are absent, most patients with supportive families or social networks may be treated in their place of residence. Patients who are alone may require day-patient care or hospitalization. The first step in treatment is rarely ECT unless rapid improvement is required due to life-threatening symptoms. Rather, medical diseases would be optimized, drug therapy would commence, a pleasurable events schedule would be introduced to increase the patient's social interaction, and cognitive therapy begun to address negative thinking. Weekly treatment such as this would continue for 6–8 weeks in typical cases.

EXERCISE AND DEPRESSION

RATIONALE FOR THE USE OF EXERCISE TO TREAT DEPRESSION

The rationale for the use of exercise as an antidepressant is based on its potential risk benefit advantage over current therapies. There is little point in exploring a treatment for depression unless it offers some potential benefit over current standard therapy. In geriatrics we like to think about treatment holistically, in terms of the effect treatment will have on the target symptoms, as well as on the patient's other co-morbidities, functional status, and quality of life.

A large literature supports the antidepressant effect of exercise.[19] If we accept the data that exercise has an antidepressant effect similar to current standard therapy, then by applying the above rationale (as illustrated in Table 2), there is a potential benefit advantage over current drug therapy.

What about the risk of therapy? While improvements in side-effect profiles of drugs used to treat depression continue to occur, it is apparent from drug trials that approximately one-third of patients still find these newer agents intolerable.[20] Data on effectiveness and side-effect profiles of these drugs in the elderly are limited with as yet no convincing evidence of a reduction in falls risk[21,22] compared to older agents. Given these observations about risk of therapy, and referring to Table 3, again there is a potential advantage in the use of exercise.

The rationale is well illustrated by comparing a 30-year-old who presents with depression vs. a 75-year-old. The 30-year-old woman is unlikely to suffer from major co-morbidities such as heart failure, arthritis, diabetes or be at risk for delirium, falls, and functional decline. Therefore, the risk benefit advantage for the use of exercise over a drug is minimal. In contrast, a 75-year-old woman presenting with depression may have difficulty with mobility and shopping because of osteoarthritis, osteoporosis, recurrent falls, and a previous hip fracture; she suffers with diabetes, hypertension, and constipation as well. In this patient there is a clear risk benefit advantage with exercise as a treatment for depression vs. pharmacotherapy.

TABLE 2
Comparison of Benefits of Standard Therapy vs. Exercise for Depression

Potential Benefit	Standard Therapy[a]	Exercise
Relief of psychological symptoms	Yes	Yes
Relief of somatic symptoms	Yes	Yes
Treatment of co-morbid conditions	No	Yes[b]
Improved fitness and function	No	Yes
Improved quality of life	Yes	Yes
Application to a larger number of depressives	?	?

[a] Standard therapy means antidepressant drug treatment for depression.

[b] Obesity, hypertension, hyperlipidemia, cardiovascular disease, diabetes, peripheral vascular disease, chronic obstructive pulmonary disease, arthritis, osteoporosis.

TABLE 3
Comparison of the Potential Risk of Standard Therapy vs. Exercise in Depression

Potential Risk	Standard Therapy[a]	Exercise
Cardiac arrhythmia	Yes	Yes
Cardiac ischemia	No	Yes[b]
Musculoskeletal injury	Yes	Yes
Fall risk	Yes	Yes[b]
Overdose	Yes	No
Dry mouth and eyes	Yes	No
Orthostatic hypotension	Yes	No[b]
Nausea, constipation, diarrhea	Yes	No[b]
Delirium	Yes	No
Sedation, agitation	Yes	No[b]
Unintended weight change	Yes	Yes[b]

[a] Standard therapy means antidepressant drug treatment for depression.

[b] Indicates risk may also be reduced by exercise.

Exercise may also be a useful adjunctive treatment to standard therapy, although to date this has only been shown to augment response in younger adults. In the elderly, in particular, if exercise augments the antidepressant effect of drugs while counteracting their side effects, it will produce a very favorable shift in the risk/benefit ratio of treatment. Theoretically, side effects may be diminished because necessary drug dosages or durations are lessened by the addition of exercise, or because exercise directly affects the risk factor(s). For example, fall risk from antidepressants may be reduced by the ability of exercise to improve postural hypotension, muscle weakness, and/or poor balance.

THE EFFECT OF EXERCISE ON DEPRESSION

The theoretical mechanisms by which exercise may exert an antidepressant effect fall into two broad groups.

1. Biological theories that include hormonal and neurotransmitter changes as well as functional and health improvements.[23]
2. Cognitive behavioral theories that are based on the fact that exercise may catalyze a transformation in a maladaptive cognitive set.[24] This interrupts the negative downward thought spiral of the depressed individual by making them feel more positive about circumstances.

It is generally accepted that exercise works by multiple mechanisms, and individual responses may depend more or less heavily on a single mechanism depending on the characteristics of the individual, the life circumstances, and the depressive illness itself.

EVIDENCE FOR A PHYSICAL ACTIVITY AND DEPRESSION LINK

Several large epidemiological studies have now found a relationship between self-reported activity level and self-reported depressive symptoms.[25,26] The cross-sectional relationship is strong, with less active individuals experiencing the highest prevalence of depressive symptoms. The longitudinal data suggest that those who are free of depression at baseline and physically active have much lower rates of depression prospectively compared to those who are free of depression at baseline and sedentary. This relationship exists for both men and women and is independent of age, chronic illness, education, income, and social support. While the issue of which came first is not clear from cross-sectional studies, there is now growing evidence from the above longitudinal research that being active may prevent the onset of depression and be an important public health strategy.

There is a large literature (over 1000 studies) exploring the relationship of exercise to mood,[27] the majority of which have been conducted in normal populations. The literature appears to have been dominated by the controversy of whether or not exercise improves mood in normal people, and there is as much evidence for an effect as against an effect. When one's mood is normal, it is hardly surprising that exercise doesn't always show an antidepressant effect. The anxiolytic effect of exercise is more clearly established in the normal population.[27] There is, however, reasonable evidence in habitual exercisers with normal mood of a deterioration in mood following withdrawal of exercise.

EXERCISE IN THE YOUNG WITH CLINICAL DEPRESSION

In clinical depression there are fewer studies, most of which have methodological problems. Examination of the better designed studies (14 randomized controlled trials) all draw similar conclusions.[28] Exercise is better than placebo and is of roughly equal efficacy to various forms of group and psychotherapy in selected populations. There is currently no study directly comparing exercise to drug treatment in young subjects although the magnitude of reduction in depression scores achieved by exercise approximates that of drugs.[28-30] There is currently work proceeding in this area comparing running treatment vs. drug therapy. Additional benefit of exercise is demonstrated when combined with standard therapy (psychiatric counseling with or without drugs) vs. standard therapy alone in inpatient depressed subjects.[31]

The majority of studies have used aerobic exercise as the intervention, as early work suggested that an aerobic training effect was required to elicit depression reduction.[31-33] There are two subsequent studies in young subjects comparing aerobic to non-aerobic training, both showing equivalent antidepressant effects.[34,35] Upon review of current data, it appears that both forms of exercise are effective in the young, clinically depressed patient.

EXERCISE IN THE CLINICALLY DEPRESSED ELDERLY

In subjects over the age of sixty, there are only three published randomized trials.[29,36] In McNiel's study, subjects (mean age 72 years) were chosen by self-reported scores of >12 on the Beck Depression Inventory (BDI) and may or may not have fulfilled diagnostic psychiatric criteria for depression. Over a 6-week intervention of walking social contact vs. wait list, the BDI was reduced approximately 33% in the walking group, not significantly different from the social contact group, but significantly different from the wait list. In our trial of clinically depressed elderly over 60 years of age (mean age 72), we demonstrated a reduction of 60% in both therapist and self-rated scales of depression in comparison to 30% in the attention control group after twenty weeks of weight training.[29] Blumenthal[37] recently repeated the results of a trial directly comparing antidepressants, aerobic exercise, and combination treatment in 156 adults of mean age 57. All three treatments had equally potent ability to relieve depression after 4 months (approximately 65% effective).

EVIDENCE FOR A NUTRITION AND DEPRESSION LINK

The majority of evidence for a nutritional link with depression is centered on the theory that dysregulation of one-carbon metabolism may be related to the pathogenesis of depression. The compounds B_{12}, folate, tetrahydrofolate, and homocysteine interact to produce S-adenosylmethionine, a major donor of methyl groups in brain chemical formation and transmission.

FOLATE

Of all the potential links in the methylation hypothesis of mood disturbance, the most data exist on folate. Depressive symptoms are the most common neuropsychiatric manifestation of folate deficiency. Borderline low or deficient serum or red blood cell folate levels are detected in 20–40% of adults diagnosed with depressive disorders.[38] In comparison to normal controls or other psychiatric patients, depressed patients have significantly lower folate levels. Within depressed patients there are several studies demonstrating a correlation between depressive severity and folate levels, with lower levels associated with more severe depression.[38] The lower levels of folate have been associated with a significantly lower likelihood of response to antidepressant treatment.[39]

These associations do not, of course, imply causality, as a reduced folate status may be secondary to the development of depression, due to changes in food intake or metabolism. However, experimental evidence for the effects of folate on mood exists as well. Intervention studies have been conducted in folate-deficient psychiatric inpatients, those with gastrointestinal disorders resulting in folate malabsorption, and epileptics whose anti-seizure medications may increase folate needs. In all of these populations, folate administration has been shown to result in mood improvement.[40] There is, however, minimal experimental evidence in depressed people who are deficient in folate. There is one double-blind placebo-controlled trial of methylfolate, 15 mg per day for six months, in addition to standard antidepressant medication. In this trial there was a minor clinical improvement and statistically better outcome on therapist rating of depression at six months in those taking methylfolate. Compelling evidence for the use of folate in any other context is lacking at this stage.

Why folate levels are reduced to such an extent in depression is not clear, but it has been suggested that it cannot be entirely accounted for on the basis of dietary intake.[41] Deficiencies of folate have important implications for the incidence of fetal malformations in young women, as well as coronary artery disease and cerebrovascular disease in the elderly. Therefore, depressed patients should be viewed as an extremely high-risk group for folate deficiency, which should be screened for and treated if present, due to health risks in other areas, if not specifically as a means to mood elevation.

S-ADENOSYLMETHIONINE

S-adenosylmethionine (SAM) is synthesized in the body and is a major source of methyl groups in the brain.[42] It can be administered orally or intravenously and several open trials of the use of SAM have been encouraging regarding its antidepressant effect. The unique property of SAM is that its onset of antidepressant action appears to be between 7 and 14 days, which is faster than all other current treatments.[43] It appears to be more effective in more severe depression and is a physiologic substance relatively free of severe side effects. There are randomized controlled trials underway whose results are awaited before any recommendations regarding its use can be supported in the elderly.

RECOMMENDATIONS FOR SCREENING ASSESSMENT AND TREATMENT OF THE OLDER WOMAN

There is overwhelming evidence that individuals with depression are being seriously undertreated. The reasons for this include patient-related factors such as under reporting severity, limited access, non-compliance, and reluctance to see a psychiatrist because of the social stigma attached to it. Health professional-related factors include poor education about depression, limited training in interpersonal skills, and failure to provide adequate treatment, both psychotherapeutic as well as pharmaceutic.[44] There is evidence that the vast majority of depression may be alleviated when appropriately treated.

The efficacy of mass or population screening of individuals for a condition relates to the prevalence of the condition and the ability to improve it once identified. Based on current epidemiological data, it is advisable to screen elderly women in nursing home settings and those at high risk of depression in outpatient practice settings, including people who have poor social supports, chronic illness, recent bereavement, disability, or are housebound with limited access to health care services.

The best form of screening for patients seen regularly is to incorporate questions about their mood during regular contact visits by asking specifically about sadness, loss of interest or pleasure in activities, and changes in sleep patterns. Suicidal thoughts should be inquired about if there is any suggestion of depression, as they may be present even if depression severity is moderate. An alternative or additional method is to combine this approach with a screening tool. Of the many screening tools available for depression, the Geriatric Depression Scale (GDS) is the preferred measure in the elderly as it is validated in the community, nursing home, and acute hospital setting. It is a series of 30 yes/no questions (score 0–30), with higher scores reflective of worse depression,[45] as shown in Table 4. With a score of 14 or above, there are 100% specificity and 80% sensitivity to detect major depression. The GDS can be self- or interviewer-administered in less than 5 minutes in most cases and is validated in a shorter form and for use over the phone as well. Ideally, screening in the high-risk group of older women should be done by whichever health professional sees them most frequently, on a yearly basis at least.

THE HISTORY AND PHYSICAL EXAMINATION OF THE DEPRESSED OLDER WOMAN

A thorough medical and psychiatric history is essential in the depressed patient. The following discusses a few key features to consider in the depressed older woman.

TABLE 4
Geriatric Depression Scale

Instructions: Choose the best answer for how you have felt in the past week.

1.	Are you basically satisfied with your life?	YES/NO
2.	Have you dropped many of your activities and interests?	YES/NO
3.	Do you feel that your life is empty?	YES/NO
4.	Do you often get bored?	YES/NO
5.	Are you hopeful about the future?	YES/NO
6.	Are you bothered by thoughts you can't get out of your head?	YES/NO
7.	Are you in good spirits most of the time?	YES/NO
8.	Are you afraid something bad is going to happen to you?	YES/NO
9.	Do you feel happy most of the time?	YES/NO
10.	Do you often feel helpless?	YES/NO
11.	Do you often get restless and fidgety?	YES/NO
12.	Do you prefer to stay at home, rather than going out and doing new things?	YES/NO
13.	Do you frequently worry about the future?	YES/NO
14.	Do you feel you have more problems with memory than most?	YES/NO
15.	Do you think it is wonderful to be alive now?	YES/NO
16.	Do you often feel downhearted and blue?	YES/NO
17.	Do you feel pretty worthless the way you are now?	YES/NO
18.	Do you worry a lot about the past?	YES/NO
19.	Do you find life very exciting?	YES/NO
20.	Is it hard for you to get started on new projects?	YES/NO
21.	Do you feel full of energy?	YES/NO
22.	Do you feel that your situation is hopeless?	YES/NO
23.	Do you think that most people are better off than you are?	YES/NO
24.	Do you frequently get upset over little things?	YES/NO
25.	Do you frequently feel like crying?	YES/NO
26.	Do you have trouble concentrating?	YES/NO
27.	Do you enjoy getting up in the mornings?	YES/NO
28.	Do you prefer to avoid social gatherings?	YES/NO
29.	Is it easy for you to make decisions?	YES/NO
30.	Is your mind as clear as it used to be?	YES/NO

Scoring Instructions: Add up the number of wrong (depressed) answers.

Coding is as follows in relation to psychiatric diagnoses obtained by structured interview:

Scores 0–8 Not depressed
Scores 9–14 Mild depression
Scores 15–23 Moderate depression
Scores 24–30 Severe depression

Yesavage, J. A. and Brink, T. L., *J. Psychiatr. Res.*, 17, 37–49, 1983. With permission.

MEDICAL HISTORY AND EXAMINATION

Certain disorders such as stroke or dementia are associated with higher rates of depression and should increase the vigilance of the health professional when present by history. Symptoms or signs of hypothyroidism, alcohol or drug abuse, and chronic pain syndromes should be actively sought, as these conditions may present as depression. A complete review of medications (both prescribed and over-the-counter) and their side effects is essential. Assessment of other co-morbidities is important in terms of treatment side effects, including a history of previous falls, balance problems, muscle weakness, weight loss, dietary intake, and constipation.

PSYCHIATRIC HISTORY AND EXAMINATION

Formal psychiatric assessment and examination are beyond the scope of this chapter but are available in any standard psychiatric textbook. History should include risk factors for depression, family history, social support network, current stressors, the current symptoms of depression and their impact on the patient's life, and previous effective treatments. It is important to talk to someone who knows the person and ask him/her independently about any changes, the patient's compliance with medications, and dietary intake. The assessment of suicidal risk is an important yet imprecise skill. Factors associated with suicide attempts in the elderly include higher socioeconomic status, evidence of more past suicide attempts, and never having achieved remission from the index depression episode. At hospital admission, the patients who later attempt suicide evidence more suicidal tendencies than those who did not attempt suicide. Questioning how far along the continuum of suicidal ideation, plans, or acts they have progressed assesses this, i.e., questions regarding how frequently and intrusive their thoughts of suicide are, or have they made a plan as to how they would commit suicide, what preparations have they made to die, have they written a note, bought a gun, visited the proposed site of suicide, etc. These are difficult questions to ask and the responses are not easy to assess in a depressed person but, in general, the more advanced along this continuum, the more likely is a suicide attempt. Approximately 8–10% of people admitted to a hospital with a major depression will commit suicide at one year, thus targeting an extremely high-risk group for assessment and close follow-up. As these figures indicate, even hospitalization may not prevent the truly suicidal patient from taking his or her own life.

In examination by health professionals, two aspects are most helpful in diagnosis. The first of these is body language during contact with the patient. The person's posture, an obvious withdrawn, apathetic, stooped or disinterested appearance, tearfulness, and inability to make or sustain eye contact are often indicative of depression. In addition, extremes of body movements during the interview, known as the level of psychomotor agitation or retardation, are important. Depressed people tend to be at the ends of this spectrum, either slow and retarded or agitated.

The second aspect is to pay particular attention to how you feel when you leave the person. Are you sad and low or frustrated and angry? Both pairs of feelings may be signs of depression in the patient. The patient may be feeling this way about herself, and without talking about it explicitly, may have communicated these feelings to you. In examination, these two broad areas can often tell you as much about how the patient is feeling as direct questioning, especially if you have known a person over time.

RECOMMENDATIONS FOR THE TREATMENT OF DEPRESSION WITH EMPHASIS ON PHYSICAL ACTIVITY PRESCRIPTION FOR DEPRESSION

PREVENTION

Longitudinal studies suggest that increasing physical activity may prevent the onset of depression. Whether or not the world-wide public health efforts to increase physical activity over the last decade will see declining rates of depression in the community in the future is unknown. It appears that things that protect you from depression revolve around being active mentally, physically, and socially. The recommendation that exercise can prevent depression is premature but appears sensible, in combination with other means to increase societal and interpersonal involvement.

TREATMENT IN CLINICAL DEPRESSION

Modality

The majority of trials have used aerobic exercise as their treatment for depression; however, there are two published studies comparing weight lifting exercise to aerobic exercise in depression,[34,35] both in young individuals under 60. These suggest that both forms of exercise are effective in reducing depression, but weight lifting had higher compliance and in meta-analysis of normals and depressed patients, possibly a greater antidepressant effect.[19] Theoretically there are advantages to resistance training rather than aerobic training for an older population. These include

1. It specifically addresses the physiologic accompaniments of frailty, including loss of lean muscle mass and strength (sarcopenia);
2. It has fewer contraindications than aerobic exercise,
3. It is proven safe and feasible with high compliance in the frailest of elderly, including non-ambulatory individuals; and
4. It may directly counteract the fall risk associated with antidepressant medications.

In the elderly there are only three randomized trials of the effect of exercise on depression. McNeil conducted the first in a group of 30 individuals with self-rated depressive symptoms with a mean age of 72. They were randomized to a supervised progressive walking regimen over 6 weeks, social contact visits at home, or a wait list group. Both the social contact and exercise groups improved in their depression scores by about 30% which was significantly greater than no treatment, but about the amount seen in placebo groups in drug trials. In our study, we explored weight lifting at high intensity vs. an attention control group over 10 weeks in a randomized controlled trial in 32 subjects with a mean age 72, fulfilling DSMIV criteria for major or minor depression or dysthymia. We found a 60% reduction in depression vs. a 30% reduction in the attention control group. The exercise was safe, well tolerated, and continued in both home and gym settings with high compliance.[30] Even at 2 years one third of participants[30] were still weight lifting at least twice a week. We saw improvements in sleep quality, strength, quality of life, and both somatic and psychological symptoms of depression. Blumenthal[37] reported significant improvements in clinically depressed subjects randomized to either aerobic exercise, traditional treatment, or exercise plus traditional treatment.

Based on the current available evidence, therefore, a trial of aerobic exercise vs. weight lifting is required to definitively resolve the issue as to which modality is more effective or feasible in older women. Aerobic exercise in studies where it has been shown effective was usually jogging, although brisk walking has also been employed in some studies. In light of this, information on prescribing both types of exercise for depression is given below.

Dose: Intensity, Frequency, and Duration

Exercise programs of duration greater than 16 weeks have the greatest benefits. Clinical response can be seen in the majority by six weeks, which is approximately the same time course as seen with drug treatments of depression.[19] There is now wide acceptance of major depression as a recurrent disorder for which chronic treatment is required to maintain response and decrease relapse rates.[46] It is also known that long-term adoption and adherence to an exercise program is best if it can be performed regularly for at least six months. Therefore, recommendation for exercise duration is *lifelong* with full behavioral technique support for at least six months.

In his first inpatient study of 43 subjects with major depression, Martinsen found a relationship between an increase in aerobic capacity and a reduction in depression. This finding and those of earlier studies using running fueled the idea that aerobic capacity change was required and the larger the change the better the antidepressant effect.[31,47] A larger subsequent study found no such relationship[34] and reviews of the aerobic exercise and depression literature[48] have consistently found no relationship between gain in aerobic capacity and reduction in depression. All trials have used standard aerobic training methods, either walking or jogging at 60 to 75% of maximal heart rate reserve [.60–.75(maximal heart rate – resting heart rate) + resting heart rate] for 20 to 50 minutes per session. The duration of training has typically been 3 to 5 times per week. In the older woman free of cardiac contraindications, a prescription of brisk walking at 60% of maximal heart rate reserve 3 to 5 days a week for 20 minutes minimum is therefore recommended.

The two weight-training studies in young subjects did not publish the details of their methods of training, other than it was of low intensity to avoid aerobic benefit. No strength gains were reported to allow assessment of the relative resistances that may have been used. In our study in the elderly, we found that intensity of weight training (the relative loads which were lifted during training sessions as a percent of peak capacity) correlated closely with improvement in depression, such that high intensity trainers achieved the greatest reduction in depression. We have subsequently tested this in a randomized controlled study of training at 80% of maximum strength vs. training at 20% of maximum strength in 38 subjects over age 60 with major depression. Using blinded assessment of the GDS by a psychiatrist, we found a 65% reduction in depression after high intensity training, compared to reductions of 35% after low intensity care and 15% after general practitioner follow-up. The high-intensity weight lifting was significantly more beneficial than the other two treatments, which were not statistically different from each other (see Figure 1). Therefore, our recommendation regarding resistance training is high intensity training 3 days a week at 80% of maximal capacity in a balanced program of all large muscle groups for approximately 45 minutes each session. Whether or not a less frequent regimen may be as effective is unknown at present. Larger studies will be needed to determine if there is a clinically important effect of low intensity resistance training, (i.e., a greater magnitude than that seen with placebo treatments).

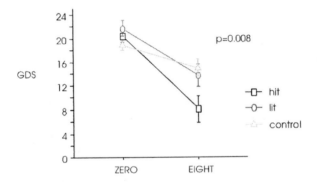

FIGURE 1   Results of high-intensity progressive resistance training (hit), n = 13 vs. low-intensity resistance training (lit), n = 13 vs. general practitioner care (control), n = 14. The GDS is the Geriatric Depression Score with higher scores reflecting more severe depression. The horizontal axis is time in weeks.

BEHAVIORAL TECHNIQUES

The depressed population is no more difficult to train than other populations. The general principles outlined elsewhere in this book to encourage participation rates apply, and in clinical trials retention rates and compliance are high. However, the depressed person will often suffer with hypersensitivity to all interactions, which may be a prominent feature of their disease, and careful watching and shaping are important in the early phase of training. As lack of motivation is also a hallmark of the disease, particular attention should be paid to reasons for exercising and barriers to adherence, as this is key to maintenance of the exercise prescription.

SETTING

It has been a commonly held belief that exercise works through socialization and requires a group setting to be effective. There is strong evidence that socialization is *not* required for people to benefit from exercise in terms of depression, just as is the case for other kinds of physiologic adaptation. The effectiveness of exercise in depression has been demonstrated in nursing homes, hostels, and community dwelling elderly as well as inpatient psychiatric hospitals. Compliance is as high at home as in group settings and the choice of setting in which the patient wishes to exercise is most important in regard to long-term adherence. In clinical depression there have been no direct comparisons between two similar exercise regimens done in different settings (e.g., at home vs. a gymnasium, or supervised vs. unsupervised programs). Our current recommendation, based on the experimental evidence available, is that exercise be commenced in a supervised way for a period until confidence allows transition to the patient's unsupervised setting of choice.

SPECIAL CONSIDERATIONS

Depression is a chronic disorder and can be viewed in various stages of response or relapse. There is an acute or ill phase, which is either followed by partial response or full response when the patient returns to normalcy. This is known as a remission if it is transient or a recovery if it is of many months' duration. If symptoms return during a remission, it is called a relapse, and if during a recovery, it is known as a recurrence. Acute treatment is aimed at bringing about a remission of the index episode, and continuation treatment is to keep someone in remission until they reach recovery. Treatment after this is known as maintenance treatment, its aim being the prevention of recurrence over the long term.

In which treatment phases is exercise beneficial? Data are available for the use of exercise in the acute and continuation phases of treatment, but the data on maintenance therapy with exercise are sparse and methodologically unsound. The current literature suggests pharmacotherapy and psychotherapy in combination are the best treatments for the maintenance phase of the disease.[13] The drugs are most effective when continued in the dose at which their index case of depression responded. This dose should be maintained throughout the maintenance phase.[46] While this whole area remains unstudied in relation to exercise, theoretically, exercise could work in this phase of treatment, and until more is known should be continued at the same dose used during acute and continuation treatment.

COMBINATION THERAPY

Exercise has been tried in combination with standard therapy (primarily psychotherapy) in depressed psychiatric inpatient units with evidence that its addition induces a significant improvement in outcomes.[31] The clinical use of exercise in inpatient psychiatric facilities is widespread in some countries such as Holland and Norway. Martinsen et al.[31,34] examined subgroups of patients (51 in total) receiving both antidepressants and aerobic or resistive exercise found no significant additive effects of the exercise. Direct comparisons of aerobic exercise and standard therapy or combinations of these interventions in elderly depressed patient populations have been published for the first time by Blumenthal[37] as noted earlier. Similar comparisons of resistance training vs. standard treatment remain to be published.

HOW TO MONITOR DEPRESSED PATIENTS

The key to monitoring the depressed patient is regular contact with continual questioning regarding mood and suicidal ideation. Typically, in someone with a major depression you initially undertake weekly contact. You should not expect any major improvement for about four weeks, regardless of treatment strategy. During this time you are really monitoring the patient for increased suicide risk. If by six weeks there is no evidence of response, a change in management is warranted. The most important part of monitoring is to ensure as complete a return to normalcy as possible. If using the GDS as a monitoring instrument, scores below 9 generally indicate mild to no depressive symptoms. The important maintenance phase of treatment will require monthly to semi-monthly contact. With no active maintenance phase treatment, at least 80% of elderly patients will relapse over the following three years,[46] pointing out the need for ongoing monitoring and care.

FUTURE RESEARCH AND CLINICAL APPLICATION QUESTIONS

The use of physical activity in the treatment of depression in the elderly woman remains in its infancy, and the mechanism of its efficacy in depression is a crucial area of future research. Questions regarding modality, setting, supervision, and dose of exercise require refinement, as do patient characteristics and disease subtypes that make response to exercise more likely. Whether or not exercise is a useful adjunct to medication or an equipotent alternative treatment, and its role in both preventative and maintenance phases of this chronic disease remain to be clarified in the future, particularly in the very old or those with chronic disease.

REFERENCES

1. Unutzer, J., Patrick, D. L., Simon, G., Grembowski, D., Walker, E., Rutter, C. et al., Depressive symptoms and the cost of health services in HMO patients aged 65 years and older, *JAMA*, 277(20), 1618–23, 1997.
2. Gurland, B. J., Wilder, D. E., and Berkman, C. E., Depression and disability in the elderly, *Int. J. Geriatr. Psych.*, 3, 163–179, 1988.
3. Cole, M. G., The prognosis of depression in old age, *Canad. Med. Assoc. J.*, 1990. 143, 633–639.
4. American Psychiatric Association, *Diagnostic and Statistical Manual of Mental Disorders*, Fourth ed. Vol. 323, American Psychiatric Association, Washington D.C., 1994.
5. Gallo, J., Anthony, J., and Muthen, B., Age differences in the symptoms of depression: A latent trait analysis, *J. Gerontol.: Psychol. Sci.*, 49, 251–264, 1994.
6. Caine, E. D., Lyness, J. M., and King, D., Reconsidering depression in the elderly, *Am. J. Geriatr. Psychiatr.*, 1(1), 4–20, 1993.
7. Blazer, D., Hughes, D. C., and George, L., The epidemiology of depression in an elderly community population, *The Gerontologist*, 27(3), 281–287, 1987.
8. Wallace, J. and O'Hara, M. W., Increase in depressive symptomatology in the rural elderly: results from a cross-sectional and longitudinal study, *J. Abnormal Psychol.*, 101(3), 398–404, 1992.

9. Parmelee, P. A., Katz, I. R., and Lawton, M. P., Depression among institutionalized aged: assessment and prevalence estimation, *J. Gerontol.*, 44, M22–29, 1989.
10. Weissman, M. M., Advances in psychiatric epidemiology: rates and risks for major depression, *Am. J. Publ. Hlth.*, 77(4), 445–451, 1987.
11. Weissman, M. M., Bland, R. C., Canino, G. J., Faravelli, C., Greenwald, S., Hwu, H. G. et al., Cross-national epidemiology of major depression and bipolar disorder, *JAMA*, 276(4), 293–299, 1996.
12. Stokes, P., Current issues in the management of depression, *J. Clin. Psychopharmacol.*, 13(suppl. 2), 2s–9s, 1993.
13. Reynolds, C. F., Frank, E., Perel, J. M., Imber, S. D., Cornes, C., Miller, M. et al., Nortriptyline and interpersonal psychotherapy as maintenance therapies for recurrent major depression, *JAMA*, 281(1), 39–45, 1999.
14. Tannock, C. and Katona, C., Minor depression in the aged. Concepts, prevalence and optimal management, *Drugs Aging*, 6(4), 278–292, 1995.
15. Pearson, J., Yeates, C., and Lyness, J., Late-life suicide and depression in the primary care setting, *Develop. Geriatr. Psychiatr.*, 76, 13–38, 1997.
16. Salzman, C., Schneider, L., and Lebowitz, B., Antidepressant treatment of very old patients, *Am. J. Geriatr. Psychiatr.*, 1, 21–29, 1993.
17. Edzard, E., Rand, J., and Stevinson, C., Complementary therapies for depression: an overview, *Arch. Gen. Psychiatr.*, 55, 1026–1032, 1998.
18. Linde, K., Ramirez, G., Mulrow, C., Pauls, A., Weidenhammer, W., and Melchart, D., St. John's Wort for depression: an overview and meta-analysis of randomized clinical trials, *BMJ*, 313, 253–258, 1996.
19. North, T. C., McCullagh, P., and Tran, Z. V., The effect of exercise on depression, *Exer. Sport Sci. Rev.*, 18, 379–415, 1990.
20. Cohn, C., Shrivastava, R., Mendels, J., Cohn, J., Fabre, L. F., Claghorn, J. L. et al., Double blind, multicenter comparison of sertraline and amitryptyline in elderly depressed patients, *J. Clin. Psychiatr.*, 51(12), 28–33, 1990.
21. Liu, B., Anderson, G., Mittman, N., To, T., Axcell, T., and Shear, N., Use of selective serotonin-reuptake inhibitors or tricyclic antidepressants and risk of hip fractures in elderly people, *Lancet*, 351, 1303–7, 1998.
22. Thapa, P., Gideon, P., Cost, T., Milam, A., and Ray, W., Antidepressants and the risk of falls among nursing home residents, *N. Engl. J. Med.*, 339, 875–82, 1998.
23. Ransford, C. A., A role for amines in the antidepressant effect of exercise: a review, *Med. Sci. Sports Exer.*, 14, 1–10, 1982.
24. Bandurra, A., Toward a unifying theory of behavioral change, *Psychol. Rev.*, 84, 191–215, 1977.
25. Camacho, T. C., Roberts, R. E., Lazarus, N. B., Kaplan, G. A., and Cohen, R. D., Physical activity and depression: evidence from the Alameda County Study, *Am. J. Epidemiol.*, 134, 220–230, 1991.
26. Farmer, M. E., Locke, B. Z., Moscicki, E. K., Danneni, A. L., Larson, D. B., and Radloff, L. S., Physical activity and depressive symptoms: the NHANES1 epidemiological follow-up study, *Am. J. Epidemiol.*, 128, 1340–1351, 1988.
27. Hughes, J. R., Psychological effects of habitual aerobic exercise: A critical review, *Prev. Med.*, 13, 66–78, 1984.
28. Martinsen, E. W., Physical activity and depression: clinical experience, *Acta Psychiatr. Scand.*, Suppl. 377, 23–27, 1994.
29. Singh, N. A., Clements, K. M., and Fiatarone, M. A., A randomized controlled trial of progressive resistance training in depressed elders. *J. Gerontol*, 1997. 52A(1), M27–35.

30. Singh, N. A., Clements, K. M., and Fiatarone, M. A., Exercise as a long-term anti-depressant in the elderly. The 16th Congress of the International Association of Gerontology, Inc., Bedford Park, S. Australia, 1997: 343, Abstract no. 1042.

31. Martinsen, E. W., Medhus, A., and Sandvik, L., Effects of aerobic exercise on depression: a controlled study, *Br. Med. J.*, 291, 109, 1985.

32. Doyne, E. J., Chambliss, D. L., and Beutler, L. E., Aerobic exercise as a treatment for depression in women, *Behav. Ther.*, 14, 434–440, 1983.

33. Martinsen, E. W., Sandvik, L., and Kolbjornsrud, O. B., Aerobic exercise in the treatment of nonpsychotic mental disorders, *Nord. J. Psychiatr.*, 1989. 43, 411–415.

34. Martinsen, E. W., Hoffart, A., and Solberg, O., Comparing aerobic and non-aerobic forms of exercise in the treatment of clinical depression: A randomized trial, *Comp. Psychiatr.*, 30, 324–31, 1989.

35. Doyne, E. J., Ossip-Klein, D. J., Bowman, E. D., Osborn, K. M., McDougall-Wilson, I. B., and Neimeyer, R. A., Running versus weight lifting in the treatment of depression, *J. Consult. Clin. Psychol.*, 55(5), 748–754, 1987.

36. McNiel, K., LeBlanc, E., and Joyce, M., The effect of exercise on depressive symptoms in the moderately depressed elderly, *Psychol. Aging*, 3, 487–488, 1991.

37. Blumenthal, J. A., Babyak, M. A., Moore, K. A. et al., Effects of exercise training on older patients with major depression, *Arch. Intern. Med.*, 159, 2349–2356, 1999.

38. Alpert, J. E. and Fava, M., Nutrition and depression: the role of folate, *Nutr. Rev.*, 55(5), 1997.

39. Fava, M., Borus, J. S., Alpert, J. E., Nierenberg, A. A., Rosenbaum, J. F., and Bottiglieri, T., Folate, vitamin B_{12}, and homocysteine in major depressive disorder, *Am. J. Psychiatr.*, 154(3), 426–28, 1997.

40. Godfrey, P. S. A., Toone, B. K., Carney, M. P., Flynn, T. G., Bottiglieri, T., Laundy, M. et al., Enhancement of recovery from psychiatric illness by methylfolate, *Lancet*, 336, 392–395, 1990.

41. Reynolds, E. H., Preece, J. M., Bailey, J., and Coppen, A., Folate deficiency in depression, *Br. J. Psychiatr.*, 117, 287–92, 1970.

42. Carney, M. W. P., Toone, B. K., and Reynolds, E. H., S-adenosylmethionine and affective disorder, *Am. J. Med.*, 83(suppl. 5a), 104–106, 1987.

43. Fava, M., Giannelli, A., Rapisarda, V., and Patralia, A., Rapidity of onset of the antidepressant effect of parenteral S-adenosyl-L-methionine, *Psychiatry Res.*, 1995, 56(3), 295–97.

44. Hirschfeld, R. A., Keller, M., Panico, S., Arons, B. S., Barlow, D., Davidoff, F. et al., The national depressive and manic-depressive association consensus statement on the undertreatment of depression, *JAMA*, 277(4), 333–40, 1997.

45. Yesavage, J. A. and Brink, T. L., Development and validation of a geriatric depression screening scale: A preliminary report, *J. Psychiatr. Res.*, 17, 37–49, 1983.

46. Frank, E., Kupfer, D., Perel, J., Cornes, M. D., Jarrett, D. B., Mallinger, A. G. et al., Three year outcomes for maintenance therapies in recurrent depression, *Arch. Gen. Psychiatr.*, 47, 1093–1099, 1990.

47. Griest, J. H., Klein, M. H., Faris, J., Gurman, A. S., and Morgan, W. P., Running as a treatment for depression, *Comp. Psychiatr.*, 20, 41–54, 1979.

48. LaFontaine, T. P., Dilorenzo, T. M., Frensch, P. A., Stucy-Romp, R. C., Bargman, E. P., and McDonald, D. G., Aerobic exercise and mood, *Sports Med.*, 13(3), 160–170, 1992.

20 Sleep

Peter A. Cistulli and Nalin A. Singh

CONTENTS

INTRODUCTION

Dissatisfaction with the amount and quality of sleep is a common complaint, particularly with advancing age. It has been estimated that in the U.S. sleep disturbances affect more than 50% of community dwelling individuals over 65 years of age as well as an estimated two thirds of institutionalized elderly persons.[1] Although sleep problems are not generally life threatening, we do spend one third of our lives in sleep and this time may profoundly influence our quality of life. Furthermore, problems with sleep have been associated with increased risk of accidents, falls, nursing home placement, and an increased mortality.[2] There are many potential causes of disturbed or unrestful sleep in the elderly, and an overview of these will be presented in this chapter. Some relate to changes in sleep physiology with aging, while others relate to specific sleep and medical disorders. The aim of this chapter is to provide an understanding of the factors which impair sleep quality in women as they age and provide a framework for their clinical management.

Insomnia can be simply defined as difficulty falling asleep, remaining asleep, or the belief that one is not getting enough sleep. Insomnia is a symptom, not a disease. It can be classified according to the part of the sleep cycle most affected, i.e., sleep initiation, sleep maintenance (frequent awakenings), or early morning wakening. In the elderly, sleep maintenance insomnia is the most common sleep complaint, affecting some 27 to 33% of individuals aged over 50 years, followed by initial insomnia (10 to 17%) and early morning wakening (13 to 17%), and the rest consisting of mixed patterns of insomnia.[3] Insomnia is more prevalent in women than men.

NORMAL HUMAN SLEEP

The function of sleep in large part remains unexplained, although it is appreciated that sleep is ubiquitous among the animal kingdom. Sleep has been largely studied and defined by polysomnography, consisting of simultaneous recording of the electroencephalogram (EEG), electro-oculogram (EOG), and electromyogram (EMG). The correlation between the EEG in sleep and the subjective report of sleep quality is not strong. The EEG remains the gold standard of sleep measurement, but it may be not entirely reflective of the function and quality of sleep, as an EEG of the awake brain reflects little of the function and quality of thought.

Two separate states of sleep have been defined by EEG, viz., rapid eye movement (REM) sleep and non-rapid eye movement (NREM) sleep. NREM sleep is subdivided into four stages, 1–4, reflecting increasing "depth" of sleep. Stages 3 and 4 are collectively termed *slow wave sleep*. NREM sleep is usually a quiescent stage in terms of mental activity. In contrast, REM sleep is a stage of cerebral activation, within a paralyzed body. Atonia of postural muscles is the result of descending inhibition from the brainstem. Dreaming is a feature of REM sleep.

Normal adults enter sleep through NREM sleep, progressing from stage 1 to 4, before entering into REM sleep. NREM sleep and REM sleep alternate cyclically through the night with periods of approximately 90 minutes occurring in 4 to 6 discrete episodes. REM sleep episodes generally become longer as the night progresses. In young adults, slow wave sleep dominates NREM sleep periods in the first third of the night, and REM sleep tends to be greatest in the last third of the night. NREM sleep typically accounts for 75 to 80% of sleep, while REM sleep accounts for 20 to 25%.

Since the length of sleep is under both biological and volitional control, it is difficult to define a normal pattern. Most young adults report sleeping 7.5 to 8.5 hours per night; however, this is highly variable. There also appears to be a genetically determined sleep need.[4]

A number of factors are known to modify sleep stage distribution during the night, and these include age, prior sleep history, circadian rhythms, temperature, drugs, and sleep disorders. Many of these factors are implicated in the etiology of age-related changes in sleep physiology and pathophysiology.

AGE-RELATED CHANGES IN SLEEP

CHANGES IN NORMAL SLEEP PHYSIOLOGY WITH AGE

A number of reasonably well-documented changes are observed as we age, and these are detailed below. However, chronological age alone often does not correlate with a higher prevalence of sleep disturbance, implicating other medical or psychological factors in the sleep disturbance seen in the elderly. Evidence now points to the important role of medical diseases and chronic illness in much of what was previously defined as *age-related* changes in sleep. A number of common co-morbid conditions which lead to nocturnal awakening (e.g., nocturia, headache, gastroesophageal reflux, paroxysmal nocturnal dyspnea, orthopnea, leg cramps, and menopausal symptoms) occur more frequently in the elderly, often resulting in an increase in daytime sleepiness and napping.

Changes in EEG and Sleep Architecture

A number of non-specific changes in waking EEG activity associated with normal aging have been reported. These include focal slow activity, decreases in alpha frequency, and increased occurrence of beta (fast) activity.[5,6] A consistent age-related change in sleeping EEG is an attenuation of the delta waves that characterize stages 3 and 4 NREM sleep (slow wave sleep). Changes in sleep spindle activity, characteristic of stage 2 NREM sleep, have also been observed, with a reduction in the amplitude and frequency.[7]

Accompanying these EEG changes are also changes in sleep architecture in otherwise normal elderly individuals. Nocturnal sleep efficiency, the ratio of total sleep time to time spent in bed, decreases and the percentage of stage 1 sleep increases in the elderly, although there is wide variability. The most consistent and easily recognized age-related change in sleep stages is the reduction in slow wave sleep. The precise age at which slow wave sleep declines has yet to be determined conclusively, but some studies suggest that this reduction begins at about age 20, and appears to be more pronounced in men than women between the ages of 30 and 40 years.[8] Slow wave sleep may disappear completely by the age of 90. There may be gender differences in this reduction, as a number of studies have shown that older women have better preserved slow wave sleep than men.[9] This contrasts with the subjective complaints that are reported more commonly by elderly women, again raising questions about the relevance of sleep EEG changes to sleep quality itself. Controversy exists over the proportion of sleep spent in REM sleep with advancing age. There may be a reduction in the amount and intensity of REM sleep with normal aging,[10] but the magnitude is quite small. A reduction in REM sleep latency (the time taken to reach the first REM stage) is more consistently observed.[11] Interpretations about the significance of these changes have varied from the contention that such changes reflect maturational processes related to declining cortical metabolic rate and increased dendritic pruning to the hypothesis that the changes represent an extremely early biomarker of aging within the central nervous system.[12]

Changes in Circadian Sleep-Wake Rhythm

A complex array of chronobiological changes in sleep and other physiologic systems (e.g., temperature regulation, endocrine system) occurs with aging. In fact, some have postulated that these changes in circadian physiology represent the fundamental characterization of the aging process.[13] Age-related increases in nocturnal wakefulness are mirrored by increased daytime hypersomnolence and napping, resulting in a shift from the normal adult biphasic sleep-wake cycle to a polyphasic rhythm similar to that seen in neonates. Phase changes are also noted, with a tendency to fall asleep and to awaken earlier, as well as a tendency to be less tolerant of phase shifts of the sleep-wake schedule (e.g., time zone changes).[14]

The suprachiasmatic nucleus of the anterior hypothalamus appears to be the central controller of circadian rhythms. This region has been shown to decrease in size with aging, especially above 80 years of age, and this may be more pronounced in women.[15] However, the precise nature of the deficiency in entrainment mechanisms is not well characterized.

Neuroendocrine output and thermoregulatory function decline with age. In particular, there is a decline in production of the pineal hormone melatonin,[16] and a reduction in circadian core body temperature amplitude.[17] Healthy elderly women appear to have a larger amplitude and higher temperature peak than their male counterparts, suggesting that aging may affect the circadian timing system of men and women differently.[18] A number of observations suggest that these changes are causally related to the deterioration in sleep maintenance associated with aging. For example, nocturnal core body temperature is elevated in the elderly;[17] elderly insomniacs have reduced melatonin levels;[19] and nocturnal exogenous melatonin appears to improve sleep in elderly insomniacs.[20] However, these observations are not uniformly seen, casting some doubt about the efficacy of exogenous melatonin in the treatment of elderly insomnia.[21]

Alterations in the circadian rhythm of other hormones have also been observed. For example, significantly reduced nocturnal levels of prolactin and growth hormone, and higher levels of cortisol have been recorded in the elderly compared to young controls. A reduced sensitivity of the hypothalamo-pituitary-adrenal axis to steroid feedback has also been noted. The changes correlate with age, and appear to be more pronounced in demented elders.[22] It is postulated that these changes represent markers of the brain aging, ascribable to structural and neurochemical changes within the central nervous system.

Changes in Sleep Need

There is considerable uncertainty as to whether or not sleep need changes with aging. Although some laboratory-based studies and surveys have shown reduced total sleep time in the elderly,[23] others suggest no change or even increases in sleep time with age. Some studies include napping in their totals, and therefore imply a redistribution of sleep around the 24-hour day. Hence, if net sleep duration does not change with aging, the need for sleep may be unchanged, but that need appears to be met differently in old age. Physiologic studies of daytime alertness in the elderly have demonstrated increased sleepiness,[24] providing additional support for the notion of an altered expression of sleep need compared to younger individuals.

EFFECT OF MENOPAUSE ON SLEEP

In women, the physiologic changes associated with the menopause provide an additional potential impediment to normal sleep processes. Elderly women report more sleep disturbance and use more sedatives than elderly men.[25] There is a rapid increase in prevalence of sleep disturbance at the onset of menopause, suggesting that the decline in endogenous estrogen has an impact on sleep.[26] In addition to vasomotor symptoms such as hot flushes and sweats, which typically occur at night, poor sleep quality is one of the most common symptoms of menopause.[27] The primary feature of menopausal insomnia is the presence of repeated nocturnal awakenings, associated with "hot flushes" or "night sweats" in a woman with other signs and symptoms of menopause. A sleep-onset disturbance is not a prominent feature. Mood disturbance is also frequently encountered in postmenopausal women.[28] It is known that sleep disturbance is commonly associated with depression and anxiety,[29] and this may partly explain the sleep disturbance associated with menopause. However, it has also been suggested that mood disturbance in menopause may be mediated by sleep disruption itself.[30]

The prevalence of sleep-disordered breathing increases after menopause,[31] and this could also explain the sleep disturbance associated with menopause. One hypothesis is that female hormones protect women from developing sleep-disordered breathing in the premenopausal state. However, a number of studies cast doubt on this hypothesis. Hormone replacement therapy, either with estrogen alone or in combination with progesterone, does not improve breathing during sleep in postmenopausal women with obstructive sleep apnea.[32] Other studies suggest that obesity and facial structure are more important than hormonal factors per se.[33] Hence these studies suggest that increases in body mass or changes in body composition and adipose tissue mass associated with menopause may promote sleep-disordered breathing, which in turn leads to sleep disturbance. From a clinical point of view, it is worth noting that sleep-disordered breathing is frequently under-recognized in women, in part because they under-report symptoms (particularly daytime hypersomnolence).[34]

ETIOLOGY OF AGE-RELATED CHANGES IN SLEEP

Biology of Aging

With age, in most organ systems there is increasing physiologic abnormality. These changes, while asymptomatic, bring the aged individual closer to the threshold of clinical symptoms. This reduced physiologic reserve means they often cannot withstand even minor stressors previously handled without precipitating clinical symptoms or illness. Factors such as inactivity, less light exposure, decreased arousal threshold, elevated autonomic activity, and circadian rhythm changes diminish the functional reserves for quality sleep as we age.[35,36] Increased frequency of disease such as heart failure, respiratory complaints, sleep disordered breathing, nocturia, pain, polypharmacy, headache, depression, and functional decline have all been shown to reduce subjective sleep quality.[26,37–40] The combination of increasing disease burden with the reduced physiologic reserve with aging leads to the high prevalence of poor sleep quality.

Environmental Changes

A range of environmental changes that accompany aging are likely to contribute to changes in sleep. For example, it is uncertain whether the circadian changes referred to above are the result of reduced exposure to relevant environmental cues (e.g., light exposure) or to an actual dysfunction of the central controller. Institutionalized elderly often have sleep problems, and it is thought that this is the result of a lack of exposure to environmental cues. This is supported by evidence that bright light exposure can improve sleep quality in this setting. The natural light–dark cycle entrains our circadian timing system to the 24-hour day. It is generally believed that intensities of 2000 lux (equivalent to outdoor sunlight soon after dawn) or above are required to produce circadian rhythm shifts. Healthy young adults receive around 2 hours a day of such exposure, community living elderly receive less than an hour; many institutionalized elders may receive none at all. Apart from insufficient light exposure itself, it is possible that impoverished time cues in the house-bound, socially isolated elder contribute to the development of circadian changes as well. Hence it appears that psychosocial factors such as isolation and residential setting may assume importance as mediators of environmental cues in old age, even though there appears to be an underlying deterioration of the central controller of circadian rhythm.[41]

Behavioural Changes

Decreased Physical Activity

As we age one of the most obvious accompaniments is a decline in physical activity levels. During this century, urbanization and technology have meant major changes in activity patterns of the entire society. While the functions of sleep continue to be elucidated, both the restorative and energy conservation theories of sleep propose that sleep is in large part a compensatory mechanism following catabolic processes of daytime activity.[42,43] Decline in activity as we age presents one of the potentially reversible contributants to sleep quality reduction. Inactivity and bed rest, so common in the nursing home setting, have been shown to disrupt sleep in younger subjects, and avoidance of daytime napping and bed rest improve sleep in the elderly.

Epidemiological evidence to support the relationship between decreased activity and sleep disturbance is lacking. Factors which make such a study difficult include the complex and interdependent relationships between age, disease, activity, and sleep. A decrease in activity with aging and an associated decline in sleep quality may be related to physical illness, psychological distress, or functional decline. Despite the lack of convincing epidemiological data, it is clear that most people identify activity as a key factor in how well they sleep. In a Finnish survey of 1600 people, exercise was described by one third of men and women as the most important factor in promoting falling asleep and improving its quality.[44] In a subset of people who had increased their exercise habits in the prior 3 months, 43% reported better subjective sleep following the change and 1% suggested worsening. For those who had decreased their exercise in that time period, 4% reported better sleep and 30% a worsening of their sleep.

Poor Sleep Hygiene

Sleep hygiene factors are those activities that interfere with normal sleep and can therefore contribute to the development of insomnia. These factors can be broadly divided into 4 classes: circadian factors, age-related changes in sleep physiology, factors that increase sleep-related arousals, and drug-related factors. Patients with poor sleep hygiene usually spend too much time in bed awake, have difficulties initiating sleep, and have variable wake-up times. When this pattern becomes habitual and chronic, it is termed psychophysiological insomnia. The frustration associated with inability to sleep may lead to more maladaptive behaviors such as the consumption of alcohol or medication to promote sleep.

Psychological Changes

Psychological changes accompanying aging may profoundly affect the sleep of the older individual. Psychological stress occurs at every age; however, several stresses are either unique to or more prevalent in the elderly. Factors relevant for geriatric populations include retirement and the loss of personal identity, disruption of daily routines, death of a spouse, family members, and friends, changes in social circumstances, financial concerns, a perception of poor health and fear of dying, and the psychological effects of chronic or terminal illness involving the patient or loved ones. These can all adversely affect sleep.

Nutritional Factors

Body Composition

As we age there is a marked change in body composition with decreases in lean and increases in fat mass. This is seen both cross-sectionally and longitudinally. The relationship between body composition and sleep is unclear. There are several studies suggesting that absolute or relative proportions of lean body mass or muscle mass are positively correlated with slow wave sleep and REM sleep duration. Lean body mass has been positively correlated with slow wave sleep in both athletes and anorexics gaining weight. This relationship does not seem to hold for obese people losing weight: a clinical situation where losses of lean tissue which would be detrimental may be balanced by losses of adipose tissue which improve sleep disorders. How the changes of body composition with aging affect sleep physiology remains to be elucidated. The one clear secondary consequence of the development of obesity is an increase in obstructive sleep apnea.

Alcohol

The use of alcohol is a common and often overlooked cause of sleep disturbance. It is commonly self-prescribed to initiate sleep, but when taken in large, but socially acceptable, quantities it results in sleep maintenance difficulties. The decline in blood alcohol levels that occur after moderately heavy consumption (30 to 80g, i.e., 3 to 8 standard drinks of beer, wine, or spirits) leads to a sympathetic arousal state, which in turn inhibits sleep. Furthermore, the effects of alcohol on respiration are well documented, particularly with regard to the development of snoring and sleep apnea, and this leads to further sleep disruption.[45]

Caffeine

The deleterious effects of caffeine on sleep are well described in the literature.[46] The mechanism relates to its effect on adenosine receptors, resulting in an overall loss of inhibition. The end result is an increase in awakenings and a reduction in total sleep time, an effect that can last as long as 8 to 14 hours.

Fluid Excretion

The elderly have a reversed pattern of fluid excretion, passing the majority of their urine in a 12-hour period nocturnally. This is related to changes in the renin-aldosterone system and antidiuretic hormone secretion. This, combined with prostate enlargement in men and weakening of the pelvic floor in women after childbirth and with the postmenopausal withdrawal of estrogen influence on pelvic musculature, leads to increased urinary excretion at night, along with the possibility of incontinence and disturbed sleep.

DISEASE-RELATED DISTURBANCES IN SLEEP

Sleep disturbance in the elderly is associated with many medical disorders, and is often multifactorial. Table 1 lists the common medical causes of sleep disturbance, giving rise to the symptom of insomnia. This list is by no means exhaustive, but gives an indication of the diversity of clinical causes that should be suspected in an older insomniac. In clinical practice, the majority of sleep disturbance associated with medical illness is secondary to the medical or psychiatric disease. The primary sleep disorders constitute a serious but minor etiologic subset of sleep complaints dealt with by primary care clinicians, although they may represent a larger proportion of those referred to a sub-specialty sleep clinic.

MEDICAL CAUSES OF SLEEP DISTURBANCE

Disease can disturb sleep in many ways, through symptoms arising from the disease, through treatment instituted for the disorder, or via its precipitation of depressive symptoms, decreased activity, and functional decline. Pain is the best example of a symptom directly affecting sleep. The most common causes of pain in elderly women are the musculoskeletal disorders. Osteoarthritis, back pain, bursitis, and fibromyalgia are particularly disruptive to sleep, and specific treatment of the cause and relief of pain will restore sleep quality. If pain becomes chronic the sleep pattern

---

TABLE 1
Common Medical Causes of Insomnia

I. Medical

       Cardiac (e.g., congestive cardiac failure, ischemic heart disease)

       Gastric (e.g., gastroesophageal reflux or regurgitation, peptic ulcers)

       Infections (e.g., tuberculosis, AIDS)

       Musculoskeletal (e.g., arthritis, myalgias, fibromyalgia, cramps)

       Neurological (e.g., strokes, dysesthesia)

       Renal (e.g., prostatism, bladder dysfunction, nocturia)

       Respiratory (e.g., asthma, chronic airflow limitation)

       Sleep disorders (e.g., sleep apnea, periodic limb movement disorder)

II. Psychiatric

       Anxiety disorders

       Cognitive impairment

       Depression

III. Medications/Pharmacological Agents

       Non-prescription medications (e.g., decongestants, antihistamines, stimulants)

       Prescription medications (e.g., diuretics, corticosteroids, some anti-depressants)

       Social drugs (e.g., alcohol, caffeine, nicotine, other)

       Withdrawal syndromes (e.g., rebound from sedatives, other)

---

becomes polycyclic in nature, such that several sleep-wake cycles occur within a 24-hour period. This polycyclic pattern is similar to the normal sleep pattern of infants, and is especially prevalent in the nursing home setting. As a result, many elderly experience a significant decrease in sleep efficiency (the ratio of total time asleep to total time spent in bed) and sleep satisfaction.

Angina or chest pain has been shown to independently cause difficulty in sleeping,[47] as has gastroesophageal reflux. Difficulty breathing related to infection or progressive lung or heart disease will disturb sleep. Frequent urination or incontinence at night will result in sleep maintenance problems.

Poor control of several medical problems can worsen sleep. For example, in the poorly controlled diabetic, high blood sugar can lead to nocturia, as will worsening heart failure and peripheral edema from any cause, as the supine position will lead to intravascular redistribution of fluid. In postmenopausal women, the incidence and prevalence of congestive heart failure is equivalent to that in men, and this disorder increases exponentially with advancing age. Thus, particularly in women over the age of 70, nocturnal symptoms related to systolic dysfunction should be searched for in those presenting with sleep disturbance.

PSYCHIATRIC DISORDERS

Psychopathology is a very powerful risk factor for the development of insomnia. Both cross-sectionally and longitudinally depression appears to be the factor most strongly related to disturbed sleep with age,[47] even more so than health status.[48]

Depression affects both the subjective and objective measures of sleep. Whether the sleep disturbance causes the depression or the reverse is a subject of some debate.[49]

The incidence of depressive symptoms in the elderly community has been estimated as high as 30%[50] and within institutions up to 50%.[51] Major depression affects about 2% of the community dwelling older population, but represents only a small portion of those suffering with depressive symptoms. In longitudinal studies depression is more common in women than men, with advancing age. The onset of menopause is not infrequently accompanied by depressive symptoms in women, coincident with the appearance of insomnia and disturbing nocturnal vasomotor symptoms. In a large U.S. study,[49] 14% of persons complaining of insomnia had major depression, compared to a 1% rate in those without sleep complaints.

Depression is usually associated with terminal insomnia or early morning awakening, but may also cause hypersomnolence. Some depressed patients experience agitation as well, which can make falling asleep difficult. Because of the strong association between depression and sleep difficulties, health care providers should consider underlying depression in every case of insomnia.

Other psychiatric problems associated with insomnia are in large part related to anxiety. Anxiety and associated disorders often result in difficulty falling asleep and frequent nocturnal awakenings. Their onset in late life is frequently related to the onset of a depressive disorder.

COGNITIVE IMPAIRMENT

The incidence of dementia increases rapidly with age to almost one third of those aged 85 and above. Patients with dementia often have significant sleep-wake cycle disturbances,[52] including a disrupted and sometimes polycyclic sleep-wake cycle. Nocturnal awakening episodes may be quite common and are associated with wandering. The degree of disturbance parallels the severity of the dementia. The altered sleep pattern may not trouble patients themselves; however, this is a serious problem for caregivers and other residents. The demands of caring for a demented person during the day are stressful enough but once this is extended to night time it is usually the straw that breaks the caregiver's back and may lead to elder abuse, long-term care placement, or caregiver illness. The sleep rhythm of the cognitively impaired elder may not match the daily routine of the caregivers or the institution. This mismatch may culminate in the prescription of hypnotic medications, virtually all of which can further impair cognition or precipitate falls, and may have adverse effects on the sleep EEG itself, such as decreased REM sleep.

PHARMACOLOGICAL AGENTS

The elderly are the greatest consumers of medications, and unfortunately, the changes in both pharmacokinetics and pharmacodynamics combined with polypharmacy lead to high rates of adverse drug reactions. The principle of drug elimination is a primary tenant in the elderly because of the high rates of such adverse events. The range of drugs which commonly cause insomnia in the elderly includes sympathomimetics, corticosteroids, thyroxine, neuroleptics, and certain antidepressant medications (particularly selective serotonin re-uptake inhibitors), beta-blockers, and methyl-dopa. Other non-prescription pharmacological agents such as alcohol, caffeine, and nicotine are also important causes of insomnia. Unfortunately, the use of hypnotic medications as a treatment for poor sleep increases with age, particularly among elderly women, despite the fact that these drugs have no real demonstrable efficacy in chronic insomnia. Sedatives can cause daytime hangover effects, leading to an increase in daytime sleepiness and further disruption of the normal sleep pattern. They can cause neuromuscular impairment, falls, and confusion. The abrupt cessation of these drugs will cause a withdrawal state, which is commonly seen in hospital after an admission for unrelated disease.

PRIMARY SLEEP DISORDERS

Aging is associated with an increased prevalence of specific sleep-related disorders, such as sleep apnea and periodic limb movement disorder, which can cause marked sleep disturbance in their own right, usually associated with daytime hypersomnolence.

Obstructive Sleep Apnea

Obstructive sleep apnea is a common disorder affecting all age groups, and is particularly prevalent in the elderly. The reported prevalence of sleep-disordered breathing, with or without symptoms, in community-dwelling elders is estimated to be 24%.[53] The disorder is characterized by snoring with repeated brief episodes of partial or complete collapse of the pharynx, with resultant oxygen desaturation and sleep disruption.[45] Sleep apnea is an important, and often overlooked, cause of daytime hypersomnolence. Additional symptoms may include depression, nocturnal polyuria, headaches, and cognitive impairment.[54] It is important to note that the elderly often interpret their symptoms differently than younger patients, and therefore fail to recognize the problem. There is also growing evidence of an association with cardiovascular morbidity, such as hypertension, ischemic heart disease, arrhythmias, and stroke.[54] Sleep apnea is important to diagnose since it can usually be treated effectively. The mortality rate of elderly with severe sleep disordered breathing is fifteen times higher than for those with no or mild sleep disordered breathing.[53]

It is pertinent to point out gender differences in the epidemiology and presentation of obstructive sleep apnea. Older surveys of sleep clinic populations have emphasized the marked male predominance of the disorder, with estimates of the male:female ratio of 10:1 or higher.[55] However, recent epidemiological studies involving community-based samples indicate that this may have been vastly overestimated, and that the ratio is of the order of 2:1.[56] Hence, sleep apnea is not rare in older women, and must be considered in any woman presenting with sleep complaints. Compared with men, women with sleep apnea consistently under-report symptoms of snoring and apnea, as well as daytime hypersomnolence, and this almost certainly accounts for the fact that it is less frequently recognized clinically in women.[34]

Restless Leg Syndrome

Restless leg syndrome is a relatively common problem in the elderly, with a reported prevalence of up to 15%. It is characterized by an irresistible urge to move the lower extremities, associated with unpleasant sensations.[57] Movements such as walking around usually provide some, albeit transient, relief. Patients may have difficulty initiating sleep as a result of the unpleasant sensations, as well as frequent awakenings. The disorder is usually idiopathic, but can occur in association with iron deficiency anemia, uremia, and neuropathies. The idiopathic form may exhibit a hereditary pattern.

Periodic Limb Movement Disorder

Periodic limb movement disorder or nocturnal myoclonus is probably related to restless leg syndrome, as more than 90% of patients with this syndrome also have periodic limb movements during sleep. Nocturnal myoclonus is also prevalent in the elderly, with rates ranging up to 45%. However, the relationship of nocturnal myoclonus to subjective sleep complaints is not entirely clear, particularly in the elderly. The condition is characterized by repetitive, brief, jerking movements of the lower, and less commonly, upper extremities.[57] These typically occur every 20 to 40 seconds, and can occur as discrete episodes that last minutes to hours or can be present for the entire night. The movements may be associated with an arousal or awakening, resulting in unrefreshing sleep. Patients who are unaware of the sleep interruptions may have daytime hypersomnolence. There is often significant night-to-night variability. The course is variable, but periods of stability are not uncommon.

DIAGNOSING AND TRIAGING WOMEN WITH SLEEP COMPLAINTS

TAKING A SLEEP HISTORY

The history is crucial in establishing the cause of the patient's sleep complaint. Only after this is undertaken should treatment be contemplated and directed whenever possible to the underlying cause. Initial questioning should focus on whether or not a sleep disorder is present. For example, is the patient satisfied with their sleep? Does sleepiness affect their daily activities? Does the bed partner report any unusual behavior during sleep (e.g., snoring, breathing pauses, abnormal movements)? If the responses suggest a sleep disorder, then it is important to take a more detailed history (Table 2). One should elicit details of the patient's typical sleep pattern, including the characteristics of nocturnal awakenings, sleep latency, satisfaction with sleep, and effects on daytime performance. Wherever possible, the history should be corroborated from the bed partner or care-giver. The general medical history should specifically focus on other relevant diseases and their control, any cause of pain, and a thorough review of all medications. The amount and timing of fluids, caffeine, nicotine, alcohol, sunlight exposure, and physical activity are all relevant. A specific search for the symptoms of depression should be made in all cases with inquiry

---

TABLE 2
Useful Questions to Ask as Part of a Sleep History

General

What is your usual sleep pattern?
How long have you had sleep problems?
How many hours do you sleep on an average night?
Are your sleep pattern and amount of sleep different now compared to past?
What time do you go to sleep and why?
How long do you think it takes you to fall asleep?
Do you sleep right through the night, or do you awaken; if so what wakes you?
What time do you awaken?
How do you feel when you wake up?
Do you experience drowsiness during the day?
Do you ever fall asleep during the daytime, while reading or watching TV, during meetings, during conversations, or driving?
Do you take naps during the day? For how long?
When was the last time that you had a good night's sleep?
What do you think the cause of your insomnia is?
Has anyone ever mentioned that you snore or stop breathing during sleep?
Has anyone said you kick or jerk your legs at night?
Has anyone said you talk or walk in your sleep?
Do you feel depressed or anxious?

Medication Use

What medications are you currently taking and for what reason?
Do you use any over-the-counter medicines and why?
When do you take your medications?
Do you use medications to help you sleep, and if so for how long?

Behavior Patterns/Sleep Environment

How much time do you spend in bed awake?
What time do you get out of bed and why?
What do you do when you can't sleep: do you stay in bed, watch the clock?
Do you consume alcohol, caffeine, nicotine; if so, when?
What time is your evening meal?
Are you anxious or unable to relax at night?
Do you have a bedtime routine?
What is your sleeping environment like in relation to noise, light, bedding?
Do you do any habitual exercise? What type and time of day?

---

about loss of interest in activities, sadness, guilt, lack of concentration, low self-esteem, weight loss, psychomotor agitation or retardation, and thoughts of suicide.

PHYSICAL EXAMINATION

A thorough directed physical examination should be performed, as indicated from the history. Of particular relevance are obesity, muscle and joint pain, deformity, and/or inflammation, nasopharyngeal exam looking for inflammation of pharyngeal tissue resulting from vibratory trauma of snoring (redness and swelling of the uvula), narrownesss or crowding of the pharynx, a bull-necked appearance, central or periph-eral evidence of fluid overload, pulmonary abnormalities including rales or wheez-ing, prostatic hypertrophy, incontinence with stress manuevers such as standing, coughing, sneezing, straining, or laughing, venous stasis with edema, psychomotor retardation or agitation, and cognitive deficits.

WHEN TO REFER FOR SLEEP INVESTIGATION

The majority of women who present with sleep complaints will only require a thorough history and examination for a diagnosis and management plan to be instituted. Even in the minority in whom a primary sleep disorder is suspected, treatment can usually be commenced in the primary care setting. In women with known cardiovascular disease who you suspect have sleep apnea, or in those who have occupations where falling asleep suddenly may be hazardous or fatal (such as drivers or machine operators), immediate referral to a sleep physician is recom-mended. Referral to a physician specializing in sleep disorders should be considered when the diagnosis remains uncertain after careful history and examination, when a sleep study is considered necessary, or if symptoms persist despite treatment. The use of polysomnography in this setting should be reserved for confirmation of diagnoses that are clinically suspected, or to assess the need for and effectiveness of treatment.

MANAGEMENT OF THE OLDER WOMAN WITH SLEEP COMPLAINTS

The underlying principle in the management of sleep complaints is to make a diagnosis of the primary cause and usual multiple contributors, and direct treatment to correct the causes rather than simply aim for symptomatic control with sedatives. A detailed review of management is beyond the scope of this chapter, but an overview of strategies is presented below.

SLEEP HYGIENE

Regardless of the underlying cause, it is often wise to address sleep hygiene in the management of patients with chronic sleep complaints (Table 3). The patient needs to understand the importance of maintaining good sleep practices, and modifying behaviors which are considered to be hindering satisfying sleep. This means creating a quiet and relaxed environment for sleep, establishing a regular sleep pattern, avoiding staying in bed awake for long periods of time, refraining from reading or watching television in bed, not looking at the clock during the night, avoiding consumption of caffeine, alcohol, and nicotine in the late afternoon or evening. For patients in whom anxiety is a contributing factor, behavioral interventions such as relaxation training and stress management may have a role.

The importance of this form of non-pharmacological therapy cannot be over-emphasized, particularly in the elderly where the use of medications is associated

---

TABLE 3
Some Sleep Hygiene Suggestions

Go to bed only when ready to sleep

Establish a bedtime ritual

Avoid foods, beverages, medications which may contain stimulants

Regularly exercise each day, but not after 6 p.m.

Avoid daytime naps

Do not eat or drink excessively for 3 hours before bedtime

Avoid alcohol, caffeine, and nicotine at night

A hot bath to raise core body temperature may help sleep initiation

Use the bedroom only for sleep, and sexual activity if it is relaxing

Avoid emotional or mental stimulation before bed

Set aside a "worry time" in the evening

Do not worry if you cannot sleep

Learn behavioral/relaxation techniques which will assist with physical and mental relaxation

Keep clock faces turned away, and do not find out what time it is when you wake up during the night

Do not stay in bed if you cannot sleep

Establish a good sleep environment in terms of lighting, noise, temperature, and comfort

Avoid unfamiliar sleep environments

If sensory impaired, provide adequate light and stimulation during the daytime hours to establish proper sleep/night cycles

---

with potential problems. Even in situations where the use of medications cannot be avoided, the use of behavioral therapies may reduce the dose required. Cognitively impaired patients present particular management problems since they may not be able to comprehend or cooperate with behavioral therapies.

Treatment of the Underlying Medical Cause

The general principle of optimization of chronic medical and drug minimization is recommended. The intersection of many diagnoses and syndromes in the final common pathway to insomnia must be recognized. For example, a woman may present with insomnia related to nocturnal incontinence by history. Clearly, the precipitating incontinence must be treated to improve her sleep, but the practitioner must recognize that the incontinence treatment will depend on the reduction of her peripheral edema related to her worsening heart failure, and that the depression resulting from her mounting disabilities may require specific treatment as well, before her symptom of insomnia can be fully resolved. Depression must be aggressively looked for and treated when suspected, as it is so often present in conjunction with a high burden of chronic disease and functional decline.

Prescription and non-prescription drug use is highest in the elderly; therefore, careful review of all medications including over-the-counter and caffeine-containing compounds is recommended.

PHYSICAL ACTIVITY RECOMMENDATIONS

Overview

It is generally accepted that exercise will enhance sleep although the evidence for such claims is only beginning to accumulate. The rationale for its use as a treatment is related to its risk benefit potential over drug therapy (Table 4.) The majority of the experimental evidence for an effect of exercise on sleep has been in normal individuals and of poor methodological quality. This has caused great controversy as to whether or not an effect exists at all.[58] This research has often concentrated on theories of how exercise may work rather than whether or not it would work in people with sleep problems.

TABLE 4
Rationale for Exercise as a Treatment for Sleep Disturbance

Treatment	Sleep	Co-morbidities	Function	Side Effects
Exercise	*	****	**	—
Sedative/hypnotics	*	—	—	xxxx
Non-drug therapy	*	—	—	—

* = Desirable effect, strength of association indicated by number of asterisks; — = No known effect in this domain; x = Undesirable effect (falls, confusion, fractured hip, etc.), strength of association indicated by number of x's.

In relation to the elderly who are sleep disturbed, the evidence is sparse but convincing that exercise is a viable treatment for sleep disturbance, with demonstrated efficacy for subjective sleep problems.[59,60] Exercise has the added advantage of having an effect on sleep disturbance in elders with and without depression. It may be able to simultaneously address a number of conditions contributing to sleep disturbance including inactivity, obesity, depression, physical functioning, and a range of co-morbidities such as arthritis, cardiac disease, and diabetes. Evidence in terms of objective change in sleep with exercise in the elderly is limited to one 6-month study where aerobic exercise marginally increased slow wave sleep. From a clinical perspective, whether or not exercise changes the EEG representation of sleep may be less relevant than the reported improvement in subjective sleep disturbance.

Modality

In the older woman, there is evidence for the effectiveness of both aerobic and nonaerobic exercise for sleep disturbance. Two randomized controlled trials in elders with moderate sleep impairment have been published. In a clinically depressed group, it was demonstrated that over 10 weeks weight lifting exercise significantly improved sleep quality compared to an attention control group. While the improvement in sleep was in part explained by improving depression, sleep quality was not altered in controls despite their improved depression. In contrast, the exercise group had a marked reduction in subjective sleep disturbance. This lack of change in controls suggests that the improvement in sleep was not mediated primarily via an antidepressant mechanism. The improvement in reported sleep quality was clinically meaningful,[60] and associated with increased activity, improved quality of life, morale, and physiology. In a study using aerobic exercise, King et al.[59] targeted a group free of clinically diagnosable sleep disorders or a medical or psychiatric condition responsible for sleep complaints. Controls were simply wait listed for an exercise program. Global sleep quality, total sleep time, and sleep onset latency were significantly improved by 16 weeks of aerobic exercise. Therefore, both anaerobic and aerobic exercise have been shown in community-dwelling, sleep-impaired elders to improve subjective sleep quality. A direct comparison of the two forms of exercise would be required to determine which is most effective, has higher compliance and feasibility, or lower rates of injury.

When choosing a modality of exercise for sleep disturbance, the etiology of the sleep disturbance, other co-morbidities, and place of dwelling will impact on choice. The factors in favor of a weight lifting program include a desire or need to increase lean body mass, co-existence of depression (it is a proven treatment for clinical depression in the elderly at an intensity and frequency achievable with safety and high compliance both in groups and at home), its feasibility in the nonambulant, and its relatively fewer contra-indications than aerobic exercise. An eighty-year-old woman with a gait disorder, frailty, osteoporosis, and recurrent falls, with depression as the cause of her sleep disturbance, for example, would likely be able to comply with and benefit from a weight training regime rather than aerobic prescription. The choice of an aerobic program of walking would be more appropriate in a sixty-year-old overweight woman with hypertension, hyperlipidemia, and peripheral claudication, both because of feasibility as well as co-morbidities which may also benefit from this prescription.

Dose

Based on the restorative theories of sleep, one would expect that intensity and duration of exercise would be important elements in changing sleep through exercise. Data in normals of varying levels of fitness, testing different intensities of aerobic exercise suggest moderate intensity exercise appears to be optimal, with exhaustive exercise appearing to increase sleep fragmentation.[61] Comparable data on intensity for weight-lifting exercise do not exist.

In studies of acute effects of exercise on objective sleep measures it is clear that exercise duration needs to be at least 1 hour with an even greater increase in total sleep time evident after 2 hours.[62] Once again the literature is largely in normals of varying fitness and never the sleep disturbed or elderly. Current recommendations for the use of exercise in elderly women can only be based on the two studies previously mentioned in sleep disturbed elders[59,60] in which aerobic exercise was effective as four 30 to 40 minute sessions a week at 60 to 75% of heart rate reserve (moderate intensity), and weight lifting exercise improved sleep when practiced for three 45 to 60 minute sessions per week, at 3 sets of 8 repetitions using a load of 80% of the one repetition maximum (high intensity).

Timing

It has been consistently found that the time exercise is performed in relation to bed time is a significant factor in reducing sleep-onset latency. Exercise is optimal when performed between 4 and 8 hours before desired sleep time. Less than 4 hours and greater than 8 hours lead to an attenuation of its effect and possibly a worsening of sleep. However, this response pattern is heterogeneous, and once again it was generated in people who had no sleep complaints.[61,62]

Location

Less exposure to light is postulated as one reason why the elderly may not sleep as well as the young. In young normals there appears to be a sleep benefit to outdoor exercise compared to indoor exercise, but whether or not this is related to increased light exposure is unknown. In the two positive trials in symptomatic elderly, exercise classes were performed indoors with undefined light exposure, suggesting that increased light exposure was not the primary mechanism of the exercise-induced improvement in sleep. Thus, when planning programs for institutionalized or home-bound elderly, or in residential settings, one should not have to depend upon the availability of outdoor or sun-exposed exercise venues for success.

NUTRITIONAL RECOMMENDATIONS

Some nutritional recommendations for someone with sleep disturbance will differ based on etiologic diagnosis; others apply to most presenting individuals. For example, caffeine is both a stimulant and a diuretic and its use should be minimized or eliminated, and restricted to morning and early afternoon, no matter what the cause of the insomnia. It should be remembered that caffeine is present in chocolate products, teas (even some herbal teas), coffee, some sodas, headache preparations, and certain diet pills. Similarly, the timing of all fluid intake should be aimed at early in the day so that less urine is passed in the evening hours, regardless of etiologic diagnosis. The reduction and regulation of alcohol intake are recommended for all insomniacs as it has a specific effect on upper airway collapsibility, thus worsening sleep apnea; it increases sympathetic state and arousability; it lowers esophageal sphincter pressure, worsening reflux; it acts as a diuretic, causing or worsening nocturia; and it may worsen depressive symptoms. If it cannot be completely eliminated, it should be pointed out that the closer to bed time it is consumed, the more disruptive it will be to sleep. Thus the common misperception of an alcoholic nightcap as a sleeping aid should be actively discouraged. Some cough syrups contain significant amounts of alcohol, and since these products are typically taken at bedtime to prevent nocturnal symptoms, they may aggravate insomnia instead.

Maintenance of a more ideal body weight is another common nutritional recommendation for sleep disturbed elders. Those who are overweight with sleep apnea would require a hypocaloric diet for weight loss, and such weight loss directly improves sleep-disordered breathing. The mechanism here is thought to relate to an increase in airway caliber and reduced collapsibility. Those with nocturnal osteoarthritis pain would similarly require a weight reduction diet if obesity is complicating the degenerative changes in their weight-bearing joints (hips, back, and knees).

If sleep disturbance is related to gastroesophageal reflux, then the consumption of small meals with the last at least 6 hours prior to going to sleep is of primary importance. In addition, benefit will be seen from a reduced fat content in meals and the avoidance of foods and drugs that lower the esophageal sphincter pressure such as tea and coffee, other sources of caffeine, alcohol, peppermint, smoking, and specific foods that cause symptoms for an individual (such as highly spiced foods). Other mechanical aids to relieve reflux such as the raising of the head of the bed on blocks may be necessary in severe cases.

SPECIFIC THERAPIES

Pharmacological Treatment of Insomnia

Unfortunately, medications are used far too frequently in the treatment of insomnia, often without due consideration of the underlying cause. Medications only have a role in the management of acute insomnias, or as a temporary measure in patients with chronic insomnia. The chronic and inappropriate use of sedatives is a large problem in our society. These medications may actually worsen the insomnia and make subsequent management more difficult. Furthermore, the use of sedative and hypnotics is particularly fraught with hazards in the elderly. There are several classes of drugs used to treat insomnia.

Benzodiazepines can be classified into long, intermediate, or short acting according to their duration. An important principle when managing the elderly is to use short-acting medications to avoid sedation, cognitive impairment, dependency, and withdrawal symptoms. In addition, elderly patients are prone to develop agitation on such medications. Long-acting benzodiazepines are associated with an increased risk of falls and hip fractures in the elderly.

Because of their sedative side effect, antihistamines are often inappropriately used to promote sleep. Their overuse is compounded because they are available without prescription. The side effects of antihistamines are wide and varied, making them a poor choice for use in the elderly. These include confusion, agitation, orthostatic hypotension, arrhythmias, and urinary retention.

Most tricyclic antidepressants have a sedative action, and are often used as hypnotics. They have a clear role in patients with coexistent depression, although newer classes of antidepressant drugs have become more popular. Again, side effects limit the usefulness of tricyclic antidepressant drugs as hypnotics, e.g., constipation, orthostatic hypotension, urinary retention, confusion, and cardiac arrhythmias. There is some evidence of an increase in the risk of falls and hip fracture in nursing home patients receiving tricyclic antidepressants.

Melatonin has been demonstrated to have hypnotic and hypothermic effects and has been proposed as a treatment for insomnia. Melatonin is produced by the pineal gland at night, and has a role in the regulation of the sleep-wake cycle. Reduced melatonin production has been associated with sleep disorders in the elderly.[19,20] The therapeutic effects of exogenous melatonin for circadian sleep disorders associated with jet lag, delayed sleep-phase syndrome, and blindness are reasonably well established. Some studies suggest a role for melatonin in the treatment of insomnia in the elderly, in cases where melatonin deficiency is established. Further work is required to clarify the efficacy and safety of melatonin in this setting.

Therapy for Sleep Apnea

The initial approach is to consider conservative measures, focusing on weight reduction, and modification of alcohol and sedative use. Avoidance of sleeping in the supine posture may be helpful in patients with mild sleep apnea occurring predominantly when supine. Nasal Continuous Positive Airway Pressure (nasal CPAP), a system for pressurizing the upper airway and thereby preventing collapse, is the treatment of choice for patients with moderate to severe sleep apnea.[45] Nasal CPAP is very effective and safe, but it is not curative. Tolerance and compliance are not always optimal, and therefore other alternatives need to be considered for some patients. Surgery to the nose or soft palate is a consideration, although evidence for the efficacy of these surgical procedures is conflicting. Dental appliances which result in mandibular advancement have been demonstrated to be an effective treatment in some patients, particularly with mild to moderate sleep apnea.[45]

Treatment of Restless Legs Syndrome and Periodic Limb Movement Disorder

Because of the similarities between RLS and periodic limb movement disorder, their treatment is also similar. Treatment should be restricted to symptomatic cases, either related to unpleasant sensory symptoms, sleep disruption, or daytime hypersomnolence. Treatment is often frustrating, and requires a balance between clinical benefit and unwanted side effects. L-dopa is frequently used as first-line therapy because of its low side-effect profile. This makes it an ideal choice in elderly patients. Clonazapam is also frequently used, but because it has a prolonged half-life in the elderly, it is best restricted to more refractory cases. Other drugs which have been used include Quinine, and opioids such as oxycodone and propoxyphene, but they are generally ineffective or associated with unacceptable side effects.

Bright Light Therapy

Light is known to be an important modulator of circadian rhythms. It is known that properly timed exposures to bright light (7000 to 12,000 lux) for 2 to 3 days can shift the circadian phase. To relate this to day-to-day natural light exposure, typical indoor room light is less than 500 lux, early morning sunlight soon after dawn produces 2500 lux, and midday sunlight is in the 100,000 lux range. The direction of the shift depends on the timing of exposure; morning bright light results in phase advance (going to sleep and waking up earlier) and evening exposure leads to phase delay (going to sleep and waking up later). Bright light therapy may be effective for a number of circadian sleep disorders, e.g., shift work, jet lag, advanced or delayed sleep-phase syndrome. In addition, bright light has an immediate arousing effect, and coupled with social interaction, can be used to reduce sleepiness and facilitate changes in the circadian rhythm.

In the clinical and research setting the light is administered via a light box consisting of a bank of fluorescent lamps behind a plastic diffusing screen within a metal box placed at eye-level and facing the subject. Indoor bright light administered during the day appears to improve the circadian rest-activity rhythm disturbance typically seen in demented patients,[63] and has also been reported to improve sleep efficiency in elderly sleep maintenance insomniacs.[64] It would appear prudent to recommend exposure to bright light during the day to older adults with little or no sunlight exposure, both for prevention and treatment of sleep disturbances. Further research is required to more clearly define the methods by which bright light therapy can be effectively administered in the home or nursing home environment. However, recommendations which may be made at this time are as follows:

1. Light, either through direct outdoor sunlight exposure or indirect (e.g., through glass or artificial lighting) exposure, may be effective for insomnia.
2. Persons must be facing the light so that it strikes their retina, although there is no need to look directly at the light source whether it be the sun or artificial lighting.
3. Exposure times of at least 30 minutes, but preferably up to 2 hours are effective.
4. Morning exposure to sunlight or artificial bright light is useful for insomniacs who go to bed late and have difficulty waking in the morning, as it will shift them toward more normal sleeping times.
5. Evening exposure to artificial bright light is useful for insomniacs who go to bed too early and wake up very early in the morning; this is particularly useful if their sleeping behavior is disruptive to family, caregiver, or institutional routines.

Other benefits of sunlight exposure in the elderly which should be kept in mind are production of vitamin D from its precursors in the skin, and treatment of seasonal affective disorder. Therefore, its use for insomnia has a very favorable benefit-to-risk ratio in the elderly woman who may also be at risk for osteoporosis and depression.

MONITORING PROGRESS

A sleep log or diary may be very helpful, particularly in patients with insomnia or circadian disturbances. It can help clarify inconsistencies or uncertainties in the history. A variety of logs are in existence, but in general the patient records the bedtime, approximate time of sleep onset, timing and duration of awakenings during the sleep period, final awakening time, and nap times during the day. The timing of meals, exercise, sunlight exposure, and medication use is also noted. It is useful for the log to cover a period of 2 to 4 weeks. Not infrequently the log unmasks previously unknown characteristics of the patient's sleep pattern, providing a new perspective for both the patient and the clinician.

If weight loss was recommended and other dietary changes suggested, then logs recording progress in these areas should be kept as well. Focusing on small short-term goals one at a time (such as the elimination of a single habit or dietary component) is more likely to be effective than attempting to achieve all changes simultaneously.

In summary, the management of most sleep disturbance in the elderly woman requires an understanding of possible causes and their treatment, optimization of medical conditions, minimization of drugs, appreciation of psychosocial precipitants, and a prescription for sleep hygiene, environmental change, physical activity, and an appropriate diet. Achieving this clearly requires an integration of traditional medical practice and lifestyle and behavioral changes in the context of a partnership between the older woman and her health care provider.

REFERENCES

1. National Institutes of Health Consensus Development Conference Statement. The treatment of sleep disorders of older people, *Sleep*, 14, 169, 1991.
2. Pollack, C. P., Perlick, D., Linsner, J. P., Wenston, J., and Hsieh, F., Sleep problems in the community elderly as predictors of death and nursing home placement, *J. Community Health*, 15, 123, 1990.
3. Foley, D. J., Monjan, A. A., Brown, S. L., Simonsick, E. M., Wallace, R. B., and Blazer, D. G., Sleep complaints among elderly persons: an epidemiologic study of three communities, *Sleep*, 18, 425, 1995.
4. Karacan, I. and Moore, C. A., Genetics and human sleep, *Psychiatr. Ann.*, 9, 11, 1979.
5. Wang, H. S. and Busse, E. W., The EEG of healthy old persons—a longitudinal study, I: Dominant background activity and occipital rhythm, *J. Gerontol.*, 24, 419, 1969.
6. Hughes, J. R. and Cayaffa, J. J., The EEG in patients at different ages without organic cerebral disease, *Electroencephalogr. Clin. Neurophysiol.*, 42, 776, 1977.
7. Feinberg, I., Koresko, R., and Heller, N., EEG sleep patterns as a function of normal and pathological aging in man, *J. Psychiatr., Res.*, 5, 107, 1967.
8. Ehlers, C. L. and Kupfer, D. J., Slow-wave sleep: do young adult men and women age differently?, *J. Sleep Res.*, 6, 211, 1997.
9. Rediehs, M. H., Reiss, J. S., and Creason, N. S., Sleep in old age: Focus on gender differences, *Sleep*, 13, 410, 1990.
10. Feinberg, I., Braun, M., and Koresko, R., Vertical eye-movement during REM sleep: Effects of age and electrode placement, *Psychophysiology*, 5, 556, 1969.
11. Feinberg, I., Changes in sleep cycle patterns with age, *J. Psychiatr. Res.*, 11, 513, 1974.
12. Feinberg, I., Thode, H. C., Chugani, H. T., and March, J. D., Gamma distribution model describes maturational curves for delta wave amplitude, cortical metabolic rate and synaptic density, *J. Theor. Biol.*, 142, 149, 1990.
13. Samis, H. V., Aging: The loss of temporal organisation, *Perspect. Biol. Med.*, 12, 95, 1968.
14. Casale, G. and de Nicola, P., Circadian rhythms in the aged: A review, *Arch. Gerontol. Geriatr.*, 3, 267, 1984.
15. Czeisler, C. A., Dumont, M., Duffy, J., Steinberg, J. D., Richardson, G. S., Brown, E. N., Sanchez, R., Rios, C. D., and Ronda, J. M., Association of sleep-wake habits in older people with changes in output of circadian pacemaker, *Lancet*, 340, 933, 1992.

16. Sack, R., Lewy, A., Erbe, D., Vollmer, W., and Singer, C., Human melatonin production declines with age, *J. Pineal Res.*, 3, 379, 1986.

17. Weitzman, E. D., Moline, M. L., Czeisler, C. A., and Zimmerman, J. C., Chronobiology of aging: temperature, sleep-wake rhythms and entrainment, *Neurobiol. Aging*, 3, 299, 1982.

18. Moe, K. E., Prinz, P. N., Vitiello, M. N., and Marks, A. L., Healthy elderly women and men have different entrained circadian temptertature rhythms, *J. Am. Geriatr. Soc.*, 39, 383, 1991.

19. Haimov, I., Laudon, M., Zisapel, N., Souroujon, M., Nof, D., Shlitner, A., Herer, P., Tzischinsky, O., and Lavie, P., Sleep disorders and melatonin rhythms in elderly people, *BMJ*, 309, 167, 1994.

20. Garfinkel, D., Laudon, M., Nof, D., and Zisapel, N., Improvement of sleep quality in elderly people by controlled release melatonin, *Lancet*, 346, 541, 1995.

21. Hughes, R. J., Sack, R. L., and Lewy, A. J., The role of melatonin and circadian phase in age-related sleep-maintenance insomnia: assessment in a clinical trial of melatonin replacement, *Sleep*, 21, 52, 1998.

22. Magri, F., Locatelli, M., Balza, G., Molla, G., Cuzzoni, G., Fioravanti, M., Solerte, S. B., and Ferrari, E., Changes in endocrine circadian rhythms as markers of physiological and pathological brain aging, *Chronobiol. Int.*, 14, 385, 1997.

23. Gillin, J. C., Duncan, W. C., Murphy, D. L., Post, R. M., Wehr, T. A., Goodwin, F. K., Wyatt, R. J., and Bunney, W. E., Jr., Age-related changes in sleep in depressed and normal subjects, *Psychiatry Res.*, 4, 73, 1981.

24. Hoch, C. C., Reynolds, C. F., Jennings, J. R., Monk, T. H., Buysse, D. J., Machen, M. A., and Kupfer, D. J., Daytime sleepiness and performance among healthy eighty and twenty year olds, *Neurobiol. Aging*, 13, 353, 1992.

25. Bliwise, D. L., King, A. C., Harris, R. B., and Haskell, W. L., Prevalence of self-reported poor sleep in a healthy population age 50–65, *Soc. Sci. Med.*, 34, 49, 1992.

26. Ballinger, C. B., Subjective sleep disturbance at the menopause, *J. Psychosom. Res.*, 20, 509, 1976.

27. Erlik, Y., Tataryn, I. V., Meldrum, D. R., Lomax, P., Bajorek, J. G., and Judd, H. L., Association of waking episodes with menopausal hot flushes, *JAMA*, 245, 1741, 1981.

28. Smith, R. N. J. and Studd, J. W. W., Estrogens and depression in women, in *Treatment of Postmenopausal Woman: Basic and Clinical Aspects*, Lobo, R. A., Ed., Raven Press, NY, 129, 1994.

29. Morin, C. and Gramling, S. E., Sleep patterns and aging: Comparison of older adults with and without insomnia complaints, *Psychol. Aging*, 4, 290, 1989.

30. Baker, A., Simpson, S., and Dawson, D., Sleep disruption and mood changes associated with menopause, *J. Psychosom. Res.*, 43, 359, 1997.

31. Block, A. J., Wynee, J. W., and Bayson, P. G., Sleep-disordered breathing and nocturnal oxygen desaturation in postmenopausal women, *Am. J. Med.*, 69, 76, 1980.

32. Cistulli, P. A., Barnes, D. J., Grunstein, R. R., and Sullivan, C. E., Effect of short-term hormone replacement in the treatment of obstructive sleep apnea in postmenopausal women, *Thorax*, 49, 699, 1994.

33. Caskadon, M. A., Bearpark, H. M., Sharkey, K. M., Millman, R. P., Roenberg, C., Cavallo, A., Carlisle, C., and Acebo, C., Effects of menopause and nasal occlusion on breathing during sleep, *Am. J. Respir. Crit. Care Med.*, 155, 205, 1997.

34. Redline, S., Kump, K., Tishler, P. V., Browner, I., and Ferrette, V., Gender differences in sleep disordered breathing in a community-based sample, *Am. J. Respir. Crit. Care Med.*, 149, 722, 1994.

35. Zepelin, H. and McDonald, C. S., Effects of age on auditory awakening thresholds, *J. Gerontol.*, 39, 294, 1984.

36. Zepelin, H. and McDonald, C. S., Age differences in autonomic variables during sleep, *J. Gerontol.*, 42, 142, 1987.

37. Mant, A. and Eyland, E. A., Sleep patterns and problems in elderly general practice attenders: An Australian survey, *Community Health Stud.*, 12, 192, 1988.

38. Gislason, T. and Almqvist, M., Somatic diseases and sleep complaints, *Acta Med. Scand.*, 221, 475, 1987.

39. Yunus, M. B., Holt, G. S., Masi, A. T., and Aldag, J. C., Fibromyalgia syndrome among the elderly: Comparison with younger patients, *J. Am. Geriatr. Soc.*, 36, 987, 1988.

40. Cook, N. R., Evans, D. A., and Funkenstein, H., Correlates of headache in a population based cohort of elderly, *Arch. Neurol.*, 46, 1338, 1989.

41. Zarcone, V. P., Sleep hygiene, in *Principles and Practice of Sleep Medicine*, 2nd ed., Kryger, M. H., Roth, T., and Dement W. C., Eds., WB Saunders, Philadelphia, 1994, 542.

42. Adam, K. and Oswald, I., Protein synthesis, bodily renewal and the sleep-wake cycle, *Clin. Sci.*, 65, 561, 1983.

43. Berger, R. J. and Phillips, N. H., Comparative physiology in sleep, thermoregulation and metabolism from the perspective of energy conservation, *Prog. Clin. Biol. Res.*, 345, 41, 1990.

44. Vuori, I., Urponen, H., Hasan, J., and Partinen, M., Epidemiology of exercise effects on sleep, *Acta Physiol. Scand.*, 574, 3, 1988.

45. Cistulli, P. A. and Sullivan, C. E., Pathophysiology of sleep apnea, in *Sleep and Breathing*, Saunders, N. A. and Sullivan, C. E., Eds., Marcel Dekker, New York, 1994, 405.

46. Curatolo, P. W. and Robertson, D., The health consequences of caffeine, *Ann. Intern. Med.*, 98, 641, 1983.

47. Newman, A. B., Enright, P. L., Manolio, T. A., Haponik, E. F., and Wahl, P. W., Sleep disturbance, psychosocial correlates and cardiovascular disease in 5201 older adults: The cardiovascular health study research group, *J. Am. Geriatr. Soc.*, 45, 1, 1997.

48. Rodin, J., McAvay, G., and Timko, C., A longitudinal study of depressed mood and sleep disturbances in elderly adults, *J. Gerontol.*, 43, 45, 1988.

49. Ford, D. E. and Kamerow, D. B., Epidemiologic study of sleep disturbances and psychiatric disorders, *JAMA*, 262, 1479, 1989.

50. Blazer, D., Hughes, D. C., and George, L., The epidemiology of depression in an elderly community population, *Gerontologist*, 27, 281, 1987.

51. Parmelee, P. A., Katz, I. R., and Lawton, M. P., Depression among institutionalized aged: assessment and prevalence estimation, *J. Gerontol.*, 44, 22, 1989.

52. Bliwise, D. L., Sleep in normal aging and dementia, *Sleep*, 16, 40, 1993.

53. Ancoli-Israel, S. and Coy, T., Are breathing disturbances in elderly equivalent to sleep apnea syndrome?, *Sleep*, 17, 77, 1994.

54. McNamara, S. G., Cistulli, P. A., Sullivan, C. E., and Strohl, K., Clinical aspects of sleep apnea, in *Sleep and Breathing,* 2nd ed., Saunders, N. A. and Sullivan, C. E., Eds., Marcel Dekker, New York, 1994, 493.

55. Guilleminault, C., Quera-Salva, M. A., Partinen, M., and Jamieson, A., Women and the obstructive sleep apnea syndrome, *Chest*, 93, 104, 1988.

56. Young, T., Palda, M., Dempsey, J., Skatrud, J., and Weber, S., The occurrence of sleep disordered breathing in middle-aged adults, *N. Engl. J. Med.*, 320, 1230, 1993.

57. Coleman, R., Periodic movements in sleep (nocturnal myoclonus) and restless legs syndrome, in *Sleep and Waking Disorders: Indications and Techniques*, Guilleminault, C., Ed., Menlo Park, CA, 1982, 265.

58. Trinder, J., Montgomery, I., and Paxton, S. J., The effect of exercise on sleep: the negative view, *Acta Physiol. Scand.*, 133, 14, 1988.

59. King, A. C., Oman, R., Brassington, G. S., Bliwise, D., and Haskell, W., Moderate-intensity exercise and self-rated quality of sleep in older adults, *JAMA*, 277, 32, 1997.

60. Singh, N. A., Clements, K. M., and Fiatarone, M. A., A randomized controlled trial of the effect of exercise on sleep, *Sleep*, 20, 95, 1997.

61. Youngstedt, S. D., O'Connor, P. J., and Dishman, R. K., The effects of acute exercise on sleep: A quantitative synthesis, *Sleep*, 20, 203, 1997.

62. Taylor, S. R. and Driver, H. S., Is sleep affected by physical exercise and fitness?, *Crit. Rev. Phys. Rehabil. Med.*, 7, 131, 1995.

63. van Someren, E. J., Mirmiran, M., and Swaab, D. F., Indirect bright light improves circadian rest-activity rhythm disturbances in demented patients, *Biol. Psychiatr.*, 41, 955, 1997.

64. Murphy, P. J. and Campbell, S. S., Enhanced performance in elderly subjects following bright light treatment of sleep maintenance insomnia, *J. Sleep Res.*, 5, 165, 1996.

21 Thirst and Dehydration

Paddy A. Phillips and Barbara J. Rolls

CONTENTS

WHY DO WE NEED THIRST?

Water is the elixir of life. All the chemical reactions in our bodies that keep us alive have to occur in water. Therefore, it is essential to maintain a normal body content of water.

As children, our bodies are about 80% water, which decreases as we get older due to increased weight of the skeleton and the amount of fat in the body. Because women have a higher fat content in the body than men, they have slightly less of their body weight as water. By adulthood, roughly 60% of the body is made up of water. Of this, about two thirds is inside the cells of the body (the intracellular fluid). The other third is outside the cells (the extracellular fluid) and is divided into plasma in which blood cells are suspended, and interstitial fluid outside the blood vessels and surrounding the cells. The intracellular fluid and extracellular fluid are in osmotic equilibrium. This means that when the overall concentration of fluid in one compartment changes, water moves from the more diluted compartment to the more concentrated one thus equalizing the osmotic pressure in the two compartments.

Not only is water important for the chemical processes in the body, but also in excretion of waste products in urine as well as regulating body temperature through sweating. Our airways also lose water to the air we breathe, and water is lost through the skin by evaporation. Water is lost by the airways and skin constantly and cannot be regulated. Our bodies do, however, regulate sweat production according to body temperature. Water loss in the urine is also regulated.

Because of the need to humidify the air we breathe, excrete waste products as urine, and evaporatively cool the skin through sweating, the body has an ongoing water loss problem, and has to be replaced. The replacement water comes from liquids we drink and the water in food. Obviously, if we take in too much water for some reason, we also have to be able to get rid of the excess. For our bodies to function normally, the osmotic pressure and concentrations of various salts (especially sodium) need to be maintained within a narrow range. To achieve this our bodies regulate the amount of water (i.e., the intracellular fluid and extracellular fluid volumes) and concentrations of various salts, etc. (i.e., the osmotic pressure) very closely (Table 1).

TABLE 1
Ways the Body Takes in and Loses Water

Water Intake	Water Losses
Drinking (~1500 ml)	Urine
Water in food (~700 ml)	Sweat and skin
Water in oxidation of food (~200 ml)	Feces/diarrhea
	Breast milk
	Lungs and airways
	Saliva
	Vomiting
	Bleeding

REGULATORY CONTROLS OF THIRST AND BODY FLUIDS

The regulation of the concentration and volume of the intracellular and extracellular fluid compartments within a narrow range is controlled mainly by two mechanisms: thirst and water intake, as well as the kidneys and urine output.

THIRST

Without the sensation of thirst there is no signal to tell us when our bodies need to replace a water deficit. As mentioned above, water loss through the kidneys, skin, and lungs is ongoing. While the kidneys can reduce water losses in urine to a minimum, the sensation of thirst is very important in detecting a water deficit and making us seek out extra water to replace that deficit.

What is thirst? Thirst is generally described as a cluster of sensations that increases with dehydration. These include a dry, scratchy mouth and throat with a bad taste, chapped and dry lips, light-headedness, dizziness, tiredness, irritability, headache, loss of appetite, and empty stomach. These are relieved when we drink.

Despite the number of the thirst sensations centered around the mouth and throat, an area in the brain called the hypothalamus (Figure 1) is the main control center for thirst. The hypothalamus also performs other important functions including regulation of certain hormones, reproduction, the thyroid and adrenal glands and growth, temperature, feeding and sleep/wake cycles. Thirst is stimulated by two main mechanisms.

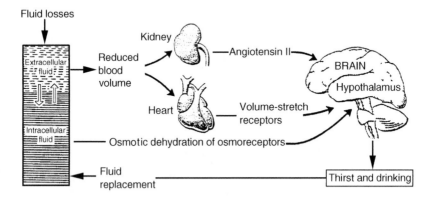

FIGURE 1   How fluid losses influence thirst and drinking.

When water is lost from the extracellular fluid compartment, for example, through sweating, the osmotic pressure and concentration of sodium in that compartment rise. This rise in the osmotic pressure is detected by certain osmoreceptor brain cells in the hypothalamus as water is drawn from them (and the other cells of the body) to equalize the osmotic pressure in the intracellular fluid and extracellular fluid. Direct evidence that this occurs and that the hypothalamus is involved is that minute injections of concentrated salt solutions in specific brain regions stimulate thirst, and injections of water (which should cause the osmoreceptors to swell) inhibit thirst. Also, certain diseases affecting the hypothalamus (e.g., tumors) can either stimulate thirst or cause an absence of thirst, which results in problems with fluid balance.

Not only must the body maintain the concentration of salts and osmotic pressure accurately but it also must maintain the volume of water (Figure 1). This is achieved by the body monitoring blood volume. Reduced blood volume stimulates thirst and drinking which then helps to replace the volume lost. The sensors that detect changes in blood volume as well as blood pressure are located in the walls of the heart and in the main arteries (aorta and carotid arteries). They are stretch receptors that pass information about blood volume to the brain via the vagus and glossopharyngeal nerves. These volume/stretch receptors inhibit thirst to a greater or lesser degree; when blood volume increases, the receptors are stretched and thirst is inhibited; when blood volume falls, there is less stretch and less inhibition. Relatively large changes (more than 10%) in blood volume are needed to stimulate thirst by this mechanism (for example, severe degrees of hemorrhage, diarrhea, or vomiting).

Reductions in blood volume may also affect thirst via the hormone angiotensin II. When the blood supply to the kidney falls as part of a general decrease in circulating blood volume, the kidneys release an enzyme called renin which activates a series of chemical reactions to produce the hormone angiotensin II. Angiotensin II has many actions that help to maintain blood volume and blood pressure. These include direct constriction of arteries, salt retention, and stimulation of the antidiuretic hormone vasopressin. However, it also stimulates thirst by acting in specific brain regions in the hypothalamus.

Another hormone, atrial natriuretic peptide, is released from the heart when blood volume increases. This hormone acts on the kidneys to increase salt and water loss. It also relaxes blood vessels, which results in a reduction in blood volume toward normal. Another action of atrial natriuretic peptide is to inhibit thirst and vasopressin secretion, again acting on the hypothalamus.

In these ways thirst is stimulated or inhibited to control the volume and composition of the intracellular fluid and extracellular fluid within a narrow normal range.

Vasopressin

The kidneys are also very important in regulating the amount of water in the body. This is achieved by filtering the blood and then chemically modifying that filtrate to retain essential chemicals and excrete waste products. Water is recycled through the kidneys by absorption with certain essential salts (for example, sodium). However, the main mechanism regulating the amount of water excreted is the antidiuretic hormone vasopressin.

Vasopressin is made in the hypothalamus and secreted into the bloodstream through the pituitary gland. As with thirst, vasopressin secretion is stimulated by increases in blood concentration or decreases in blood volume. Vasopressin acts on the kidney so that water can be retained and recycled into the bloodstream. Thus when we are dehydrated, vasopressin is released and water excretion in urine is reduced. When we are overhydrated, for example, after drinking a lot of water, vasopressin release is inhibited and excess water is excreted. Although vasopressin makes our lives more convenient through reducing urine volume and water losses, and thus not needing to drink or urinate very frequently, it is not an essential hormone. Some people do not make vasopressin for various reasons and yet they maintain their normal body water content within a narrow range by making sure they have enough to drink. However, their urine volume may be more than 10 liters per day. If such people also lack thirst (and therefore, the signal indicating they have a body water deficit), then they develop major problems with fluid balance and significant swings in the volume and composition of the intracellular and extracellular fluids. These people illustrate how important thirst is.

Satiety

Switching off thirst and vasopressin secretion is not just removal of the original stimulus. Interestingly, the simple act of drinking acts as a signal to switch off thirst and water intake as well as vasopressin secretion even before the water is absorbed and the water deficit replaced. Mechanisms that sense the ingested fluid are in the back of the throat and gullet. Colder fluids are more efficient at stimulating these mechanisms than warm fluids. Furthermore, cold water increases saliva flow compared with warmer water. These findings help to explain why colder fluids are more satisfying when we become thirsty. Distention of the stomach also plays a role in stopping drinking and switching off thirst. If the gullet is re-routed so that water/food does not enter the stomach, animals keep drinking without satiety.

BEHAVIORAL AND OTHER INFLUENCES

In our society we do not drink just when we become thirsty; nor do we always respond to our thirst as soon as it becomes apparent. There are many social and environmental factors that can influence our thirst (Table 2).

TABLE 2
Some Influences on Drinking Behavior

Palatability of liquids (temperature, sweetness, flavor)
Ease of access to fluids
Cultural/religious habits
Degree of dehydration (affected by environmental temperature, exercise)
Pharmacological effects of the fluid (caffeine, alcohol)
Eating dry food
Social situation (cocktail party)
Physical incapacity, medications, general health
Avoidance of night or frequent urination

SOCIAL FACTORS

Not only is fluid intake essential to replace water deficits, but drinking is also a pleasurable activity. We drink liquids for many reasons, including the palatability of liquids (e.g., soft drinks), associated effects (e.g., caffeine, alcohol), as a social "lubricant," and to help chew and swallow dry foods. All of these may mean we take in more water than we really need. This is when switching off thirst and vasopressin secretion to get rid of this excess becomes important.

Problems with incontinence and having to get up at night to urinate can also influence fluid consumption. Some older people voluntarily limit their fluid intake during the late afternoon and evening to avoid having to get up at night to pass urine. This may not be wise in hot, humid weather especially when exercising vigorously, as limiting water intake during such activity can lead to dehydration and reduced work capacity.

ENVIRONMENT

The environment will obviously influence the amount of water we lose. In a hot climate we use extra water as sweat to help regulate our body temperature through evaporation. In colder climates there is less need for this form of water loss. The same influence is applicable when we work hard or are relaxing.

The environment can also influence our thirst and drinking through the ease or difficulty of obtaining drinks. When drinks are hard to get or are unpalatable, then animals and humans limit their intake to just the amount that is necessary, and drink on fewer occasions.

PALATABILITY OF DRINKS

The taste of drinks is a major determinant of the amount we drink. Some of the factors that influence our perception of the taste of drinks include cultural background, previous experience with the drink, and time of day and is not always the same. Dehydration can increase the pleasantness of drinking and rehydration can decrease it. This decrease in pleasantness can be specific to the drink being consumed. Therefore, if the goal is to increase overall fluid consumption, changing to different drinks will help to increase the amount consumed. Sweetness, bitterness, acidity, temperature, and carbonation also influence the palatability of drinks and fluid intake.

MEDICATIONS

Medications such as diuretics, used to treat edema and high blood pressure, or excess laxative use can also increase salt and water loss and increase the risk of dehydration. Again, care should be taken if exercising in hot, humid weather while taking these. Discussion of these issues with your patients may be worthwhile, as most such problems are avoidable with a little advance planning of activities and fluid intake.

CHANGES WITH AGING IN THIRST AND KIDNEY FUNCTION

As people grow older a number of changes occur with regard to water balance (Figure 2). As mentioned previously, the percent of body weight that is water falls as the percentage of body fat increases. Also the regulatory mechanisms involving thirst and the kidneys change. It is well known that the excretory and recycling functions of the kidney for water and different salts get less efficient with age. This means that the kidneys cannot excrete excess water as quickly and efficiently as in younger people. Although the osmotic stimulation of the release of vasopressin remains intact, the kidneys of elderly individuals are relatively insensitive to the action of vasopressin so they cannot conserve water as efficiently and easily. Similarly, the elderly do not get as thirsty as younger people and do not replace body water deficits as efficiently or as quickly.

Several studies have now shown that otherwise healthy elderly men and women do not become as thirsty as young people when the osmotic pressure of their blood and extracellular fluid rises. Eventually they do replace the water deficit through a combination of slow water intake secondary to thirst, and water in palatable liquids

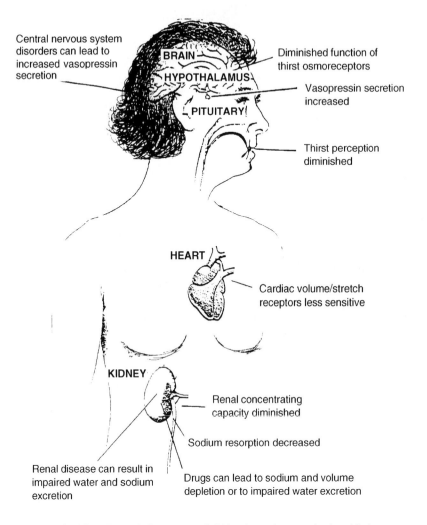

Central nervous system disorders can lead to increased vasopressin secretion

BRAIN

HYPOTHALAMUS

PITUITARY

Diminished function of thirst osmoreceptors

Vasopressin secretion increased

Thirst perception diminished

HEART

Cardiac volume/stretch receptors less sensitive

KIDNEY

Renal concentrating capacity diminished

Sodium resorption decreased

Renal disease can result in impaired water and sodium excretion

Drugs can lead to sodium and volume depletion or to impaired water excretion

FIGURE 2 Some influences on fluid intake and output in the elderly.

and food. However, when physical disability limits their access to water, they can become chronically dehydrated.

The mechanism for the reduction of thirst with age is not clear. However, at least part of it centers around changes in the function of the hypothalamus. As mentioned above, the elderly do not respond to increases in osmotic pressure as efficiently as the young. This suggests that the osmoreceptor function may be diminished. Abnormalities in hypothalamic function are also suggested since the elderly do not regulate body temperature as efficiently as younger people. When elderly men or women exercise in the heat, their body temperature rises to a greater extent than younger people, and they become less thirsty and do not replace body fluids as efficiently as younger people. Also the volume/stretch receptors that stimulate thirst are less efficient in the elderly.

SIGNIFICANCE OF CHANGES IN THIRST: DEHYDRATION

Reduced thirst in response to a water deficit and reduced sensitivity of the kidneys to the water-retaining effect of vasopressin mean that the elderly are predisposed to dehydration. This is especially the case if they have illnesses that cause extra water loss (such as diarrhea or vomiting) or have physical incapacity limiting their ability to access water and fluid replacement.

A body water deficit (dehydration) can affect people in various ways. In its milder forms, reduced blood volume leads to reduced ability of the blood to deliver oxygen and nutrients to different parts of the body. This can cause feeling generally unwell, dry mouth, sunken eyes, lethargy, reduced urine output, and, as dehydration becomes more severe, drowsiness, very low blood pressure, impaired kidney function and absence of urine production, and ultimately, coma and death. However, early dehydration may be easily missed especially in older people. The more severe symptoms are obviously associated with larger body water deficits and occur when body water is reduced by more than 20%. Even so, mild dehydration may still reduce the ability to exercise or perform normal daily duties. This is recognized now by athletes who constantly replace water and electrolytes, but especially water, during exercise, thus maintaining intracellular and extracellular fluid compartment volume and composition which leads to improved performance. "Sports drinks" have developed to help speed the absorption of water. The formulation of sports drinks is based on oral rehydration formulae (glucose/salt drinks) which are the best way to replace gastrointestinal fluid losses as in diarrhea and vomiting in children. The reason is that pure water is passively absorbed by the gut; however, glucose and salt are actively and more quickly absorbed. When glucose and sodium are reabsorbed by the gut, water also is reabsorbed as a "copassenger" to maintain osmotic equilibrium. This means that oral glucose/salt solutions (either as oral rehydration solutions for diarrhea and vomiting in children, or as sports drinks) lead to more efficient replacement of salt and water. Obviously if there is too much salt in the liquid, then problems can occur. This is why the solutions that have been developed have very specific amounts of water, glucose, and sodium. Even so, some of the sports drinks do contain large amounts of sugars, which should be taken into account when calculating calorie intake and assessments of diets.

STRATEGIES TO MAINTAIN FLUID BALANCE

The best strategy to maintain fluid balance is to avoid dehydration (Table 3) or overhydration. Becoming dehydrated is more of a risk than becoming overhydrated. Overhydration is usually not too much of a problem unless people have kidney damage or are taking medications that limit their ability to excrete excess water and salts, which some arthritis/painkilling medications can do. In people taking these medications, extra intravenous fluid, for example, in association with surgery, can lead to overhydration. Similarly, excessive amounts of palatable drinks can be a problem when excretion is impaired.

TABLE 3
Preventing Dehydration

PREVENTION IS BETTER THAN CURE!

Avoid exercise in very hot humid weather—put it off until cooler parts of the day

Wear light-colored clothing to reflect heat

Drink extra fluids—before, during, and after the exercise

Do not voluntarily limit fluid intake

Avoid alcoholic drinks

Be careful if taking diuretics or laxatives

Do not ignore feeling thirsty

Dehydration is more of a risk for the majority of elderly people; they should avoid exercising in extremely hot and humid weather and make sure that fluid intake occurs regularly in hot weather or when exercising. Because our bodies are extremely efficient in regulating salt excretion and our diets are normally very high in salt, it is not always necessary to use sports drinks; rather, regular water intake in association with a normal diet will usually be sufficient.

Water requirements vary with age and exercise. Average water intake in beverages is about 1.5 liters per day. However, extra water comes from water in food (e.g., fruit and vegetables may be 90% water) and by the body burning food to produce energy (oxidation). The amount in food varies with type, but the amount from oxidation is usually only about 200 ml. This means that drinking 6 to 8 glasses of water is enough in a mild climate, but not during intensive or prolonged exercise.

In hot or humid weather, we lose extra water through the skin due to evaporation (which is not controlled) and through extra sweating (controlled by the hypothalamus) to increase heat loss and reduce body temperature. Because of the extra water loss, when working in hot, humid weather it is important to increase water intake. Up to 500 ml per hour of work in that environment may be necessary. Not taking enough fluid and exercising in hot weather can lead to heat stroke. Heat stroke causes very high body temperature, absence of sweating, and can cause severe muscle damage, kidney failure, and death. In the elderly heat stroke can be a real risk as they already have reduced ability to control elevated body temperature.

An easy way to ensure plenty of fluid is to drink the equivalent of a couple of glasses of fluid with every meal. Also, if working in the heat, schedule drink breaks every hour.

Diarrhea or vomiting also cause extra fluid loss and increasing fluid intake is important then, too. Although it may seem that vomiting will cause the fluid to be immediately lost again, drinking small amounts frequently will result in some of it being absorbed with less of the stomach distension which aggravates nausea and vomiting.

Alcoholic drinks can also be a problem. Alcohol inhibits the secretion of vasopressin, and a reduced blood level of vasopressin leads to reduced water retention by the kidneys and excessive urine production. This is why we urinate more after drinking alcohol and why, after ingesting large amounts of alcoholic beverages, we can become dehydrated the next day. Avoiding alcoholic drinks, especially in hot weather, can also help prevent dehydration. Drinking a couple of glasses of water to replace any urine passed will help to limit alcohol induced dehydration.

As mentioned above, limiting water intake for any reason during hot, humid weather especially when exercising vigorously can be a problem. Although people may do it to reduce the need for getting up at night to pass urine, it can cause dehydration. When dehydration occurs, the body's ability to regulate temperature is also compromised.

CONCLUSIONS

The regulation of the volume and composition of the intracellular and extracellular fluids within a narrow range by thirst and the kidneys allows us to lead normal healthy lives. When dehydration or overhydration occurs, the functioning of many body systems is compromised. As we grow older these control mechanisms change, and often become less responsive to environmental stressors. By being conscious of these changes and taking appropriate preventative action, we reduce the risk of fluid balance problems.

REFERENCES

Chernoff, R., Thirst and fluid requirements, *Nutr. Rev.*, 52, S3–S5, 1994.

Ferry, M. and Vellas, B., Prevention and treatment of dehydration in the elderly, in *Hydration Throughout Life*, International Conference Vittel (France), June 9–12, 1998, Arnaud, M. J., Ed., John Libbey Eurotext, Montrouge, France, 137–149, 1998.

Greenleaf, J. E., Stress, aging and thirst, in *Hydration and Aging. Facts, Research and Intervention in Geriatrics*, Vellas, B., Albarede, J. L., and Garry P. J., Eds., Springer, New York, 47–57, 1998.

Morley, J. E., Miller, D. K., Zdrodowski, C., Gutierrez, B., and Perry, H. M, III, Fluid intake, hydration and aging, in *Hydration Throughout Life*, International Conference Vittel (France), June 9–12, 1998, Arnaud, M. J., Ed., John Libbey Eurotext, Montrouge, France, 107–115, 1998.

Naitoh, M. and Burrell, L. M., Thirst in elderly subjects, in *Hydration and Aging. Facts, Research and Intervention in Geriatrics*, Vellas, B., Albarede, J. L., and Garry P. J., Eds., Springer, New York, 33–45, 1998.

Rolls, B. J. and Phillips, P. A., Aging and disturbances of thirst and fluid balance, *Nutr. Rev.*, 48, 137–144, 1990.

Section IV

Integrating the Exercise, Nutrition, and Wellness Prescription into Health Care Practice

In the previous three sections of this book, much specific information has been provided to describe the important role of lifestyle, exercise, and nutrition in the health and well being of older women. If this knowledge were all that were needed to change behavior at the individual or societal level, however, we would not be experiencing such enormously high rates of obesity, sedentariness, and smoking, which realistically represent a public health epidemic of poor lifestyle choices related to all of the major chronic diseases of western society. Consider that approximately 30 to 40% of Americans are overweight, 60 to 70% are mostly sedentary, 80 to 90% not optimally active, 25% smoke, and 10% or more have chronic problems with excess alcohol intake. In contrast to the infectious disease epidemics which have often driven public health policy in the last century, the challenge for the next century is the management of these lifestyle factors that are in part responsible for the growing burden of disability, chronic disease, premature mortality, and health care expenditures in the ever-expanding older population. Women form the majority of the very old due to their longer lifespan, and this demographic fact is likely to continue well into the next century. For older women, heart disease, breast cancer, colon cancer, arthritis, osteoporosis, gait and balance disorders, obesity, diabetes, hypertension, frailty, and functional decline, among other diseases, are related in many ways to lifestyle choices, as well as genetic influences. Thus, prevention of the diseases of older women, including attention to behavioral choices, will need to occupy a primary place in the philosophy and goals of any health care system of the future.

Many years of research have made it clear that simply knowing the risks of a given behavior is insufficient to change that behavior or effect long-term adherence to a new habit. This is as true for individuals who are trying to change themselves as it is for practitioners who are meant to prescribe such new behaviors. For example, most physicians currently do not actively seek out sedentary individuals among their older patients to provide them with comprehensive physical activity programs that are feasible and effective, despite the wealth of scientific data documenting the hazards of inactivity, and the health benefits which would accrue. Similarly, most individuals are inappropriately underactive, despite widespread public health campaigns to promote active lifestyles over the past several decades.

Therefore, in this section, we have attempted to provide some practical tools that can be used to translate the previous information and guidelines into actions needed for *adoption of* and *adherence to* nutritional and physical activity goals. Simple ways in which older women or their health care practitioners can evaluate their current levels of nutritional adequacy and fitness are presented. Practical ideas for turning nutritional guidelines and exercise recommendations into daily habits and choices are given. An overview of behavioral change theory is provided, as an understanding of the stages of behavioral change is integral to the operationalizing of any lifestyle prescription. Tips on the implementation of effective programs of exercise in the home or in a variety of aged care and residential settings are offered. Suggestions for the kinds of medical screenings appropriate for older adults prior to adoption of new exercise patterns are outlined. A new paradigm of environmental design and safety is described, one which addresses both the need to encourage positive behavioral adaptations as well as ensure safety and universal access for the elderly or impaired.

We hope that this range of tools and approaches will allow better utilization of the information presented in the previous three sections of this book, within an integrated prescription for wellness in older women.

22 Preventive Health Strategies: Evaluating Current Information on Exercise and Nutrition

Christina D. Economos

CONTENTS

QUACKERY — CAN YOU SPOT IT?

As far back as records indicate, foods have been touted as "cures for things that ail you." Some things never change—we still hear claims about the miraculous benefits of food and nutrition every day. The difference is that in the past, when the diet lacked variety, the claims were more likely to be true. The inclusion of a food or nutrient may have cured a deficiency. Today, the diet is quite varied and nutritional deficiencies are uncommon, except in special groups such as impoverished, homebound, institutionalized, elderly, or ill individuals. Nevertheless, the claims we hear are quite provocative, creating the illusion that without a particular product, health is sure to decline. Distinguishing between scientifically based information and misinformation or "quackery," can be a challenge for the consumer.

    Quackery is rampant. Companies are telling consumers whatever it takes to sell a product; the media sensationalizes false information; and millions of victims fall prey to the techniques of health quacks every year. The fact is that almost any product, device, regimen, or program that promises what sounds "too good to be true," is most likely just that. Always be skeptical of quick, dramatic, and miraculous promises. Promoters know how to sell by playing on fear and manipulating the emotions of the vulnerable customer; they give us hope, offer pain relief, and promise a longer, healthier, more active life. They often use scientific terms trying to make it seem as though they are quoting scientific references. Often most enticing is that they ask for little effort on the part of the consumer—simply popping a pill or following a seemingly effortless program.

In contrast to the work of quacks, scientists are making important discoveries that are helping to shape the way we eat and exercise for optimal health. These findings you want to know about. Becoming a resource for your elderly clientele will help them to become educated consumers who can assess sources of health information and identify reliable advice. This is your best defensive against quackery.

ARMING YOURSELF TO DEFEND AGAINST QUACKERY

BEWARE OF MELODRAMA

Promoters of fallacies are fond of making severe statements like "you can't get adequate nutrients from foods, everybody needs to take supplements" or "lose 10 pounds of fat in 1 week." Because the media captures its audience through dramatic narration, the truth is usually exaggerated and shamelessly false as in the above claims.

RECOGNIZE THE TACTICS

Quacks know how to radiate assurance. They try to convince consumers of their products' benefit through confidence and enthusiasm, even when their methods have not been scientifically proven. They may offer a money-back guarantee, especially if it is a mail order, even when they have no intention of returning your investment. They can lead you to believe that you are getting the first crack at a secret remedy that will soon be breakthrough medicine. Beware of seductive tactics that are used to play on your emotional side, making you believe that you are genuinely being cared for.

DO YOUR HOMEWORK

Research the claim and read the actual studies from which it is being drawn. Note whether the studies were funded and carried out by the company that made the claim under investigation or by an objective research institution. If the funds were from the company, but the research was performed at an objective research institution, the results are more likely to be believable. Ideally, the study would be funded by a non-profit organization or by the federal government and performed at an objective research institution, which is what generally happens if the claim was worth evaluating to begin with. Also find out whether conclusions are being drawn or recommendations are being made based on a single study. Preliminary evidence is not regarded as substantial until it is put into context with other research. Solid recommendations are based on a body of evidence that has evolved over time.

EVALUATING THE VALIDITY OF CLAIMS

UNSOUND SOLUTIONS

Magazines. These are the principal sources of diet, nutrition, and fitness information in the American home, yet surveys consistently find that less than half of the magazines are reliable sources of health information. If you read something intriguing in a magazine, confirm the accuracy of the information with reputable professionals, nutrition or exercise physiology textbooks and journals, or professional organizations.

Nutritionist or fitness specialist. These terms do not mean anything, since their use is not regulated in any way. To have significance, genuine credentials from an accredited institution must support them.

Health food, fitness, and sports store employees. These people need not have any formal training and many of them are pushers of supplements and radical exercise programs.

Health care personnel. Some are trained and some are not. Don't assume that a chiropractor, a pharmacist, a physician, or a homeopath has an adequate background in nutrition or fitness; ask them about their training.

Testimonials and anecdotes. A friend who believes that he/she has been helped by an unconventional method and shares his/her success story does not mean he/she knows about nutrition or fitness. It is impossible to evaluate a health product or program on the basis of personal experience.

Front-page headlines. These often get distorted in an effort to capture audience attention—read the whole article and look for reference to the original research to get to the real source. Frequently when you go beyond the headlines, you will find language analogous to: "don't change your life just yet, more research is needed."

Advertisements. If you read about a health benefit on a label or a brochure, or you hear about it through a commercial, be skeptical and check it out.

The Internet. Although a wonderful way to transfer information and communicate, it is not policed for content. There is no guarantee that what you read is reliable. For a rating of nutrition information, visit www.navigator.tufts.edu

SOUND SOLUTIONS

Reputable professionals. People trained in nutrition science, with appropriate credentials and memberships in relevant professional organizations are the best sources of information. A registered dietician (R.D.), licensed dietician (L.D.), or a practitioner with a nutrition-related Bachelor of Science (B.S.), Master of Science (M.S.), or Doctorate (Ph.D.) from an accredited institution who belongs to a relevant organization such as the American Dietetic Association, the Society for Nutrition Education, or the American Society for Clinical Nutrition can provide you with reliable nutrition advice. Fitness experts are exercise physiologists or exercise scientists with a B.S., M.S., or Ph.D. from an accredited institution, or certified personal trainers or fitness instructors, with up-to-date certification from an accredited organization such as the American College of Sports Medicine (ACSM), the National Strength and Conditioning Association (NSCA), or the American Council on Exercise (ACE).

Professional journals and newsletters. Professional journals cannot be substituted as the best source for accurate information, but they are generally limited to academic libraries. Subscriptions to a professional, responsible newsletter, on the other hand, can keep you up-to-date with nutrition research. A few of the publications that are excellent choices can be found at the end of this section.

Textbooks. Not generally regarded as pleasurable reading, a good textbook will go a long way in dispelling myths and clearing up mixed messages. A general nutrition or fitness textbook designed for an upper-level high school or introductory college-level class is your best bet. A couple of tried and true textbooks are listed at the end of this section.

Books. The bookstores are flooded with new books on nutrition and exercise—choosing one can be very intimidating. Seek advice from a health professional you trust and take time to read about the author. Usually a reputable author is one whose educational background and/or present affiliation is with a nationally recognized university or medical center that offers programs or courses in the fields of nutrition, medicine, exercise physiology, or a closely allied specialty. Buy a recent edition, as things are constantly changing and being updated. A few recommended books are listed at the end of this section.

Public Libraries. Full of information on health, medicine, nutrition, and exercise. Get to know your local librarians and let them know what your interests are.

PROFESSIONAL ORGANIZATIONS

This list is not exhaustive by any means, but provides national organizations that can assist you in obtaining reliable information. Inquire about position statements or summary statements produced by most of the organizations on controversial, "hot," topics. These are critical aids in helping you see the big picture and sort through the confusion.

Nutrition
   The National Center for Nutrition and Dietetics
   American Dietetic Association
   216 W. Jackson Boulevard
   Chicago, IL 60606-6995
   (800) 366-1655
   www.eatright.org

National Agricultural Library
Food Nutrition Information Center (FNIC)
Public Services Division, RM. 111
Beltsville, MD
(301) 504-5414
www.nalusda.gov

The Center for Science in the Public Interest
1875 Connecticut Avenue N.W.
Suite 300
Washington, D.C. 20009-5728
(202) 332-9110
www.cspinet.org

Food Research and Action Center
1875 Connecticut Avenue N.W.
Suite 540
Washington, D.C. 20009-5728
(202) 986-2200
http://essential.org/afj/frac.html

Community Nutrition Institute
910 17th St., N.W.
Suite 413
Washington, D.C. 20006
(202) 776-0595
www.iglou.com/why/resource/1013.html

Exercise

Aerobics and Fitness Association of America
15250 Ventura Blvd
Suite 200
Sherman Oaks, CA 91403
(818) 905-0040
(800) YOUR-BODY [968-72639]
www.cybercise.com/affa.html

American College of Sports Medicine
P.O. Box 1440
Indianapolis, IN 46206
(317) 637-9200
www.acsm.org

American Council on Exercise (ACE)
5820 Oberlin Dr.
Suite 102
San Diego, CA 92121
(800) 529-8227
www.sandiegoinsider.com/community/groups/ace/index.html

Center for Disease Control
Public Inquiries
1600 Clifton Road, N.E.
Atlanta, GA 30333
(404) 639-3534
www.cdc.gov

Cooper Institute for Aerobics Research
12330 Preston Road
Dallas, TX 75230
(214) 701-8001
www.cooperinst.org

International Health, Racquet and Sportsclub Association
263 Summer St.
Boston, MA 02210
(800) 228-4772
www.ihrsa.org

National Association of Governor's Councils on Physical Fitness & Sports
201 S. Capitol Ave., Suite 560
Indianapolis, IN 46255
(619) 534-3547
www.fitnesslink.com/Govcouncil

National Coalition for Promoting Physical Activity
P.O. Box 1440
Indianapolis, IN 46206-1440
(317) 637-0349
Fax: (317) 634-7817
E-mail: natcoal@ncppa.org

The Melpomene Institute for Women's Health Research
1010 University Avenue
St. Paul, MN 55104
(612) 642-1951

WHERE TO COMPLAIN ABOUT QUACKERY AND HEALTH FRAUD

We do not have to tolerate deception in advertising. Make the effort to oppose quackery—it may save others from being hurt. National offices are provided below, but regional offices can also be found on the blue page of telephone directories.

The National Council Against Health Fraud
P.O. Box 1276
Loma Linda, CA 92354
www.hcrc.org/ncahf/ncahf.html

The National Fraud Information Center
(800) 876-7060
www.fraud.org

Quackwatch
www.quackwatch.com

FTC Bureau of Consumer Protection
Washington, D.C. 20580
www.ftc.gov

Federal Drug Administration (FDA)
5600 Fishers Lane
Rockville, MD 20857
www.fda.gov

Chief Postal Inspector
U.S. Postal Service
Washington, D.C. 20260-1100
www.usps.gov

You can also contact
- The local public health department
- Medical societies
- Other professional organizations (see above)
- The medical or nutrition department of a university or college

WHAT EXERCISE CAN AND CANNOT DO FOR YOU

Decades of scientific investigation can be summarized in some very basic health recommendations. Eat moderate amounts of food from each of the food groups in the *Food Guide Pyramid* to get the amounts and types of nutrients your body needs and accumulate 30 minutes of moderate-intensity physical activity on most days of the week. Adopting and adhering to these recommendations at any age help maintain health and independence. Studies show that good nutritional and fitness habits are associated with a reduction in age-related declines in cognitive and physical function, enhanced immune function, and lower risk of infectious and chronic disease (cardiovascular disease, colon and breast cancer, arthritis, diabetes, and osteoporosis). Maintaining a lifestyle change does require certain key ingredients such as knowledge, motivation, and dedication. Soliciting social support from family, friends, and health professionals is a proven method to help adhere to health-enhancing protocols.

There are several major contributors to our overall health: genetics, chance, and lifestyle factors (diet, exercise, alcohol consumption, and tobacco use). Our genes dictate what we will look like, and to some extent, whether or not we will end up with an inheritable disease. Chance is another factor in life that we are forced to endure. There is always a chance that something will go wrong even if you have taken all precautions to avoid misfortune. Lifestyle factors, on the other hand, are very controllable throughout life—even in the face of life's ups and downs. Exerting control over these factors is one of the most important things that a woman can do for herself.

The main types of physical activity or exercise are aerobic and anaerobic. Aerobic exercise includes activities that raise your heart and breathing rates and increase the body's demand for oxygen; for example, fast walking, jogging, biking, dancing, swimming, tennis, and rowing are all aerobic forms of activity. Anaerobic exercise requires intense muscular exertion and is generally performed in short bouts; for example, weight training, sprinting, or swinging a golf club are all forms of anaerobic activities. Both forms of exercise are important. Aerobic exercise helps to keep the cardiovascular system in shape while anaerobic exercise conditions the musculoskeletal system. Regular physical activity or exercise, supported by a healthy diet, can affect many of the risk factors for chronic disease and functional deterioration.

Weight loss and long-term weight management are enhanced with regular bouts of caloric expenditure achieved through physical activity. When weight is lost through physical activity, it tends to be primarily fat mass rather than the metabolically active lean mass. The change in body composition has important repercussions including maintenance of metabolic rate, strength, and physical function.

Blood glucose or blood sugar is better regulated when regular physical activity is part of the lifestyle. Individuals prone to non-insulin-dependent diabetes or glucose intolerance may prevent the onset with regular activity, while the severity of a diagnosed disease can decrease with a supervised exercise program.

Blood lipids (cholesterol, HDL, LDL, and triglycerides) are generally within the desirable range in physically active individuals, while those with undesirable levels will see improvement by adopting an exercise program.

Muscle strength, function, and mobility will improve with a regular exercise program. These variables are among the strongest predictors of whether an individual will maintain his/her independence. In addition, arthritis sufferers will find decreased stress, pressure, and pain in the joints, which will improve their ability to get up and about.

Psychological benefits from exercise can extend to combat the depression that is often seen with aging, especially when there are feelings of isolation from living alone. Exercise has also been shown to instill confidence and improve self-efficacy.

Energy level typically increases when individuals adopt an exercise program. As physical endurance increases, the ability to perform tasks becomes easier. This often translates into an increase in overall activity level—feeling better encourages movement!

Sleep patterns improve with regular physical activity and exercise. People fall asleep more quickly, sleep better through the night, and tend to sleep longer and deeper.

Immune function improves, with regular physical activity providing the means to battle illness, infection, and disease more effectively.

Bone mass can increase from weight bearing exercise like walking or weight training and helps slow the development of osteoporosis.

Balance and coordination generally improve with regular physical activity, which can ultimately prevent falls and injuries.

Regardless of age or physical condition, it is never too late to assist the older women in your practice to take control of their lives and reap the benefits of physical activity and good nutrition.

WHERE TO FIND ADDITIONAL INFORMATION

Newsletters
Tufts University Health and Nutrition Letter
53 Park Place
New York, NY 10007
(800) 274-7581
www.healthletter.tufts.edu

University of California at Berkeley Wellness Newsletter
Health Letter Associates
P.O. Box 420148
Palm Coast, FL 32142
www.enews.com/magazines/ucbwl

Nutrition Action Healthletter
Center for Science in the Public Interest
1875 Connecticut Ave. N.W., Suite 300
Washington, D.C. 20009-5728
www.cspinet.org/nah

Textbooks
Contemporary Nutrition: Issues and Insights
Gordon Wardlaw, Paul Insel, and Marcia Seyler
Mosby Publishers
www.mosby.com

Understanding Nutrition
Eleanor Ross Whitney and Sharon Rady Rolfes
West Publishing
www.westpub.com

Modern Nutrition in Health and Disease
Maurice Shils and Vernon Young
Williams & Wilkins
Philadelphia, PA

Exercise Physiology: Energy, Nutrition and Human Performance
William D. McArdle, Frank I. Katch, and Victor L. Katch
Williams & Wilkins
Philadelphia, PA

Professional Journals
  American Journal of Clinical Nutrition
  Journal of the American Dietetic Association
  International Journal of Sports Nutrition
  Journal of Nutrition Education
  Nutrition in Clinical Care
  Nutrition Reviews
  Medicine in Science Sports and Exercise
  Journal of Applied Physiology
  Sports Medicine

Books
  ADA's Complete Food and Nutrition Guide
  American Dietetic Association, 1998
  Chronimed Publishers

  The Wellness Encyclopedia of Food and Nutrition
  Sheldon Margen, M.D. and the editors of the University of California at
    Berkeley Wellness Letter, 1992

  ACSM Fitness Book
  American College of Sports Medicine, 1997
  Human Kinetics Publishers

  The Wellness Guide to Lifelong Fitness
  Timothy P. White, Ph.D. and the editors of the University of California
    at Berkeley Wellness Letter, 1993

Other Websites
    Nutrition Links
    Sponsor: USDA Cooperative Extension Service, Kansas State University
    www.oznet.ksu.edu/dp-fnut/Nutlink/n2.htm

    Tufts University Nutrition Navigator
    www.navigator.tufts.edu

    Shape up America
    www.shapeup.org

    Fitness Links - Fitness Associations and Organizations
    www.fitnesslink.com

23 Nutritional Assessment

*Maria A. Fiatarone Singh and
Helen Rasmussen*

CONTENTS

INTRODUCTION

It has been quite a while since we have experienced epidemics of nutrition-related diseases due to a deficiency of a nutrient, although perhaps it is possible to view the prevalence of osteoporosis, cancer, and heart disease in this light because of the strong linkage of these chronic diseases with nutrient imbalances or deficiencies in part. Infectious and pure nutritional deficiency diseases, while not eliminated, are not as widespread as they were in the beginning of the 20th century. Rather, the nutrition-related diseases we focus on currently are more those of excess and imbalance. Degenerative and chronic diseases are the major causes of death and disability. Due to the lengthening of life expectancy, the pursuit of health and well-being has been many an individual's focus. In the year 2000, the American population has a median age of more than 36 years, compared to 29 years in 1975. The population of the "oldest old" (over 85 years) will have increased by 30% in this time period, and this cohort will accumulate a significant burden of disease before death. Therefore, dietary and health advice is needed more than ever as a preventive strategy against chronic disease.[1] It is the purpose of this chapter to present ways in which you can assess the quality of the older woman's diet, and evaluate the adequacy of nutritional status on this basis.

NUTRITIONAL ASSESSMENT

If you were to inventory all factors that impact nutritional health, the list of physical, psychological, social, economic, spiritual, and environmental influences would be quite large. However, using simple techniques, the following framework may be a useful tool by which to judge nutritional history. The importance of this knowledge is that it can be passed directly to women who can then take more control of their nutritional behavior rather than continually deferring to others for direction.

Evaluating the Diet and a Nutrition History

It is important to determine the role of food in the woman's life, and how she relates to food, before determining the adequacy of the current diet or attempting to change it. Questions to ask in the primary assessment would include

What roles do food and drink play in your life?

How do you think of your next meal—with annoyance, relish, guilt?

How important have food and drink been in interactions with your family and friends?

How much does eating affect your social life?

What is it about your behavior and attachment to eating and food that you want to change, or celebrate?

Diet Restrictions and Special Diets

After determining general attitudes toward food and eating behavior, specific questions about dietary practices should be asked. These would include

What are your special restrictions with respect to your diet?

Do you follow a diet which has been prescribed by a health practitioner, such as a low sodium, diabetic, or fat-restricted diet? How compliant are you with these dietary restrictions?

Are you a vegetarian?

What foods will you probably never entertain the idea of eating? Why?

Is your diet complicated in any way by the way you must eat it (such as trouble with your teeth, requiring adaptation of your food to more soft, well-cooked, easier to chew foods)?

Are your financial resources so stretched that although you need to follow a special diet, you end up eating whatever you can afford at the end of the month?

Previous Dietary Counseling

Progress in understanding diseases has made some diets easier to follow, and less restrictive, and has relegated diet to a more primary position in chronic disease prevention. Often it is important, however, to counter previously held beliefs and myths that have been propagated over many years in order to give new information or change long-standing behaviors. It may help to ask

What kind of dietary counseling and advice have you been given in the past? Was it useful?

Could you understand it?

Did the counselor turn you off so completely from changing your diet that you gave up on the whole idea?

Did you just get a pamphlet from your health care provider and no other support?

How long ago did you obtain any dietary counseling?

What social factors would make it difficult for you to change your diet in any way (e.g., cooking for spouse, other special diets of family members, difficulty cooking, dislike of food preparation, financial constraints, lack of interest, lack of belief that diet is related to health status, lack of time, etc.)?

Are you at a time in your life when you need an update on previous nutrition and dietary information?

FOOD ALLERGIES AND INTOLERANCES

There are many misconceptions in this realm as well. Find out

Are there certain foods which are better for you to avoid because they cause distress?

Can you properly digest certain foods? What symptoms tell you that foods are not being digested properly?

Are there foods that you used to be able to eat that you cannot now? Why?

What reactions are truly allergies as opposed to dislikes?

GENERAL NUTRITION KNOWLEDGE

Gather some information on the overall knowledge base of the woman.

How much do you know about nutrition?

How much do you feel you need or want to know?

Do you get all your information from tabloid headlines in the supermarket, news reports, the internet or library, friends and relatives, health care professionals?

Would you like to become more nutrition literate?

DRUG–NUTRIENT INTERACTIONS

Information about medications that may interact with diet should be obtained by asking

What are the medications that you take?

Are these self-prescribed, or prescribed by your health care provider?

Are there certain pills you take that you have been told may be better absorbed depending on how you take them, i.e., with or without food?

Do you take any nutritional supplements of any kind?

DIET ASSESSMENT

The overall nutritional quality of the diet is usually determined by one of four methods of dietary recall. Obviously this requires reasonable memory and compliance on the part of the woman to provide accurate information, and can only be used in settings where this is a realistic expectation. It has been recommended that dietary assessment instruments used in older individuals should include items that are representative of the cohort's usual diet; should provide both qualitative and quantitative information on food items; should be specific with respect to food items, serving sizes, cooking methods and frequencies; and should be validated (to determine test-retest reliability and relationship to other measures of nutrient intake if possible) prior to use in the specific population (gender, ethnicity, health status) in which they are to be used. Administration is usually aided by the inclusion of food models, pictures, measuring cups and spoons, and scales when possible. Each of these methods will be described briefly in the following sections.

The 24-Hour Recall

This method involves asking the woman what she ate during the previous day. The question usually asked is " What did you eat yesterday?"

The list of foods is created, and then the real detailed information of this intake is probed—the quantity and state of the food (i.e., fresh, canned, raw), the brand names, cooking methods, beverages, snacks, and vitamin and mineral supplements. The food items are then calculated based on food composition tables that are available in many standard references. An excellent and inexpensive food table, "Bowes and Church's Food Values of Portions Commonly Used," can be found in most local bookstores.[2] There are also many diet calculation software programs currently available for computer-assisted calculations. The analyses are only as good as the data provided and the database used, and may be inaccurate if answers are vague or inaccurate or many food items eaten (such as ethnic or regional specialties) are not included in the database of the program or the written tables.

Food Records

In this more comprehensive method, the client is asked to write down all foods and beverages at the time they were eaten. Obviously, the food record can be done with varying levels of precision. As with the above recall method, detailed descriptions of the food are recorded, but unlike the recall, the food is measured and a notation is made on the record as soon as possible. The measurements can vary from putting the food directly on a household scale, or in measuring cups and spoons, to asking the waiter at the restaurant, "How many ounces is that piece of chicken?" Detailing of food records can be based on common sense—if you buy a food item ready to eat, and it has the nutrition label and weight of each serving available, the information only needs to be transcribed onto the record. If you are eating a serving of a dish which has many ingredients (such as homemade minestrone), the details of the recipe should be listed for the entire dish, and the total yield (e.g., "this soup recipe made 8 cups of minestrone") should be measured, then the amount of the soup that was eaten should be entered in the record. Once this record is completed, the food items can be calculated as in the 24-hour recall, with food tables or computer software. Food records are useful in measuring the actual foods eaten over the specified period. If the food record is extended over a long enough period of time, habitual food intake (such as always having coffee with cream in the morning) can be determined. Providing that the diet is truly represented and nothing is omitted, a food record is a very useful tool in understanding dietary habits, and where there may be opportunity for change.

What problems are encountered in using this tool? Individuals who don't participate in the actual food preparation, such as students who frequent the dining room, clients who travel extensively and cannot accurately describe food eaten in transit, and individuals who are not literate or numerate, are examples of challenging situations of recording and assessing the food actually eaten. Obviously this is a relatively time-consuming and cumbersome task to ask of an individual, and accurate information is only likely with a very compliant and committed client who has been given excellent instructions before beginning to collect data.

FOOD FREQUENCY QUESTIONNAIRES

This method is most often used in surveys and epidemiological studies because of its relative ease of administration and focus on long-term patterns of intake rather than specific points in time that may be poorly representative of habitual intake. There are many ways of obtaining information about how frequently certain foods or groups of food are eaten. This method of assessing diet is regarded as a quality measure of dietary adequacy. The time frame for asking this is defined: "During the last 6 months, how often did you drink milk?", for example. Quantity of the certain foods or groups of foods can also be asked: "Each time you drank the milk, what was the amount?" This approach provides only an estimate of foods or groups of foods eaten over time. This type of dietary assessment can obtain broad categories of amounts: low, medium, or high intakes of food(s). From these amounts it can provide estimates of what particular nutrients may be deficient. Using the above example of milk, if all answers to the milk intake question are low (one specific food), and additional questions of consumption of other foods from the dairy group such as yogurts and cheese are also low, then an individualized assessment of the nutrients that this group provides in rich amounts (calcium and Vitamin D) will be low. Asking the additional question of type of milk ("I only drink skim milk"), cheese ("I only eat non-fat cottage cheese") or yogurt ("I hate yogurt") can also estimate the intake of other nutrients (such as fat).

To make this method of estimating dietary intake as accurate as possible, as many foods and groups of foods need to be represented in the questionnaire as possible. The diversity of the population for which the questionnaire is intended must also be reflected in the questionnaire for it to be a valid measurement of intake, for example, certain ethnic foods may not be asked about at all in some versions. Calculation of nutrients using this type of tool is more difficult than the way food records or recalls are calculated. Let's illustrate roast beef as an example. The nutrient value of the beef needs to be calculated by the size of the portion (a large serving of roast beef), frequency of consumption (such as eating roast beef once a week), and then divided by the frequency into a daily consumption figure: one large serving (X amount) of beef eaten once a week (divided by 7) will give a daily amount of beef. A nutrient value can then be assigned to the estimated daily intake (~2 ounces per day).

This questionnaire procedure has been very useful in determining if there are any relationships between the consumption of certain food groups and the incidence of a disease in large epidemiological studies. Its usefulness in assessing individual nutritional status or change over time is more questionable. It should also be remembered that there are seasonal variations in dietary intake due to availability of certain food items, particularly fresh fruits and vegetables. Therefore, timing of food frequency questionnaires or interpretation of their results must always take into account seasonal differences as well.

DIETARY HISTORY

This method of diet assessment is the most complete, and encompasses some components of all of the above methods: the 24-hour recall (of actual intake), an interview of the client's overall eating patterns, and a food frequency questionnaire to verify information from the interview. In the interview, the following questions need to be considered:

How could you describe a typical day's food intake for yourself? What about in-between meal snacks? Alcoholic beverages?

How would you describe a typical Saturday's food intake? Do you eat any of these meals out? What about in-between meal snacks? Alcoholic beverages?

Repeat the questions for Sunday.

Calculate the nutrient intakes from the estimated food recalls using the food tables.

This method can provide insight into habitual intake without a large burden on the client to compulsively record daily food intakes. Notice that weekends are also covered separately from weekdays. It is recognized that the majority of individuals have separate and distinct ways of enjoying these days, which include a different eating pattern. Obviously, individuals who have problems with memory, or clients with very erratic routines, make this, and all methods of dietary recall assessment, unreliable.

Calculation of food intake requires the use of a food composition database. The reference in the 24-hour recall section is a widely used food composition book. It contains the majority of nutrients for all commonly consumed foods obtained in the United States. An excellent reference for software products is "Byting" in the '95-'96 Software Buyers Guide, which lists computer programs designed for nutritional analysis. For more information, contact: Meta Media, P.O. Box 689, Chesterton, IN 46304; (800) 654-8106.

CHARTS FOR RECORD KEEPING

There isn't anything magic about the way in which food intake is recorded. What should be included is shown in Table 1. Many people skip meals or eat snacks between meals, so space should be allocated for these patterns, particularly if this information will be used to guide recommended changes in behavior as part of the nutritional prescription. The food needs to be recorded specifically in terms of type and amount, as well as method of cooking, particularly for estimation of fat intake and nutrient retention. The recipes, if any, should be included at the bottom of each daily record and should have a place to record the total yield of the dish. If it is felt to be important in an individual, it may be useful to record additional cues, such as psychological state when eating, the location, and any other salient factors. These pieces of information are useful in modifying eating behavior, and are discussed in more detail in Chapter 24.

TABLE 1
Food Intake Record

Date:	Breakfast Time of Day:	Snack Time of Day:	Lunch Time of Day:	Snack Time of Day:	Dinner Time of Day	Snack Time of Day:	Snack Time of Day:
Food eaten, amount, how cooked							
Food eaten, amount, how cooked							
Food eaten, amount, how cooked							
Food eaten, amount, how cooked							

EVALUATING THE RESULTS OF DIETARY ANALYSIS

All any of us have to do to become confused with how healthy we believe our diet is is to read the local newspaper after a dietary study has hit the press. In a period of one week we can go from believing that butter is bad; margarine is good, but some margarine is bad; red wine is the answer; and reach for the olive oil! Fortunately, there are some basic guidelines that have been assembled by scientific boards, professional organizations, and government panels over the past several decades, and they may be the most reliable overall guides to assessing dietary adequacy in individuals and in populations. These guidelines are being constantly revised, and the newest, which have not been released in complete final form at the time of this writing, are *Healthy People 2010* and *The Dietary Reference Intakes*, preliminary drafts of which will be described at the end of this section.

The major sources of currently available, reliable nutritional information for Americans are outlined below. The repetition of common themes and overlap between all of these various guidelines is obvious and expected, given the similar body of scientific literature upon which they have each been formulated. For many general education purposes, behavioral programs, and assessment of basic food group choices, the simple Dietary Guidelines for Americans or the Food Pyramid may suffice. For more detailed dietary analysis and counseling on specific nutrient intakes, the Recommended Dietary Allowances or Dietary Reference Intakes will be more appropriate.

Recommended Dietary Allowances (RDA)

Beginning in 1941, the Food and Nutrition Board published standards (most recently in 1989) for adequate nutrient intakes for each recognized nutrient, known as the Recommended Dietary Allowances, or RDA,[3] and these were the most widely used guidelines until 1997, when a new series of recommendations and definitions of adequacy began to be released (see below). It should be stressed that this assessment is based on recommendations for *groups* of people. What does that mean? If you look at the chart of the most recent Recommended Dietary Allowances, and look at the heading "category," you will notice how the population is grouped. Under the Female category, the ages are grouped with consideration of certain growth characteristics important to that age group. The corresponding recommendations for all nutrients are amounts that are intended to be eaten as part of a normal diet. The derivation of adequate levels of nutrients is from extensive scientific documentation of nutritional research; these recommendations are neither minimal, nor are they considered for some individuals as "optimal." Rather, they are *safe and adequate* estimates of nutrient amounts, which have incorporated safety margins for that nutrient to cover individual variability for 95% of the population.

Dietary Guidelines for Americans, 2000

This set of guidelines (revised in 1999) was established by the U.S. Department of Agriculture and the U.S. Department of Health and Human Services.[4] These guidelines, while seemingly simplistic, represent extensive scientific input initially based on the 1988 Surgeon General's Report on Nutrition and Health;[5] the National Research Council's 1989 document "Diet and Health: Implications for Reducing Chronic Disease Risk";[6] and the 10th Edition of the Recommended Dietary Allowances.[3]

The guidelines are arranged into an ABC-type presentation:

Aim for fitness.
    Aim for a healthy weight.
    Be physically active each day.
Build a healthy base.
    Let the Pyramid guide your food choices.
    Eat a variety of grains daily, especially whole grains.
    Eat a variety of fruits and vegetables daily.
    Keep food safe to eat.
Choose sensibly.
    Choose a diet that is low in saturated fat and cholesterol and moderate in total fat.
    Choose beverages and foods that limit your intake of sugars.
    Choose and prepare foods with less salt.
    If you drink alcoholic beverages, do so in moderation.

The full document is easy to read, and full of tips about planning a healthy diet which are useful in counseling individuals. It is available free of charge from the Human Nutrition Information Service, Home and Garden Bulletin No. 232, Superintendent of Documents, Washington, D.C. 20402.

THE USDA FOOD GUIDE PYRAMID

In 1992, after much deliberation, the United States Department of Agriculture issued a new graphic interpretation of the Dietary Guidelines (see above). The pyramid shape (as shown in Chapter 4) is an attempt to illustrate the proportionality of the food choices recommended, in opposition to the older concept of a "balanced diet" in which all food groups appeared to be ideally represented equally on a daily basis. The foods that are recommended for the most consumption are at the bottom of the pyramid. They are bread, cereal, rice, and pasta, and the servings recommended are 6 to 11 per day. The foods at the top of the pyramid are fats, oils, and sweets, and the advice is to use these foods "sparingly." To order a copy of "The Food Guide Pyramid" booklet, contact the Superintendent of Documents at Consumer Information Center, Department 159-Y, Pueblo, Colorado 81009.

Recently, a "Modified Food Guide Pyramid for People over Seventy Years of Age" has been recommended by researchers at the USDA Human Research Center on Aging in Boston[6] for healthy, active older adults. This suggested modification continues to be based on the second edition of the Dietary Guidelines,[4] but contains some changes based on nutrient and energy needs of older adults. The conceptual change is to narrow the shape of the pyramid to reflect the decreased total energy intake and needs of the elderly, and, second, to emphasize nutrient density (foods with a high ratio of nutrients to energy), so that micronutrient and protein requirements can be met within this reduced total volume of food. In addition, a suggestion is made to add a small supplement flag to the top of the pyramid, and symbols for water and fiber. The nutrients which should be considered in the supplement area are calcium, vitamin B_{12}, and vitamin D, which may be problematic because of physiologic or disease-related conditions to supply from diet alone. Calcium (1200 to 1400 mg/d) and vitamin D (600 IU/d) needs are based on the recently released Dietary Reference Intakes rather than the older RDA values and may exceed what can be consumed in dairy or fortified products in some individuals. Vitamin B_{12} supplements may be required in those who have atrophic gastritis or take acid-blocking drugs chronically and cannot absorb food-bound B_{12}. Fiber intake is suggested at 20 g/d for optimum health. Fluid intake (apart from alcohol and caffeinated beverages) is recommended at 2 liters per day in normal circumstances.

The emphasis on nutrient density means that in addition to suggesting a number of servings of bread, grains, etc. per day, a recommendation is made to choose whole grain rather than refined flour products because of their nutrient density and fiber content. Similarly, fortified cereals would be preferred to non-fortified varieties. Fruit and vegetable choices among the deeply colored and cruciferous varieties are advocated, to enhance antioxidants, carotenoids, vitamin C, folic acid, and other nutrient densities. Selection of whole products rather than juices will increase fiber intake. Within the dairy group, at least 3 servings per day of low-fat, lactose-free (if necessary), and vitamin D-fortified products are recommended. In the meat group, at least 2 servings per day, emphasizing variety, and increased consumption of fish, lean cuts, and vegetable substitutes (beans, legumes) are desirable. In terms of fat intake, it is still recommended to limit this to 30% or less of dietary calories, as in younger individuals, and the amount from saturated and *trans* hydrogenated sources should be limited. Thus the modified food pyramid expands upon the basic dietary guidelines with new emphasis areas relevant to altered physiology, activity level, and intakes likely in older adults.

HEALTHY PEOPLE 2000

In 1979, one of the missions of the Surgeon General's office was to map out a health strategy to formulate an agenda of disease and disability prevention for the U.S. population of all ages.[1] Since then, there have been guidelines for this agenda which targeted the year 2000 as a chance to articulate fully the goals of the disease prevention campaign. A list of the health status objectives with respect to nutrition, formulated for the general population, and the means which were suggested to achieve these goals, are as follows:

1. Reduce coronary heart disease deaths to no more than 100 per 100,000 people. By recommending a reduction of dietary fat intake to an average of 30% of calories or less and average saturated fat intake to less than 10% of calories among people aged 2 and older.
2. Reverse the rise in cancer deaths to achieve a rate of no more than 130 per 100,000 people. The recommendation is to increase complex carbohydrate and fiber-containing foods in the diets of adults to 5 or more daily servings for vegetables (including legumes) and fruits, and to 6 or more daily servings for grain products.
3. Reduce overweight to a prevalence of no more than 20% among people aged 20 and older, and no more than 15% among adolescents aged 12 through 19. By encouraging those people who are overweight to adopt sound dietary practices combined with regular physical activity.
4. Increase calcium intake so at least 50% of youth aged 12 through 24 and 50% of pregnant and lactating women consume 3 or more servings daily of foods rich in calcium, and at least 50% of people aged 25 and older consume 2 or more servings daily.
5. Decrease salt and sodium intake so at least 65% of home meal preparers prepare foods without adding salt, at least 80% of people avoid using salt at the table, and at least 40% of adults regularly purchase foods modified or lower in sodium.
6. Reduce iron deficiency to less than 3% among children aged 1 through 4 and among women of childbearing age.
7. Increase to at least 85% the proportion of people aged 18 and older who use food labels to make nutritious food selections.

The success with which these goals have been met, and the resultant formulations of new goals are discussed below in the section on *Healthy People 2010*.

HEALTHY PEOPLE 2010

The fifth revision of this report, *Healthy People 2010*, is due to be released in 2000 jointly by the Department of Health and Human Services and the USDA. At this time, success in achieving the goals of the previous report is being analyzed in preparation for the development of recommendations to be included in this newest version. The report covers all major areas of health and prevention for various demographic groups within the U.S., including the elderly and women. Topics include nutrition, physical activity, chronic diseases, drug and tobacco use, and environmental hazards, among others. As the co-lead agencies in the area of nutrition, the Food and Drug Administration and the National Institutes of Health have reviewed progress on the goals of reducing overweight status, and increased prevalence and consumption of fruits and vegetables. The draft nutritional recommendations and others are available for comment in pre-publication format (at http://web.health.gov/healthypeople).

This report includes a summary of current nutritional assessment of the U.S. population. Items relevant to older women include

1. The prevalence of overweight has increased since 1980 for nearly all age, ethnic, and gender groups. For example, from 1976–1980 to 1988–1994, overweight prevalence (body mass index [BMI]>27.3) in adult women 20 to 74 years of age increased from 27 to 37%. The year 2000 target was 20% for adult men and women, a goal which is now farther from reach. Obesity is often a lifelong problem, and this rising prevalence in adult women is unfortunately heralded by an alarming increase in overweight status, even in very young children. While there were no year 2000 objectives for reducing overweight in children, data show that overweight in girls aged 4 to 5 increased from 7.6% in 1976–1980 to 11.2% in 1988–1994.
2. There has been modest progress toward the year 2000 targets of 30% fat and 10% saturated fat calories in the diet. Between 1989 and 1996 average fat intake has gone from 34 to 33% of total calories and saturated fat from 12 to 11% for Americans over 2 years of age. More importantly, in 1994–1996, 33% of people met the goal for fat intake (baseline: 22%) and 35% met the goal for intake of saturated fat (baseline: 21%), which is progress toward the 50% target.
3. The proportion of the population aged 20 and over that met the Dietary Guidelines for American's recommendation of 5 or more servings of fruit and vegetables daily has increased from 32% in the baseline period 1989–1991 to 40% in 1994–1996, compared to a goal of 50%. In 1994–1996, the population aged 20 years and over consumed an average of 4.9 daily servings of fruits and vegetables, the highest of any age group (baseline: 4.3).

4. In 1995, 18% of worksites with 50 or more employees offered nutrition or cholesterol education programs and 14% offered weight management programs. The year 2000 target was for 50% of these worksites to provide such programs.

5. In 1992, the percentages of primary care providers who provided nutrition assessment and counseling and/or referral to 81 to 100% of patients were as follows: pediatricians, 53%; nurse practitioners, 46%; obstetricians/gynecologists, 15%; internists, 36%; family physicians, 19%. The year 2000 target for each specialty was 75%.

Further interpretation of the findings of relevance to older women that has been offered by the members of the review panel is as follows:

1. Increasing Body Mass Index (BMI) carries increased risks of heart disease, diabetes, and other chronic diseases in all populations, although there is some variation in absolute risk among different ethnic groups.

2. Research on the mechanisms that control food intake and energy balance is increasing the understanding of the roles that genetic, behavioral, and physiologic factors play in the development of obesity.

3. The 5-A-Day for Better Health Program is a multi-level (national, state, and local) nutrition education program and public-private partnership that encourages the daily intake of at least 5 servings of healthful fruits and vegetables. Data suggest that nutrition education must be continued over time to achieve lasting success; when suspended, consumption of fruits and vegetables drops.

4. Fruit and vegetable consumption varies by meal and day of the week. It is higher on Mondays and Tuesdays, lower on Fridays and Saturdays. Eating away from home also influences consumption.

Finally, based on the current progress toward goals, and the health risks associated with poor nutrition, the following draft list of recommendations has been put forth for public comment prior to finalizing *Healthy People 2010*:

1. Forge stronger partnerships among federal, state, local, and private agencies that conduct programs to promote healthier eating habits as part of a healthy lifestyle.

2. Emphasize the close linkage between diet and physical activity in health promotion messages. Ensure the consistency of positive, reinforcing messages to the public on nutrition, allowing for varying emphases depending on the particular population group targeted.

3. Explore the feasibility of a Surgeon General's Report on obesity.

4. Investigate ways to enhance funding to initiate, sustain, and broaden efforts to promote fruit and vegetable consumption and other healthful behaviors, especially at the state and community levels.

5. When setting agendas for research on changing dietary behavior, explore behavioral and social intervention strategies based on lifestyles.

6. Encourage the Department of Education to promote greater emphasis on public school programs in nutrition and physical activity.
7. Seek ways to integrate and leverage funding for programs to promote healthful behaviors after school as well as in school.
8. Achieve greater integration of current food consumption surveys with a view to increasing the compatibility of data sets.
9. Develop consistent measures in federal reporting on nutritional status, including those reported in strategic plans and budget documents developed under the Government Performance and Results Act.

Several things are notable in this draft report. First, older adults are continuing to have increased obesity, despite better performance in fat intake and fruit and vegetable consumption than previously, as well as relative to younger adults and children. This suggests strongly that decreased physical activity levels contribute to the energy imbalance over time that results in obesity, and ultimately nutritional intake and physical activity patterns must always be linked in both research and clinical practice to fully understand and treat this epidemic. Second, suboptimal performance in terms of nutritional counseling was seen in physicians who were likely to treat older adults, highlighting the need for better efforts at nutritional education among health care practitioners in this field. Third, there is very little mention of general undernutrition in the elderly, despite the evidence that there is much preventable disability and disease exacerbation which could be prevented by attempts to avert this poor nutritional state. The emphasis on obesity and childhood nutrition is clearly indicated for the long-term health of the nation, and a reduction in cancer and cardiovascular disease, but current demographic trends also indicate the need for preventive medicine goals with applicability to the fastest growing segment of the population, the oldest old. These individuals are unlikely to suffer from obesity like their younger counterparts, and may instead develop health problems centered around weight loss, undernutrition, and sarcopenia, which are equally in need of targeted plans of action.

DIETARY REFERENCE INTAKES

Dietary Reference Intakes (DRIs) is a generic term used to refer to at least three types of reference values: Estimated Average Requirement, Recommended Dietary Allowance, and Tolerable Upper Intake Level. In the past, the Recommended Dietary Allowances (RDAs), published by the Food and Nutrition Board of the National Academy of Sciences,[3] have served as the benchmark of nutritional adequacy in the United States. The traditional role of the RDA is described by its definition adopted more than 20 years ago: The levels of intake of essential nutrients that, on the basis of scientific knowledge, are judged by the Food and Nutrition Board to be adequate to meet the known nutrient needs of practically all healthy persons.[3] Scientific knowledge regarding the roles of nutrients has expanded dramatically since the inception of the RDAs. Contemporary studies address topics ranging from the prevention of classical nutritional deficiency diseases, such as rickets, to the reduction of risk of chronic diseases such as osteoporosis, cancer, and cardiovascular disease. This expansion has extended the fundamental basis for the development of Dietary Reference Intakes.

In partnership with Health Canada, the Food and Nutrition Board has responded to these developments by making fundamental changes in its approach to setting nutrient reference values. The new title, Dietary Reference Intakes (DRIs), is the inclusive name being given to this new approach. They are a series of standards designed to be the new framework for guiding federal agencies about nutrient needs. The Dietary Reference Intakes are more comprehensive than the RDAs in that they provide 3 levels of intake rather than a single level, and for the first time separate older adults into over 50 and over 70 age groups, who are in fact likely to be quite different in terms of nutritional requirements in some cases. Where the scientific evidence is sufficient, the reports will ultimately recommend for each nutrient.

1. The Recommended Dietary Allowance (RDA) is the dietary intake level that is sufficient to meet the nutrient requirements of nearly all individuals in the group.
2. The Estimated Average Requirement (EAR) is the intake value that is estimated to meet the requirement defined by a specified indicator of adequacy in 50% of an age- and gender-specific group. At this level of intake, the remaining 50% of the specified group would not have its needs met.
3. The Tolerable Upper Intake Level (UL) is the maximum level of daily nutrient intake that is unlikely to pose risks of adverse health effects to almost all of the individuals in the group for whom it is designed.

When not enough scientific evidence was available to derive EAR and RDA values, the Adequate Intake (AI) is provided. Adequate intake is defined as the observed average or experimentally set intake that appears to sustain a defined nutritional state, circulating nutrient value, or other functional indicator of health. The AI is expected to likely exceed EAR and RDA values, when these ultimately emerge.

The Dietary Reference Intake project has been divided into seven nutrient groups and two subcommittees, each of which reports to the Standing Committee on the Scientific Evaluation of Dietary Reference Intakes. The seven nutrient groups are

- Calcium, vitamin D, phosphorus, magnesium, fluoride
- Folate and other B vitamins
- Antioxidants (e.g., vitamins C and E, selenium)
- Macronutrients (e.g., protein, fat, carbohydrates)
- Trace elements (e.g., iron, zinc)
- Electrolytes and water
- Other food components (e.g., fiber, phytoestrogens)

The report on calcium and related nutrients, B vitamins, and choline (see below) was released in August, 1997 at the National Academy Press Website (www.nap.com), but the other nutrient reports are not yet available at the time of this writing, although they are expected in the near future.

Calcium and Related Nutrients

The Institute of Medicine (IOM) established a panel under its Food and Nutrition Board (FNB)'s Standing Committee on the Scientific Evaluation of Dietary Reference Intakes to review the scientific literature on calcium, phosphorus, magnesium, vitamin D, and fluoride metabolism in humans throughout the lifespan, and data on intakes in the U.S. population. Such analysis included a review of the metabolism of related nutrients and of non-nutrients, such as phytosterols and fiber, as they relate to bioavailability. The panel drafted recommendations for nutrient intakes of calcium, vitamin D, phosphorus, magnesium, and fluoride for each stage of the lifespan, where adequate data were available, and which may result in decreased risk of chronic disease. The fluoride, calcium, and vitamin D recommendations are for adequate intakes (AI) only, as insufficient evidence was felt to be available at this time for more definitive recommendations. However, the AIs have been set substantially higher than the 1989 RDA levels for older women (from 800 to 1200 mg/day for calcium, and from 200 to 400–600 IU/day for vitamin D), based primarily on data from bone density changes and fracture rates with supplementation, and normalization of 25-OH vitamin D and PTH levels.

ANTHROPOMETRIC ASSESSMENT OF NUTRITIONAL ADEQUACY

ESTIMATING IDEAL BODY WEIGHT

Desirable or ideal body weight is usually defined as the average weight or weight range associated with minimal mortality for a specific demographic group. The most common of these reference tables are those created by insurance companies, such as the Metropolitan Life Insurance Company.[7] These figures represent self-report of height and weight among insured individuals, and therefore cannot be said to be representative of those who are uninsured due to health status, disability, socioeconomic factors, etc. Frame sizes (small, medium, large) that are used to further specify weight ranges within age and gender categories in these tables were never directly measured when this information was gathered. The most recently published Metropolitan Life Insurance Company tables from 1983 provide a higher weight range than those tables previously published in 1959 (reflecting the trends for increased average body weight over this period), and for that reason, there has been some hesitation by health care professionals to use the newer tables, despite their relationship to mortality as a "gold standard" guide. It should be recognized that apart from mortality, overweight is associated with much morbidity which would not necessarily be completely reflected in excess mortality in such tables, including an increased prevalence of arthritis, mobility impairment, diabetes, hypertension, cancer, cardiovascular disease, sleep apnea, and low self-esteem, for example. It is the combination of excess morbidity and mortality which describes the true health costs of obesity in a population, but a method of defining ideal weight based on all of these considerations has not yet been developed. See Chapter 17 for the specifics of the current weight guidelines.

Body Mass Index

Measures of weight adjusted for height are commonly applied in clinical settings. The Consensus Development Conference on the Health Implications of Obesity sponsored by the National Institute of Health in 1985 recommended that the body mass index (Table 2) (commonly referred to as BMI) be used to evaluate the health status of patients.[8,9] The idea behind this ratio is a measurement of body weight corrected for height. As a measurement of overweight and obesity, it is the most accepted measurement correlated with mortality risk. To calculate body mass index, the following formula should be used:

$$BMI = Weight(kg)/Height(m)^2$$

If metric measurement tools are not readily available, a simple formula for determining BMI using a calculator is

1. Multiply weight in *pounds* by 700.
2. Divide this figure by height in *inches*
3. Divide the figure you get in #2 AGAIN by height in *inches*.

Body mass index nomograms or charts are also readily available to avoid the above calculations, if desired. Using this method, obesity is usually defined as a BMI greater than 27 kg/m^2, and severe obesity as greater than 40kg/m^2. Underweight is defined as a BMI of less than 20.

Ideal body mass index for older adults appears to plateau within the range of about 24 to 27 kg/m^{2,10} with excess mortality on either side of this level resulting in a U-shaped relationship between BMI and mortality, in contrast to a more typical J-shape in younger individuals. This implies that the risks of being underweight are accentuated in the elderly in contrast to lean, younger individuals. This likely reflects the fact that extreme leanness or unintended weight loss in older adults often indicates undernutrition or pre-clinical or clinical disease rather than athleticism as it might in the young.

There are several problems with the measurement and use of BMI in the elderly that should be recognized. First, there are little data on mortality relationships in individuals over the age of 80 or ideal BMI in the nursing home population. Second, there are changes in height with aging that will affect the BMI calculation independent of changes in weight, and disease-related factors (arthritis, osteoporosis) that make the accurate measurement of height difficult or impossible in some cases. Various approaches have been suggested to overcome these problems, including the use of peak adult height, segmental lengths, arm span, demi-span, or knee-height, as substitutes for current height.[11] None of these approaches is ideal, however, and currently it is recommended to measure standing height without shoes using a wall-mounted stadiometer if possible, to the nearest 0.5 cm, with the head in a plane parallel to the ground (Frankfort plane), at full inspiration. Knee-height or demi-span seems the most reasonable substitute, and can be performed even in frail nursing

TABLE 2
Body Mass Index (BMI)

Height		Good Weights							BMI						Increasing Risk							
	19	20	21	22	23	24	▶	26	27	28	29	▶	31	32	33	34	▶	36	37	38	39	▶
4'10"	91	96	100	105	110	115	119	124	129	134	138	143	148	153	158	162	167	172	177	181	186	191
4'11"	94	99	104	109	114	119	124	128	133	138	143	148	153	158	163	168	173	178	183	188	193	198
5'	97	102	107	112	118	123	128	133	138	143	148	153	158	163	168	174	179	184	189	194	199	204
5'1"	100	106	111	116	122	127	132	137	143	148	153	158	164	169	174	180	185	190	195	201	206	211
5'2"	104	109	115	120	126	131	136	142	147	153	158	164	169	175	180	186	191	196	202	207	213	218
5'3"	107	113	118	124	130	135	141	146	152	158	163	169	175	180	186	191	197	203	208	214	220	225
5'4"	110	116	122	128	134	140	145	151	157	163	169	174	180	186	192	197	204	209	215	221	227	232
5'5"	114	120	126	132	138	144	150	156	162	168	174	180	186	192	198	204	210	216	222	228	234	240
5'6"	118	124	130	136	142	148	155	161	167	173	179	186	192	198	204	210	216	223	229	235	241	247
5'7"	121	127	134	140	146	153	159	166	172	178	185	191	198	204	211	217	223	230	236	242	249	255
5'8"	125	131	138	144	151	158	164	171	177	184	190	197	203	210	216	223	230	236	243	249	256	262
5'9"	128	135	142	149	155	162	169	176	182	189	196	203	209	216	223	230	236	243	250	257	263	270
5'10"	132	139	146	153	160	167	174	181	188	195	202	209	216	222	229	236	243	250	257	264	271	278
5'11"	136	143	150	157	165	172	179	186	193	200	208	215	222	229	236	243	250	257	265	272	279	286
6'	140	147	154	162	169	177	184	191	199	206	213	221	228	235	242	250	258	265	272	279	287	294
6'1"	144	151	159	166	174	182	189	197	204	212	219	227	235	242	250	257	265	272	280	288	295	302
6'2"	148	155	163	171	179	186	194	202	210	218	225	233	241	249	256	264	272	280	287	295	303	311
6'3"	152	160	168	176	184	192	200	208	216	224	232	240	248	256	264	272	279	287	295	303	311	319
6'4"	156	164	172	180	189	197	205	213	221	230	238	246	254	263	271	279	287	295	304	312	320	328

From Bray, G. A. and Bray, D. S., *West J. Med.*, 149(5), 555–571, 1988. With permission.

home residents in most cases, with regression equations used to estimate peak adult height from these measurements for use in BMI calculations.[11]

In a joint effort, the USDA and the U.S. Department of Health and Human Services published the document "Dietary Guidelines for Americans"[4] mentioned earlier. This publication stresses the concept that each individual has a healthy weight and discusses how both underweight and overweight carry health burdens, regardless of age; these tables for healthy weight do not have an allowance for age. Obesity has been strongly linked to a higher risk of coronary heart disease, certain cancers, diabetes, and premature death. The most compelling of all evidence comes from a study of over 115,000 middle-aged women who have been followed in a longitudinal study from the Harvard School of Public Health, The Nurses' Health Study.[12] This study reported that being of average weight, which in this investigation was a body mass index of 25 to 26.9 kg/m^2, increased a woman's risk of premature death by 30%. Notably, one vital piece of information not measured in the Nurses' Study was physical activity level. Since inactivity is an independent and potent cardiovascular risk factor, it is therefore likely that the attributable risks of obesity may have been partially due to low levels of physical activity commonly seen in women who are overweight. This study omission could have the effect of making it appear that the mortality risk associated with BMI begins at a lower level or is greater than it actually is (25 instead of 27 kg/m^2, for example, as other studies seem to indicate). In any case, whatever the exact cut-off at which risk increases, a gain of just 15 to 20 pounds after age 18 will put middle-aged and older women at substantially increased risk based on data in this and other studies (see also Chapter 17).

REGIONAL FAT DISTRIBUTION

Mapping body fat and recognizing gender differences in its distribution is actually not a new phenomenon, exemplified by many ancient statues and works of art. However, descriptions of the typical fat distribution of men (android, central, or abdominal obesity) vs. women (gynoid, lower body obesity) took on more scientific scrutiny after the 1947 description of the higher metabolic complications associated with android obesity.[13] Cross-sectional studies have shown android obesity to be associated with cardiovascular disease risk factors of hypertension, insulin resistance, and hyperlipidemia, as well as cardiovascular disease, diabetes, and overall mortality.[14] Gynoid obesity doesn't carry the same risk factors that abdominal obesity does, and is not associated with excess mortality at all. It seems that fat distributed around the abdomen is more metabolically active than fat below the waist.

In terms of nutritional assessment, the way to estimate the amount of central obesity present, without the precise assistance of computerized tomography or magnetic resonance imaging, is to measure circumferences of the waist and the hip. The results may be expressed as the waist circumference alone as an absolute number, or by calculating the ratio between these two circumferences. To measure the waist-to-hip ratio

1. Locate the narrowest part of the waist between the last rib and the iliac crest (the natural waist).
2. While the person is relaxed and not holding his/her breath, measure circumference to the nearest 0.5 cm, using a flexible anthropometric tape held firmly against the skin, and following but not compressing the natural contours of the body.
3. Repeat step 2 for the hips, defined as the widest area over the buttocks, with the tape held parallel to the ground.
4. Divide the waist measurement by the hip measurement to calculate the waist-to-hip ratio.

Any waist-to-hip ratio greater than 0.80 for women or 0.95 for men is categorized as high risk. A waist measurement alone of greater than 80 cm in women is associated with elevated levels of visceral adiposity and cardiovascular disease risk.

There are several advantages to the use of the waist circumference alone as an index of central obesity. First, it is more closely related to actual measurements of visceral fat than is the ratio.[15] Second, it simplifies the measurement technique and improves accuracy, as it is often difficult to reproducibly locate the widest hip circumference. Third, improvements (i.e., reductions) in waist-to-hip ratio may occur *either* because the waist circumference is decreasing, *or* because the hip circumference is increasing. Obviously, only the first of those two scenarios is indicative of successful weight loss efforts and thus improved health status in the obese woman. Fourth, repeated measurements of waist circumference at monthly intervals is a simple but powerful behavioral tool, which is more likely to reinforce eating and exercise habits than following the slow weight loss on a scale. This is because visceral fat is preferentially lost first when energy balance is negative or exercise is initiated in older adults, and thus the most rapid changes in anthropometric measurements will occur in this region.

OTHER MEASURES OF OBESITY AND BODY COMPOSITION

Techniques of determining fat in the body may also be carried out using more sophisticated methods, such as computed tomography (CT scan), and magnetic resonance imaging (MRI). Briefly, these methods give regional estimates of subcutaneous and intra-abdominal fat amounts. While these methods are not widely available to the general public, a technique which is becoming more available is called bioelectrical impedance analysis (BIA). This method of measuring human body fat is most widely used in assessing grades (i.e., fat content) of meat, and has only recently been applied to human beings. Bioelectrical impedance measurements are derived from differences in electrical conductivity of fat-free mass and fat, measured by connecting electrodes to both the wrist and the ankle. An electrical signal measuring total body resistance is used in a regression equation with age, weight, and height of the person to estimate total body water. Total body water will be proportional to fat-free mass and therefore non-hydrated (fat) tissue can be derived by subtraction. These regression equations are derived from validation studies in which independent measurements of total body water from stable isotopes or fat from hydrodensitometry are made in addition to BIA. Difficulties with this technique include the need to standardize test conditions (hydration status, meals, exercise, time of day, placement of electrodes, skin conductivity) and specificity of populations (regression equations for prediction of fat-free mass tend to be valid only in populations similar to the one in which they were derived).

LABORATORY TESTS

It would be ideal if there was a simple biochemical indicator of how well someone is eating. Unfortunately, most tests of an individual's health, particularly with respect to overall diet, do not detect subtle nutrient deficiencies. Instead, most commonly, the manifestations will be in chronic diseases such as diabetes, heart disease, cancer, osteoporosis, and from any of these diagnoses the nutrients which are specifically related can then be targeted. In light of the desire to prevent disease, subclinical deficiency states are now often measured by laboratory determinations. These tests provide objective measurements of nutritional assessment. However, many tests of individual nutrients are what are called static measurements. This implies that the tests carried out are subject to many factors at the time of gathering the sample. Below are some of the problems associated with these tests.

HORMONAL STATUS

Tests on women can be harder to interpret since there haven't been enough studies on how particular nutrients behave in various stages of a woman's life. Premenopausal women have different hormonal states depending on the menstrual cycle, postmenopausal women have another, and perimenopausal women are additionally confounding.

EXERCISE

Extremely vigorous exercise such as running a marathon in 90-degree heat or prolonged military marching can cause a variety of laboratory abnormalities, such as march hematuria (the appearance of red blood cells in the urine) and myoglobinemia (the release of muscle enzymes into the blood stream). Elevated levels of creatine phosphokinase (CPK) can be seen after one bout of moderate-to-high intensity weight lifting or aerobic exercise on the previous day.

RECENT DIETARY INTAKE

Many laboratory tests reflect an individual's most recent intake, and may not accurately capture a long-standing nutrient deficiency. For some assays, particularly lipids, glucose, and insulin levels, fasting is essential to interpretation. Fasts of at least 12 hours are suggested for cholesterol and triglyceride determinations. If creatinine excretion is being used to estimate total body muscle mass from measurements of 24-hour creatinine excretion in the urine, then a meat-free diet must be consumed for 3 days beforehand, as well as during the collection period, to eliminate contribution from the breakdown of animal muscle protein, which will add to the excreted creatinine pool and falsely elevate estimates of muscle mass.

LABORATORY METHODS

Precision of the measurement, collection procedures, and the specificity and sensitivity of the procedure are all important aspects in the internal workings of a reputable lab. The laboratory analyzing your specimen should be state accredited. Some nutritional tests, such as vitamin levels that are not routinely performed in clinical laboratories, may be best done in dedicated research laboratories where adequate quality assurance procedures and the latest assay techniques are in place. Some blood samples must be protected from ultraviolet light (vitamin D, for example) to prevent breakdown prior to measurement, and others must be stored at specific temperatures for accuracy.

MEDICATIONS

Many tests can give a different reading based on a medication being taken. A laboratory test may show a positive or a negative result based on a drug-nutrient interaction, but it may not reflect the actual health status. A complete drug ingestion history needs to be ascertained when obtaining blood or urine samples for nutritional analysis.

BIOLOGICAL FLUIDS AND TISSUES USED FOR LABORATORY TESTING

BLOOD

Blood levels of nutrients are tightly regulated to provide the body with necessary amounts in relation to current metabolic needs, which may change rapidly in the face of stressors such as exercise. Thus, even when other body storage tissues are severely depleted of nutrient concentrations, the serum or plasma tests of the same nutrient may remain fairly normal until deficiency states are quite advanced. Abnormalities in blood tests for red blood cell counts, glucose, and lipids are the most common findings in blood for which there are nutritional therapies. Elevated blood glucose levels may prompt dietary changes, such as spacing of meals, careful measuring of the macronutrients fat, carbohydrates, and protein, as well as weight control and exercise. Elevated cholesterol levels may be treated with a diet restricting fat and energy and exercise. Low body stores of iron, folate, or B_{12} can result in anemia. Food high in these nutrients as well as nutritional supplements are commonly prescribed to correct the anemia, if it is not due to a definable source of occult blood loss.

TISSUE STORES

Any assessment of body tissues would require a biopsy, and for this reason, it is too invasive for routine testing. Certain tissues are repositories for nutrients, such as calcium in bone, or fat soluble vitamins (like vitamin A or E) in adipose tissue.

Sometimes, blood cells isolated from whole blood can provide a closer prediction of tissue stores (e.g., red blood cell magnesium, white blood cell zinc) and are recommended over standard blood tests when earlier degrees of deficiency are to be diagnosed. Again, these more specialized tests are likely to be available only in research laboratories at this time.

HAIR AND NAILS

Trace elements of nutrients have been studied in sampling cuttings of human hair and in finger and toenails. The theory behind these analyses is that these trace elements, specifically minerals such as chromium, selenium, and manganese, are more concentrated in hair and nails than in blood or urine. Heavy metal exposure and toxicity are also studied from hair analysis. Nutrient analysis by hair and nail sampling seems almost too good to be true; these are body parts that are easy to donate without trauma. However, there are many problems related to interpretation of the laboratory tests. Hair and nail cosmetic treatments, shampoos, geographical locations, and environmental contaminants can markedly confound the test results. As is the case for all laboratory testing, the laboratory doing the testing must be reputable, and this is often not the case for private companies advertising nutritional analysis by these methods, followed by counseling, and predictably, subsequent treatment with proprietary vitamin products.

URINE

In the absence of renal insufficiency, urine can be used to assess certain nutrients: water soluble vitamins (those in the B-vitamin family and vitamin C), protein, and minerals. These nutrients all reflect the individual's most recent dietary intake and have certain limitations, particularly in the methods of collecting the sample. Complete 24-hour samples are needed for calculations, which can be substantially altered by missed or lost samples, incontinence, etc. Such collections are difficult to make in free-living individuals. Urine samples may be also used to estimate rates of bone resorption from markers of bone turnover that may be elevated in vitamin D deficiency. Urine samples can be used to assess compliance with dietary prescriptions in some cases, such as salt restriction in those with hypertension or edema, or protein restriction in chronic renal failure (via urinary urea nitrogen excretion analysis).

ENZYME AND METABOLIC PRODUCT TESTS

So many of our nutrients are interrelated in metabolic processes that the product of some of these processes are measured and evaluated to determine what nutrient must be limited to the body. A common example would be hemoglobin determination for iron assessment. Certain enzyme activities are dependent on vitamins or minerals as co-factors in their reactions, and thus level of enzymatic activity may be substituted for direct measurements of the nutrient itself. Examples of this would include measurement of glutathione reductase in place of vitamin B_6 and lipid peroxidation for vitamin E.

COMMON DISEASES AND SYMPTOMS THAT MAY REQUIRE NUTRITIONAL COUNSELING

Treatment or counseling by a qualified nutrition specialist is recommended for certain conditions, because they are disorders which require close attention to dietary intakes. Some of the most important considerations are outlined below.

DIABETES MELLITUS

In the over 60 age group, diabetics make up about 15% of the population. In the quest for good diabetic control, which has been shown to reduce the risk of microvascular complications and improve cognitive functioning, diet plays a major role, coupled with medication and a regular exercise program. Poorly controlled diabetes can result in devastating long term physical sequelae. Compared to the general population,

1. Diabetics are twice as likely to suffer from coronary artery disease.
2. Aside from limb amputations due to accidental injury, diabetics comprise half of all other amputations.
3. In analyzing the causes of the end-stage renal failure, 25% of these patients are diabetics.
4. Diabetes is the leading cause of blindness in adults.

Specific dietary suggestions for diabetics are outlined in Chapter 12.

ARTHRITIS

A special diet for the symptoms of arthritis would be a merciful blessing to all of the many sufferers. People have traveled to special mineral baths, worn copper bracelets, ingested herbal remedies, taken huge amounts of oils, including cod liver oil, and moved to a warmer climate in search of relief. Many of these claims of cures are poorly documented in the scientific literature. Osteoarthritis is the most common form of arthritis found in the older population, and affects women more than men.[16] Although there is no universal diet for treating osteoarthritis, there are a few caveats for a sensible diet. Extra body weight can add stress to the weight-bearing joints, and therefore the primary intervention is to work with the arthritic toward achieving a body weight that is closer to ideal. Even small amounts of weight loss have been shown to provide symptom relief, and may make feasibility and compliance with an exercise program greater as well. See Chapter 10 for a more detailed discussion.

Arthritis may be secondary to gout, in which case dietary restriction of foods high in purine, such as organ meat, some fish such as mackerel and sardines, and dried legumes, coupled with the addition of a medication to decrease uric acid, can help alleviate or prevent gouty attacks. Reduction in alcohol intake, total fat intake, and weight loss also appear to be beneficial in individuals genetically predisposed to high uric acid levels.

Coronary Artery Disease

Women, particularly postmenopausal women, are not exempt from heart attacks. Dietary management of this disease is the cornerstone to successful prevention and and aid to treatment of this chronic condition. Younger women are less prone to heart attacks than men, but once they pass menopause, they actually suffer heart attacks at the same rate as men, as discussed further in Chapter 14. Lifestyle alterations that are suggested for improving this disease and its risk factors are beneficial regardless of age. Achieving or maintaining a healthy weight, avoiding high fat diets, increasing fruit and vegetable intake, increasing fiber, and including adequate folate and vitamin E in the diet are the nutritional principles that are complementary to advice to abstain from smoking, perform moderate daily exercise, and practice stress management techniques.

Osteoporosis

The two major causes of osteoporosis in older women are lack of estrogen and a diet that lacks nutrients important in maintaining bone health, as described in Chapter 18. The primary dietary risk factors for this disease include low vitamin D and calcium, low body weight, alcohol abuse, protein deficiency, severe vitamin C deficiency, and perhaps other trace element deficiencies.

Obesity

Obesity has many causes, but the bottom line is excess fat, most simply defined as being 20% over the desirable weight designated for an individual (see also Chapter 17). The causes are many: genetic, endocrine, neurological, psychological, and environmental. Managing this condition is fraught with failure and recidivism. Efforts can involve diet, exercise, surgery, behavioral modification, use of specially modified foods, appetite suppressing or other medications, or a combination of these approaches, and must be individualized for success. As the preliminary *Healthy People 2010* report summarizes, this is truly a modern epidemic, now affecting 37% of the adult population in the U.S. over the age of 20. This is a substantial increase from the 27% prevalence rate noted in *Healthy People 2000*, indicative of the failure of public health campaigns so far to effectively deal with this problem in the nation's health. Efforts at controlling and preventing obesity have substantial rewards, from decreasing morbidity and mortality, to improving psychological well-being, and new recommendations for achieving these goals are due to be released in the year 2000.

Signs and Symptoms That May Indicate a Nutritional Deficiency

There are ways that nutritional deficiencies can manifest themselves, and health care practitioners should keep these symptoms in mind when evaluating older women. Many signs of nutritional deficiencies can represent an underlying disorder or disease which needs to be addressed. Unintentional weight loss (10% or more of usual weight) is often a sign of a change in a body's metabolic state, and can be a result of a gastrointestinal disorder, endocrine abnormality, occult malignancy, psychological abnormality, functional or cognitive decline, or an acute illness, for example. One of the common causes of fatigue and weakness is anemia, and depending on the kind of anemia, can be treated with vitamin and mineral therapy. The anemia of chronic disease, a normochronic, normocytic anemia often diagnosed in the elderly, is now thought instead to represent protein or calorie undernutrition in most cases. Protein calorie undernutrition will result in losses of lean body mass, with resultant fatigue and weakness as well. A severe nutrient-deficient diet will cause skin and hair abnormalities. A well-balanced diet replete with all nutrients should help these conditions. Vitamin A is well-known for its role in good vision and healthy skin and membranes. Severe forms of skin disease, such as psoriasis or acne, can be controlled quite remarkably with vitamin A derivatives. Large doses of the vitamin, although available without a prescription, can cause severe hepatic toxicity, so treatment should be monitored by a specialist in all cases. Common signs of vitamin and mineral deficiencies are burning tongue, cracks in the corners of the mouth, and sores, hemorrhages, or bleeding in the gums, and should be looked for on physical examination of individuals at nutritional risk. Water-soluble vitamins (the B-vitamin family) can be low in syndromes or diseases that cause these problems, but a diet low in all nutrients can display the same picture. Other considerations for the causes of oral problems include poor dentition or oral hygeine, immune dysfunction, smoking, lack of saliva secondary to anticholinergic medications, or use of medications that prevent the body from properly absorbing nutrients.

NUTRITIONAL INTERVENTION AND COUNSELING

People who need to obtain very specific dietary advice other than the broad public health recommendations that have been put forth here should seek the advice of a nutrition professional in consultation with their primary health care professional, as nutritional counseling is generally not the primary focus of traditional medical practice. The specialty of nutrition is becoming more recognized as one path for medical doctors, and some do complete more extensive training after completing internship and medical residency training. Chiropractors and osteopaths also get some nutritional training, as do those individuals obtaining Ph.D.s in nutritional science. But like any specialty, if it isn't the primary focus of their practice, or if they haven't really studied the clinical aspects of nutrition and disease, they may not be fully qualified to give specific dietary advice. The best option therefore is generally a registered dietitian, who is trained in both the specific nutritonal requirements relevant to disease prevention and treatment, as well as behavioral management techniques critical for successful adherence to dietary recommendations (see also Chapter 24).

Many states offer a licensure process which defines the qualifications and requirements for persons offering nutrition and dietetic services. The American Dietetic Association is the organization that provides the registration of individuals who have met the following criteria:

1. A Bachelor of Science or higher from an accredited college or university has been obtained. The major fields of study are human nutrition, nutrition education, foods and nutrition, dietetics, nutritional biochemistry, public health nutrition, or equivalent study.
2. There is an examination by the Commission on Dietetic Registration after a documented experience. Registered Dietitians are thus charged with assessing nutritional needs of individuals and groups of individuals based upon all nutritional data collected (such as the tests and measurements outlined in this chapter). They then translate these needs into actual food choices, or recommendations.

"Nutritionist" is a title which describes someone who also may perform nutritional assessments and provide counseling; however, no specific credentials are implied in this title. A Registered Dietitian may call her or himself a "Nutritionist," as there are no criteria set up for the legislation of this title, but a "Nutritionist" may not call themselves a Registered Dietitian unless they have the credentials above.

What about referring an individual for treatment by someone who has nontraditional training? Not everyone needs the same kind of nutritional intervention, and medical nutrition therapy as is suggested (and probably reimbursed by managed care plans) by the traditional route, may have been tried and not been found effective in some situations. Alternative therapy is slowly becoming a legitimate health care option as scientific research validates claims for some products and techniques. It wasn't until 1995, for example, that the United States Department of Agriculture and the Department of Health and Human Services Dietary Guidelines[4] stated that carefully planned vegetarian diets are good for you. Currently, there are intervention studies to evaluate the benefits of a multitude of novel therapies to prevent symptoms of diseases, or even to stop disease progression. Many of these programs involve testing foods or purified food components in human intervention trials.

Americans still spend billions of dollars on products or services that are unproven and even potentially harmful, however, as discussed in Chapter 22 in more detail. Some of the warning signs of such health fraud to be aware of include

1. Claims of a quick and painless cure.
2. A "special," "secret," "ancient," or "foreign" formula, available only through the mail and only from one supplier.
3. Testimonials or case histories from satisfied users as the only proof that the products work.
4. A single product effective for a wide variety of ailments.
5. A scientific "breakthrough" or "miracle cure" that has been held back or overlooked by the medical community.

Agencies which may help evaluate such claims and products include the Federal Trade Commission (Washington, D.C. 20580), the Food and Drug Administration, or the local Postmaster or the Postal Inspection Service.

REFERENCES

1. *Healthy People 2000*. U.S. Department of Health and Human Services Public Health Service, Washington, D.C. DHHS Publication No. (PHS) 91–50213.
2. Pennington, J. A. T., *Bowes and Church's Food Values of Portions Commonly Used*, 16th ed., J.B. Lippincott, Philadelphia, 1994.
3. Food and Nutrition Board, *Recommended Dietary Allowances*, 10th ed., National Academy Press, Washington, D.C., 1989.
4. Dietary Guidelines for Americans, 4th ed., U.S. Department of Agriculture and Department of Health and Human Services, Home and Garden Bulletin, No. 232, 1995.
5. The Surgeon General's Report on Nutrition and Health, U.S. Department of Health and Human Services, Washington, D.C. DHHS (PHS) Publication No. 88–50210, 1988.
6. Russell, R. M., Rasmussen, H., and Lichtenstein, A. H., Modified food guide pyramid for people over seventy years of age, *J. Nutr.*, 129(3), 751–3, 1999.
7. 1983 Metropolitan height and weight tables, in Stat. Bull. Metro. Life Insur. Co. 1984, 64, 2–9.
8. Foster, W. R. and Burton, B. T., Health Implications of Obesity: National Institutes of Health Consensus Development Conference, *Ann. Int. Med.*, 103(6, part 2), Dec. 1985.
9. Bray, G. A. and Gray, D. S., Obesity. Part 1 Pathogenesis, *West. J. Med.*, 149, 429–41, 1988.
10. Nutrition Intervention Manual for Professionals Caring for Older Americans, Washington, D.C., Nutrition Screening Initiative, 1992.
11. Mitchell, C. O. and Chernoff, R., Nutritional assessment of the elderly, in *Geriatric Nutrition: A Health Professionals Handbook*, 2nd ed., Chernoff, R., Ed., Aspen Pub., Galthersburg, MD, 1999, 382–415.
12. Manson, J. E., Willett, W. C., Stampfer, M. J., Colditz, G. A., Hunter, D. J., Hankinson, S. E., Hennekens, C. H., and Speizer, F. E., Body weight and mortality among women, *N. Engl. J. Med.*, 333(11), 677–685, 1995.
13. Vague, J., La differenciation sexuelle-facteur determinant des formes de l'obesite, *Presse Med.*, 30, 339–40, 1947.
14. Kissebah, A. H., Vydelingum, N., Murray, R. et al., Relation of body fat distribution to metabolic complications of obesity, *J. Clin. Endocrinol. Metab.*, 54, 254–60, 1982.
15. Despres, J.-P., Body fat distribution, exercise and nutrition: Implications for prevention of atherogenic dyslipidemia, coronary heart disease, and non-insulin dependent diabetes mellitus, *in Perspectives in Exercise Science and Sports Medicine: Exercise, Nutrition and Weight Control.*, Vol. 11, Lamb, D. and Murray R., Eds., Carmel, IN, Cooper Publishing Group, 1998, 107–150.
16. Maurer, K., Basic Data on Arthritis Knee, Hip and Sacroiliac Joints in Adults Ages 25–74 years, United States 1971–74. Hyattsville, MD, U.S. Department of Health, Education and Welfare, Public Health Service, Office of Health Research, Statistics, and Technology, National Center for Health Statistics, 1979.

24 Practical Implementation of Nutritional Recommendations

Sharon Bortz and Maria A. Fiatarone Singh

CONTENTS

0-8493-0258-0/00/$0.00+$.50
© 2000 by CRC Press LLC

INTRODUCTION

There are many nutritional guidelines that provide general principles for what adults should be eating. The most important of these are

The U.S. Dietary Guidelines, which give general recommendations for maintaining a healthy diet.
- Eat a variety of foods
- Maintain healthy weight
- Choose a diet low in fat, saturated fat, and cholesterol
- Choose a diet with plenty of vegetables, fruits, and grain products
- Use sugars only in moderation
- Use salt and sodium only in moderation
- If you drink alcoholic beverages, do so in moderation

The Food Pyramid, which describes how many servings an individual should be consuming from each food group.
- 6 to 11 servings bread, cereal, rice, and pasta group
- 3 to 5 servings vegetable group
- 2 to 4 servings fruit group
- 2 to 3 servings milk, yogurt, and cheese group
- 2 to 3 servings meat, poultry, fish, dry beans, eggs, and nuts group
- Sparingly use fats, oils, and sweets

The Recommended Daily Allowances (RDAs) outline minimum amounts of nutrients required to prevent nutritional deficiency states based on sex and age. For women who are 51 years of age or older, the basic recommendations are
- 1800 calories
- 46 g protein
- 4000 international units (IU) or 800 retinol equivalants (RE)
- vitamin A
- 200 IU vitamin D
- 8 mg or 30 IU vitamin E
- 60 mg vitamin C
- 400 µg folacin
- 12 mg niacin
- 1.1 mg riboflavin
- 1.0 mg thiamin
- 2.0 mg vitamin B_6

- 3.0 µg vitamin B_{12}
- 1000 mg calcium
- 800 mg phosphorous
- 150 µg iodine
- 10 µg iron
- 300 mg magnesium
- 15 mg zinc

Specific nutritional guidelines for people over 50 have been in development over the past several years to optimize health, rather than merely prevent deficiency states. Some of these are as follows:

- 1000 mg calcium if premenopausal or postmenopausal on estrogen replacement therapy; 1500 mg calcium if postmenopausal not on estrogen replacement therapy
- 100 to 400 IU vitamin E
- 500 to 1000 mg vitamin C
- 1 cup fluid/20 pounds body weight
- 600 to 800 IU vitamin D.

Additional guidelines will be available for those over 50 and over 70 when the Daily Recommended Intakes (DRIs) are released over the next 1–2 years (see Chapter 23), and will supercede the above RDAs.

ASSESSING DIETARY COMPLIANCE WITH GUIDELINES

The best way to assess dietary adequacy is to compare the current dietary patterns and food choices of your patients or clients with the above guidelines. This can be done by the individual herself, which may be the best way of reinforcing her control over appropriate food choices for the long term. For example, you may instruct her to

1. Compare the values obtained from nutritional assessment (see Chapter 23) to the values stated above.
2. Place check marks next to each guideline that is met with the current diet.
3. Keep a chart (Table 1) to write the changes needed in the diet (i.e., 400 mg more calcium, 2 more servings of vegetables, 20 grams less fat, etc.).

In the pages of this chapter which follow practical recommendations for planning meals, shopping, cooking, storing, and assessing food intake are provided in a format meant to be used directly by older women in your care.

DEVELOPING INDIVIDUAL NUTRITION GOALS

After reviewing compliance with general guidelines, the next step is to turn these dietary changes into personal nutrition goals. It is important to remember that people choose and eat food, not vitamins, minerals, protein, and fat. So micronutrient and macronutrient goals must be ultimately translated into dietary patterns. Review the list generated in Table 1 and see if there are any changes that are similar to each

TABLE 1
Chart of Dietary Goals

Dietary Goals Met	Dietary Goals Not Met	Changes Needed to Meet Goals
Iron		—
	Calcium	400 mg calcium; 2 more servings dairy products/day
	Fruits and vegetables	3 more servings per day

other. Then try to devise one or a small number of food choice goals that will satisfy them all, rather than initiating a long list of changes that will be overwhelming and difficult to sustain. For example, some dietary changes may include one more serving of vegetables, 400 mg more calcium, and one more serving of dairy products. These can be combined into the one nutrition goal of incorporating one more serving each of a calcium-rich vegetable and dairy product. If goals include reduction of fat content as well as increasing servings of fruits and vegetables, then a goal of replacing a serving of meat with a vegetable-based protein serving once a day may be the only change needed to satisfy both goals.

ALTERNATIVE SOLUTIONS TO INDIVIDUAL NUTRITION GOALS

The bridge between making goals and actually achieving them can be crossed by breaking each goal into at least three possible solutions. For instance, if one of the goals established is to incorporate one more serving each of a calcium-rich vegetable and dairy product into the diet each day, three possible solutions can be

Yogurt as an afternoon snack;
Dark green lettuce instead of iceberg;
Utilize more vegetable/calcium-rich recipes, such as broccoli pizza or vegetable quiche.

With at least three possible solutions to chose from, based on preferences, medical or allergic restrictions, and ethnic or cultural background, the likelihood of someone meeting these nutrition goals on a consistent basis is increased. Flexibility is a key to dietary modification. If one solution does not work as a means to meet the nutrition goals, then alternatives can be tried. A chart can be filled out as shown in Table 2 to assist in breaking down the dietary behaviors in this way.

PUTTING SOLUTIONS INTO ACTION

Once the goals and behaviors have been outlined as illustrated in the sections above, they must be put into action to succeed. The next sections give suggestions on healthy

TABLE 2
Developing Alternative Solutions to Dietary Goals

Use the space below to create at least three possible solutions for each of your nutrition goals:

Nutrition Goal #1:
    Solution #1: _____
    Solution #2: _____
    Solution #3: _____

Nutrition Goal #2:
    Solution #1: _____
    Solution #2: _____
    Solution #3: _____

Nutrition Goal #3:
    Solution #1: _____
    Solution #2: _____
    Solution #3: _____

food group choices, meal planning, recipes, and grocery shopping to put individually tailored solutions into action.

HEALTHY FOOD GROUP CHOICES

Often there is a need to come up with better food choices from certain food groups. Use the list below to select from healthy choices commonly consumed at each meal.

Breakfast
    Grains: whole wheat bread, bagels, English muffin, bran flakes, puffed dry cereal, cooked whole grain cereal
    Fruits: fruit juice (not "ade," "drink," or "cocktail" which contain large amounts of sugar and sometimes only 10% actual juice), orange, banana, peach, nectarine, pear, grapefruit, berries
    Dairy: skim milk, nonfat yogurt, part-skim mozzarella cheese, nonfat cottage cheese

Lunch
    Grains: Whole wheat bread, whole wheat pita (pocket) bread, whole wheat pasta, whole wheat tortilla, tabouli
    Fruits: apple, orange, banana, grapes, peach, nectarine, plum, pear fruit juice (not "ade," "drink," or "cocktail")
    Vegetables: carrot sticks, celery sticks, sliced bell peppers, broccoli and cauliflower flowerettes, radishes, cucumber rounds, sprouts, vegetable juice
    Meats: chicken, turkey, water-packed tuna, lowfat cheeses, hard-boiled egg, lentil soup, split pea soup, 3-bean salad

Dinner
  Grains: brown rice, bulgur, cracked wheat, barley, whole wheat pasta, baked potato
  Meats: chicken, turkey, fish, chile sans carne (with beans), lean cuts of red meat
  Vegetables: broccoli, cauliflower, string beans, zucchini, tomato, salad-type vegetables; cucumber, dark green lettuce, sprouts
  Dairy: nonfat milk, cream-based soup, nonfat frozen yogurt, ice milk

Snacks
  Grains: whole-grain crackers, rice cakes, unsalted pretzels, air-popped popcorn, graham crackers
  Fruits: apple, orange, banana, grapes, peach, nectarine, plum, pear, dried fruit, fruit juice (not "ade," "drink," or "cocktail")
  Vegetables: carrot sticks, celery sticks, sliced bell peppers, broccoli and cauliflower flowerettes, radishes, cucumber rounds, vegetable juice

Note: the emphasis on low fat foods in the above lists is appropriate for those who are overweight, with heart disease, diabetes, hypertension, arthritis, etc. For women who are of normal weight or underweight, whole milk dairy products and moderate use of monounsaturated or other vegetable oils are appropriate.

Menu Planning

Once armed with general food ideas as above, the woman should be encouraged to plan a typical daily menu that adheres to her goals by listing food group choices for each meal or snack (see sample for breakfast in Table 3). If any meals are typically eaten on the run, be sure to consider food choices that are portable.

Breakfast

This should include at the minimum one whole grain, a fruit or juice, and a low/nonfat dairy product. These choices will provide good sources of complex carbohydrates, fiber, calcium, and vitamin C. If someone is a hearty breakfast eater, include a meat or meat alternate as well. If she is typically rushed in the morning, consider the Power Breakfast Shake below that combines these food groups into one tasty and convenient drink.

POWER BREAKFAST SHAKE

½ cup plain nonfat yogurt	½ banana
½ cup sliced strawberries, blueberries, peaches, or crushed pineapple (in its own juice)	½ cup nonfat milk
	1 tbsp. nonfat dry milk
	1 tbsp. wheat bran
½ tsp. vanilla	ice cubes

Put all ingredients into a blender and whir until smooth. Try different combinations of yogurt, juice, and fruit for variety. Provides 1.5 gram fat, 555 mg calcium. Servings: 2 Milk + 2 Fruit + 1 Bread/Starch

---

TABLE 3
Typical Menu Plans

Breakfast

Breakfast grains I like: _____

_____

_____

_____

Breakfast fruits (juices) I like: _____

_____

_____

_____

Dairy products I like: _____

_____

_____

_____

Put these breakfast foods together to create 3 breakfasts combinations.

_____   _____   _____

_____   _____   _____

_____   _____   _____

Lunch and Snacks

If lunch is frequently eaten away from home, consider packing a lunch. This way, one remains in total control of this meal. Food choices must be portable in this case, however. Include snacks as well, so that good intentions at lunch are not undone by trips to the vending machine at mid-morning or afternoon (see snack list). Lunch and snacks combined should consist of at least two whole grains, one meat or meat alternate, and two fruits and/or vegetables.

Dinner

We tend to have the most time to prepare dinner, so this meal is typically larger and more varied than the others. For these reasons, planning dinners is not as simple as planning lunches. Try to get women in the habit of having enough dinner supplies to last one week. This does not mean they have to plan every dinner of the week, but instead have the necessary supplies to pick and choose meals each evening, depending on mood and time. This method also helps avoid unnecessary trips to the grocery store where impulsive purchases can occur. Dinner should consist of at least one whole grain, one meat or meat alternate, one fruit and/or vegetable, and one low/nonfat dairy.

ALTERING RECIPES

Some of the solutions to nutrition goals may need some creative alterations of recipes. For example, you know a good solution to consuming more vegetables and calcium would be to eat more dark green leafy vegetables. Yet the thought of eating a cup of collard greens every day does not sound too appealing. Table 4 outlines some common dilemmas such as this and some creative recipe alteration solutions which can be offered.

TABLE 4
Altering Recipes to Meet Goals

Nutrition Goal	Recipe Alteration
Increase calcium intake	Add ¼ cup nonfat dry milk to casseroles with cream-based sauce
	Use evaporated skim milk in recipes in place of regular skim milk
	Puree dark green leafy vegetable and add to spaghetti or tomato-based sauce
	Have a high calcium drink 3 mornings a week
Increase fiber intake	Add bran to casseroles, chilis, thick soups, ground meat mixtures, and coating mixtures for chicken or fish of white flour in baking
	Substitute refined bread products with whole grain foods (brown instead of white rice, whole wheat instead of white bread)
	Incorporate legumes into soups and casseroles
Decrease fat intake	Use low/nonfat plain yogurt instead of sour cream in recipes
	Use lowfat or part-skim cheeses in recipes
	Use lean cuts of meat such as flank, rump, or London broil
	Substitute roasting, baking, broiling, stir-frying, or grilling for frying
	Skim fat off meat juice before adding to gravies or stews
	Substitute applesauce in place of fat in baked goods

CREATING A GROCERY LIST

Organizing shopping trips can greatly increase the efficiency and nutritional value of the selections. Some general tips to offer are

1. Limit food shopping to no more than once a week. Shopping more often than this leads to extraneous purchases (and temptations!), not to mention the extra time, money, and energy involved.
2. Plan the food supply. Think about how many times a week meals are usually eaten at home and write down what is likely to be wanted for that week. Consider both meals and snack foods.
3. Read the grocery store circulars that are in the newspaper for specials on items frequently eaten. Buy at least a two weeks' supply of these items. If the item is perishable, freeze what will not be using immediately.
4. Clip coupons from the Sunday paper. Use for only those items that are eaten frequently. They may not seem like much of a savings, but over a year can save a considerable amount of money.

5. Plan food shopping lists. Make a list of items needed based on the planned menus and snacks, newspaper specials and coupons. Stick to the list.
6. Eat before going. Food shopping on an empty stomach can lead to extraneous purchases.
7. Use unit pricing which tells the cost per unit of volume (e.g., .25/oz). Often a product on sale or with a coupon is still not as good a bargain as others.
8. Use open dating information to assure quality and freshness. This is particularly helpful in purchasing perishable items such as meat, poultry, fish, dairy products, and fresh bakery goods.
9. Buy large sizes for items that can be stored a long time (rice, cereal, canned foods). They cost less per unit volume.
10. Buy only what can be consumed before the next shopping trip for items that are perishable and cannot be frozen (e.g., eggs, cheese). Otherwise, it's food (and money) wasted.
11. Compare the prices of the store brand to other brand names. Most often, the store brand costs significantly less.

The next step in food planning is to put meal choices and recipe ideas into a grocery list. For each of the food choices, figure how much will be need for at least a one week supply. Be sure to add extra if there are others for whom you shop. Make an initial list by randomly listing what is needed, then write a second list organizing foods by where they are in the grocery store. This extra step could actually save time going back and forth between aisles. A shopping list could look something like this:

Breads
    1 loaf whole wheat bread
    1 package whole wheat bagels
    1 package whole wheat pita bread
    1 prepared pizza crust

Cereals
    wheat germ
    1 box shredded wheat
    1 box raisin bran

Canned goods
    2 cans water packed tuna
    6-pack V-8 juice
    2 cans cream soup

Dry goods
    1 package low-sodium pretzels
    1 box granola bars

1 package rice cakes
1 box brown rice
3 boxes pasta
1 package lentils
nonfat dry milk
low fat salad dressing
peanut butter
jelly or jam
dried fruit (raisins, prunes, apricots)

Dairy
1 qt. nonfat milk
5 8 oz. containers nonfat fruited yogurt
part-skim mozarella cheese
1 package Neufchatel cheese
parmesan cheese
tub margarine
eggs

Produce
carrots, green peppers, celery for snacks
1 bunch bananas
3 apples, oranges, or peaches
salad fixings: Romaine lettuce, 3 tomatoes, cucumber, etc.
broccoli
zucchini

Meats
2 packages boneless, skinless chicken breasts
1 lb. extra lean ground beef
½ lb. deli turkey breast

Frozen
frozen yogurt
3 cans frozen orange juice concentrate
healthy frozen entrees

DECIPHERING FOOD LABELS

Whether a woman plans menus in advance or fixes meals at the last minute, what is bought at the supermarket probably determines most of the ultimate food intake. Shopping in today's supermarkets is a real challenge. Consumers are faced with thousands of new products every year that often lure us with their health claims, such as "cholesterol free," "high fiber," "low fat," and "reduced sodium." It is often difficult to know what these labels actually mean, and labeling information can sometimes be misleading. Fortunately, much of the confusion has been swept away with the passing of the 1990 Nutritional Labeling and Education Act.[3] Below are listed the constituents of today's food labels and what they mean.

INGREDIENTS

Each ingredient on a food product is listed in descending order by weight: heaviest (first), down to the lightest (last). Ingredients that make up two percent or less of a food are listed at the end of the ingredient listing in no particular order. However, for the small proportion of Americans with sensitivities to particular substances in foods, ingredient lists have become more specific. All certified food colors, sweeteners, and flavorings, for instance, are listed by name.

In the past, some foods did not have an ingredient list because they have mandatory ingredients (e.g., ice cream, cheddar cheese, ketchup, and mayonnaise). These foods are now required to fully list the ingredients of the food in the package. Another bygone is having to depend on the ingredient list for the nutritional content, since providing nutrition information was considered voluntary.

Today, food labels must include nutrition information, thereby downplaying the role of the ingredient list in deciphering the nutritional content of a food. Even so, it is still important to recognize certain ingredients in light of which food group they are from, especially in the world of synthesized ingredients. For instance, we all know common sources of fat such as butter and oil, but there are other sources of fat added to processed foods by manufacturers that cannot easily be recognized from reading the list of ingredients. Table 5 lists other words for ingredients that are solely or mainly fat. Those with a "*" contain saturated fat, which may be of animal or vegetable origin.

In addition to hidden fats, labels can also tell about hidden sugars. Hidden sugars are usually fat free, but can be a main source of empty calories or foods that provide calories but no nutrients such as vitamins, minerals, or fiber. The words listed in Table 6 are other names for sugars that are used on ingredient labels.

TABLE 5
Ingredient Names for
Sources of Fat

Cocoa butter*
Coconut or coconut oil*
Cream and cream sauce*
Egg and egg yolk solids*
Glycerin
Glycerol esters
Hydrogenated vegetable oil*
Lard*
Mono- or di-glycerides
Palm or palm kernel oil*
Shortening*
Suet*

* Contain saturated fat.

TABLE 6
Ingredient Names
for Sources of
Sugar

Corn syrup
Corn syrup solids
Dextrose
Fructose
Glucose
Honey
Lactose
Maltose
Mannitol
Maple syrup
Molasses
Sorbitol
Sucrose

NUTRITION INFORMATION PANEL

Before the change took effect, nutrition labeling was only required if a food was fortified, or a nutrition claim was made (e.g., no cholesterol). Otherwise, label information was still considered voluntary. Today, however, shoppers will find nutrition information about virtually all the foods they want to buy. The plus side is that the list of nutrients now includes those most important to the health of today's consumers, many of whom need to worry about getting too much of certain items (fat, for example). The down side is that much of the vitamin/mineral information from the old labels has been discontinued.

Below you will find a sample of what a food label looks like now. What follows is a guide to the specific changes from the old labels.

SAMPLE FOOD LABEL
Nutrition Facts
Serving Size ¹/₂ cup (114 g)   Servings Per Container 4

Amount Per Serving

Calories 260   Calories from Fat 120

	% **Daily Value**[a]
Total Fat 13g	20%
Saturated Fat 5 g	25%
Cholesterol 30 mg	10%
Sodium 660 mg	28%
Total Carbohydrate 31 g	11%
Dietary Fiber 0 g	0%
Sugars 5 g	
Protein 5 g	

SAMPLE FOOD LABEL (continued)

	% Daily Value[a]
Vitamin A	4%
Vitamin C	2%
Calcium	15%
Iron	4%

[a] Percent Daily Values are based on a 2,000 calorie diet. Daily values may be higher or lower depending on individual calories needs:

	2,000	2,500
Calories	2,000	2,500
Total Fat	Less than 65 g	80 g
Sat. Fat	Less than 20 g	25 g
Cholesterol	Less than 300 mg	300 mg
Sodium	Less than 2,400 mg	2,400 mg
Total Carbohydrate	300 g	375 g
Fiber	25 g	30 g

Calories per gram:
  Fat 9
  Carbohydrates 4
  Protein 4

STANDARDIZED SERVING SIZES AND NUTRIENT CONTENT

Formerly, if a product was high in fat, for example, a company could make a serving size smaller to reduce its fat content. In addition, consumers could take a hefty serving of a food, assuming that their serving size was the same as the one described on the nutrition label, but in reality, using two or three times the amount of food described in the label information. With the new labels, serving sizes are standardized based on food consumption surveys to reflect the amount people actually eat. This way, one can easily compare two products without having to go through the mental gymnastics of comparing products with different serving sizes. Even so, this information should still be compared to actual serving size.

Calories From Fat

It is no longer necessary to multiply the grams of fat by 9 to figure the calories from fat. To get the percent calories from fat though, the calories from fat need to be divided by the total calories.

Saturated Fat

Labels have to list not only the grams of total fat, but the grams of saturated fat as well. This is in response to the fact that saturated fat bears the most dietary responsibility for increasing blood cholesterol, contributing to atherosclerosis, and predisposing to cardiovascular and cerebrovascular disease.

Dietary Fiber

Fiber is important to health, especially at older ages. The current labels, which are required to list fiber content, will help assess whether individuals are meeting fiber goals, and allow them to choose more fiber-rich options with ease.

% Daily Values

This addition reveals the percentage of fat, saturated fat, carbohydrate, protein, and dietary fiber for a 2,000 calorie diet that is in the food. For example, if a product has a % Daily Value of 25% for total fat, this means that the product contains 25% of the fat that a person needs in the whole day, if she consumes 2,000 calories a day. Assuming this person wishes to stay within the guidelines of consuming no more than 30% of her calories from fat, she would be consuming 25% of the 30%. In other words, if she ate this product four times in one day and had no other sources of fat, she would meet her fat needs for the day. This may sound a bit confusing at first, especially if one is eating less than 2,000 calories. In this case, you could just use a the Daily Values as a guide; too many servings of foods that contribute 25% of the Daily Value for fat, for example, would exceed the fat limit.

The current label also gives the % Daily Value for other nutrients that are the same for everybody regardless of calorie intake. These include cholesterol, sodium, vitamins A and C, calcium, and iron. For example, if a product states it contains 15% calcium, this means it contains 15% of the USRDA for calcium of 800 mg., or 120 mg.

The reasoning behind % Daily Values is to provide a good idea of how different foods fit into the overall diet. These numbers can also be used to comparison shop. For instance, if a serving of Brand X's macaroni and cheese has a % Daily Value of 27 for total fat, compared to Brand Y's 45, it's obvious that Brand X is far lower in fat, regardless of the number of calories typically consumed.

Calories Per Gram

To give one less number to be memorized, the number of calories per gram of fat, carbohydrate, and protein can be found at the bottom of the Nutrition Information Panel.

Label Terms

Terms such as "cholesterol free," "light," and "low sodium" now have specific definitions. Review Table 7 for these terms and their definitions.

Label Traps

Even with the current food labels, food manufacturers may still be able to trap someone into believing that their product is the healthiest. Be aware of the possible traps listed below:

Trap 1: With the current labels, % fat free can only be used on foods that are low fat or fat free initially. Therefore, this claim is no longer seen on foods such as meats and some dairy foods. Even so, this claim can easily be interpreted to mean % fat free calories, not weight. Be sure to read the Nutrition Information Panel for a more accurate look at the fat content.

Trap 2: With the current label, a food labeled "low cholesterol" must also be low in saturated fat; however, it still can be high in total fat, if there are sources of fat from oil, for example. This is where reading the Nutrition Information Panel for "Calories from Fat" is important.

Trap 3: Watch for products claiming they are "cholesterol free." Cholesterol free does not mean fat free. Since cholesterol is only in products of animal origin, any vegetable fat does not contain cholesterol. With the current labels, a product claiming to be cholesterol free must also be free of saturated fat. So even though olive oil, safflower oil, and Wesson oil claim to be cholesterol free (and saturated fat free), they are still 100% fat.

Trap 4: When products are labeled light, be careful. A nondairy creamer labeled light may be relatively lower in fat and calories than the original product, but it may still be high in fat and calories. Again, look over the Nutrition Information Panel for better information.

TABLE 7
Label Definitions

Label Term	Required Definition
Free	Contains none or only negligible amounts of fat, saturated fat, cholesterol, sodium, sugar and/or calories
Low fat	< 3 grams per serving
Low saturated fat	< 1 gram per serving
Low sodium	< 140 mg per serving
Very low sodium	< 35 mg per serving
Low cholesterol	< 20 mg and no more than 2 gms saturated fat per serving
Low calorie	< 40 calories per serving; or < 120 calories per 100 grams
Lean	< 10 grams of fat, 4 grams of saturated fat, and 95 mg of cholesterol per serving
Extra lean	< 5 grams of fat, 2 grams of saturated fat, and 95 mg of cholesterol per serving
High	Contains 20% or more of the Daily Value for a particular nutrient
Good Source	Supplies 10 to 19% of the Daily Value for a particular nutrient
Reduced	Contains 25% less of a nutrient than the regular product
Less/Fewer	Contains 25% less of a nutrient than a comparable food (e.g., pretzels as 25% less fat than potato chips)
More	One serving contains at least 10% more of the Daily Value for a nutrient than the regular food
Light	Calories have been reduced by at least a third, or the fat or sodium content by at least half of what they were in the regular product
% fat free	Only on foods which are low fat or fat free to begin with (this is % fat free by weight and is not the same as by calories)
Implied claims	Prohibited if it misleads the consumer into believing a food contains or does not contain significant amounts of certain nutrients (e.g., "no tropical oils" or "made with oat bran")

Calculating % Fat

As mentioned above, food labels now state the number of calories from fat. Unfortunately, they do not have to state the percent of calories from fat. To do this, divide the calories from fat by the total calories. For example, if a label says that the product contains 45 calories from fat and has 90 calories total, the product has 50% of its calories from fat (45 ÷ 90 = .50). Not all calculations will obviously be this easy. So by just comparing how close the calories from fat are to the total calories, the consumer will at least be able to get a ballpark idea whether the product is low or high in fat.

Don't be confused into thinking that because total calories should contain no more than 30% of calories from fat, individual foods must also contain no more than 30% fat. Eating healthfully is more of a balancing act; having some olive oil (100% fat) with vegetables and rice (less than 5% fat), for example, will balance out to far less than 30% fat.

TIPS FOR CHOOSING FOOD PRODUCTS

The following contains information that will help in choosing food products in the grocery store.

THE DAIRY CASE

- Milk. Nonfat milk has 0 grams of fat/cup; lowfat has 5 grams/cup; whole milk has 9 to 10 grams/cup. Note that the front label tells you 1% fat, 2% fat, etc., and that this refers to the weight, not the calories from fat. Nonfat dairy products provide the most calcium for their calories.
- Cheeses. It takes about a gallon of milk to make one pound of cheese. Most cheeses are made with whole milk. Since there are almost two pats of butter in every cup of whole milk, there are about 32 pats in a gallon—as well as in one pound of cheese. That's why many cheeses, such as cheddar, Monterey Jack, and Swiss, are high in fat. There are many lowfat cheeses available which give nutrition information. With the current label rules, remember, any product labeled "lowfat" must be 3 grams of fat or less per serving. "Reduced" fat, on the other hand, means that a product contains at least 25% less fat than the original product. Most cheeses that are low in fat have about 5 grams of fat per ounce, which is considered a standard serving size for cheese. Thus, labels that once read lowfat may now read reduced fat.
- Yogurt. There are many nonfat varieties. Natural yogurt may not be better if the goal is to minimize fat intake; many natural yogurts are made with whole milk. Look for nonfat milk at the top of the ingredient list. Adding fruit to plain yogurt is likely to provide fewer calories and less sugar than commercial types made with sweetened fruit or preserves.
- Nondairy Creamers. Mocha mix has 320 calories/cup (vs. 90 for nonfat milk) and 9 teaspoons of sugar/cup. It has no calcium, low protein, and

contains partially hydrogenated oil. It is good for people with lactose intolerance, but not good for people who want to lose weight.
- Sour Cream. Generally a high fat product. "Light" sour creams have half the fat as regular. To lower fat and calories even further, look for the new "fat-free" sour creams, or try substituting plain nonfat yogurt.
- Margarine. Make sure that the first ingredient listed on the label is liquid oil, and that the P:S ratio (the ratio of polyunsaturated fats to saturated fats) is greater than or equal to 2:1. Like butters and oils, all margarines are 100% fat, even the "light" versions. The difference is the addition of water or air to the lower calorie ones, so there is less margarine, or fat per tablespoon.

THE MEAT COUNTER

The United States Department of Agriculture (USDA) regulates nutrition labeling for meat, poultry, and eggs. Because of the way that meats and poultry are sold, it is often impractical to have nutrition labels on each food package. The nutrition information may therefore be presented in the store in posters, brochures, or other displays.

- Poultry. Boneless, skinless chicken or turkey are the best bets. The lowest-fat poultry is light meat turkey without the skin, which gets only about 8% of its calories from fat. Light meat chicken without the skin is also a relatively good choice, but still gets more than 20% of its calories from fat. Dark meat is higher in fat. To really cut the fat, remove the skin—it can more than double the fat calories. Some companies now offer a "Fitness" line of chicken and turkey thighs and breasts, which have lowfat recipes included in each package.
- Seafood. Fish and seafood are naturally lower in fat than almost all meat and poultry—unless fat is added in preparation and cooking. While 48% of the fat in beef and 36% of the fat in pork is saturated, the percentage for fish and shellfish ranges from 11 to 27, depending on the species. Be sure to avoid seafood which has been breaded and/or fried, since it tends to be high in fat and sodium. With canned seafood, look for salmon with the bones to boost calcium intake. And when selecting canned tuna, remember that tuna packed in water has less fat than tuna packed in oil.
- Meats. The rule of thumb when looking for a lean cut is to look for the words "loin," "round," "tip," or "flank." When looking at grades of meats, "prime" and "choice" are the highest in fat. Generally, the lower the grade ("select" being the lowest), the less fat it contains. To keep the meat moist, cook it in liquid. Another way to cut fat from meats is to remove all visible fat before cooking. Cut away the white fat surrounding steaks, roasts, and other cuts as close as possible to the lean part. To stretch the meat servings, stir fry small amounts of meat with lots of vegetables, or add it to a pasta dish. When using broth or stock, chill it, then skim the fat off the top (each tablespoon of fat that you skim off saves 100 calories). For ground

beef, buy only the leanest types, labeled as containing no more than 15% fat. When cooked, there is very little difference in the fat content of 20% fat and 30% fat ground beef. To further lower the fat content, see the section on "How To Lower the Fat Content of Ground Meat."

- Luncheon Meats. Ham, corned beef, turkey breast, and chicken breast are better choices than regular cold cuts, but they are still high in sodium. A luncheon meat is considered lean if it has less or than equal to 4 grams of fat per 2 ounce serving (2 slices). Some luncheon meats list a serving as one ounce, so be sure to double the grams of fat from the label information to see if it is really lean. Watch for lean-sounding luncheon meats like turkey salami and chicken bologna, which can have up to 18 grams of fat per 2 ounce serving.

THE PRODUCE SECTION

Nutrition labeling of fresh fruits and vegetables is voluntary, since these foods are often sold unpackaged. As with meats, the nutrition information may be available as posters, brochures, or other displays. It is very hard to go wrong in the produce section, but variety is important. Buy fruits and vegetables that are high in vitamins A and C. Vitamin A-rich fruits are dark yellow or orange in color, such as papaya, apricots, cantaloupe, and mango. Vitamin A is widely distributed in dark green leafy or yellow-orange-red vegetables. Vitamin C-rich fruits and vegetables include citrus, tomatoes, peppers, and cruciferous vegetables. Avocados are 80% fat, though it is mostly mono-unsaturated fat, a type of fat that has the least effect on serum cholesterol levels. Dried fruits are good snack foods; they are high in iron and good for people who want to eat less meat. Dried fruits, however, are higher in calories per unit weight than fresh fruit.

GRAINS

- Bread. The breads with the most fiber say whole wheat on the label vs. just wheat flour. Wheat flour is refined flour and is the same as white flour. True, the breads may not be white, but often caramel coloring is added to make it brown. "Light" bread usually has half the calories per slice mainly because the slices are half as thin as regular bread. If this helps a person to stay within the allotted starch servings for the day, then this type of bread is worth it; otherwise, the shopper is better off just buying regular whole wheat bread.
- Cereal. Watch for hidden fat, high sodium, and high sugar. The serving sizes listed on the package vary between brands. Hot cereals are good choices, especially those without added flavoring. On many boxed or ready-to-eat cereals, carbohydrate information is listed. How much sugar is in each serving can be calculated by knowing that 4 grams of "sugars" equal one teaspoon. Choose cereals where sugar is not one of the first

ingredients. Comparing labels can help choose a cereal that's low in sugar and high in fiber.

- The Supermarket Bakery. Sweet baked goods (cakes, pastries, muffins) provide more fat and sugars than plain breads, rolls, and bagels. Croissants and biscuits are higher in calories and fat than most other breads and rolls.

THE FROZEN FOOD SECTION

- Beverages. Look for the word "juice" to ensure receipt of 100% nutrition. If the words "ade," "cocktail," "drink," "punch," or "beverage" are used, it contains empty calories. The same applies to bottled fruit juices. Try calcium-fortified orange juice to boost your calcium intake, especially if lactose intolerance is a problem.
- Frozen Desserts. Gourmet ice creams have as much as 10 teaspoons of fat per cup. In contrast, most fat-reduced frozen desserts have only ½ to 3 ½ teaspoons of fat per cup. This is mostly due to the use of skim milk in place of heavy cream, as well as a higher proportion of air. The differences between most store-bought frozen yogurts and ice milk are the name and the price. Otherwise, these products are virtually identical. The nonfat frozen yogurts found at specialty stores can have even less fat and calories. Sorbets are also a good bet, with virtually no fat. Even though some are lower in fat than most ice cream, they can have about the same number of calories due to a high sugar content.
- Frozen Dinners. Read the labels carefully. The light frozen dinners are about 300 calories. So just remember that if there are 10 grams of fat in those 300 calories, that means that 30% of the calories come from fat. In other words, look for those that have 10 grams or less fat. Many low-calorie frozen dinners are higher in fat, but are able to keep the calories down by keeping the serving size small. So it is often better to choose the dinner with 20 more calories if the fat content is significantly lower. This way the healthiest calories are being chosen, not just the fewest.
- Frozen Fruits and Vegetables. These are great to have during the winter months when the fresh selection is not at its prime. Usually, produce is frozen directly from the field, so nutrient retention is very good. When choosing frozen produce, choose those without anything added. With the addition of cream sauces, heavy syrups, and flavorings, extra calories are being added that can be done without.

SNACK FOODS

Any package smaller than 12 square inches (such as a small candy bar) does not have to provide nutrition information on the label. It does, however, have to provide an address or telephone number for consumers who wish to obtain it.

Most cookies, brownies, and other sweets contain a lot of fat, as well as sugar. Watch out for hidden sources of fat, especially animal shortening (lard). The average cookie gets about 40% of its calories from fat, and another 30% from sugar. Lowfat commercial cookies have less than or equal to 30% fat. Lowfat cookies include vanilla wafers, fruit bars, ginger snaps, graham crackers, and animal crackers.

Crackers vary quite a bit in fat content. Generally, crackers that feel greasy to the touch are higher in fat than other types. Look at the source and amount of fat. No fat crackers include Wasa Crispbread, Matzos, Ry-Krisp, Melba Toast, and rice cakes. Also try unsalted pretzels.

PRE-PREPARED ITEMS

- Salad Dressings and Mayonnaise. Choose those that have no more than 2 grams of fat per two tablespoon (one ounce) serving. Most dressings list a serving size of one (level) tablespoon—about half what most people use. So when shopping, be sure to double the fat.
- Canned and Packaged Foods. These aisles contain old standbys like canned vegetables and fruit juices, as well as newer items like dry soups, packaged dinners, and sauces. If looking for convenience, easy storage, and a long shelf life, canned and packaged foods can be a good choice. The rule of thumb here is to choose products with the least added to them. Typically, the more "doctored" the product, the more empty calories it contains, not to mention the additional cost. For example, choose canned whole potatoes (or fresh!) rather than a box of scalloped potatoes with cream sauce.

ANALYZING SHOPPING BEHAVIOR

Most people have a routine when shopping for food. Check the blanks in Table 8 that best describe what you do before, during, and after each trip to the supermarket. Small changes in shopping habits may make it easier to prepare healthy meals at home.

HOW TO LOWER THE FAT CONTENT OF GROUND MEAT

Ground meats are quite versatile in cooking, and are used throughout the world. In addition, they are excellent sources of iron and zinc, two minerals which are often deficient in the diet. Unfortunately, most ground meats (beef, pork, lamb) contain a high amount of saturated fat and cholesterol, the two types of fat that are the leading dietary culprits indicated in heart disease. The traditional method of reducing fat from cooked meats is to drain the fat. Unfortunately, only a small percentage of saturated fat can be removed this way (6 to 17%) and even less of the cholesterol (1 to 4%). Less cholesterol is extracted because it is bound in the muscle of the meat, not the fat. Fortunately, researchers at Boston University have developed a method for extracting larger amounts of saturated fat and cholesterol from ground meat without sacrificing much flavor.[6] With this method, approximately 68% of the

TABLE 8
Shopping Behavior

Behavior	Hardly Ever	Sometimes	Most of the Time
Before shopping, I...			
Check to see what foods I have on hand	_____	_____	_____
Plan meals to include a variety of foods from each of the major food groups	_____	_____	_____
Plan food purchases to keep amounts of fat and sugars moderate	_____	_____	_____
Consider how much money I have to spend on food	_____	_____	_____
Make a shopping list	_____	_____	_____
While shopping, I...			
Read ingredient labels, watching for ingredients that provide fat and sugars	_____	_____	_____
Use nutrition labels to help select food products	_____	_____	_____
Use unit pricing to compare prices	_____	_____	_____
After shopping, I...			
Store foods promptly and properly to maintain their nutritive value and quality	_____	_____	_____
Place newer foods in the back of refrigerator, freezer, and cabinet shelves, so older foods will be used first	_____	_____	_____
Use perishable foods promptly to avoid food waste	_____	_____	_____

Note: If "most of the time" is your answer to the majority of these questions, you are a healthy shopper! Read the section below for more tips on how to shop healthfully.

---

fat and 39% of the cholesterol can be removed from lean ground beef. The de-fatted meat is granular and is, therefore, not intended to be used plain. Instead, use it for dishes such as spaghetti sauce, chili con carne, and taco filling. To make meatloaf, or some other kind of ground beef dish that requires binding, reduce the broth and stir it back in with egg whites and bake it. It may look like quite a process to de-fat your meat, but it actually takes less time than you think. You can also de-fat large amounts of ground meat, then freeze it in portion sizes you will most likely use.

The method is as follows:

1. Put 1½ cups of vegetable oil (olive oil or vegetable oil) in a pan and turn on the burner.
2. Add 2 lbs of ground beef, pork, lamb. Break up well with potato masher. Set the pan over moderate heat and cook for about five minutes until water in meat starts to boil. The oil should not be boiling.

3. Continue to cook for 5 or 10 minutes, or until the meat is cooked through. Transfer meat to strainer and let drain for 2 minutes into a bowl. Wash well with 1½ cups of boiling water, draining liquid into the same bowl.
4. Separate oil from the broth by skimming, or refrigerate until fat solidifies and remove it as a cake.
5. Reduce broth by cooking and add it to the meat, or, if making a sauce that will be cooked, add broth without reducing.

FOOD PREPARATION

Purchasing and Storing

Some tips for organizing the food supply to make nutritious and varied meals easier to prepare are listed below.

- Buy staples that can be stored for extended periods of time (pasta, cereal, rice) in bulk.
- Perishable items such as milk, fish, and many fresh fruits and vegetables should be purchased in smaller quantities. Even though it costs more per unit weight to buy small containers of foods (i.e., single serving soups, 4 oz. sour cream), not eating more is worth it.
- Avoid purchasing specialized ingredients not ordinarily used. For instance, it makes little sense to purchase a whole can of water chestnuts if only two will be used. Experiment with recipes to learn which ingredients can be changed without drastically altering the basic flavor of the recipe.
- Large quantities of meat and milk can be stored in the freezer for future use. Be sure to divide it into usable portions.
- When handling raw meat, wash hands thoroughly before and after. Also clean counter space or cutting boards with a bleach and water solution.

Portion Sizes

- Many recipes that normally make four or more servings can be altered to yield a smaller number of portions, but keep in mind that cooking times and pan sizes may change, too.
- If making smaller portions is unrealistic (such as when making a lasagna), portion foods into usable servings and freeze for later use.

Food Preparation Tips

When preparing food

- Use the three Bs: bake, broil, and boil (steam);
- Cut vegetables as close to cooking time as possible;

- Save cooking water from steamed vegetables as a nutritious broth to add to other dishes; and
- Store orange juice and other citrus juices in closed containers to help retain vitamin C.

When storing food

- Put food away immediately. To prevent bacterial growth, do not allow hot food such as cooked meats or cold foods such as potato salad to remain at room temperature for too long;
- Freeze portioned foods for another meal.

FOOD PLANNING/PREPARATION WORKSHEET

After reading the tips above for food planning and preparation, complete the worksheet below to rate your habits. Check off those habits you have or need improving.

Food Planning/Preparation
Habits That Need Improving

No breakfast	_____
Incomplete breakfast	_____
No lunch	_____
Incomplete lunch	_____
Junk food snacks	_____
No dinner	_____
Incomplete dinner	_____
Buy food too frequently	_____
Do not make grocery list	_____
Buy staples in small amounts	_____
Buy too large so part wasted	_____
Do not plan for leftovers	_____
Do not use "3 Bs" often	_____
Other	_____

LONG-TERM NUTRITIONAL HEALTH

Now that have the know-how for improving your nutritional health is available, the next and final task is to keep it that way, forever. Sure, you know why it is important to keep nutritional health at an optimum, but there can be several additional factors that can make even the most carefully devised eating plan fall apart. Frequent dining out, for example, can mean a limited selection of healthy foods on a regular basis. The habit of responding to stress with a bag of tortilla chips can also sabotage efforts. What follows are some techniques to help maintain long-term nutritional health.

RESTRUCTURING THE ENVIRONMENT

The environment is made up of many things; the actual: surroundings such as a person's home, people with whom she socializes, and her thoughts and feelings. Ideally, the environment influences the person in a positive way, strengthening a healthful lifestyle. If she falls into this category, it will be easier to maintain new habits. If not, realize that some basic changes to the environment can be advantageous.

A particular situation that faces many older women is living alone, since most women will outlive their spouse. Additionally, many women have outside commitments such as working full-time, volunteer activities, or caring for grandchildren. Together, these lifestyle factors may challenge one's ability to eat healthfully. This does not mean healthy eating is impossible, just that it will require a little more foresight to become practical. For instance, if someone tends to eat whatever is quickest and easiest because she eats alone, invite a friend over for dinner once in awhile to make the food choices fun to prepare. Another solution would to be to get involved or create a dinner club, where people can get together regularly with others in a potluck fashion. In other words, if a women finds herself in an eating rut because of a living or working situation, try thinking of solutions to enhance healthy eating.

In the paragraphs below, we look at the environmental influences a little closer to see how they influence a particular way of eating. There will then be an opportunity to analyze the environment and restructure it in a way to enhance nutritional health.

PHYSICAL ENVIRONMENT

Where people live, work, and play make up their physical environment. How they appear influences different people in different ways. For example, a kitchen like Old Mother Hubbard's with bare cupboards may make one person not even think about food—out of sight, out of mind. In another person, bare cupboards may trigger an opposite response—a feeling of desperation. Therefore, learn responses to the physical environment, and try to change features which trigger negative behaviors or choices.

SOCIAL ENVIRONMENT

There are probably some people who conjure up images of food and good times, while others may do the opposite. There may also be social situations that support poor eating habits, such as eating dinner alone, and those which support good eating habits, such as dinner with a good friend.

COGNITIVE ENVIRONMENT

Our emotions, thoughts, and feelings can have a powerful effect on our nutritional health. Negative thoughts, for example, can undermine attempts at self-improvement. On the other hand, positive thinking can do wonders for making the world seem like a better place, and stimulate efforts to improve one's health.

After increasing awareness of what aspects in the environment influence nutritional health, the aspects that contribute to good eating habits can be strengthened, and those that contribute to poor eating habits reduced. The answers may be as simple as removing the poor food choices from the kitchen, yet as complex as changing attitudes about life in general. The bottom line is to come up with solutions to restructure the environment in ways to enhance nutritional health. For the more complicated solutions, incremental steps may need to be designed to accomplish the task. Shaping behavior with such small steps is as important in nutrition as it is in exercise or any other new habit to be adopt.

RECORD KEEPING

As with most aspects of health maintenance, a regular check-up can help us stay healthy and handle any problems while they are still small. Record keeping is an easy way to give yourself a nutritional health check-up. It only needs to be done occasionally (once a month at most) and requires writing down everything eaten for a day or two. Most people who do this are amazed how this task improves their ability to observe and analyze their environment as well as recognize their cues to eating. Record keeping also may have the instantaneous effect of foregoing unhealthy foods that may have slipped into the regular eating plan (Who wants to write them down?). A sample food diary is shown in Table 9.

Another option for record keeping is self-contracting. This is a good option for those who may have specific nutrition goals to achieve by a certain time. For example, more fiber may need to be incorporated into the diet, but increasing the amount overnight leaves a bloated feeling. Opt for a plan of gradually increasing the fiber content over a month. Have a witness or friend sign a self-contract as well if this will help with compliance in meeting the goal. A sample contract is shown below.

SELF-CONTRACT

I _____ ,

now _____ .
(write down the undesirable behavior/food habit you want to change)

By _____ , I will _____ .
     (short-range goal date)   (short-range goal step)

By _____ , I will _____ .
     (half-way goal date)   (half-way goal step)

By _____ , I will _____ .
     (long-range goal date)   (long-range goal step)

_____   _____
      (sign your name here)   (witness sign here)

_____   _____
         (date)   (date)

TABLE 9
Food Diary

DATE _____

Breakfast

Item	Food Group	Servings
_____	_____	_____
_____	_____	_____
_____	_____	_____
_____	_____	_____

Lunch

Item	Food Group	Servings
_____	_____	_____
_____	_____	_____
_____	_____	_____
_____	_____	_____

Dinner

Item	Food Group	Servings
_____	_____	_____
_____	_____	_____
_____	_____	_____
_____	_____	_____

Snacks

Item	Food Group	Servings
_____	_____	_____
_____	_____	_____
_____	_____	_____
_____	_____	_____

Actual Servings

	Desirable	More/Fewer Needed
Bread/Grain	_____	_____
Fruit/Veg	_____	_____
Dairy	_____	_____
Meat	_____	_____
Fat	_____	_____
Other	_____	_____

MAINTAINING A COMMITMENT TO LONG-TERM NUTRITIONAL HEALTH

Now that the necessary tools for long-term nutritional health are available, the last task is to keep using these tools to maintain commitment. Some ways to do this are

1. Focus on successful experiences. Don't dwell on mistakes or feel guilty about eating foods you want to eliminate. It is the larger picture that counts, not the occasional blunders.
2. Tell family members and friends about your nutrition goals. Since these are the people you are around the most, their knowledge of your goals will serve to strengthen your commitment.
3. Anticipate the kinds of problems that are likely to occur in trying to achieve your goals. If you see yourself forgetting to drink fluids regularly, for example, try keeping a glass of water nearby—just the sight of it will remind you to drink.
4. Focus on foods that can be eaten rather than should not be: seeing the world as a limited place may deflate your commitment. Take the opposite stance and look at all the new things you now can enjoy (e.g., new vegetables, new recipes).

Changing a diet cannot be achieved overnight, but taking small steps while keeping nutrition goals in sight will soon lead to a nutritionally healthier lifestyle.

Resources for Consumers

1. The American Dietetic Association
   216 W. Jackson Blvd., Chicago, IL 60606-6995
   312-899-0040 ext. 5000
   > Large-print food tip instruction sheets:
   >> When You Need to Eat More
   >> To Cut Down on Fat
   >> When You Have High Blood Pressure
   > Staying Healthy - A Guide for Elder Americans
   > ADA Hotline: (800) 366-1655
   > Can provide names of dietitians in local area specializing in geriatric nutrition.

2. American Association of Retired Persons
   AARP Fulfillment, 601 E St. N.W., Washington, D.C. 20049
   > Nutrition booklets
   >> #D12994: How Does Your Nutrition Measure Up
   >> #D12164: Eating for Your Health

3. The National Dairy Council
   (708) 803-2000: ask for the number of your local dairy council
   > Spice of Life (video)
   > For Mature Eaters Only: Guidelines for Good Nutrition (brochure)
   > Getting Along with Milk: For People with Lactose Intolerance

4. The National Council on Aging
   NCOA Publications, Dept. 5087, Washington, D.C. 20061-5087
   > Eating Well to Stay Well

5. Books on geriatric nutrition
   > *Food for Fitness after 50: A Menu for Good Health in Later Years*
   > Frederick J. Stare and Virginia Aronson
   > George F. Stickley Co., Philadelphia, PA, 1985
   >
   > *The Nutrition Game: The Right Moves if You're Over 50*
   > Edna Langholz et al.
   > Bristol Publishing Enterprises, Inc., San Leandro, CA, 1990
   >
   > *Over 50 and Still Cooking: Recipes for Good Health and Long Life*
   > Edna Langholz et al.
   > Bristol Publishing Enterprises, Inc., San Leandro, CA, 1990
   >
   > *The Real Life Nutrition Book*
   > Susan Finn, Ph.D., RD and Linda Stern Kass
   > Penguin Books, New York City, NY, 1992

REFERENCES

1. Departments of Agriculture and Health and Human Services. Nutrition and Your Health: Dietary Guidelines for Americans. 1990.
2. Departments of Agriculture and Health and Human Services. The Food Guide Pyramid. Home and Gardens Bulletin No. 252. U.S., 1992.
3. The Food and Drug Administration. Code of Federal Regulations, 1990.
4. Food and Nutrition Board Committee on Dietary Allowances. Recommended Dietary Allowances, 10th ed., National Academy of Sciences, Washington, D.C., 1989.
5. Foreman, J., "Can You Find Health in a Vitamin Bottle?," The Boston Globe, December 9, 1991, 21, 24. (nutrient value sources from Jeffrey Blumberg as "optimal dose for disease prevention").
6. Small, D. M., Chemistry in the kitchen: making ground meat more healthful, *NEJM*, 324, 73–7, 1991.

25 Practical Implementation of Exercise Prescriptions

Maria A. Fiatarone Singh

CONTENTS

INTEGRATION OF THE EXERCISE PRESCRIPTION WITH OTHER ASPECTS OF HEALTH CARE

Ideally, the exercise prescription should be integrated into all other components of an older woman's health care plan, since it will impact functional capacity, health status, nutritional requirements, psychological status, and other lifestyle changes which may be addressed by other members of the health care team. Physicians should be aware of any new exercise prescription that has been implemented by others that may impact medication requirements (see Chapter 3) or potentially cause exacerbation or improvement of underlying conditions.

Coordination of exercise and nutritional prescriptions is particularly important, as there are many misconceptions in this area propagated by the lay media as well as some sports medicine practitioners. Many women will start an exercise regimen when they are advised to lose weight, and the incorporation of sound nutritional recommendations with activity suggestions is critical to the success of such attempts, as exercise alone is minimally effective at reducing body weight, as described in Chapter 17. Often, patients will have questions about what to eat when exercising or the need for special drinks, supplements, or protein sources. Guidelines for commonly encountered exercise-nutrition interactions are outlined in Table 1, and discussed further in Chapter 3. In general, food sources are preferable to packaged supplements, and education regarding the often overstated advertising claims for many of these expensive products should be given to patients who might better spend their money on good athletic shoes or home exercise equipment.

TABLE 1
Nutritional Recommendations for Exercising Older Women

Nutrient	Recommendation
Water requirements	Encourage extra water intake (500–1000 ml) on exercise days; particularly important in those • on diuretics • low sodium diets • in high temperature or humidity • after recovery from febrile or dehydrating illness
Weight loss/energy restriction	Balanced hypocaloric diet (approximately 500 kcal deficit per day), and supplement with multivitamin at RDA levels
Weight maintenance/energy balance	Increased energy intake • normal ratios of fat/carbohydrate/protein) as food rather than supplements • encourage dietary diversity to fulfill energy requirements and supply micronutrient needs
Weight gain/positive energy balance	Increased energy intake • add nutrient and calorically dense food snacks between meals and after exercise sessions • maintain normal ratios of fat/carbohydrate/protein
Protein requirements	Needs met by 1.0–1.2 g/kg/day • should be achieved with diverse dietary sources rather than unbalanced amino acid or protein supplements • resistance training decreases protein requirements • increased balanced diet with increased energy intake to maintain weight will provide all the necessary protein
Glucose control	In diabetics and glucose intolerant • time exercise sessions for the post-prandial peaks in blood glucose (1.5–2 hours after a meal) • keep high carbohydrate and concentrated sugar snacks available during exercise sessions for brittle or insulin-dependent diabetics • don't exercise after prolonged fasting or skipped meals if on oral hypoglycemics or insulin • combine with hypocaloric diet for best control in obese, insulin-resistant diabetic • exercise increases urinary excretion of chromium (needed for insulin action); increase consumption of whole grain food sources to replace losses
Minerals	Increase dietary or pharmacological sources of potassium and magnesium if serum levels are marginal or low, particularly in • coronary artery disease • arrhythmia-prone patients • those on diuretics or digoxin

If exercise is to become truly integrated into the overall care plan, health care practitioners must be fully committed to the idea, as outlined in Table 2. Time must be made for discussions of physical activity participation in team meetings; medical records, assessment forms, and other official documentation from the practitioner's office must be re-designed to include space for vital exercise-related data. Discussions of physical activity patterns should take place in team conferences and discharge planning meetings. Make available easily completed forms for patient assessment in terms of exercise history, physical fitness testing, exercise prescription, and activity logs. Add to the health library references on major exercise techniques and videotapes which can be viewed in the waiting room or borrowed from the library for home use.

TABLE 2
Role of the Caregiver in Exercise Programming

Role model
Exercise trainer
Cheerleader
Integration into overall health care plan
Monitoring benefit and risk
Involvement of family members and other social supports
Supporting institutional/policy changes that reward and facilitate such programs

---

The emphasis on appropriate physical activity levels may be enhanced by attention to the physical design of office and exam space as well. Consider replacing several chairs in the waiting room or lobby of the facility with stationary exercise equipment along with tables of educational materials to read. Make sure that stairways are accessible, well-lighted, have sturdy handrails, and are marked clearly to encourage use. Provide incentives for exercise adherence in the form of reduced fees, free exercise equipment, or educational materials, lottery tickets, or whatever is meaningful to the clientele in a particular setting. Practice good exercise habits yourself, as your prescription will carry a lot more credibility if your patient sees you following it in the workplace. Most environments can be creatively modified to encourage rather than restrict activity; this is as true of the doctor's or nutritionist's office as it is of the nursing home. Many small spaces in such settings can be converted to mini-gyms with little capital investment, and may be the seed from which much larger programs develop.

ASSESSMENT OF EXERCISE NEEDS AND GOALS

Once the commitment is made to integrate exercise prescriptions into general practice, protocols and systems need to be established to operationalize these prescriptions. The first step is to complete a targeted history and physical assessment which will identify potential needs for specific modalities of exercise, as well as current conditions or limitations which may impact upon exercise risk and adverse events. This process may be divided into three component parts.

1. The medical history and physical activity habit profile
2. The physical exam
3. The current level of physical fitness.

Each of these components will be considered in turn.

THE MEDICAL HISTORY AND PHYSICAL ACTIVITY HABIT PROFILE

The purpose of the history in the pre-exercise assessment of the older woman is to elicit current and prior physical activity patterns and preferences, history of exercise-related injuries, chronic diseases which may preclude exercise, chronic diseases or risk factors which are indications for specific exercise recommendations, and presence of new symptoms which require evaluation prior to initiating a change in physical activity pattern. Some of the important considerations relevant to the medical history are listed in Table 3.

TABLE 3
Screening for Exercise Participation: The Medical History

Domain	Recommendations
Cardiovascular disease	• Refer for evaluation of new or uncontrolled symptoms • Determine presence of symptoms during exercise including angina (or anginal equivalent such as jaw pain), claudication, arrhythmias, dizziness, weakness, dyspnea • Keep nitroglycerin available during exercise • Stop if unsure of any new symptom
Chronic pulmonary disease	• Determine symptoms at rest and during exercise • Determine need for supplemental oxygen • Plan use of inhalers prior to exercise • Keep inhalers available during exercise • Avoid exercise during flares of disease or infection
Mental status	• Avoid exercise if there are signs of acute drug or alcohol intoxication • Acute change in mental status/inattentiveness suggestive of delirium • Aggressive or disruptive behavior • Severe withdrawal or lethargy
Podiatric problems	• Determine presence of ulcers, fungal infections, neuropathy, edema, ischemia, skin breakdown, calluses, bunions, painful areas in foot and ankle • Wear shoes with lowest comfortable heel, non-slip soles, thick socks • Avoid high impact activities
Visual impairment	• Those with active or newly treated proliferative retinopathy, ophthalmologic surgery, or retinal detachment should not raise blood pressure, or intraocular pressure with any form of exercise until stable • Exercise in best possible lighting and wear corrective lenses at all times to avoid falls

---

It is important to note that this history taking goes far beyond the usual screening for participation in exercise, which is focused on identifying individuals who may be at higher risk for exercise-related adverse events, and therefore require supervision or modified activity levels. A broader use and definition of medical screening for exercise for the older woman are suggested. Rather than asking yourself "Is this woman safe to exercise?," instead you might pose the question "Is this woman safe to be sedentary?" It is important to keep in mind that sedentariness is the lethal condition, and that habitual exercise protects against many major chronic diseases, as well as being indicated in their treatment. In this broader concept of screening, therefore, the practitioner should be alert to the presence of sedentariness itself as a risk factor for disease and disability, chronic diseases that are amenable to physical activity, readiness to change behavior, and finally exacerbations of chronic diseases which should be brought to the attention of a physician, regardless of whether or not an exercise prescription is about to be given. In general, hypertension, angina, diabetes, pulmonary disease, obesity, neurological disease, and arthritis are indications *for* exercise as long as they are under control, rather than contraindications to physical activity.

Some specific areas of concern in the medical history of the older woman include cardiopulmonary status, musculoskeletal integrity, mental status, podiatric problems, and vision. It is important to know an individual's pattern of angina or shortness of breath, and what level of exertion produces it. Any change in chronic patterns warrants referral to a medical practitioner. For most cardiopulmonary symptoms, activity should be stopped or slowed down at their onset. The notable exception to this is claudication, where evidence indicates that walking a little farther once the pain begins is the most effective way to extend the time to claudication and improve pain-free walking distances. Cardiac stress testing should be done for standard medical indications in consultation with the patient's physician, and not simply because an asymptomatic older adult wants to begin a moderate exercise regimen. Requiring such testing before any exercise could be undertaken would pose an enormous psychological and financial disincentive to physical activity, and would likely result in false positive tests in many asymptomatic women which would then require further medical testing such as thallium stress testing or angiography to resolve the findings.

For patients with pulmonary disease, symptoms at rest and with exertion should be elicited, as well as determination of the need for supplemental oxygen during exercise. Plan the use of inhalers if needed for 15 to 30 minutes prior to exercise, to allow maximum effect, and keep on hand during all sessions. During febrile episodes or acute flares of disease, exercise should be avoided as the risk of cardiac arrhythmias and pulmonary edema is high during this time in the older adult. Some patients may not tolerate aerobic activity at all, but can perform resistance, balance, and flexibility exercises, which are less consumptive of oxygen, without much difficulty. It is important to remember that the catabolic effects of chronic pulmonary disease, often accompanied by anorexia, malnutrition, and corticosteroid treatment produce severe losses of lean tissue (muscle and bone). Such losses cannot be counteracted by cardiovascular endurance training alone, but require the adaptive response to resistive exercise (along with better nutrition) to reverse this wasting process. Therefore, patients with the most severe lung disease, who are least likely to be able to tolerate aerobic activities, are in fact more likely to benefit in terms of body composition and function from weight lifting exercise.

Identification of depression, anxiety, or insomnia on screening is important as these conditions all benefit from both resistive and aerobic exercise. Severe withdrawal or lethargy may require additional diagnosis and treatment and make an unsupervised exercise prescription unlikely to succeed, or unsafe if acute delirium is responsible for these symptoms. Cognitive impairment is not a contraindication to exercise, but may necessitate close supervision, group exercise, and safety precautions. Often a nonimpaired spouse or home care worker can be helpful as a walking partner or exercise trainer for those living at home. In an institutional setting with adequate staff-to-patient ratios, demented patients can successfully participate in all kinds of exercise. Aggressive or disruptive behavior, poor safety awareness and judgment, or uncontrolled alcohol intake should be screened for, as these will dictate the feasibility of group or isolated activity.

Many exercise-related injuries are related to the foot and ankle, although most are preventable with proper foot care, well-built shoes, thick socks, properly fitted orthotics, use of necessary assistive devices, and avoidance of high impact activities. Look for ulcers, fungal infections, peripheral neuropathy, infections, edema, ischemic changes, skin rashes or breakdown, calluses, bunions, ingrown or long toenails, and painful points on the ankle, heel, and foot. Those patients with peripheral vascular disease or neuropathy should be particularly careful about sudden increases in weight-bearing activities. If ulcers develop on the foot or ankle and ambulation is restricted temporarily, advise the patient to substitute seated weight-lifting exercises to prevent disuse atrophy from occurring during this period of reduced activity. It is wise to have a family member or caregiver check the feet, particularly of diabetics who may also have visual impairment that prevents them from seeing early problems as they develop. Shoes with the lowest comfortable heel and non-slip soles are important, particularly in those with balance impairment who are at risk for falls.

Visual problems are common in the older woman, and optimal lighting, exercise in the daylight hours, and use of corrective lenses at all times will minimize safety problems. Those with active or newly treated proliferative retinopathy, retinal detachment, or cataract surgery should not perform any exercise which raises the blood pressure or intraocular pressure or lift weights until cleared by their ophthalmologist. Substitution of stationary bikes, rowers, and steppers for other aerobic activities allows even completely blind individuals to exercise vigorously without supervision, and these patients should not therefore be automatically denied an exercise prescription, as many such alternatives are now available.

The physical activity history should be taken as follows:

- History of athletic participation in youth and middle age
- General recreational physical activity pursuits in mid- and older adult years
- Work-related physical activity patterns and year of retirement
- Any change in physical activity patterns over the past year
- Current (last 7 days) listing of all physical activities.

Current household, work-related, and recreational activities should be solicited, and quantified in terms of days per week, weeks per year, average length of each session or activity, and how long this pattern has been followed. In addition, specific questions about distances walked per week (in miles or blocks) and number of flights of stairs climbed per week will provide useful information on which to build the prescription, as well as provide an index of current capacity. Scales such as the Harvard Alumni Questionnaire[1] can be used to score this information in standardized formats, which have been linked to chronic disease outcomes and longevity itself.[2-4] This quantification of current exercise habits is important for several reasons. It provides a means of comparison to other older adults from epidemiological studies that have reported such figures. For example, the risk of stroke, heart disease, and diabetes is markedly reduced in those who expend about 2000 kcal/week in physical activities, compared to those who expend only 500 kcal. Second, a specific description of current habits can be used to set realistic and specific goals that can be tracked over time, such as increasing walking from 30 to 60 minutes per week.

Questions about the need for human or mechanical assistance with activities of daily living and household tasks will also point out where the greatest deficits in physiologic capacity lie. Individuals should also be asked about their preferred modes of exercise, specific dislikes or fears, preferences for lone or group activity, and potential limitations to increased activity levels imposed by spousal care, transportation, finances, etc.

If a history indicates that physical activity has declined over the past year, this is a very important observation to follow with additional questions. It may be a sign of early dementia, depression, functional impairment, arthritis of weight bearing joints, fear of falling, gait and balance difficulties, accelerating angina or peripheral vascular disease, or worsening valvular heart disease or pulmonary disease. Too often it is assumed that older people should become less and less active with aging, and this finding is not evaluated further. It is not unusual for older adults to gradually restrict their physical activities in response to real or perceived impairments, so that symptoms are minimized. For example, if the only question asked is "Do you get claudication when you walk?" and the woman denies this symptom, the practitioner may miss the fact that she no longer walks more than 2 blocks at a time or up hills, in order to avoid this symptom and, in fact, has progressive peripheral vascular disease. Risk factors for disease that are particularly important to identify in the history of the perimenopausal woman include obesity, glucose intolerance, hypertension, hyperlipidemia, osteopenia, and family history of diabetes, premenopausal heart disease, breast cancer, colon cancer, and osteoporotic fracture, as exercise is important as a preventive measure to reduce the future incidence of heart disease, diabetes, cancer, and hip fracture in these women. Current diseases and symptoms that should provoke a specific exercise recommendation, in conjunction with other medical treatment, are discussed in Chapter 1 and the disease-specific chapters in this book.

A complete medication history should be taken, and if any drugs with potential exercise interactions are identified, they can be handled as described in detail in Chapter 3. Certainly the most important class of agents to consider in this regard is chronic corticosteroid therapy, which results in severe atrophy of muscle and bone within a few months of initiation at high doses.[5,6] Patients maintained chronically on these drugs are at high risk for clinically significant muscle weakness, osteopenic fracture, and avascular necrosis of the femoral head, and include transplant patients (renal, cardiac, lung), those with chronic obstructive pulmonary disease, and rheumatologic diseases (rheumatoid arthritis, systemic lupus erythematosis, polymyalgia rheumatica), and other chronic inflammatory conditions. All women on chronic corticosteroid therapy should be on a regimen of progressive resistance training and calcium and vitamin D supplementation, which have been shown to counteract the steroid-induced myopathy and osteoporosis, unless there are very good reasons to prohibit these effective measures.

It is also important to elicit symptoms that are currently present during exertion, as they may be exacerbated by a new exercise prescription. This would include angina, palpitations, claudication, dyspnea on exertion, postural symptoms or dizziness with change in position or activity, pain in muscles or joints, aching or protrusion of a hernia or hemorrhoids, seizures, headaches, or urinary incontinence. The exact level of effort required to produce these symptoms should be noted for two reasons. First, the exercise prescription (except in the case of claudication) will generally be set below this symptom-limited threshold for safety. Second, as the woman adapts physiologically to prescribed training, her exercise tolerance should improve; she will be able to complete more intense activities before symptoms begin. This feedback is important as a behavioral tool to reinforce compliance and as a way to monitor the adequacy of training intensity and volume.

The Physical Exam

The physical exam relevant to the exercise prescription is used to corroborate information obtained by history, as well as to identify previously unknown problems that may require exercise for optimal management, or would alter or preclude the exercise prescription. The major relevant findings and actions suggested by each finding are listed in Table 4. As with findings from the medical history, the general rule is that uncontrolled disease or new symptoms require medical evaluation and treatment, not *because* the woman wishes to exercise, but simply because they indicate a need for better health maintenance.

Physical Fitness Level

In addition to the standard medical history and physical examination, the exercise prescription is logically guided by an assessment of the current exercise capacity in four major domains.

- Muscle strength, power, and endurance
- Aerobic capacity
- Flexibility
- Balance

Most health care practitioners will not have access to sophisticated exercise physiology laboratories where precise measurements can be made in these areas. However, for the purposes of guiding the exercise prescription and monitoring progress over time, it is often sufficient to conduct simple bedside or field tests which serve as proxies for the gold standard assessments, and require minimal equipment and training. A series of tests useful for assessment in these domains is suggested in Table 5. Rather than comparing the older woman to an arbitrary standard that may be difficult to interpret, it is best to simply record the results of these tests at periodic intervals (every 2 to 3 months) after training. Progression is fairly predictable if training principles (see Chapter 2) are adhered to, unless illness has intervened. Therefore, in relatively healthy women, lack of progress usually indicates non-compliance or insufficient intensities of training in the relevant modality.

IDENTIFY BEHAVIORAL READINESS TO CHANGE

The determination of exercise goals appropriate to the current health status and physical fitness level of the older woman must be followed by an assessment of her readiness to change sedentary habits, as discussed in Chapter 26. Sometimes, the priorities and advice of the health care practitioner will be enough to move someone to the point where they begin to exercise, but often more than this is required. A health care crisis (myocardial infarction, hip fracture) can sometimes serve as the crucial turning point, but obviously it is desirable to effect change long before health status deteriorates if at all possible.

When attempting to implement an exercise program on an institutional level, as opposed to an individual level, additional barriers arise, particularly financing the program, providing adequate staffing, finding time within busy activity/therapy schedules, buying or placing exercise equipment, integration into existing activities, maintaining commitment and quality of programming, and expanding participation beyond a few enthusiastic residents. In settings such as long-term care facilities, it is usually staff and institutional barriers that dictate the ultimate level of involvement of residents. This is because many of the individual barriers seen in the community (transportation, cost, fear, access) have been addressed by the institutional setting itself. Therefore, behavioral efforts must focus on administrators and staff who may not be used to considering physical activity a mandatory part of the long-term care setting and health care needs of their residents. We have often found it necessary to supplement staff with volunteers to provide adequate staff:patient ratios in exercise programming. Maintaining staff motivation is critical, and may be facilitated by anticipating relapse, giving public rewards and recognition for participation as exercise leaders or coordinators, involving staff leaders directly in the planning sessions, and encouraging innovation and modification of existing programs to incorporate new fitness goals for the residents.

TABLE 4
The Physical Exam Findings Relevant to Exercise Prescription

Finding	Responses
Body mass index < 21 kg/m²	• Evaluation for undernutrition • Resistance training in combination with increased energy intake
Body mass index > 28–30 kg/m² Waist circumference > 90 cm Waist:hip ratio > 0.85	• Evaluation for causes of weight gain • Evaluation for the presence of hypertension, hyperlipidemia, elevated fasting insulin or glucose, glucose intolerance • Resistance or aerobic training in combination with hypocaloric diet will aid in weight loss and reduction in visceral adiposity
Kyphosis	• Evaluation of risk factors for osteopenia • Resistance training including back extensor muscles • Avoidance of back flexion activities • Weight-bearing aerobic exercise • Balance training if impaired prior to aerobic exercise
Tachycardia (HR > 100 bpm at rest); irregular pulse	• Evaluation for dehydration, fever, arrthymias, thyrotoxicosis, drug effects, etc. prior to exercise prescription
Bradycardia (HR < 50 bpm at rest)	• Evaluation for heart block, drug toxicity, other prior to exercise prescription
Hypertension	• Evaluation of drug and dietary management for adequate control before initiation of adjunctive exercise prescription • Retinal evaluation for the presence of active hypertensive retinopathy • Aerobic and resistance training will produce small decreases in systolic and diastolic blood pressure chronically; reevaluate medication needs after adaptation
Fever, acute systemic infection or severe local infection	• Avoid all exercise until resolved

Postural hypotension (drop of 20 mm or more in systolic pressure on standing; failure of pulse to rise on standing); may or may not be associated with dizziness, lightheadedness, dysequilibrium	• Evaluation for disease- or medication-related causes prior to exercise prescription • Ensure hydration status is adequate prior to and during exercise • If symptomatic and severe, avoid standing exercises until treated • Both aerobic and resistive exercise can minimize postural hypotension in response to stressors, and may help in the chronic management of this condition • Avoid exercise in first 30 minutes after meals when postural hypotension may worsen (post-prandial hypotension) • Add balance training to offset increased risk of falls due to postural hypotension • Attempt to substitute exercise for drugs which cause postural hypotension (e.g., tricyclic antidepressants)
Delirium, psychosis, alcohol intoxication Cognitive impairment	• Evaluate and treat appropriately prior to initiating exercise prescription • Evaluate if etiology unknown • Prescribe supervised exercise for safety and compliance
Depressed affect; psychomotor retardation	• Refer for evaluation of possible clinical depression • High intensity progressive resistance training and aerobic exercise have been shown to be approximately as effective as drug therapy in clinical depression
Ophthalmologic exam abnormalities (elevated intraocular pressure, proliferative retinopathy, retinal hemorrhage, retinal detachment; recent surgery)	• Exercise of any kind contraindicated until evaluation and treatment by a specialist • Avoid Valsalva maneuver, putting head below heart • Resumption of exercise on advice of ophthalmologist (usually 2–6 weeks after surgery) • All older adults (particularly patients with diabetes and hypertension) should have had a retinal exam within the previous 12 months
Aortic stenosis murmur	• Evaluation of aortic valve disease status prior to initiation of exercise • Exercise precluded if severe aortic stenosis is present and/or angina, syncope, or drop in systolic blood pressure occur with exertion
Pericardial rub	• Exercise precluded until evaluation and treatment of pericardial effusion/pericarditis completed

TABLE 4 (CONTINUED)
The Physical Exam Findings Relevant to Exercise Prescription

Finding	Responses
Abnormal pulmonary exam (wheezing, dullness to percussion, rales, etc.)	• Evaluation and treatment of chronic or new cardiac or pulmonary disease indicated prior to exercise prescription
	• Chronic stable asthma and obstructive lung disease, congestive heart failure benefit from aerobic training
	• Resistance training indicated in undernourished patients with chronic lung disease to treat sarcopenia and osteopenia from drugs and disease; also in stable congestive heart failure to treat skeletal muscle myopathy
	• Time bronchodilators for 15–20 minutes prior to aerobic training sessions if needed
	• Use supplemental oxygen during exercise to increase exercise tolerance and training progression in hypoxemic patients
	• Resistance training may be better tolerated than aerobic training in those with low threshold for hypoxia
Abdominal bruits, aneurysm	• Evaluate presence and size of aortic aneurysm
	• Exercise of any kind precluded in aneurysm > 5 cm in transverse diameter or expanding until treated
	• Exercise may be initiated after successful recovery from aortic bypass surgery
Hemorrhoids	• Evaluate need for treatment prior to exercise prescription in large or symptomatic hemorrhoids
	• Avoid Valsalva maneuver, resistance training in significant disease until treated
	• Resistance training may be prescribed in those with small or asymptomatic hemorrhoids with careful avoidance of breath holding, Valsalva at moderate intensities (60–70%) of the 1RM
Abdominal or inguinal hernias	• Evaluate need for surgery prior to exercise prescription in large or symptomatic hernias
	• Avoid Valsalva maneuver, resistance training in significant hernias
	• Resistance training may be prescribed in those with repaired or small asymptomatic hernias with careful avoidance of breath holding, Valsalva at moderate intensities (60–70%) of the 1RM
Testicular atrophy	• Evaluate and treat cause
	• Resistance training will counteract skeletal and muscle atrophy in addition to hormone replacement

Joint inflammation, instability, pain
- Evaluate and treat medically/surgically if needed prior to exercise prescription
- Delay exercise until stabilization of unstable joints
- Aerobic, resistance, and flexibility training improve symptoms in chronic arthritis
- Avoid weight-bearing endurance exercise until muscles and ligaments are strengthened by resistance training in severe cases
- Medicate for pain prior to exercise sessions to increase tolerance of activity in chronic stable disease

Degenerative disease of lumbar spine, spinal stenosis
- Resistive exercise for back extensor muscles

Decreased joint range of motion
- Both flexibility training and resistance training will increase range of motion
- Most effective when tissue temperature is increased by prior activity such as aerobic exercise

Peripheral vascular disease
- Evaluate presence of claudication or rest pain; treat medically or surgically if indicated.
- Prescribe aerobic exercise, continuing for 30–60 seconds after the onset of claudication; rest, then repeat for optimal benefit

Deep venous thrombosis, superficial phlebitis
- Avoid exercise until resolved or stabilized on anticoagulant therapy for several weeks

Venous stasis; peripheral edema
- Aerobic or resistive exercise involving the calf muscles will reduce peripheral edema and stasis
- Minimize time spent with feet dependent, hips flexed

Peripheral sensory neuropathy, decreased proprioception
- Evaluate and treat underlying cause if possible
- Protect feet during weight-bearing exercise
- Avoid high impact activities
- Prescribe balance/strength training to counteract increased risk of falls due to neuropathy

Parkinsonian signs
- Prescribe exercises to counteract the orthostatic hypotension, constipation, depression, muscle atrophy, decreased range of motion, and balance impairments that are part of the disease
- A combination of resistive, flexibility, and balance exercises would likely be most helpful

Muscle atrophy and weakness
- Evaluate underlying cause, treat as necessary
- Resistance training at moderate to high intensity will increase muscle size and strength

Urinary incontinence on standing, Valsalva, cough, sneeze; weakness of levator ani muscle on pelvic exam
- Evaluate for presence of infection, glycosuria, other bladder problems
- Prescribe isometric resistance exercise for levator ani muscles (Kegel exercises)

TABLE 5
Measurements of Physical Fitness in Health Care Settings

Domain of Assessment	Test	Comments
Muscle strength	Maximum amount of weight that can be slowly lifted one time with a particular muscle group	Record in pounds Requires a series of incrementally heavier objects, such as dumbbells; ability depends on muscle mass and training status
Muscle power	Time taken to rise from a chair as fast as possible without using arms	Normal power indicated by rising without assistance from arms in about 1–2 seconds
Muscle endurance	Time taken to rise 10 times in a row from a chair, without using arms if possible	Times of greater than 15–20 seconds indicative of impairments in muscle endurance
Cardiovascular endurance	6-minute walk test (maximal distance that can be covered in 6 minutes)	Distances less than 500 meters/6 minutes indicate increasing degrees of limitation
Flexibility	Range of motion of specific joints	Measured in degrees with goniometer; less than full extension, flexion, etc. is abnormal
Static balance	Ability to hold semi-tandem, tandem, and one-legged stand for 15 seconds each	Less than 15 seconds indicative of impairment
Dynamic balance	Tandem walk over 3–6 meters	Errors and prolonged time taken to complete indicate impairment

PRIORITIZE PHYSICAL ACTIVITY NEEDS IN RELATION TO RISKS

It is quite likely that after the assessment many deficits and needs will be identified in the typically sedentary individual. Therefore, it becomes important to know how to deliver the prescription in logical stages that are palatable and feasible, and have some likelihood of successful implementation. In most cases, it is recommended to start with only one mode of exercise (balance, strength, endurance, flexibility) and let the woman get used to the new routine of exercise before adding other components. This approach obviously requires attention to risk factors, medical history, physical exam findings, and personal preferences, and will be different for each individual. However, there are a few generalizations that can be made.

If significant deficits in muscle strength or balance are identified, then these should be addressed prior to the initiation of aerobic training. A simple way of helping with the decision-making process is the following modification of the "Get Up and Go" test: Ask the woman to sit in a chair with her arms folded and then on your command, stand up, place feet in a tandem position and hold for 15 seconds, and then walk as rapidly as possible around the corridor 1 to 2 times.

- If she cannot stand up quickly without using her arms, or cannot rise independently at all, then resistance training is the first modality of exercise which must be initiated.
- If she rises quickly from the chair, but has difficulty maintaining the tandem stand position, then start with balance training; otherwise, standing aerobic exercise may be risky.
- If she has no difficulty with standing up or balance, but finds one to two minutes of rapid walking causes fatigue, dyspnea, angina, claudication, or other symptoms, then start with aerobic exercise.

Demonstrating difficulty with these simple tasks will reinforce the need for the prescription that is offered, and thus is likely to enhance compliance. If deficits in all three areas are identified, follow the progression: resistance training, balance training, aerobic training in sequence for the most effective and safe increase in function and mobility. Attempting to prescribe progressive aerobic training in the absence of sufficient balance or strength is likely to result in knee pain, fear of falling, falls, and limited ability to progress aerobically, and is not recommended. There is sometimes a tendency in therapy settings to treat ambulation as the primary goal by encouraging walking as the first kind of exercise after recovery from surgery or other illness. However, attempting to ambulate those who cannot lift their body weight out of a chair or maintain standing balance is a suboptimal approach. An approach that pays attention to the physiologic determinants of transfer ability and ambulation, and specifically targets these with the appropriate exercise prescription when reversible deficits are uncovered is more likely to succeed.

In some cases, the woman may benefit equally from resistance or aerobic training (for the treatment of depression, for example) but the decision is made based on her ability to tolerate one form of exercise over another. Severe osteoarthritis of the knee, recurrent falls, and a low threshold for ischemia may make resistance training safer than aerobic training as an antidepressant treatment. Prioritization requires careful consideration of the risks and benefits of each mode of activity, as well as the current health status and physical fitness level.

PRESCRIBE THE SPECIFIC EXERCISE MODALITY AND DOSE DESIRED

Once the prescription has been decided upon, it is most effective to prescribe it as specifically as possible, using the guidelines in Chapter 2. Often the mistake is made of giving only vague, general advice about being more active, but this is insufficient if real change in behavior and physiologic adaptation is expected in a previously sedentary woman. As with any other medical prescription, the kind of exercise, dose, frequency, expected benefits, and possible side effects should be given in written form. If a lifestyle approach to integrating physical activity into the daily routine is decided upon in lieu of structured exercise, this should be accompanied by specific relevant examples in written form as well.[7] A comparison of the pros and cons of these two approaches to the exercise prescription is presented in Table 6. Experimental data comparing these two approaches are thus far available only for aerobic exercise in middle-aged adults,[8] and it appears that adherence rates are similar (about 20% of participants exercising at target levels long term). As noted in Chapter 2, it is likely that the treatment of disease may require a different dose of exercise than the prevention of disease, and all of these factors should be kept in mind when planning the approach to an individual woman.

TABLE 6
A Comparison of Structured Exercise vs. Lifestyle Prescription

Feature	Structured Exercise	Lifestyle Prescription
Specificity of prescription	High	Low
Physiologic adaptation likely	Moderate to high	Low to moderate
Ability to track behavior	High	Low to Moderate
Compliance usually observed	Low-moderate	Low-moderate
Health benefits	Dependent on compliance	Dependent on compliance
Relevance to resistance training	High	Unknown[a]
Relevance to aerobic training	High	Moderate
Relevance to balance training	High	Unknown[a]
Relevance to flexibility training	High	Unknown[a]
Cost	Low-high	Low
Safety	Moderate to high	High
Relevance to treatment of established disease	Moderate to high	Low to moderate
Extra time incurred by exercise	Moderate	Little to none

[a] Only aerobic training has been reported as a lifestyle intervention compared to structured exercise sessions.[8]

Some elderly patients will have medical problems that place them at higher risk for exercise-related adverse events. Examples include visual impairment, balance disorders, osteoarthritis of the shoulder or weight-bearing joints, low thresholds for ischemia or bronchospasm, peripheral vascular disease, or peripheral neuropathy. In general, problems can be avoided by providing monitoring if needed, exercising in adequate lighting, strengthening muscles around arthritic joints prior to weight-bearing exercise, and keeping intensity levels below those which produce cardiopulmonary symptoms. If an older runner who likes competition is getting into difficulty with knee and ankle injuries, substituting a lower impact yet intense activity such as race walking can provide all of the physical and psychological benefits desired without the risk of musculoskeletal trauma. If the risk of ischemia is very high with aerobic exercise, then prescribing resistance exercises may offer similar benefits in terms of health and functioning with less potential to provoke cardiac symptoms.[9-11] In all cases, it is important to balance the pleasurable components of exercise for the individual with the health maintainance aspects important to the practitioner, or the prescription is likely to be unheeded in the long term. Anticipating both benefits and risks and discussing them with the older woman at the time the prescription is given is the best way to avoid injuries and adverse events.

PROVIDE OR REFER FOR SPECIFIC TRAINING

The prescription must be accompanied by realistic options for training and access to equipment. It is ideal if training can take place by personnel within the same health care practice, in person, or with a combination of hands-on training, videotapes, and written materials. Many older adults with chronic diseases will require more training than can be provided by the average health care professional without special exercise knowledge. Therefore, a referral to a qualified fitness instructor or physical therapist is often needed, along with explicit graphic instructions or videotapes. Such materials provide both knowledge and motivation for the novice exerciser, and having them on hand in the waiting room or office setting reinforces the power of the prescription and emphasizes the commitment of the practitioner to healthy lifestyle principles. If it is necessary to refer to an outside facility, make sure the trainers are experienced in the principles of exercise you are advocating, and comfortable with older adults with chronic illness. It is helpful to be quite specific in the referral about the medical concerns underlying the referral, and the modalities of training desired.

All modalities of exercise can be carried out at home, and the benefits of this approach as opposed to supervised or unsupervised sessions in a gym or fitness center should be discussed. The most important issues are transportation, cost, sense of security, need for medical monitoring, desire for group support, and flexibility in scheduling. Whatever approach results in optimal safety and compliance is the one to choose. Aerobic, flexibility, and balance training can be carried out without equipment, so home training is easily accomplished in these domains. Resistance training does require the purchase of free weights or a weight stack system, but many good options for home use are now available in sporting goods stores.

SET UP BEHAVIORAL PROGRAM FOR ADOPTION, ADHERENCE, RELAPSE PREVENTION

Simply identifying the appropriate exercise goals is not sufficient to ensure a change in behavior. It is equally important to identify in what stage of behavioral change the person is currently, if the counseling is to have any effect. In the transtheoretical model of behavior, individuals advance through stages of pre-contemplation, contemplation, action, regular activity, and maintenance in regard to any behavioral choice. Offering a pre-contemplator a free membership to a gym will be unlikely to induce exercise adoption for example, while the same incentive given to someone who has advanced to the contemplation or action stage may be just the motivation needed to start a regular new habit of physical activity. Once someone is in a regular pattern of behavior, techniques such as positive reinforcement, record keeping, external reminders of the desired behavior, goal-setting, and relapse prevention all work to keep the behavior ongoing. Maintenance is a phase indicating at least 6 months of continuous adherence to the new behavior, whether it is exercise, dietary change, smoking cessation, or other lifestyle habits, and evidence indicates that recidivism is quite low if you can get patients to this point. Most failures in any new behavior occur long before the 6-month interval has passed, so it makes sense to put in place rigorous behavioral programs in this critical initial period. These may take the form of supervised classes, logs to send in, rewards, telephone calls, financial incentives, group support mechanisms, etc.

There are many barriers to the initial adoption of physical activity in the elderly, as outlined in Table 7. Questioning the older woman about the specific barriers most relevant to her, and addressing them in the beginning are necessary or the prescription will fail. Some of these barriers are at a societal level (expectations, grandparent roles), others involve local regulations or geographical features, and others are personal in nature (fear of injury, boredom, time constraints). In all cases, it is important not to assume that all old people are alike or function with similar reasoning in regard to exercise participation. For some, offering exercise in a group setting may relieve fears and provide social support; for others, embarrassment over disabilities or skill level may make exercising at home a much more appealing option. Creativity in exercise planning is a key factor. If transportation is a major barrier, then exercise classes at a meal site where elderly vans are already in service can efficiently overcome this barrier. Perceived lack of time is a barrier frequently cited even by nursing home residents when asked why they don't exercise. It is helpful to go through a daily schedule, pointing out times when watching television or other sedentary activities can be combined with flexibility, resistive, or even stationary aerobic exercise or, for example, when stairs can be substituted for elevators and escalators.

TABLE 7
Barriers to Physical Activity in the Older Woman

- Acute and chronic medical problems and disabilities
- Caregiving role for sick spouse or family member
- Disinterest
- Exaggerated perception of risk
- Financial constraints
- Geographical limitations and environmental design features
- Institutional/residential policies restricting activity
- Lack of advocacy by family and health care community
- Lack of appropriately designed exercise equipment
- Lack of health care professional/caregiver/family education about exercise
- Perceived or real lack of time
- Psychological issues (depression, dementia, bereavement, self-efficacy, fear of falling, low self-esteem, social isolation)
- Reduced appreciation of benefit
- Societal norms/expectations of sedentariness

Set up the behavioral program to encourage long-term adherence at the same time the prescription is generated by giving the client an exercise calendar or diary to fill out each week, motivational tokens, and a plan for feedback on their progress at frequent intervals. A successful method we have used in the community that takes very little time is to ask participants to fill out an exercise log or diary that is mailed in at the end of each week or month. The receipt of this log is followed by a brief phone call from a staff member to discuss issues of compliance, progression, adverse events, illness, or other problems. Without such adherence measures in place, the likelihood of long-term adoption, particularly in frail elders or those with chronic disease, is quite low.

If relapse is likely because of intercurrent illness, caregiving responsibilities, travel, or other identified problems, address these concerns early and outline plans to anticipate and avoid such pitfalls. Ask about the compliance with the exercise prescription at every health care visit, as well as perceived benefits and adverse events that have occurred. Repeating the physical function testing used to generate the initial prescription can be very motivating, as the woman can be given direct feedback on the specific physical benefits attributable to her new physical activity pattern. As functional status improves and once the routine of regular physical activity has been firmly established, modify the exercise goals to emphasize new areas of fitness. Shaping behavior in small increments is more likely to be successful than overwhelming an adult who has been sedentary for 50 years with an overly ambitious plan of physical activity.

When setting up programs in facilities, behavior that must be changed and rewarded is that of caregiver and administrative staff, as well as residents. The same principles of adoption and adherence apply to this new staff behavior of teaching exercise. Some appropriate ways of rewarding staff for their efforts in this area are listed in Table 8.

TABLE 8
Staff Incentives for Participation in Exercise Programming

Money
Recognition
Time off
Relief from regular duties
Achievement of personal fitness goals
Altruism/commitment to patients
New skills acquisition

MONITOR COMPLIANCE, BENEFITS, ADVERSE EVENTS OVER TIME

When exercise is used as part of an overall medical care plan, its use by the individual should be systematically reviewed and adjusted over time (as shown in Table 9), like any other medical intervention. Periodically repeating the physical fitness assessments and reviewing activity logs will form the primary means of assessing compliance and adaptation over time. Often errors in training technique (particularly lack of regularity, progression, and appropriate intensity) will be uncovered in this way. The primary goal of the exercise prescription is to change exercise behavior and fitness itself. However, secondary goals may be improvements in specific symptoms or conditions such as arthritis pain, depression, sleep disturbance, angina, time to claudication, glucose control, or blood pressure, and appropriate measurements should be made to gauge progress in these areas as well. However, since some things are slow to change or effects are not dramatic in the short term, it is best not to overly emphasize goals such as weight loss, need for anti-hypertensive medicines, etc., as the participant may be discouraged rather than encouraged by the results.

TABLE 9
Monitoring the Outcomes of the Exercise Prescription

Define the extent of the problem (current exercise level)
Define desired behaviors/goals
Use quantitative assessments of physical fitness
Give feedback regularly
Periodically reassess progress toward goals
Redefine goals as required by change in circumstance

Appropriate exercise goals would include

"I want to exercise at least 3 days every week."
"I want to increase the weight I lift by 1 kg every 2 weeks."
"I want to walk 1 minute longer each time I exercise."
"I want to keep a record of all exercise I do each week."
"I want to stop using elevators whenever there are stairs available."

These are measurable, achievable changes in behavior that are very likely to be accomplished, and are thus the kinds of goal-setting to be encouraged by the health care practitioner.

On a facility level, success will be determined by the extent to which an overall change in activity participation is effected in the institution, as well as the perceived benefits and burdens of this new initiative. Ways in which institutional goals can be measured are listed in Table 10.

TABLE 10
**How to Evaluate Exercise Program Success
at the Facility Level**

Penetration into facility (clients and staff)
Staff acceptance/perceived burden
Change in staff exercise attitudes and behaviors
Job morale/turnover
Impact on other facility activities
Satisfaction of clients/families/community
Costs/savings
Health outcomes
Incorporation into philosophy or mission of facility
Dissemination to other health care facilities and services

Finally, care should be taken to modify the exercise prescription as health status/goal/behavioral stage changes. For example, if the plan was to start with resistance training, add balance training, and then add aerobic training, as psychological and physical status permitted, this plan needs to be implemented in incremental steps based on monitored changes in health and physical ability over time. Intercurrent illness, progressive disease, or hospitalization may dramatically alter physical capacity and health care needs, requiring a re-assessment of exercise goals and strategies for implementation. For example, a cardiac event may necessitate monitored activity in a cardiac rehabilitation setting for a period of time, before returning to a general community exercise program. The onset of dementia or functional decline may require caregiver or family training in the exercise techniques that were formerly prescribed to be carried out independently.

Participation in physical activity is not merely a medical prescription or treatment, it is a right of individuals, both fit and frail, and thus a responsibility of caregivers, family members, and volunteers to provide education, opportunity, and access in this domain to the eldest members of our communities. Health care practices and policies for the elderly should be enlarged to promote fitness, activity, and independence to the fullest extent possible for each individual as an important component of overall quality of life

REFERENCES

1. Paffenbarger, R. S., Wing, A. L., and Hyde, T. R., Physical activity as an index of heart attack risk in college alumni, *Am. J. Epidemiol.*, 108, 161–5, 1978.
2. Lee, I., Hsieh, C., and Paffenbarger, R., Exercise intensity and longevity in men: the Harvard alumni health study, *JAMA*, 273, 1179–1184, 1995.
3. Helmrich, S., Ragland, D., and Paffenbarger, R., Prevention of non-insulin-dependent diabetes mellitus with physical activity, *Med. Sci. Sports Exerc.*, 26, 824–830, 1994.

4. Paffenbarger, R. S., Jr., Hyde, R. T., Wing, A. L., Lee, I. M., Jung, D. L., and Kampert, J. B., The association of changes in physical-activity level and other lifestyle characteristics with mortality among men [see comments], *N. Engl. J. Med.*, 328, 538–45, 1993.
5. Braith, R., Mills, R., Welsch, M., Keller, J., and Pollock, M., Resistance exercise training restores bone mineral density in heart transplant recipients, *J. Am. Coll. Coariol.*, 28, 1471–1477, 1996.
6. Braith, R., Welsch, M., Mills, R., Keller, J., and Pollock, M., Resistance exercise prevents glucocorticoid-induced myopathy in heart transplant recipients, *Med. Sci. Sports Exerc.*, 30, 1998.
7. Leaf, D. A. and Reuben, D. B., "Lifestyle" interventions for promoting physical activity: a kilocalorie expenditure-based home feasibility study, *Am. J. Med Sci.*, 312, 68–75, 1996.
8. Dunn, A., Marcus, B., Kampert, J., Garcia, M., Kohl, H., and Blair, S., Comparison of lifestyle and structured interventions to increase physical activity and cardiorespiratory fitness: A randomized trial, *JAMA*, 281, 327–340, 1999.
9. Benn, S., McCartney, N., and McKelvie, R., Circulatory responses to weight lifting, walking and stair climbing in older males, *J. Am. Geriatr. Soc.*, 44, 121–125, 1996.
10. McCartney, N., Acute responses to resistance training and safety, *Med. Sci. Sports Exerc.*, 31, 31–37, 1999.
11. McKelvie, R. and McCartney, N., Weightlifting training in cardiac patients: considerations, *Sports Med.*, 10, 355–64, 1990.

26 Promoting Adoption and Maintenance of Physical Activity and Dietary Behavior Change

Bess H. Marcus, Matthew M. Clark, Beth C. Bock, Bernardine M. Pinto, and Deborah F. Tate

CONTENTS

INTRODUCTION

Research has shown that it is difficult for people to make dietary changes (Brownell and Cohen, 1995) or to adopt new physical activity habits (Dishman and Sallis,

1994) and to maintain either of these changes over time. The purpose of this chapter is to highlight strategies practitioners can use to assist their patients in making changes to dietary and physical activity practices. We will discuss how to assess your patients' readiness for change, methods of working with patients who are not ready for change, and strategies to help patients accomplish these changes. Additionally, we will provide a resource list of materials practitioners may refer to for more specific information and one which may be helpful to patients during the process of changing and maintaining their new habits. Specific information about nutrition and physical activity recommendations for women over 50 can be found in other chapters in this book.

READINESS FOR CHANGE

How does an individual know if she is ready to make a change? There are a number of ways to determine one's readiness. One way is for your patient to ask herself the question, "What will I get as a result of making this behavior change?" (i.e., What are the benefits of change?). If your patient cannot come up with at least a few compelling benefits, it is unlikely that she will be able to accomplish even short-term change. Another equally important step is determining what your patient will have to give up, or other unpleasant aspects of change. It is helpful to have your patient write down her reasons for wanting to change her eating or activity habits (the benefits for changing) and barriers or obstacles to changing (Table 1). If your patient wants to make changes in both areas, you should have her do this activity for each behavior separately.

TABLE 1
Benefits and Barriers to Behavior Change

_____ (write specific behavior)

Benefits to Change (Pros)	Barriers to Change (Cons)
Example: I will feel better once I start regular physical activity.	Example: I do not have the time to be more physically active.
1. _____	1. _____
2. _____	2. _____
3. _____	3. _____
4. _____	4. _____
5. _____	5. _____

Another way to decide whether an individual is ready to make a behavior change is to more formally assess her readiness for change or stage of behavior change. The Transtheoretical Model has been used to describe the process of change for a variety of health behaviors (Prochaska and DiClemente, 1983). This model asserts that individuals progress through a series of stages as they make behavior changes. As applied to physical activity, a person who is not physically active and does not intend to start is considered to be in the *Precontemplation* stage. A person who is not physically active but intends to start is in the *Contemplation* stage. Individuals who participate in some physical activity, but do not do so on a regular basis, are in the *Preparation* stage. Regular physical activity is defined in the joint recommendations from the Centers for Disease Control (CDC) and American College of Sports Medicine (ACSM) as an accumulation of 30 minutes or more of moderate-intensity physical activity performed on at least 5 days each week (Pate et al., 1995). The *Action* stage describes individuals who participate in regular physical activity but have done so for less than 6 months. Finally, an individual is said to be in *Maintenance* when they have been physically active on a regular basis for 6 months or longer (Marcus, Rossi, Selby, Niaura, and Abrams, 1992). These stages are conceptualized as a series of progressions or preparations for change and patients may become more or less prepared for change (progressing forward or backward) over time.

The readiness quiz (Table 2) may be used to assess your patient's level of readiness for change. Based on the item your patient selects, you can determine how ready she is to make changes in her habits and some appropriate steps you can take to provide assistance.

TABLE 2
Readiness for Physical Activity or Dietary Behavior Change

Readiness Quiz

Circle the response that best describes how you are thinking and feeling *right now*:

1. I am not thinking about changing my eating or activity habits.
2. I am thinking about changing my habits and I intend to start changing during the next 6 months.
3. I am thinking about changing my habits and I intend to start changing during the next month.
4. I am already making some changes in my habits (e.g., I walk once per week; I use 1% milk).
5. I have recently changed my behavior and I am doing what I am supposed to do (e.g., eating 30% of my calories, or less, from fat; accumulating at least 30 minutes of moderate-intensity physical activity at least 5 times per week).
6. I have successfully changed my behavior and I have maintained this new behavior for:
   _____ 6 months _____ 7 to 12 months _____ more than 12 months.

Adapted from Marcus, B. H., Rossi, J. S., Selby, V. C., Niaura, R. S., and Abrams, D. B., *Health Psychol.*, 11, 386–395, 1992.

If your patient selects item 1, she is not ready for change. These patients are in the Precontemplation stage. If your patient selects item 2 or 3, she is in the Contemplation stage and may be more ready to change in the future. It is important to continue to address the topic of changing diet or physical activity patterns at future visits. Techniques outlined in the section "Helping Patients Get Ready For Change" are appropriate for increasing motivation for change. Patients who select item 4 are in the Preparation stage. They have made some initial steps toward changing and are ready for strategies outlined in the "Initiating Dietary or Physical Activity Behavior Changes" section. If your patient has already established a regular pattern of physical activity or already eats a healthy diet, they are either in Action (item 5) or Maintenance (item 6). Review strategies in the sections entitled "Making Dietary or Physical Activity Behavior Change a Regular Habit" and "Maintaining Dietary or Physical Activity Behavior Changes" for more information about helping these patients.

HELPING PATIENTS GET READY FOR CHANGE

As practitioners you are familiar with helping people achieve certain goals such as overcoming an illness, recovering from an injury, finding a job, etc. Often patients who come to you for help are ready to take steps toward changing. Usually whatever they are seeking help for has become a problem they would like to change. Making changes to diet or activity patterns can be different because your patient may not see their current diet or activity level as causing her any problem or the consequences may be so far in the future that the individual may not be ready to take steps toward changing. It can be helpful to use motivational interviewing techniques (Miller and Rolnick, 1991) when working with patients who are not ready to change. These techniques have been developed to enhance motivation for change by helping the patient evaluate her own behavior and begin to identify how the behavior might be problematic. If your patient states that she wants to be healthy, you can help her understand how a goal of becoming healthy is inconsistent with her current diet or physical activity habits. Strategies for motivational interviewing include asking open-ended questions about the patient's diet or activity habits, validating their feelings, exploring in more detail the expected costs and benefits of changing their diet or activity, providing information about how the patient might change their diet or activity patterns and asking about their reaction to this information. When talking with patients who are not ready for change, it is important to maintain a balanced perspective—not condoning their unhealthy behaviors, but not forcing them to change either. This prevents discussions from being argumentative and may prevent your patient from becoming defensive about her behavior. Continue to discuss change with these patients during future clinical visits using the techniques described above, e.g., express your support, and show your willingness to assist them when they are ready.

In working with patients who are contemplating change, it can be useful to have them think about who in their life (at home, work, or in the community) will support them in their efforts and who will make things more difficult. Ask about how confident she is that she can make these health behavior adaptations. You can increase her confidence by helping her recognize successes she has had making other changes in her life. Ask about what worked? What did not work? Help your patient determine how to use this information for themselves now.

It is important to keep in mind that it may take your patient some time before she is actually ready to change her habits. This may be frustrating, but jumping right in when your patient is not really ready will probably be unsuccessful. When this happens, your patient's behavior change is likely to be very brief, and she may return to her old habits frustrated and may have doubts about her ability to succeed in the future.

INITIATING CHANGES IN DIET OR ACTIVITY HABITS

Most people benefit from identifying their current patterns prior to making changes in their lifestyle (NIH Technology Assessment Conference Panel, 1992). One of the foundations of behavior change is the identification of current behavioral patterns. Identifying three areas—triggers, behaviors, and results—is an important first step. After identifying patterns, your patient can avoid or modify a trigger, or work to change the result of her behavior. Triggers make it more likely that a behavior will occur. Triggers can be things, thoughts, emotions, feelings, people, places, or situations that cause (or trigger) a behavior. It will be helpful for your patient to become aware of the triggers that cause her to be inactive or eat an unhealthy diet and to work with her to develop a plan for avoiding or modifying these triggers (Table 3).

TABLE 3
Behavioral Patterns

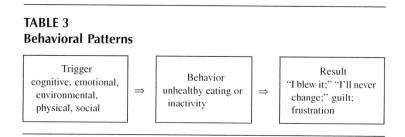

Triggers for any behavior typically fall into one of five general categories: cognitive, emotional, environmental, physical, and social. Some *thoughts* that trigger inactivity or unhealthy diets include "I'm too busy for physical activity today, think of all the time I'll save by skipping it;" "It's my birthday, anniversary, etc., therefore, I have to overeat in order to celebrate;" "I've worked real hard this week so I deserve a soup to nuts dinner;" or "Using a treadmill is so boring." A common *emotional* trigger is stress. Frequently, people overeat or skip physical activity during times of stress. However, any emotion can be a trigger, and feeling down or blue, boredom, and anger are also common triggers. *Environmental* triggers are things in the physical environment that lead to inactivity or unhealthy diets such as stopping at a doughnut shop for a cup of coffee and the aroma triggering the purchase of two jelly doughnuts. *Physical* triggers are physical sensations such as fatigue (e.g., "I'm too tired to go for a walk") or hunger (e.g., "I'm very hungry in the afternoons"). Sometimes other people can influence an individual's behavior; these are called *social* triggers; for example, family members may convince your patient to eat certain foods or to skip exercise class.

After either engaging (or not engaging) in a behavior, your patient will experience results. Help them determine how they feel? what they think? etc. Results can be positive or negative. When results are negative, such as feelings of frustration or guilt, they can become triggers for further inactivity or unhealthy eating. Negative thoughts such as: "I blew it," or "I'll never get this right" can also become triggers for the unhealthy behaviors.

SELF-MONITORING

For your patient to identify triggers for her behavior, have her continue with her current lifestyle but complete a detailed self-monitoring record. Your patient should complete either a dietary record (Table 4) or an activity record (Table 5) (Guare et al., 1989). Patients should record their food intake (amount, calories, fat grams, etc.) or their activity level (time, distance, type of physical activity, etc.). The record should also include a place to list potential triggers including places, people, feelings, time of day, sleep, thoughts, workload, hunger, energy level, etc. Many patients often state that it is difficult to identify emotional triggers. It can be challenging for some individuals to rate their mood if this is a new task. In this case, modify your patients self-monitoring record form to include a sad face, a neutral face, or a happy face for each meal or physical activity session. Your patient can check the face that reflects her mood. After completing the monitoring record for one week, look for patterns in her behavior. Does your patient overeat when she skips breakfast or attends social eating situations? Does your patient skip physical activity when she works overtime or stays up too late? Look for trends that occur over the course of the week(s). Once a pattern is identified, you can begin to set goals for change and teach her to identify specific solutions for problems she encounters.

SETTING INITIAL GOALS FOR CHANGE

Sometimes when people want to change, they set vague, poorly defined goals like: "I want to be healthier," or "I want to lose weight." The problem is that these goals do not provide a direction on how to accomplish them. In contrast, specific behavioral goals provide focus, direction, feedback, and motivation. There are six steps to goal setting (Table 6) (Murphy, 1997). If, for example, your patient wants to have healthier eating habits—the first step would be to select a specific behavior that is involved in eating a healthy diet. Eating a balanced breakfast every day and having a piece of fruit instead of a candy bar for a mid-afternoon snack are examples of behavioral goals that are part of developing healthier eating patterns. Encourage your patient to set a specific goal. For example, a specific goal is having a piece of fruit at 3:30 p.m. Monday through Friday. Next, evaluate the difficulty of the goal. Is this goal reasonable, or is it too challenging? It is helpful to break down long-term goals into small steps that are reasonable and achievable. For example, a long-term goal of achieving regular physical activity (150 minutes of moderate-intensity activity each week) can be broken down into several small goals that start simple and get progressively more challenging. After discussing a plan for beginning physical activity with their physician, your patient may set an initial goal of walking 5 minutes a day the first week, then increase to 7 minutes the next week, and so on until they reach a long-term goal of walking for 30 minutes, five days per week.

Having the patient take an active role in selecting her goals is important. If your patient feels that expectations from others are being forced upon her, she may not be as successful in initiating lifestyle changes. Your role is to guide her in this process. Targeting weekdays, when your patient's schedule may be more predict-

TABLE 4
Sample Dietary Record

	Time	Food	Amount	Fat (g)	Calories	Setting	Mood
Breakfast							
Lunch							
Dinner							
Snacks							

TABLE 5
Sample Physical Activity Record

	Type of Physical Activity (e.g., walking, biking, etc.)	Minutes
Monday		
Tuesday		
Wednesday		
Thursday		
Friday		
Saturday		
Sunday		

TABLE 6
Steps for Setting Goals

- Choose a behavioral goal.
- Choose a specific goal.
- Choose a reasonable goal.
- Choose both short- and long-term goals.
- Choose your own goals.
- Anticipate challenges and problem-solve solutions.

Adapted from Murphy, S. M., *The Achievement Zone*, Putnam, New York, 1997.

able, can be a reasonable start. As your patient sets goals it is important to help her anticipate obstacles to achieving them. When problems or barriers impede progress toward meeting goals, use problem-solving techniques to help your patient find solutions.

PROBLEM-SOLVING

After identifying a trigger or encountering an obstacle, your patient may need to avoid, manage, or change the situation in some way. Problem-solving is a five step (Table 7), structured approach your patient can use to find good solutions to problems (Chiauzzi, 1991). The first step is to help your patient clearly identify a specific problem. Your patient cannot problem-solve a solution to eating too much junk food. However, if your patient frequently eats junk food at 10:00 at night while watching TV with a friend or family member, this is a problem that can be solved. The situation is clear and well defined. Your patient may need to problem-solve many situations over time to have healthy eating habits or maintain regular participation in physical activity, but it is critical to focus on one problem at a time. The next step is to generate a list of possible solutions. In this example, your patient could read and avoid TV, drink a glass of water, plan a nutritious snack, ask the person not to snack at that time, knit or do a crossword puzzle at that time. The important thing at this step is to encourage her to generate 4 to 8 possible solutions and to be creative. The next step is to evaluate the merits of each solution. For example, your patient is too tired at 10:00 to read, and she already asked the other person in an assertive manner not to snack but he continues to do so; having a piece of fruit might work. Step four is to implement the solution and step five is to have her evaluate the success of the solution. If the solution worked, great! If not, choose another solution and try it. The advantages of problem-solving are that it focuses in on a specific problem, generates more than one solution to each problem, and if the solution doesn't work, some alternatives have already been identified.

TABLE 7
Steps for Problem-Solving

1. Clearly define the problem.
2. Brainstorm possible solutions.
3. Evaluate pros and cons of each solution.
4. Implement solution.
5. Evaluate results.

MAKING DIETARY AND ACTIVITY CHANGES A REGULAR HABIT

Many people are able to begin making behavioral changes but have difficulty incorporating them into their daily life. Unfortunately, it can be more difficult for patients to keep new habits going than it was to get started in the first place. The good news is that many of the skills that got your patient started can also be used to make new behaviors into regular habits.

TRACKING PROGRESS

As previously outlined, your patient began self-monitoring her activity and eating patterns to identify areas where she could make changes. Now your patient can use this same technique to help make these new practices more regular habits. Begin by having your patient think about which behaviors she would like to do more often. Review the steps for goal setting that we outlined earlier. Encourage her to be as clear and specific as possible. Have her avoid thinking in general terms such as "I'd like to be more physically active" or "I should eat less fat." It will be more useful for your patient to have goals like "I'd like to walk 3 times this week." Just as your patient did when she began to make changes, have her keep a log which reflects both her goal(s) for the week and the things she has done to accomplish her goal(s). Your patient should use her log to write down what happened whenever her plans were interrupted and as a tool for identifying patterns and common obstacles that get in her way.

BALANCING THE PROS AND CONS

One type of obstacle that can be a problem is lack of motivation. Many women are aware, in a general way, of the importance of leading a physically active lifestyle and eating foods that are low in fat and high in fiber. Unfortunately, wanting to do the right things for general reasons like better health is not very motivating for many people. If your patient's activity/diet log shows that her plans are frequently interrupted, and there doesn't seem to be any pattern to the disruptions, it may be that your patient hasn't identified the specific things that will keep her motivated.

One strategy that can help is to determine your patient's "Decisional Balance" (Table 8) (Marcus, Rakowski, and Rossi, 1992). This is similar to the technique you used to help your patient determine if she was ready for change. In the simplest of these methods, your patient lists all the benefits (Pros) of practicing the new behavior and then lists all the negative things, or hassles (Cons), associated with this new behavior. For example, if your patient is trying to be more regular in her physical activity, one Pro might be "exercising makes me feel more energetic;" a Con might be "it takes too much time." If your patient's Cons list is longer than her Pros list, it may explain why she is having trouble. More sophisticated decisional balance procedures consider how important each Pro and Con is to the individual. Using the decisional balance sheet shown in Table 8, instruct your patient to think of the Pros and Cons and circle the number in the right-hand column that reflects how important it is to her. Total the numbers circled for Pros and Cons separately. Subtract the Cons from the Pros (Pros minus Cons) to determine you patient's decisional balance. Decreasing the Cons can help increase motivation; however, behavior change is more likely if the number of Pros is increased and if the Pros become more salient. Refer back to the techniques for "Helping Patients Get Ready For Change" for methods you can use to enhance motivation.

TABLE 8
Determining Your Decisional Balance for Physical Activity

	How important to Me?				
	Not at all Important				Very Important
The things I like about being physically active are...					
1. ______________________	1	2	3	4	5
2. ______________________	1	2	3	4	5
3. ______________________	1	2	3	4	5
4. ______________________	1	2	3	4	5
5. ______________________	1	2	3	4	5
The things I find difficult about becoming physically active are...					
1. ______________________	1	2	3	4	5
2. ______________________	1	2	3	4	5
3. ______________________	1	2	3	4	5
4. ______________________	1	2	3	4	5
5. ______________________	1	2	3	4	5
Total for the Pros ______________					
Total for the Cons ______________					
Decisional Balance ______________ (Pros – Cons)					

Adapted from Marcus, B. H., Rakowski, W., and Rossi, J. S., *Health Psychol.*, 11, 267–271, 1992.

Longer Term Goal Setting

Once your patient has achieved some regularity in the practice of her new behavior, it's time to begin looking farther into the future. Up until now your patient has been setting goals for the day, or maybe for the week. After about 2 to 3 weeks of achieving her goals, your patient might consider her goals in terms of *regularity*. For instance, instead of setting a goal of exercising three times per week, your patient might focus on regularity by setting a goal of exercising three or more times each week for the next month. Remember to help your patient set goals in terms of things she can control (e.g., her behavior), and not results she can't control (e.g., changes in cholesterol, blood pressure, or weight). Although dietary change and regular physical activity can help women lose weight, reduce cholesterol, and lower blood pressure, these things are also affected by genetics, life stress, and other factors. For instance, weight training is a very good type of physical activity, especially for older women. It helps increase muscle strength, balance, and bone density—and as a result it reduces the number of falls and the extent of injuries incurred from falls (Fiatarone et al., 1990). While your patient could end up looking and feeling better as she builds lean muscle, these changes may not show up on the scale. If your patient has been working out regularly, she should feel proud of her accomplishments. However, if your patient had set her goal in terms of changes on the scale, instead of changes in her behavior, she may feel disappointed.

COMMON BARRIERS TO CHANGE AND EXAMPLES OF SOLUTIONS

One of the most common difficulties people have in reducing the fat in their diets is all the hidden fat in prepared and convenience foods (Sobal, 1995). Most foods available at restaurants (especially fast-food and sandwich places) and through vending machines are high in fat. Your patient may need to rely more on foods she prepares herself in order to avoid high-fat foods. This involves planning ahead. A common problem for people trying to become more physically active is finding the time (King et al., 1992). Since women tend to lead very busy lives, and often take care of many other people such as children and parents, extra time for physical activity is unlikely to happen all by itself. Two strategies for dealing with the time crunch are for your patient to exercise in several brief (10 to 15 minute) bouts each day, to accumulate to 30 minutes at least five times a week, or to schedule the time into the day just as she does for other important activities.

SOCIAL SUPPORT

Getting help and support from others is helpful to many people, but seems to be particularly important for women (Wing, 1991). Having others around who support your patient's efforts or better yet, who share their goals and participate with them can make a big difference in helping them turn behavior changes into long-term habits. Sometimes having additional support can increase an individual's confidence in her ability to change. For example, have your patient try joining a class (cooking or exercising), especially one where new skills are taught or interesting information is presented, as this will help preserve motivation and introduce her to other people who share her interests. Suggest that she arrange to meet a friend for a walk or other physical activity as a way to ensure she doesn't lose enthusiasm at the last minute. Chances are that your patient will make exercising more of a priority if someone is waiting for her.

INTERNAL AND EXTERNAL REWARDS

Rewards can be very important for making new behaviors into regular habits. Although the new things your patient is doing have their own built-in rewards (like better health), these may not be very noticeable, or may only be something that will be important years from now. It can be very helpful for your patient to give herself rewards for meeting more immediate goals. Rewards can be either *internal* or *external*. In some ways external rewards are the easiest to understand. Buying a new outfit, going to the movies, and taking some quiet time to read a book are all examples of external rewards your patient could give herself. Internal rewards are things your patient can say to herself when she achieves her goals. Examples include thinking of oneself in positive ways and congratulating oneself ("Good Job!" "Nice Going!") for doing that extra lap, walking those extra five minutes or choosing the lighter dinner option instead of the heavy fat-ridden entree.

MAINTAINING DIETARY OR PHYSICAL ACTIVITY BEHAVIOR CHANGES

One of the greatest challenges of lifestyle change is long-term maintenance of the new healthier behavior. Research has shown that people who are successful at maintaining new behaviors are those who

- Anticipate and plan for difficult times
- Recover quickly from setbacks
- Are creative and introduce variety into the new behaviors
- Are helpful to others making similar changes
- Get support from family and friends for the new behaviors
- Reward themselves for their progress

PLANNING FOR DIFFICULT TIMES

Many individuals who have made changes such as staying active or eating a nutritious diet say that they can do so during a normal routine day. Celebrations, vacations, illness, and injury are some of the events that tend to throw people off track. To help identify specific situations, have them complete the quiz on maintaining physical activity (Table 9).

TABLE 9
Determining Your Confidence for Staying Active

How confident are you that you can be physically active in each of the following situations?

	Not at all Confident		Moderately Confident		Extremely Confident
	1	2	3	4	5
a) When I am bored	1	2	3	4	5
b) When I am in a bad mood	1	2	3	4	5
c) When I'm on vacation	1	2	3	4	5
d) When I don't have time	1	2	3	4	5
e) When the weather is bad	1	2	3	4	5

Adapted from Marcus, B. H., Selby, V. C., Niaura, R. S., and Rossi, J. S., *Res. Q. Exerc. Sport,* 63, 60–66, 1992.

Your patient may have indicated that it is difficult for her to be physically active while on vacation. A key point is to anticipate and plan for these difficult times. Use the problem-solving techniques detailed in the previous section. Some solutions you may suggest are calling ahead to find out about the exercise facilities at the hotels at which she will be staying during her vacation, or packing her workout clothes and shoes to remind her to stay active while on vacation. When your patient plans ahead, she is less likely to be thrown off by the change in her normal routine. You can use the same technique to assess her confidence for maintaining healthy dietary behaviors in different situations.

GETTING BACK ON TRACK

During the process of changing a behavior and maintaining those changes, it is common for individuals to experience setbacks or slips back into unhealthy behaviors. This process is know as relapse. Relapse involves a series of events in which the individual reverts to unhealthy behaviors, temporarily or even permanently (Marlatt and George, 1998). For example, your patient may eat a high fat meal when she has not planned to do so. The key to making sure your patient does not slip into her old ways lies *not in the slip by itself, but what happens after the slip*. For example, many people on a diet, after eating cookies and cake at a party, often tell themselves that they are failures, worthless, and are now off the diet. This leads to people giving up and returning to old habits (Brownell, 1994). It is much more helpful, when a slip occurs, to review what has happened, and identify what your patient could do to prevent it if a similar situation was to occur again.

> Consider the example of Sally who has maintained a well-balanced diet for about a year. A friend was visiting and during the dinner celebration, Sally ate fried chicken, french fries, and cake. The next day, she felt miserable and thought that all her efforts over the year had been wasted. That made it difficult for her to plan her meals that day and this problem continued over the next 2 weeks. She then realized that she could learn from her slip. She tried to determine what had led to those poor choices at the dinner. She found that allowing her friend to order for both of them and being very hungry before the meal had led to the high-fat dinner. To maintain a healthy diet and prevent future slips, Sally decided to order her own meal at future celebrations and to eat a small snack before such dinners.

VARY THE ROUTINE

Maintaining new behaviors may become easier if your patient introduces some variety in her new routine. For example, if your patient has been walking every day along the same route and it has become boring, she can try to change the routine by walking a different route, listening to music while she walks, calling a friend to accompany her, or joining a walking club. Your patient may also want to think about trying different types of activities; for example, she may want to walk on weekdays and swim or play tennis on weekends. Using a variety of activities may not only prevent boredom but also prevent overuse injuries. Similarly, six months of having the same type of sandwich and salad at lunchtime can become tiresome.

REWARDS REVISITED

To keep your patient's new behaviors exciting and fun, be sure they reward themselves for being active or for staying with healthy food choices. They may not be rewarding themselves as frequently as they were during the initial period of change, but encourage them to continue to reward themselves and recognize how their bodies change in positive ways with their new habits. These rewards could be positive statements (internal rewards) your patients could say to themselves (e.g., "I've come a long way from being a couch potato."). Your patients may also want to include special rewards for meeting some of their long-term goals. Some examples include buying plants or new clothes, taking cooking classes, or getting a magazine subscription. Behaviors that bring positive internal and/or external rewards are more likely to be maintained.

SHARE THE EXPERIENCE OF CHANGE WITH OTHERS

When your patient has established these new behaviors, she can reach out to family or friends who may be thinking of becoming more active or changing their dietary intake. Your patient can discuss her experiences with them and share her tips on what helped her to become successful: in other words, she can become a *role model* for others interested in a healthy lifestyle. This technique is helpful for maintaining healthy behaviors because it can be a source of mutual social support for the new behaviors and can modify social triggers for unhealthy behaviors.

REFERENCES

Brownell, K. D., *The Learn Program for Weight Control*, American Health Publishing, Dallas, TX, 1994.

Brownell, K. D. and Cohen, L. R., Adherence to dietary regimens: 1. An overview of research, *Behav. Med.*, 20, 149–154, 1995.

Chiauzzi, E. J., *Preventing Relapse in the Addictions: A Biopsychosocial Approach*, Pergamon Press, New York, 1991.

Dishman, R. K. and Sallis, J. F., Determinants and interventions for physical activity and exercise, in *Physical activity, fitness, and health: International proceedings and consensus statement*, Bouchard, B., Shephard, R. J., and Stephens, T., Eds., Human Kinetics, Champaign, IL, 214–238, 1994.

Fiatarone, M. A., Marks, E. C., Ryan, N. D., Meredith, C. N., Lipsitz, L. A., and Evans, W. J., High-intensity strength training in nonagenarians, *J. Am. Med. Assoc.*, 263, 3029–3034, 1990.

Guare, J. C., Wing, R. R., Marcus, M. D., Epstein, L. H., Burton, L. R., and Gooding, W. E., Analysis of changes in eating behavior and weight loss in type II diabetic patients, *Diabetes Care*, 12, 500–503, 1989.

King, A. C., Blair, S. N., Bild, D., Dubbert, P. M., Marcus, B. H., Oldridge, N. O., Paffenbarger, R. S., Powell, K. E., and Yeager, K., Determinants of physical activity and interventions in adults, *Med. Sci. Sports Exerc.*, 24, S221–S236, 1992.

Marcus, B. H., Rakowski, W., and Rossi, J. S., Assessing motivational readiness and decision making for exercise, *Health Psychol.*, 11, 267–271, 1992.

Marcus, B. H., Rossi, J. S., Selby, V. C., Niaura, R. S., and Abrams, D. B., The stages and processes of exercise adoption and maintenance in a worksite sample, *Health Psychol.*, 11, 386–395, 1992.

Marcus, B. H., Selby, V. C., Niaura, R. S., and Rossi, J. S., Self-efficacy and the stages of exercise behavior change, *Res. Q. Exerc. Sport*, 63, 60–66, 1992.

Marlatt, G. A. and George, W. H., Relapse prevention and maintenance of optimal health, in *The Handbook of Health Behavior Change*, Shumaker, S. A., Schron, E. B., Ockene, J. K., and McBee, W. L., Eds., Springer, New York, 1998, 33–58.

Miller, W. R. and Rolnick, S., *Motivational Interviewing: Preparing People to Change Addictive Behavior*, New York: Guilford, 1991.

Murphy, S. M., *The Achievement Zone*, Putnam Publishing, New York, 1997.

NIH Technology Assessment Conference Panel. Methods for voluntary weight loss and control, Ann. Intern. Med., 116(11), 942–949, 1992.

Pate, R. R., Pratt, M., Blair, S. N., Haskell, W. L., Macera, C. A., Bouchard, C., Buchner, D., Ettinger, W., Heath, G. W., King, A. C., Kriska, A., Leon, A. S., Marcus, B. H., Morris, J., Paffenbarger, R. S., Patrick, K., Pollock, M. L., Rippe, J. M., Sallis, J., and Wilmore, J. H., Physical activity and public health: A recommendation from the Centers for Disease Control and the American College of Sports Medicine, *J. Am. Med. Assoc.*, 273, 402–407, 1995.

Prochaska, J. O. and DiClemente, C. C., Stages and processes of self-change of smoking: Toward and integrative model, *J. Consult. Clin. Psychol.*, 51, 390–395, 1983.

Sobal, J., Social influences on body weight, in *Eating Disorders and Obesity: A Comprehensive Handbook*, Brownell, K. D. and Fairburn, C. G., Eds., Guilford Press, New York, 1995, 73–77.

Verhoef, M. J. and Love, E. J., Women's exercise participation: The relevance of social roles compared to non-role-related determinants, *Canad. J. Publ. Health,* 83(5), 367–370, 1992.

Wing, R. R., Marcus, M. D., Epstein, L. H., and Jawad, A., A "family-based" approach to the treatment of obese type II diabetic patients, *J. Consult. Clin. Psychol.*, 59(1), 156–162, 1991.

PATIENT RESOURCE LIST

Some excellent resources for more information on programs on becoming active:

1. *Living with Exercise: Improving Your Health Through Moderate Physical Activity*, Steven N. Blair, P.E.D., American Health Publishing Company, Dallas, TX, 1991.
2. Publications by the National Institute on Aging, P.O. Box 8057, Gaithersburg, MD 20898-8057, Phone (301) 495-3455.
3. *Activating Ideas: Promoting Physical Activity Among Older Adults*, AARP, 601 E Street N.W., Washington D.C. 20049, Phone (202) 434-2230.

For eating healthy and wealth loss:

1. *The LEARN Program for Weight Control*, 7th ed., Kelly D. Brownell, Ph.D., American Health, Dallas, TX, 1994.
2. *The Weight Maintenance Survival Guide*, Kelly D. Brownell, Ph.D. and Judith Rodin, Ph.D., Brownell & Hager, Dallas, TX, 1990.
3. *Weight Loss Through Persistence*, Daniel S. Kirschenbaum, Ph.D., New Harbinger, Oakland, CA, 1994.

PRACTITIONER RESOURCE LIST

1. Department of Health and Human Services, *Physical Activity and Health: A Report of the Surgeon General*, Centers for Disease Control and Prevention, National Center for Chronic Disease Prevention, 1996.
2. Marcus, B. H. and Forsyth, L. H., Tailoring interventions to promote physically active lifestyles in women, *Women's Hlth. Iss.*, 8, 104–111, 1998.
3. Miller, W. R. and Rolnick, S., *Motivational interviewing: Preparing people to change addictive behavior*, Guilford, New York, 1991.
4. Shumaker, S. A., Schron, E. B., Ockene, J. K., and McBee, W. L., Eds., *The Handbook of Health Behavior Change*, Springer, New York, 1998.

27 Environmental Design for Health

Patricia A. Moore and Maria A. Fiatarone Singh

CONTENTS

UNIVERSAL ACCESS VS. HEALTH PROMOTION

There is a dynamic tension that exists between the equally laudable goals of assuring universal access in design and at the same time promoting optimal levels of physical activity and performance. For example, installing elevators in public buildings broadens access for the disabled and frail of all ages. Yet, paradoxically, it may have the undesirable and unforseen side effect of promoting sedentariness in the able-bodied or near-frail, thus hastening their rates of physiologic decline. A major unresolved question in this era of universal access and safety regulations is the potentially opposing forces that may result from these seemingly unrelated goals. In its extreme form, we see "falls prevention" designed into the environment of nursing homes in the form of physical restraints, "geri-chairs" which prohibit rising without assistance, locked stairwells, and environments generally unfriendly to mobility of most sorts. And yet the physiologic consequences of such "safety precautions" include muscle weakness and atrophy, loss of balance and postural reflexes, cardiovascular deconditioning, inactive minds, withdrawal from environmental stimuli, and ultimately a worsening of the fall risk profile. A more creative approach to universal access and safety can by contrast embrace a philosophy and environment that encourage rather than restrict mobility and function while adapting to underlying limitations and disabilities. This more visionary approach which integrates both access and health promotion ideals will require the collaboration of engineers, architects, psychologists, and physiologists to create building and grounds design with a suitable (accessible and safe) structure, while at the same time developing a behavioral design or plan for encouraging its appropriate usage. In this chapter we will suggest ways that this can be accomplished in the home setting, the nursing home, the health practitioner's office setting, and residential housing sites for the elderly.

THE HOME ENVIRONMENT

My mother has always enjoyed an active life and relatively good health, for which I am most grateful. Now, having passed her 70th birthday, Mom maintains a daily schedule of household chores, works in her garden, and perhaps most important to her physical well-being and personal happiness, she recreates with her two grandsons and their friends in the neighborhood. Recently retired from teaching in the grammar school a few blocks from her home, Mom begins each day by walking my nephews to school, with our family's dog. Her return trip usually includes a stop at the local convenience store, for a quart of milk or loaf of bread. After her breakfast, there is the bed to be made, laundry, vacuuming, windows to wash, perhaps some ironing, and of course, her most dreaded chore, planning dinner.

These tasks of daily living require a full range of abilities. As we age, our capacity for performing these necessary skills will determine our level of independence and our quality of life. To be able to do the things we want and choose to do, we must be properly equipped. We all seem to have a favorite utensil we rely on to make our special sauce or favorite treat. For me, it is a multipurpose grater my Mother presented to me in a basket of goodies when I left home for college. Even though, over the years I've received and purchased other things to do the job, I always reach for this much used gift. We are surrounded by such tools, the things that extend our abilities and allow us to achieve goals, simple or complex. To enhance our individual capabilities, we need to consider our homes a "tool chest" for a lifetime of good health and independence.

THE HOME AUDIT

Just as we carefully arranged our homes for the safety of our children, and now grandchildren, we need to evaluate how well our house meets the unique needs of aging with varying levels of health and function. With normal aging, our vision, hearing, balance, strength, and endurance will change, even though some of these changes can be minimized by attention to physical activity and nutritional habits over the years. In addition, some of us will deal with the effects of arthritis or a stroke. But regardless of the individual challenges that exist, we all have capacities.

Selecting the proper complement of products in our homes allows us to create an atmosphere that celebrates our uniqueness and optimizes our health and well-being.

To be sure that your home is addressing your personal needs for health and fitness, you can conduct a "Home Audit." You'll need to analyze each area and room in your house and record your findings so that you can make necessary changes and improvements in the design of your home and how it functions and meets your needs.

THE GREAT OUTDOORS

Whether you live in a private house, apartment, or complex, your entrance ways, porch, patio, and yard can put you at risk of a fall. Check to be sure that you have adequate lighting at every door, especially if there are steps. Garages, tool sheds, and utility rooms are often places where an additional light will make for safer access and use.

A door mat is a good idea to keep dirt or rain and snow out of your home, but be sure that it is secure, so you won't trip or slip. You can find a variety of very good options in home shopping catalogs, hardware stores, and through carpet dealers, as well as skid-resistant materials that will keep mats and rugs in place.

Every staircase and landing should be surrounded by a strong railing or fence, so that you can climb and descend safely, especially in inclement weather. Adding these fixtures will increase your confidence in your ability to use the stairs safely, and discourage a sense of being trapped behind these potential barriers to mobility.

If you live with snow, be sure to keep salt available, and clear a path instead of trying to maintain your balance on an icy stair. It is particularly hazardous for older adults who rarely exercise vigorously to shovel snow, as the combination of the cold air and the intense aerobic exertion may provoke angina or a heart attack. My mother enjoys shoveling the white stuff, which can be good exercise if you are consistently active, but you can always make arrangements with a neighbor or friend to assist you in the event of a storm.

If you have a gravel sidewalk or driveway, you might want to consider having a path of flat, firm bricks or flagstones added to increase your ability to walk and provide an attractive setting in which to do it. For those of us who use a cane, walker, or wheelchair, this addition also makes yards and gardens more accessible and enjoyable. Gardening is still possible for those who are wheelchair bound or unable to kneel on the ground because of arthritis or osteoporosis. Padded kneeling boards can eliminate some of the strain, and for even greater access, elevating flower and vegetable beds to boxes which are at the height of a chair or wheelchair can provide hours of outdoor activity and creative gardening without neck, back, hip, or joint pain. Even those who cannot walk at all can enjoy gardening in this way. Because forward flexion of the spine places tremendous compressive forces on the anterior portion of osteopenic vertebrae, it can lead to compression fractures in the woman with osteoporosis of the spine. So sitting upright while gardening is a good alternative in this type of person, even if she is still capable of kneeling on the ground.

FLOORS AND STAIRCASES

At any age, a slippery floor, a loose tread, or an unexpected object in our path can cause a dangerous fall. If your home has carpeting, check doorways and stairs to be sure that there are no raised edges or tears. If the pile is high or worn, you might want to consider removing it, especially from stairs. Low-gloss and skid-resistant finishes can be applied to wood floors and stairs to make walking easier and much safer.

Throughout your home, be sure electric cords do not interfere with any walkway. If you have any light cords under a rug, add an extension cord to that fixture, or have an electrician provide a more convenient outlet, so that you do not risk a fire from a frayed cord or a trip over a bump in the carpet. Floor-mounted outlets, which can be located under tables or chairs, provide a safe solution for those places where a cord would otherwise run across the floor.

Be sure that area rugs are secure. Small rugs that are typically found in kitchens and bathrooms help keep floors clean and dry, but they present a risk for tripping. Skid-resistant pads and strips should be placed under all rugs.

In the bathroom, you might consider adding a new rubberized floor. These materials are available in sheets or tiles from carpet dealers and provide an added level of skid resistance when wet, as well as a cushion, should you ever fall, which may make the difference between a bruise and a hip fracture. The bathroom is the site of many, if not most, indoor falls. Indoor-outdoor carpeting is also available in sheets and tiles. This soft surface stays warm in the winter and will make the bathroom safer for you and your grandchildren.

Staircase railings should be strong and secure. If you don't have a railing on each side of a staircase, consider having one added. As a reminder that you are approaching the top or bottom of a staircase, apply a decal or paint of contrasting color or finish so that you see or feel the difference on the handrail. Decorative skid-resistant bathtub decals are especially effective for this feature. You might also consider alternating the color or finish of one step to the next. If you have difficulty seeing, this design element will make traversing them much easier.

Stairs to basements and cellars should be well lighted and feature a rubber tread. This is especially important if your laundry area is located on this level, as you will often have your view of the steps blocked by what you are carrying. Make sure water or spilled liquids in the basement are not left to be tracked up the stairs and predispose to falls.

Check the level of lighting on all stairs. A brighter wattage of bulb might improve your ability to see each step, but if you find that areas of a staircase still don't receive adequate light, hire an electrical contractor to install additional wall fixtures or a ceiling fixture which you can easily reach when it comes time to replace a bulb.

It is good to remember that stairs represent both a safety challenge as noted above, and an opportunity for increased strength, power, endurance, and balance. With a few tips, the stairs can be transformed into safe yet challenging pieces of exercise equipment which are always at hand. For example, the bottom step can be used as a way to train for balance by hanging your heels off it, and slowly rising up on your toes as high as possible and then slowly lowering your body weight again (see also Chapter 2 for more tips). Repeat this move five to ten times whenever you start to climb the stairs. Initially this should be done while holding onto the handrail, but as you improve. you can graduate to one fingertip support and even closed eyes. Once even this is too easy, you can do it on one foot instead of two, which will give twice the stimulation to the muscles around the ankle, improving both strength and coordination. This is particularly important for the prevention of falls and as a way of rehabilitating after an ankle injury such as a sprain or fracture. Because balance is so often a problem in older women, these exercises form an important addition to any exercise routine. Initially, they should always be done with a relative or neighbor standing behind you in case you lose your balance.

Similarly, stairs can become a handy aerobic and strengthening device. For strengthening, climb slowly, lifting your whole body weight with one foot, without holding on if balance is good. Try to advance to taking two steps at a time in this way, feeling the force develop in the muscles at the front of the thigh (quadriceps) as the lift occurs, and remembering not to hold your breath. Climbing stairs rapidly, on the other hand, is a good aerobic and power-building exercise, and the aerobic intensity can be increased by carrying an extra load as you do it. Doing it once as fast as you can will increase explosive muscle power, thought to be important in the reflexes that maintain balance in the face of a sudden perturbation. Doing it slightly less rapidly, but for a period of 5 to 10 minutes without stopping will increase cardiovascular endurance. So stop avoiding that trip to the basement to bring up the laundry—this onerous chore can become an aerobic routine if you simply change your attitude toward the work to be done and conceptualize it as an opportunity to enhance fitness instead.

It is important that stairs to be used in any of the above ways are well lighted and ventilated, covered in nonslip carpeting, have a sturdy handrail on both sides, and a landing which is covered with a soft padded material. Attic and basement stairs are particularly hazardous and should not be used unless modified in this way. These stairways are often used as extra storage space, which will certainly not enhance the safety or feasibility of exploiting their exercise potential.

Once your confidence in using stairs builds, try to move some household items you need to use frequently up or down stairs so that you will have an excuse to climb to get them. A good trick to reinforce this behavior is to keep a little calendar or magnetic noteboard at the top of the stairs. Every time you climb a flight, place a checkmark on the calendar for that day. See what your normal pattern is for one week and then challenge yourself to double or triple the number of flights per day. If stairs are too painful because of knee arthritis, wait until you have strengthened the muscles around the knee with some progressive resistance training (see Chapter 2), and then try to incorporate stairs into your daily routine. One of the most common things women report after resistance training is that they can climb stairs without pain for the first time in years, and this change may be noticeable in a matter of weeks.

FURNISHINGS

Walk throughout each room in your home to determine if there is clear and easy access in every direction. Whether you are walking through a darkened room or your grandchild is romping through the house, an ill-positioned chair or ottoman could cause a fall.

If your favorite table or chair has developed a loose leg or joint, have a carpenter or friend secure it properly. When purchasing new pieces, check to be sure they are sturdy and substantial. Try to select nightstands and low tables with rounded corners and edges. In the event that you fall and strike a piece of furniture, you'll be less likely to sustain a cut or bruise.

Chair rails and furniture can provide for a natural handhold while you walk through a room or a corridor. If balance is poor or you use a cane when you walk, consider adding handrails along walls instead. These railings can be aesthetic, as well as functional. This approach is preferable to depending on furniture that may not be sturdy enough to support body weight and eliminates potential clutter created by arranging furniture as walking supports.

Chairs and sofas should provide you with a comfortable backrest and good support. If you find that a seat cushion is too deep, making it difficult to rise from a seated position, add decorative pillows for more support. When selecting new seating, look for firm cushions and a seat which does not press against the back of your knees. Such seating, especially wooden chairs, can impinge on the peroneal nerve, which will cause numbness. Also look for armrests that are easy to hold when you lift yourself from a chair. Higher seats will be helpful if osteoarthritis of the knee and hip make rising painful.

If it's time to replace a sagging mattress, you might want to consider the purchase of a contour bed. These beds operate on a remote control that allows you to adjust the mattress for a variety of sleeping options. Some individuals with cardiorespiratory problems find a seated position the only way to obtain a good night's sleep. You can also complete a routine of stretching exercises and leg lifts from the comfort of these beds, when lying on the floor is not feasible.

While not technically furniture, the presence of a portable telephone is an important addition for your home. Having a phone in close proximity to your activities provides an added sense of comfort and safety. The majority of models available today include a volume control that makes it easier to hear whether you are near the washing machine or in a noisy backyard, enjoying a swim. Many falls are reported when people with mobility difficulties or arthritis rush to answer a telephone in a remote room. Such portable phones can prevent these kinds of accidents.

Lighting

With age, our eyes require more light for reading and close work. Therefore, check each room in the home to be sure that the light sources provide even lighting, and that there are no areas of dark or shade.

If you have rooms or halls with only ceiling fixtures, you might want to add wall sconces or table lamps. Changing ceiling bulbs presents a hazard at any age, so be sure you are comfortable with the height and use a sturdy stepladder or stool; one with a handle or back that allows you to support yourself while you remove and add a bulb. An electrician can also provide you with ceiling fixtures that are on adjustable cords. These lights can be lowered and raised to create various lighting levels, as well as for ease in maintenance.

Place night lights throughout your home. When we wake at night to use the bathroom or to get a drink, our eyes require more time to adjust to darkness than when we were younger. Be sure you have flashlights and a supply of batteries placed throughout your home in key locations. Your nightstand, the bathroom, kitchen, front hall, basement, and garage should feature storage for a flashlight. Several manufacturers produce a wall-mounting bracket for their lights, so you won't have to fumble through a kitchen drawer during a power failure.

The Bathroom

In addition to replacing your current flooring with a slip-resistant, softer material, you should install grab bars in your bathtub or shower. The grab bars available today include a variety of colors and finishes that provide for a decorative and safe feature.

If you have any concerns about your balance or rising from a seated position, place another grab bar by the toilet. Although towel racks are often substituted for this function, they are meant to hold the weight of a towel, not an adult, and will loosen and create hazards if used as grab bars inappropriately. On the other hand, a properly installed grab bar can serve a dual function as a towel rack, which will disguise its more medical or utilitarian look some people may not want to introduce into their bathroom. Be sure to utilize the services of a licensed contractor or carpenter when installing grab bars, so you are certain they have been properly placed in wall studs. Hardware and home health shops that sell grab bars and other safety features for your home can typically provide you with a listing of trustworthy builders in your area.

There are also a number of bath benches and stools that are a helpful addition for those times when you might want to simply soak your feet or wash the dog. These are useful for individuals who cannot negotiate sitting down in a tub and perhaps find standing in the shower difficult because of weakness, dizziness, or poor balance. Installation of a handheld shower head provides an added range of comfort and ease when washing your hair or giving your grandchild a bath.

The Kitchen

Perhaps the biggest problem with the traditional American kitchen is that it was designed by men. With great respect for my male colleagues, this observation has resulted in a great amount of recent effort by designers and builders to better understand the use of the kitchen and the needs of both men and women and their families.

If your kitchen was built before 1990, you are likely surrounded by stationary shelving and a single counter height. Your storage cupboards require you to climb a stool or ladder to retrieve your favorite serving platter and there never seems to be enough room for everything you need in the pantry, if you are lucky enough to have a pantry.

To provide yourself, your family, and friends with an optimal variety of meals and nutritious snacks, your kitchen design must deliver a range of options for food preparation and storage. There are a number of additions, renovations, and appliances to consider that will make your time in the kitchen more productive and safer, as well as make it easier to achieve the nutritional goals set by you or your health care provider.

A visit to your local home improvement center will acquaint you with the range of adjustable shelves currently available. Some items, like lazy susan storage units and multilevel organizers don't require tools for installation. By simply re-orienting your existing storage space with these items, you can crate more room for items currently stored on higher shelves. I've undertaken this project in my own home which was built in the 1940s and now use the upper shelves for storage of collectibles, baskets, and cook books I rarely use, but can't bear to give away.

Space in your refrigerator can easily be added with clip-on trays and storage units for use under existing shelves. Transferring bottled juices to plastic containers with handles and pouring spouts makes them easier to store and use.

A mobile cart makes a welcome storage solution for everyday use and special occasions when more room is needed for a buffet or bar. When you find yourself in bed, nursing a cold, or enjoying a lazy day with a good book, your mobile cart makes a nice addition for your bedroom, with medicines, foodstuffs, and extra reading material close at hand. My mother uses an electrified cart that plugs into a nearby outlet, so she can keep her tea pot or vaporizer close at hand.

Hand tools and utensils have also been redesigned to make them easier to hold and use, such as the Good Grips™ line of kitchen utensils by OXO, for which I served on the design team. These tools feature a wide, soft grip handle that helps someone with arthritis or her granddaughter, whose inexperience makes for awkward maneuvers. OXO also makes a variety of flatware featuring this special handle and a new line of garden tools which make planting and tending to your fresh herbs and vegetables a welcome chore. The concept of these tools is particularly relevant to all adaptive design, in that the modification makes the task more comfortable for everyone, whether or not they have a disability, rather than just providing benefit to a narrow range of users. This concept may be applied to exercise equipment, walking paths, lighting design, and many other areas relevant to residential and institutional settings for older adults.

Fresh fruit and vegetable juices are much easier to prepare with electric juicers, and provide a very nutrient dense product that may make it easier to meet micronutrient nutritional goals for older women. You can select a commercial or consumer model, with prices that vary accordingly. My kitchen features one machine for fruit drinks and the other for my favorite, carrot juice.

The introduction of the microwave oven created a boon for instant popcorn and re-heated coffee, but is in fact a great way to preserve vitamins (e.g., steaming vegetables without water) or minimize fat (such as poaching fish in broth or wine). Processed food manufacturers and cook book publishers are quickly managing to catch up with the technological advance of the microwave with the creation of special meals, single-serving meals, and cooking tips that make the microwave an exceptional tool for the delivery of nutritious food. It is vital to the kitchen of functionally impaired or frail individuals who may not be able to spend the hours they formerly did preparing fresh meals from scratch, and who need to cover their nutrient requirements with small quantities of high quality food that is easily prepared.

The invention of no-heat, no-flame stoves gives us and our families the added benefit of safety, at any age. Whether you place a potholder too close to a burner or inquisitive, little fingers of grandchildren get too close, these stoves won't cause dangerous fires or burns. If you are considering the purchase of a new stove, this addition to the safety and security of your home is a worthy investment. It takes a little time to get accustomed to cooking without being able to see a flame, but with some practice, you will soon forget the stove you've had since you were a bride. The ease in cleaning will also convince even the staunchest holdouts, like my mother.

HOME GYMS AND EXERCISE EQUIPMENT

Now that you've made your home accessible, efficient, and safe, you might want to consider the ultimate addition for your lifelong health and fitness, the purchase of exercise equipment to complement your daily walk and other activities.

There are a number of stationary bicycles to chose from, but the most adaptable are those with a full semi-recumbent seat and backrest. This design allows you to sit comfortably, support your back, and pedal for an efficient cardiopulmonary workout. Ordinary upright stationary bikes have the problem of exacerbating low back pain from degenerative arthritis of the lumbar spine, as well as causing high compressive forces on osteopenic thoracic vertebrae due to the forward flexed posture they encourage. Even quite frail individuals can tolerate relatively long biking sessions with these machines due to the extra comfort and sense of security the full seat provides, which will enhance compliance with the exercise prescription as well as progression to higher levels of exertion over time.

Another investment that will promote both a good workout and the desirable physical results is a treadmill. There are two basic types for your consideration: those with a fixed handle and those with independent handles, which approximate the action of cross-country skiing. If coordination and balance permit, the arm and leg movement offers a more full-body workout that will expend more calories and enhance fitness accordingly. They can be difficult to coordinate for some individuals, however, and should be tried out in the store before committing to this relatively expensive purchase. Stair-climbers have become affordable additions to a home gym as well. These devices typically create long lines at fitness gyms, as they are easy to use and provide an excellent low impact aerobic workout and strengthening for important gluteal muscles, quadriceps, and calf muscles. Most models provide for an easy adjustment of the step tension feature and include a digital screen for monitoring your progress.

You should consider selection of any fitness equipment with an agreement for delivery and assembly, as the majority of units are heavy, bulky, and unassembled with purchase. Many major stores will also provide you with training and trade-in options, welcome features in creating a home gym that will provide you with cost-effective fitness.

Equipment for strength training has been described in Chapter 2, and the choice depends on space, financial considerations, and level of frailty.

All home exercise equipment suffers the common potential problem of becoming nothing more than an expensive coat hanger or box to be stored in the attic or under the bed, if there is no behavioral program aimed at adoption and adherence (see Chapter 26) which accompanies the purchase. Therefore, it may be best to avoid expensive purchases until steps have been taken to put exercise recommendations into action. Beginning exercise programs can be carried out using the staircases in the home, as described above, walking, and inexpensive free weights. Once a pattern has been established, reward progress and achievement of exercise goals with good, useful pieces of exercise equipment which will enhance compliance, provide new motivation, and encourage progression to more intensive levels of effort. It is usually a mistake to invest in a cheap piece of aerobic equipment, as these devices are often poorly constructed, unsuitable for prolonged or heavy use, and may not have the safety features and ability to track progress essential for lasting behavioral change.

RETHINKING TIME SPENT AT HOME

All the modifications above can only partially address the issues of optimum activity level in the home. Much of the change must come not from modifying the environment or the furnishings, but from changing the way in which the space and its contents are utilized. For example, the remote control is a wonderful invention for someone with significant disabilities, or for those times you are watching television from bed. But in daytime hours and when mobility is not problematic, take the opportunity at the end of a show to get up to change the channel instead, and include some stretches or balance exercises along the way as well. Even better, replace one of the chairs facing the television with a piece of exercise equipment, so that you can combine a sedentary pursuit with an active one, and create a new active habit without sacrificing anything. Similarly, doubling up on reading, knitting, or making the grocery list while riding a stationary bicycle can solve the universal problem of never having enough time to add exercise to an already full daily schedule.

Many other opportunities to become more physically active in the home setting present themselves if you are looking for them. When you unpack your groceries, repeat the action of reaching the top shelf with a can or box for 2 minutes instead of just once, and then do the same with your other arm. And while you're washing the dishes, hold the countertop and do leg lifts to each side, plantar flexion exercises (see Chapter 2), or alternate standing on each leg for 30 seconds at a time. The task of washing the dishes will pass rapidly when it is thought of as an opportunity to exercise instead of an unwanted chore. Walk around the house, while you talk to a friend on the phone, and use a carpet sweeper, instead of a vacuum, or if you own a tank-style vacuum cleaner, try to carry it instead of pulling it for at least part of the time. Be sure to stand upright when mopping, vacuuming, sweeping, and performing similar tasks, to avoid forward flexion of the spine. Invest in longer-handled appliances if you are using ones with inappropriately short handles that encourage poor posture and back strain. With some creativity and new ways of thinking, many other examples can be developed to integrate healthful exercise routines into the context of everyday household chores such as these.

THE HEALTH CARE FACILITY

NAVIGATING BETWEEN FLOORS

Older adults spend a good deal of time in health care facilities, including doctor's offices, clinics, hospitals, nursing homes, and rehabilitative settings. It may seem that such facilities are already designed to do everything possible to enhance health and well-being, given their primary usage, but in fact there are often major deficits in design and usage of such facilities, just as has been pointed out in the home setting.

One feature common to many such structures is a multi-story design. This immediately creates the problem of providing universal access to people of varying levels of physical ability. The obvious and usual solution is the provision of an elevator with wide doors, low-mounted buttons, Braille imprinting, no open spaces between the elevator floor and door to catch assistive devices or feet, and bells or electronic voice announcements of each floor. What is usually missed is the equally important opportunity this creates for enhancing physical fitness of staff and visitors to the building by encouraging and facilitating use of the stairs instead. This requires more than simply the existence of a staircase between floors. Some ways in which stair climbing can be encouraged in those for whom it is possible include

1. Posting signs outside the elevator suggesting that use be reserved for those with difficulty using stairs or need to traverse many flights;
2. Placement of stairs in prominent, visible locations in the building;
3. Adding attractive features to staircases such as decorative railings, open designs, bright lighting, carpeting, paintings, or other design elements which draw attention and interest in their direction;
4. Including sturdy handrails on each side of the steps;
5. Covering steps with non-slip surfaces and easily visible patterns to mark top and bottom steps and edges;
6. Minimizing very heavy doors leading to stairwells which discourage those with assistive devices, balance difficulties, or weakness from using them;
7. Where doors are needed, making them automatic and/or adding handles which can be opened by those with arthritic hands;
8. Installing landings at the top of each flight with enough space for a bench or chair to rest or place packages;
9. Adding safety bells, phones, and lights on landings;
10. Avoiding very narrow steps or sharp turns in staircases;
11. Including information plaques on the doors and walls depicting the health benefits of stair climbing, calories consumed by each flight, illustrations of proper usage of canes and handrails, motivational quotes, etc.;
12. Establishing a contest among staff or residents to reward the most number of flights climbed per week.

THE WAITING ROOM

Another feature common to many health care facilities is the waiting room, where the usual approach is to offer television and reading materials to help minimize complaints due to the inevitable delays. Another approach to this situation is to utilize the time and space in a positive and productive way, while at the same time relieving the boredom and discomfort of waiting. Such spaces could include interactive computer or video programs offering exercise, nutrition, or other health-related information. Samples of various pieces of exercise equipment (weights, bikes, etc.) could be put on display for trial usage. Healthful cooking demonstrations and samples could be offered. Patients could complete a simple self-assessment of their balance, strength, and walking speed, or other measurements such as height, weight, waist circumference, etc. in a private area, with printed information to help interpret the results obtained. Screening tools for symptoms of insomnia, sleep apnea, depression, memory loss, undernutrition, incontinence, menopausal symptoms, osteoporosis or cancer risk, etc. could be made available for those who are interested. Suggestions would be made for follow-up with the health care practitioner if warning signs for these or other conditions were thus identified. Individuals could enter into a computer records of exercise sessions completed at home between office visits, or compliance with dietary recommendations, so that graphic feedback could be provided to the patient and practitioner, and new prescriptions suggested and/or rewards for reaching target behaviors triggered.

These are just a few of the ways in which the health care practitioner's message of healthful habits and lifestyle choices could be reinforced and monitored without excessively prolonging the routine office visit. Often the waiting room time exceeds the visit time by three- to fourfold, which leads to frustration and anger on the part of the patient or families. If this is no longer considered a waste of time but instead an active, important part of the health care encounter, efficiency and satisfaction should increase enormously. Again, it is a matter of rethinking the elements of the spatial design of the facility's waiting room, but more importantly reformulating the concept of how that space and the time spent in it are utilized to maximize health and well being.

OPTIMIZING FUNCTION AND MOBILITY

Most of the concepts outlined in the section on the home setting above are applicable to health care facilities and residential housing for the elderly as well. In addition, the presence of large common areas such as lobbies, dining rooms, recreation rooms, hallways, gyms, and auditoriums provides even more opportunity to enhance physical activity levels. However, the overwhelming focus has been on safety in public buildings, with little thought as to how safety rules and prohibitions may in fact discourage mobility and encourage inactivity, which is paradoxically quite "unsafe."

Creative use of existing space is often the only option when financial resources prevent major renovations or additions of any kind. Wherever possible, hallways should be uncluttered and openly inviting of ambulation, singly or in small groups. Pathways that include outdoor walking areas protected from sun and rain, as well as indoor routes winding around interesting architectural designs, plants, or artwork are best. Changing the exhibits or artwork as frequently as feasible will also encourage walkers to explore the facility more often. Paths that include inclines, steps, ramps, and turns are desirable, as they can offer enough variety to embrace all levels of ambulation skill and include features which make the walk interesting and challenging for those who are willing to try.

Utilizing inherent design features such as hallways and steps to promote fitness can overcome the limitations of small common areas not suitable for permanent gym equipment, as is often the case in nursing homes and older facilities. Such usage of facility space will not happen automatically, however, and requires detailed planning and promoting, just as structured exercise activities do if they are to be successful. A good plan is to form a multidisciplinary staff team (including members from nursing, activities, rehabilitation therapies, psychology, building maintenance, and volunteer services, for example) to create a novel program that fits within the structure and functions of the building and directly addresses the needs of the residents or patients.

A similar approach can be taken to restructure meal services or dining room areas in geriatric facilities to encourage healthful and adequate food intake, which is as much a problem as low activity levels in many older adults. It is an unfortunate fact that the sicker and frailer individuals are, the more they are at risk of undernutrition, and yet less attention is paid to those features of eating that are known to enhance pleasure and intake of food. Again, the problem is single-minded attention to the safety law—in this case, providing a diet which is complete in all of the essential vitamins and minerals outlined by the Food and Nutrition Board (as described in Chapter 23). However, without attention to the hedonic and aesthetic elements of the diet as well (presentation, taste, smell, food preferences, ambience of the dining area, stimulation of other senses, presence of social companions, human touch while eating, etc.) older adults with limited appetites will not eat in sufficient quantities anyway, so the food's perfectly balanced proportions will not matter.

In summary, environmental design is a concept whose definition in geriatrics should be broadened to include not only the architectural features which allow access and provide safety, but also promote health and well-being in subtle and intentional ways. In concert with behavioral medicine, good design *can* and should reinforce and facilitate the concepts of healthful living delivered by health care professionals and aged care planners in other ways.

Appendix

Suggested Readings

American College of Sports Medicine, ACSM's Guidelines for Exercise Testing and Prescription, Williams & Wilkins, Philadelphia, PA, 1995.

Atkinson, R., Dietz, W. et al., Weight Cycling. National Task Force of the Prevention and Treatment of Obesity, Bethesda, MD, 1994.

Bouchard, C., Ed., Physical Activity. Fitness, and Health: International Proceedings and Consensus Statement, Human Kinetics Publisher, Champaign, IL, 1994.

Chumlea, W., Guo, S., Glaser, R., and Vellas, B., Sarcopenia, function and health, *Nutr. Health Aging*, 1(1), 7–12, 1997.

Drinkwater, B., Grimson, S., Cullen-Raab, D., and Harter-Snow, C., ACSM position stand on osteoporosis and exercise, *Med. Sci. Sports Exerc.*, 27(4), i-vii, 1995.

Fletcher, G., Balady, G., Hartley, L., Haskell, W., and Pollock, M., Exercise Standards. A statement for health care professionals from the American Heart Association, *Circulation*, 91(2), 580–616, 1995.

Fletcher, G., Exercise in prevention of stroke, *Health Reports*, 6(1), 106–110, 1994.

Joint National Committee, The fifth report of the joint national committee on detection, evaluation, and treatment of high blood pressure, *Arch. Intern. Med.*, 153, 154–183, 1993.

Kissebah, A. and Krakower, G., Regional adiposity and morbidity, *Physio. Rev.*, 74(4), 761–811, 1994.

Kuczmarski, R., Flegal, K. et al., Increasing prevalence of overweight among U.S. adults: national health and nutrition examination surveys, 1960 to 1991, *JAMA*, 272(3), 205–211, 1994.

Mazzeo, R., Cavanaugh, P., Evans, W. et al., Exercise and physical activity for older adults, *Med. Sci. Sports Exerc.*, 30(6), 992–1008, 1998.

National Institute on Alcohol Abuse and Alcoholism, 1981 Report. DHHS Publ. No. (ADM) 81-1080.

National Institutes of Health, Diet and Exercise in NIDDM. NIH - Consensus Development Conference, 1987.

Pate, R. R., Pratt, M., Blair, S. N., Haskell, W. L. et al., Physical activity and public health: A recommendation from the centers for disease control and prevention and the American College of Sports Medicine, *JAMA*, 273(5), 402–407, 1995.

Pollock, M., Gaesser, G., Btcher, J. et al., The recommended quantity and quality of exercise for developing and maintaining cardiorespiratory and muscular fitness, and flexibility in healthy adults, *Med. Sci. Sports Exerc.*, 30(6), 975–991, 1998.

Stefanick, M., Exercise and Weight Loss, in *Exercise and Sport Science Reviews*, Holloszy, J., Ed., Williams & Wilkins, Philadelphia, 1993, 452.

Stephenson, M., Levy, A. et al., 1985 NHIS findings: nutrition knowledge and baseline data for the weight-loss objectives, *Public Health Rep.*, 102, 61–67, 1987.

Index

A

Abdomen, 54, 64
Abdominal bruits, 534
Abdominal machines, 382
ACE, see Angiotensin converting enzyme
Achlorohydria, 116
Acid-blocking drugs, 476
ACSM, see American College of Sports
   Medicine
Adequate Intake (AI), 130, 481, 482
ADH, see Alcohol dehydrogenase
Adipose tissue mass, decreased, 13
Aerobic capacity, 10, 302
Aerobic dance, 5, 80
Aerobic exercise, 255
   benefits of, 82, 83
   increasing intensity of, 79
   musculoskeletal adaptations to chronic,
      11
   randomized controlled trials using, 357
   risks of, 84
   stretching prior to, 91
   types of, 386
Aerobic fitness, 214
Aerobics, step, 76, 85
Aerobic training, 17, 50, 90, 537
African Americans, heart disease mortality
      rate among, 280
Aging, see Exercise and aging
Agitation, 403
AI, see Adequate Intake
Aid to Families with Dependent Children,
      334
AIDS, 192, 327, 425
Alcohol, 236, 336, 447
   consumption, 225, 237
   dehydrogenase (ADH), 237
   intoxication, 533
   sleep disturbance and, 424
Alpha-blockers, 108
Alzheimer's disease, 188, 298
American Cancer Society, 237

American College of Sports Medicine
   (ACSM), 458, 547
American Council on Exercise, 458
American Dietetic Association, 457, 492
American Heart Association, 355
American Society for Clinical Nutrition, 457
Amino acid(s)
   essential, 147
   supplements, 151
Amputations, 247, 261, 263
Android obesity, 485
Anemia, normocytic, 492
Aneurysm, 534
Angiotensin converting enzyme (ACE), 293
Animal protein, 147
Ankle
   injury, 565
   joint, flexibility at, 91
   plantar flexion strength, 272
Anorexia, 23, 25, 140, 149, 527
Anterior deltoid, 58
Antidepressants, 406, 425, 435
Antidiabetic agents, 122
Anti-estrogens, 325
Antihistamines, 425, 435
Antioxidants and immune response,
      183–205
   antioxidant vitamins, 184–190
      how antioxidants work, 184–189
      maintaining oxidant/antioxidant
         balance, 189–190
   immune function, 190–200
      effects of vitamin E, vitamin C, and β-
         carotene on immune response,
         193–200
      immune system, 191–193
Anxiety, 111, 425
Aortic stenosis murmur, 533
Appetite, loss of, 44
Arachidonic acid, 157
ARIC, see Atherosclerosis Risk in
      Communities Study
Arm exercises, 46